Master Techniques in General Surgery

BREAST SURGERY

Edited by:

Kirby I. Bland, MD
Fay Fletcher Kerner Professor and Chairman
Department of Surgery
University of Alabama at Birmingham School
  of Medicine
Surgeon-in-Chief
University Hospital
Senior Advisor to the Director UAB
  Comprehensive Cancer Center
Birmingham, Alabama

V. Suzanne Klimberg, MD
Professor of Surgery and Pathology
Department of Surgery
University of Arkansas for Medical
  Sciences
Muriel Balsam Kahn Chair in Breast
  Surgical Oncology
Director of Breast Cancer Program
Winthrop P. Rockefeller Cancer Institute
Little Rock, Arkansas

Illustrations by: Anne Rains, Arains Illustration, Inc.

 Wolters Kluwer | Lippincott Williams & Wilkins
Health
Philadelphia · Baltimore · New York · London
Buenos Aires · Hong Kong · Sydney · Tokyo

Acquisitions Editor: Brian Brown
Product Manager: Nicole Dernoski
Vendor Manager: Alicia Jackson
Senior Manufacturing Manager: Benjamin Rivera
Marketing Manager: Lisa Lawrence
Design Coordinator: Doug Smock
Art Coordinator: Brett MacNaughton
Artists: Anne Rains/Body Scientific International, LLC
Production Service: Aptara, Inc.

Printed in China

Library of Congress Cataloging-in-Publication Data

Breast surgery / edited by Kirby I. Bland, V. Suzanne Klimberg;
Illustrations by Anne Rains.
    p. ; cm. — (Master techniques in general surgery)
Includes bibliographical references and index.
    ISBN 978-1-60547-428-1 (hardback : alk. paper)
1. Breast—Surgery.   I. Bland, K. I.   II. Klimberg, V. Suzanne.
III. Series: Master techniques in general surgery.
    [DNLM: 1. Breast—surgery.   2. Breast Neoplasms—surgery.
3. Mammaplasty—methods.   4. Mastectomy—methods.   WP 910]
    RD539.8.B74 2011
    618.199059—dc22   2010034827

DISCLAIMER
Care has been taken to confirm the accuracy of the information presented and to describe generally accepted practices. However, the authors, editors, and publisher are not responsible for errors or omissions or for any consequences from application of the information in this book and make no warranty, expressed or implied, with respect to the currency, completeness, or accuracy of the contents of the publication. Application of the information in a particular situation remains the professional responsibility of the practitioner.

The authors, editors, and publisher have exerted every effort to ensure that drug selection and dosage set forth in this text are in accordance with current recommendations and practice at the time of publication. However, in view of ongoing research, changes in government regulations, and the constant flow of information relating to drug therapy and drug reactions, the reader is urged to check the package insert for each drug for any change in indications and dosage and for added warnings and precautions. This is particularly important when the recommended agent is a new or infrequently employed drug.

Some drugs and medical devices presented in the publication have Food and Drug Administration (FDA) clearance for limited use in restricted research settings. It is the responsibility of the health care provider to ascertain the FDA status of each drug or device planned for use in their clinical practice.

To purchase additional copies of this book, call our customer service department at (800) 638-3030 or fax orders to (301) 223-2320. International customers should call (301) 223-2300.

Visit Lippincott Williams & Wilkins on the Internet at: LWW.com. Lippincott Williams & Wilkins customer service representatives are available from 8:30 am to 6:00 pm, EST.

10 9 8 7 6 5 4 3 2 1

To our families, colleagues, and mentors who have been the well of support from which the water of this atlas has been drawn.

Benjamin O. Anderson, MD
Director, Breast Health Clinic
Professor of Surgery and Global Health-Medicine
Department of Surgery
University of Washington
Seattle, Washington

Peter D. Beitsch, MD, FACS
Director, Dallas Breast Center
Department of Surgery
Medical City Dallas Hospital
Dallas, Texas

Kirby I. Bland, MD
Fay Fletcher Kerner Professor and Chairman
Department of Surgery
University of Alabama at Birmingham School of Medicine
Surgeon-in-Chief
University Hospital
Senior Advisor to the Director UAB Comprehensive Cancer
    Center
Birmingham, Alabama

Cristiano Boneti, MD
Assistant Professor of Surgery
University of Arkansas for Medical Sciences
Winthrop P. Rockefeller Cancer Institute
Little Rock, Arkansas

Kristine E. Calhoun, MD
Associate Professor of Surgery
Department of Surgery
University of Washington
Seattle, Washington

Juan C. Cendan, MD, FACS
Associate Professor of Surgery
Department of Surgery
University of Florida
Shands Cancer Hospital
Gainesville, Florida

Robert J. Cerfolio, MD
Professor of Surgery
Estes Endowed Chair for Lung Cancer Research
Department of Surgery, Division of Cardiothoracic Surgery
University of Alabama at Birmingham School of Medicine
Chief, General Thoracic Surgery
University Hospital
Birmingham, Alabama

Dean R. Cerio, MD
Instructor, Division of Plastic Surgery
Department of Surgery
University of Alabama at Birmingham School of Medicine
Birmingham, Alabama

David W. Chang, MD, FACS
Professor and Deputy Chair
Department of Plastic Surgery
MD Anderson Cancer Center
Houston, Texas

Lydia Choi, MD
Assistant Professor
Department of Surgery
Wayne State University
Karmanos Cancer Institute
Detroit, Michigan

Hiram S. Cody, III, MD
Attending Surgeon, Breast Service
Department of Surgery
Memorial Sloan-Kettering Cancer Center
Professor of Clinical Surgery
The Weill Medical College of Cornell University
New York, New York

Edward M. Copeland, III, MD, FACS
Emeritus Distinguished Professor of Surgery
    (Surgical Oncology)
Department of Surgery
Attending Physician, Shands
University of Florida
College of Medicine
Gainesville, Florida

Jorge I. de la Torre, MD, FACS
Professor of Surgery
Chief, Division of Plastic Surgery
University of Alabama at Birmingham School
    of Medicine
Section Chief, Plastic Surgery Section
Birmingham VA Medical Center
Birmingham, Alabama

Amy C. Degnim, MD
Associate Professor of Surgery
Consultant
Department of Surgery
College of Medicine
Division of Gastroenterologic and General
    Surgery
Mayo Clinic
Rochester, Minnesota

William C. Dooley, MD
Director of Surgical Oncology
Department of Surgery
OU Health Sciences Center
Surgeon
OU Medical Center
Oklahoma City, Oklahoma

Richard E. Fine, MD
Associate Clinical Professor
Department of Surgery
University of Tennessee, Chattanooga Unit
Chattanooga, Tennessee
Director
Department of Breast Surgery
Advanced Breast Care
Marietta, Georgia

R. Jobe Fix, MD
Professor
Department of Surgery, Division of Plastic Surgery
University of Alabama at Birmingham School of Medicine
Active Staff
Surgical Service: Plastic Surgery
University Hospital
Birmingham, Alabama

Sheryl G.A. Gabram, MD, MBA
Professor of Surgery
Department of Surgery
Emory University
Director
AVON Comprehensive Breast Center at Grady
Winship Cancer Institute at Grady
Atlanta, Georgia

Richard J. Gray, MD, FACS
Associate Professor of Surgery
Department of Surgery
Consultant, Section of Surgical Oncology
Mayo Clinic
Phoenix, Arizona

Stephen R. Grobmyer, MD, FACS
Associate Professor of Surgery
Division of Surgical Oncology
University of Florida
Chief
Breast, Melanoma, and Sarcoma Service
Department of Surgery
Shands Cancer Hospital
Gainesville, Florida

Virginia M. Herrmann, MD, FACS
Professor of Surgery
Department of Surgery, Division of Surgical Oncology
Medical University of South Carolina
Charleston, South Carolina
Medical Director
Breast Health Center
Hilton Head Hospital
Hilton Head, South Carolina

Kelly K. Hunt, MD
Professor
Department of Surgical Oncology
The University of Texas
MD Anderson Cancer Center
Houston, Texas

Nolan Karp, MD
Associate Professor
Department of Plastic Surgery
New York University School of Medicine
Chief, Plastic Surgery Service
Tische Hospital
New York, New York

V. Suzanne Klimberg, MD
Professor of Surgery and Pathology
Department of Surgery
University of Arkansas for Medical Sciences
Muriel Balsam Kahn Chair in Breast Surgical Oncology
Director of Breast Cancer Program
Winthrop P. Rockefeller Cancer Institute
Little Rock, Arkansas

Steven J. Kronowitz, MD, FACS
Professor
Department of Plastic Surgery
University of Texas
MD Anderson Cancer Center
Houston, Texas

Arthur G. Lerner, MD, FACS
Executive Vice President
American Society of Breast Surgeons
Columbia, Maryland

Albert Losken, MD, FACS
Associate Professor
Division of Plastic and Reconstructive Surgery
Emory University
Atlanta, Georgia

Julie A. Margenthaler, MD, FACS
Associate Professor
Department of Surgery
Division of Endocrine & Oncologic Surgery
Washington University School of Medicine
Staff Surgeon
Barnes-Jewish Hospital
St. Louis, Missouri

Elisa Perego, MD
Department of Surgery
San Gerardo Hospital
The University of Milan-Bicocca
Milan, Italy

Barbara A. Pockaj, MD
Professor
Department of Surgery
Division of Surgical Oncology
Mayo Clinic
Phoenix, Arizona

Raphael E. Pollock, MD, PhD
Professor and Chair, Division Head
Department of Surgical Oncology
The University of Texas
MD Anderson Cancer Center
Houston, Texas

Lee L.Q. Pu, MD, PhD, FACS
Professor of Surgery
Department of Surgery
University of California Davis School of
    Medicine
Sacramento, California

Geoffrey L. Robb, MD, FACS
Professor and Chairman
Department of Plastic Surgery
The University of Texas
MD Anderson Cancer Center
Houston, Texas

Virgilio Sacchini, MD
Professor of Surgery
Department of Surgery
The Weill Medical College of
    Cornell University
Attending Surgeon, Breast Service
Memorial Sloan-Kettering Cancer Center
New York, New York

Justin M. Sacks, MD
Assistant Professor
Department of Plastic Surgery
Division of Surgery
University of Texas
MD Anderson Cancer Center
Houston, Texas

Elizabeth A. Shaughnessy, MD, PhD
Associate Professor
Department of Surgery
University of Cincinnati
Surgeon
University Hospital
Cincinnati, Ohio

Edgar D. Staren, MD, PhD, MBA
Senior Vice President and Chief Medical Officer
Cancer Treatment Centers of America
Zion, Illinois
Visiting Professor
Department of General Surgery
Rush Medical College
Chicago, Illinois

Keila E. Torres, MD, PhD
Surgical Oncology Fellow
Department of Surgical Oncology
University of Texas
MD Anderson Cancer Center
Houston, Texas

Luis O. Vásconez, MD, FACS
Professor of Surgery
Division of Plastic Surgery
Vice-Chair, Department of Surgery
University of Alabama at Birmingham School of Medicine
Birmingham, Alabama

Michael S. Wong, MD, FACS
Residency Program Director
Associate Professor of Surgery
Department of Surgery
University of California Davis School of Medicine
Sacramento, California

James C. Yuen, MD
Professor of Surgery
Chief, Division of Plastic Surgery
Department of Surgery
University of Arkansas for Medical Sciences
John L. McClellan Veterans Administration
Little Rock, Arkansas

Michael R. Zenn, MD, FACS
Associate Professor
Department of Surgery
Duke University
Vice Chief of Plastic and Reconstructive Surgery
Duke University Medical Center
Durham, North Carolina

Breast cancer is the most common cancer affecting women. This cancer has a lifetime risk for one in every eight women. Surgical treatment of breast cancer has evolved from very radical debilitating surgeries to minimally invasive techniques and from disfiguring procedures to reconstructive excellence. The field of breast cancer surgery is advancing so rapidly that many of the procedures illustrated in this book are not readily available in community practice and certainly not in such a collective form.

The purpose of the First Edition of *Master Techniques in General Surgery: Breast Surgery* is to provide an atlas that covered not only traditional surgical techniques used in the diagnostic and therapeutic management of breast diseases but also those of forefront techniques in this rapidly progressive and evolving field. The content is organized into nine sections including imaging techniques, biopsy techniques, techniques of lymphadenectomy together with adjunctive techniques to prevent lymphedema, techniques of partial mastectomy, radiotherapy (brachytherapy device placement and intraoperative radiotherapy), mastectomy, advanced resections and local reconstruction, and, finally, oncoplastic surgery for lumpectomies, reduction mammoplasties as well as mastectomies. Some of these techniques are well established; others represent emerging and optional choices for the patient that surgeons should be conceptually familiar with and be able to offer such consultation options to their patients. Much effort was made to not only provide detailed anatomical and illustrative technical drawings but also to offer companion photos that are lacking in many atlases. For each chapter, the authors have made implicit effort to provide detailed coverage of the indications and contraindications of the procedure, preoperative planning, surgical technique and anatomy, pearls and pitfalls, postoperative management, complications, and outcomes of relevant research.

Lewis G. Janes stated: "Disease is war with the laws of our being. . .". Contemporary medicine requires that surgeons have multiple options in their diagnostic and therapeutic armamentarium, for no patient is like another. This book offers a detailed analysis and step-by-step instruction of a variety of procedures used in the war against breast cancer. May we incessantly strive to improve the treatment of our patients with breast cancer and ensure their rapid diagnostic and therapeutic outcomes are realized with contemporary state-of-the-art procedures.

We are indebted to each contributor for this First Edition of *Master Techniques in General Surgery: Breast Surgery.* Time was taken from already busy clinical schedules, overloaded administrative duties, and family time to carefully detail the steps of a comprehensive list of not only conventional breast surgical procedures but also newer techniques not afforded the surgeon in traditional texts. The diligent effort of each of the contributors to provide uniform step-by-step instructions as well as precise illustrations complimented by elucidatory photographs from the operating room is laudatory. Because of the collective efforts of the prestigious collection of authors, this atlas will be helpful to all who read, from the medical student to the learned professor.

We would also like to thank the staff members of Lippincott Williams & Wilkins, who have made the publication of this First Edition possible. Mr. Brian Brown has provided strong encouragement and support for the initiation and the development of this First Edition. Nicole Dernoski has been the pivotal communication link throughout planning, editing, and production of this tome. Dr. Josef C. Fischer, editor of *Mastery of Surgery,* was pivotal in convincing the editors to undertake this effort and assured Lippincott Williams & Wilkins of the intrinsic academic value of the First Edition to the broad field of breast diagnostics and oncology. Further, the editorial office is to be extolled for their advice and direction provided the contributors, illustrators, and editors to ensure timely and realistic publication schedules. In addition, Chris Miller has provided assistance in formatting and editorial review. Special appreciation goes to our project assistants, Kan Moore at UAB and Roberta Clark at the University of Arkansas, who were highly engaged and responsive to our contributors and the publication staff. We also express gratitude to Anne Rains for patiently drawing and redrawing illustrations until they were anatomically correct and complete.

Finally, the editors are highly indebted to our residents, fellows, students, and colleagues for their insightful questions that pertain to the technical management for the diagnosis and therapy of breast diseases. It is these queries that stimulated the genesis for the production and publication of *Master Techniques in General Surgery: Breast Surgery.*

Kirby I. Bland
V. Suzanne Klimberg

PART I: BREAST AND AXILLARY IMAGING

PART II: BREAST BIOPSY

PART III: LYMPH NODE MAPPING AND DISSECTION

PART VII: BREAST RECONSTRUCTION

1 Breast and Axillary Imaging for the Surgeon

Edgar D. Staren

Introduction

Dramatic and rapid change has become a common occurrence in all aspects of medicine; in few areas, however, has that change been as substantial and its implications as far reaching as in the subspecialty area of breast imaging for cancer. To put this in perspective, it is worth reflecting on the state of the art for diagnostic breast imaging in 1990, less than two decades ago. At that time, the superiority of standard roentgenographic mammography as compared with xeromammogram was being recognized. Rather than substantial attention being given toward optimizing the technique of choice, however, the bulwark of attention was focused on whether performance of mammogram of any type had value, particularly in the extremes of adult age groups. Interestingly, that debate continues even today for women 40 to 49 years of age. Also at that time, diagnostic ultrasound (US) of the breast was only rarely considered, and when performed, it was limited to straightforward differentiation of the cystic versus solid nature of a mammographically identified, nonpalpable breast lesion. Investigational techniques included scintimammography, thermography, magnetic resonance imaging (MRI), and others. Each of these has undergone significant evolution; despite that, with the possible exception of MRI, the role of scintimammography perhaps, certainly thermography, and others, remains ill defined. Evidently, therefore, the field of breast imaging remains a highly dynamic discipline.

One might rightly ask why after such a period of time a clear standard for breast imaging has not been delineated. As is the case in so many areas of medicine, the answer is simply dissatisfaction with the standard; until recently, that standard was mammography alone. Even today, conventional film screen mammography continues to be associated with an unacceptably high false-negative and false-positive rate; mammography sensitivity ranges from 66% to 91%, with specificity ranging from 88% to 96% (1,2). To put that into a more practical perspective, approximately 10% of patients undergoing a screening mammogram will be called back for a diagnostic mammogram. Approximately 1.5% (15 of 1,000) of those undergoing diagnostic studies will be referred for a biopsy; of these 15 referred for biopsy, approximately 30% or 5 of an original 1,000 will be found to have a cancer. Furthermore, at the other extreme, 20% of patients diagnosed to have a breast cancer will have had a negative mammogram within 1 year of their diagnosis (3). These results have caused investigators to persist on the search for the optimal method(s) to image the breast.

This review will address in some more detail those breast-imaging techniques deemed as "standard of care" and will also briefly consider a select number of those viewed as investigational and whose role is less well defined. Particularly for those in the former category (e.g., mammography, US, and to a lesser degree, MRI), it will focus on indications, technique, efficacy, and ongoing or anticipated updates.

"Standard of Care" Techniques in Breast Imaging

Mammography

Historical Background of Mammography

Some of the earliest work on mammography actually had its origins in the early 1900s and was summarized in an article by Gershon-Cohen in 1938; in 1913, Albert Solomon, a surgeon, reportedly used a conventional x-ray machine to image cancers from 3,000 mastectomy specimens (4). Initial radiographs of the breast had numerous technical limitations that hindered their usefulness. They utilized industrial films rather than film receptors specific for mammography. This required high-energy radiation and, therefore, was associated with substantial radiation exposure. The equipment was not able to consistently compress the breast and used large focal spots. All of the mentioned factors caused substantial blurring of the image.

Despite these limitations, the potential benefit of mammography was being increasingly recognized. Raul Leborgne was credited with identifying the significance of punctuate calcifications demonstrated on mammogram as being indicative of breast cancer. He also emphasized the importance of compressing the breast tissue as one means of optimizing characterization of the calcifications (5). Radiologist Robert Egan was credited with paying particular attention to methods that optimized the technique associated with mammogram. For example, he introduced dedicated film for mammography so as to produce detailed images that were reproducible (6,7).

While these individuals acknowledged the potential value of screening mammogram and set about to prove its value in carefully performed studies, they do not appear to have considered the potential hazards of regular radiation exposure. Ultimately, this recognition plus the relatively poor quality of film-screen studies at that time encouraged the development of various technical modifications and most notably, xeromammography (Fig. 1.1). This technique involved a photoelectric method to record a roentgenographic image on a coated metal plate. It used low-energy photon beams and dry chemicals to provide the image. A report from Kalisher and Schaffer in 1975 demonstrated it to be quite accurate in detecting breast cancer. Moreover, it was more convenient and somewhat less expensive than film-screen techniques (8). These factors plus the nearly one-third radiation dose associated with xeromammography as compared with film-screen resulted in its rapidly gaining considerable favor.

Xeromammography was considered better at imaging calcifications while film-screen held the advantage in imaging subtle breast masses (Figs. 1.2 A,B and 1.3). Despite the inherent differences in image quality, the result was of only minimal clinical import as these differences were felt to be subtle. Gradually, however, advancements continued in film-screen technology such that the radiation dose utilized decreased to a point where it was becoming less than that utilized for xeromammography; this in turn reversed the movement back in favor of film-screen (8).

In 1969 Charles-Marie Gros reported that molybdenum used as an anode with a molybdenum filter produced low energy x-rays (9). About that same time, the first dedicated mammography unit was developed, utilizing molybdenum. A more specific x-ray spectrum and tube was incorporated so as to focus on the breast tissue. Subsequent advancements included reducing the time of exposure and improved ability to compress the breast safely. Tissue compression further lowered radiation exposure by minimizing

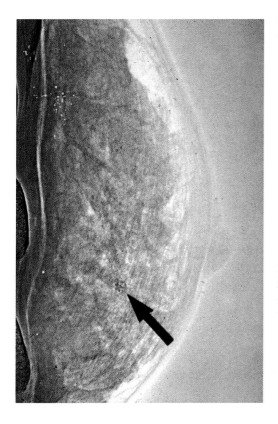

Figure 1.1 Screening xeromammogram demonstrating cluster of suspicious microcalcifications (*arrow*).

photon scatter, which would otherwise be absorbed. Ultimately, in the early 1980s, a reliable mechanical compression device facilitated the beginning of mass breast screening endeavors.

Screening Mammography

Indications and Efficacy   A number of reviews have examined the benefits associated with screening mammography (10). The positive predictive value of mammography for breast

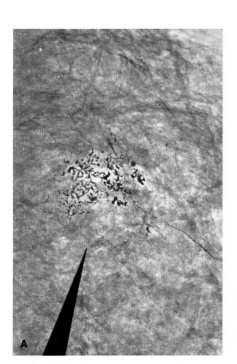

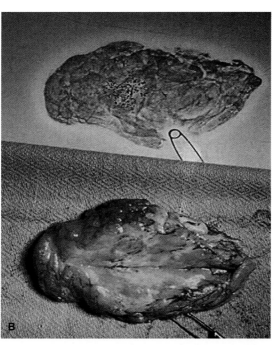

Figure 1.2 **A.** Magnified view of cluster of suspicious microcalcifications identified on screening xeromammogram noted in Figure 1.1. **B.** Lumpectomy specimen (**lower frame**) demonstrating an infiltrating carcinoma identified from a cluster of suspicious microcalcifications on screening mammogram (Fig. 1.1) and removal of same confirmed on specimen xeromammogram (**upper frame**).

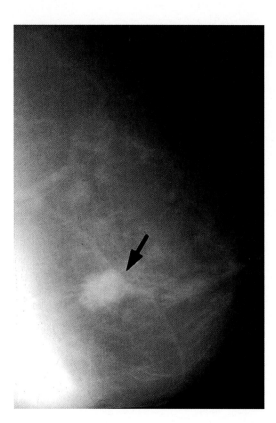

Figure 1.3 Film-screen mammogram (circa late 1970s) demonstrating an ill-defined mass lesion found to be an infiltrating carcinoma (*arrow*).

cancer ranges from 20% in women younger than 50 years to 60% to 80% in women aged 50 to 69 years. Although trials have convincingly demonstrated a 30% reduction in breast cancer mortality in women 50 to 69 years of age who are screened annually or biennially, data on women under age 50 years are less clear. Criticisms of the mammographic screening trials and which limit strong conclusions for this group of women include the following:

- Inadequately designed studies (e.g., failure of randomization and inadequate sample size),
- Low compliance in the intervention group, and
- High screening rates in the control group.

Following are among the well-reviewed trials evaluating screening mammograms:

- HIP trial performed in the United States in 1963;
- Malmo (1976), Two-County (1977), Stockholm (1981), and Goteborg trials (1982), all performed in Sweden;
- Canadian trial (1980); and
- Edinburgh trial (1978) performed in the United Kingdom.

Over several decades, these studies have been carefully scrutinized. Gotzche and Nielsen concluded that only two of these trials were randomized adequately (Malmo and Canadian) and that neither trial showed a reduction in mortality from screening mammography (12). They also noted that although the HIP, the Two-County, the Stockholm, and the Goteberg trials did show a reduced mortality associated with screening mammography, these studies were not optimally randomized. They did not include the Edinburgh trial in their analysis as it was considered to be biased. It is worth noting that although these trials examined nearly half a million women, they included few women older than 70 years and none younger than 39 years.

In a review by Armstrong et al. (13) for the American College of Physicians, they focused on screening mammography in women 40 to 49 years of age. They reviewed

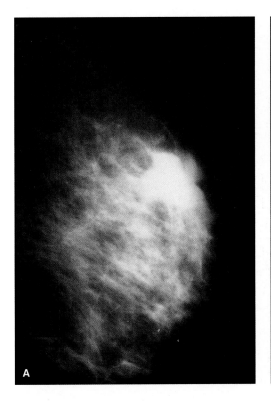
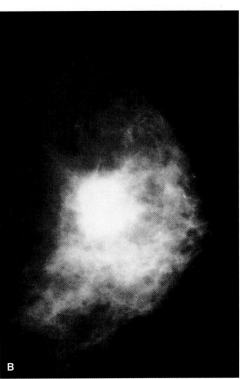

Figure 1.4 **A.** Mediolateral view film-screen mammogram of the left breast of a 38-year-old woman with a suspicious palpable mass shown on lumpectomy to be an infiltrating carcinoma. **B.** Craniocaudad view film-screen mammogram of the same breast as in Figure 1.4A.

117 other studies in addition to the above-mentioned 7 trials. They concluded that although the studies estimated a mortality risk reduction of 7% to 23% in this group of women, there was a substantial false-positive rate leading to a large number of unnecessary breast biopsies. In addition to unnecessary biopsies resulting in pain and surgical complications, other risks include radiation exposure and false-negative results. As such, it has been suggested that in women from 40 to 49 years of age, decisions regarding screening mammography should be guided by performance of periodic assessment of a patients risk for breast cancer (14,15).

Recommendations

Most experts do agree that the risk of breast cancer for asymptomatic women younger than 35 years is not enough to warrant the risk of radiation exposure. In fact, most radiologists do not generally recommend performing screening mammography in women younger than 40 years. Exceptions, however, may include women at particular risk for breast cancer. That is, if there is a positive family history, BRCA positivity, or a suspicious palpable mass, mammography may still be important (Figs. 1.4 A,B).

The American Cancer Society, the American College of Radiology (ACR), and the American College of Obstetricians and Gynecologists recommend screening mammography for women aged 40 to 49 years every 1 to 2 years and annually after the age of 50 years (16,17). The American College of Physicians recommends biennial screening for women aged 50 to 74 years. The American Academy of Family Physicians, which recommends mammography screening for women older than 50 years, is currently updating its guidelines. The Canadian Task Force on the Periodic Health Examination recommends annual mammography for women aged 50 to 69 years and recommends against mammography screening for women aged 40 to 49 years (18). Similarly, the U.S. Preventive Services Task Force recommends mammography screening every 1 to 2 years for women aged 50 to 69 years (19).

Technique

When mammography is performed as a screening study, the intent of the examination is to detect changes in the breast in women who have no clinical signs of cancer. The

Figure 1.5 A. Film-screen mammogram of a diffusely dense parenchymal pattern breast in a left mediolateral oblique view. **B.** Film-screen mammogram of the same breast as in Figure 1.5A in a left craniocaudad view.

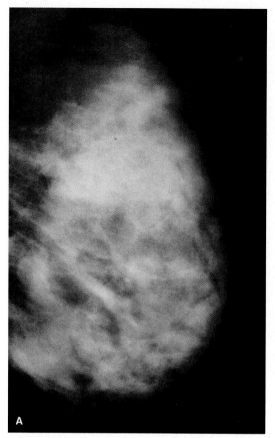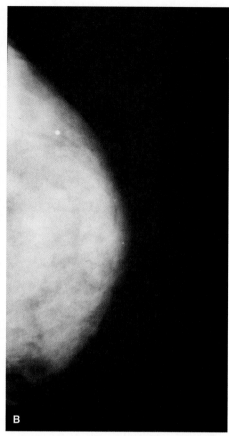

Figure 1.5 A. Film-screen mammogram of a diffusely dense parenchymal pattern breast in a left mediolateral oblique view. **B.** Film-screen mammogram of the same breast as in Figure 1.5A in a left craniocaudad view.

breast is placed in a dedicated mammographic machine gantry and compressed so as to even out the tissue and to maintain the breasts position. Screening studies involve performance of two views, mediolateral oblique and craniocaudad (Figs. 1.5 A,B). So as to decrease iatrogenic false-positive rates, women are discouraged from applying powder, deodorant, and even lotions before the study.

As with any interpretative skill, mammography "reading" requires time and experience to develop. In reading a mammogram, it is useful to proceed with a two-step strategy. In the first step, one reviews the more prominent features of the image. This will involve a qualitative assessment of either normal anatomy or distortion thereof and with identification of obvious abnormalities such as mass lesions. During the second step, a more detailed and orderly review ensues, which aims for not only identification of more subtle features including calcifications but also more detailed analysis of lesions and associated findings such as parenchymal distortion, skin thickening, asymmetry.

Diagnostic Mammography

Technique and Indications

Diagnostic mammography is aimed at providing specific analysis of patients with abnormalities of the breast detected by clinical and/or screening mammographic examination. In addition to standard views, additional angles and special views may be required; special views may include magnification to enlarge an area of the breast that was shown to contain a possible mass or calcifications. Such views may also include spot compression used to press out areas of dense or distorted breast tissue and thereby better determine whether a lesion is present (Figs. 1.6 A,B). Patients may require additional studies such as US, MRI, in the course of the diagnostic evaluation. Indications for diagnostic mammogram include the following:

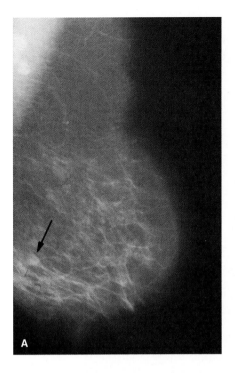

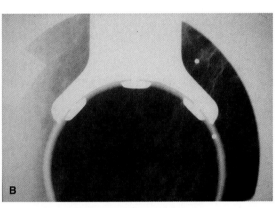

Figure 1.6 **A.** Mediolateral view film-screen mammogram demonstrating a less than 1 cm questionable nodular density (*arrow*) that led to recommendation for a diagnostic mammogram. **B.** Compression view diagnostic mammogram confirming nodular mass (*arrow*) demonstrated on screening mammogram in Figure 1.6A.

- A specific area of concern based on a suspicious breast-related symptom or sign (e.g., mass, axillary adenopathy, skin change),
- Possible lesion or abnormality identified on screening mammogram,
- Follow-up of a questionable area of concern,
- Patients with implants, and
- Patients who have been treated for breast cancer.

Digital Mammography

Although most studies are still performed with film-screen cassettes on a dedicated mammography gantry, there has been a recent migration toward performance of mammograms using digital detectors in a procedure referred to as *full-field digital mammography (FFDM)* (Figs. 1.7 A,B). First introduced by General Electric in 2000, digital mammography has been the most significant advancement in mammography in decades. With this technique, low-energy x-rays (25–40 kV) pass through the breast as with standard mammography but are recorded by an electronic digital detector rather than a film. Digital mammography offers several potential advantages over standard mammography, including the following:

- Near-instantaneous imaging,
- The ability to transmit the same image to various, even remote, locations, and
- The ability to manipulate (e.g., reverse contrast, enlarge) the image so as to optimize visualization of abnormalities (Figs. 1.8 A–D).

The Digital Mammographic Screening Trial (DMIST) included nearly 50,000 women from across the United States and Canada who had no signs of breast cancer, had no history of breast cancer, were not pregnant, and did not have breast implants (2).

Among 42,760 women analyzed in a comparison of both film-screen and digital imaging, it was found that the latter was significantly advantageous in detecting breast cancers in three groups of women

- Who were younger than 50 years,
- Who had dense breasts, and
- Who were premenopausal or perimenopausal (had their last period within a year of their mammograms).

Figure 1.7 A. Screening digital mammogram of the right breast in mediolateral view demonstrating only scattered fibroglandular tissue but no abnormal calcifications or masses. **B.** Screening digital mammogram of same breast as in Figure 1.7A in a right craniocaudad view.

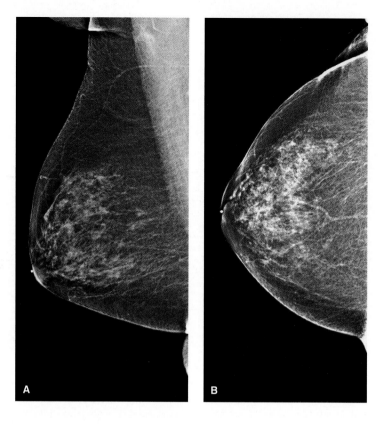

Digital mammogram provided no benefit for women older than 50 years, those who did not have dense breasts, and those who were postmenopausal. These factors held true regardless of the race or risk for developing breast cancer.

Results

Mammographic Interpretation

Mammograms are optimally reported in a standard format that recognizes the importance of clear communication between the interpreting radiologist and the clinician. Such a format is the ACR Breast Imaging Reporting and Data System (BI-RADS) classification. The ACR BI-RADS format recognizes the inherent limitations associated with variation of fatty versus parenchymal tissue in the breast and separates breast imaging into categories based on these components as follows:

1. Almost entirely fatty—in which mammogram is very sensitive,
2. Scattered fibroglandular tissue—in which there may be a minor decrease in sensitivity,
3. Heterogenously dense tissue—in which there may be a mild decrease in sensitivity,
4. Extremely dense tissue—in which there may be a marked decrease in sensitivity.

Subsequent to this description of the overall breast composition, the bulk of the report attends to description of findings, final assessment, and recommendation. In describing findings, attention is given to masses, calcifications, and associated findings.

Masses are defined according to their location, size, shape, margin, and associated findings. Benign masses are characterized by round or oval shape and well-circumscribed margins. Malignant masses are characterized by irregular shape and architectural distortion as well as indistinct or irregular margins.

Calcifications are defined according to their location, distribution, size, and shape. Benign calcifications are characterized as being coarse, large, rod-like, rounded, eggshell, or punctuate. They may also be characterized as typical of skin, vascular, or milk-of-calcium. Benign calcifications are often diffusely scattered or regional, whereas

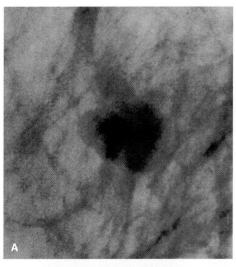

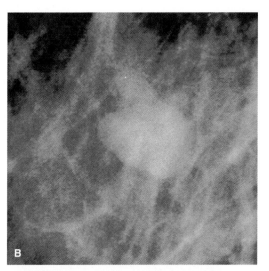

Figure 1.8 A & B. Smooth margined nodular density manipulated by digital mammography to demonstrate both zoom and reverse contrast capabilities. **C.** Diagnostic left breast digital mammogram craniocaudad view demonstrating suspicious upper outer quadrant density with spiculated appearance. **D.** Digital mammogram of density area from Figure 1.8C, manipulated with a zoom to show suspicious diffuse pleomorphic microcalcifications found on biopsy to be an infiltrating carcinoma.

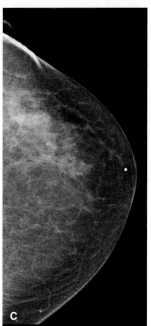

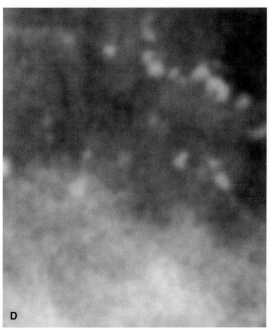

malignant calcifications are more often grouped or segmental. Malignant calcifications are characterized as indistinct, pleomorphic, and branching or linear.

Associated findings consistent with a benign diagnosis include a skin lesion, whereas skin/nipple retraction, surrounding tissue architectural distortion, and prominent axillary adenopathy are suggestive of malignancy.

Based on these findings, an assessment is made and assigned to one of six categories. These categories indicate an associated recommendation, varying from category 0 (need additional imaging evaluation) to category 5 (highly suggestive of malignancy). Such an approach greatly facilitates communication with the clinician and as such, with the patient.

- Category 0—need additional imaging evaluation.
- Category 1—negative; recommendation: routine screening mammography.
- Category 2—benign finding; recommendation: routine screening mammography.
- Category 3—probably benign finding; recommendation: follow-up in x (short-interval) months.
- Category 4—suspicious abnormality; recommendation: biopsy should be considered.
- Category 5—highly suggestive of malignancy; biopsy is strongly recommended.

Breast US

Indications

Ultrasound refers to any frequency of sound greater than 20 KHz, that is, the frequency above which humans cannot normally hear. All sound travels through different tissues at different rates of speed. When sound hits the interface between two tissues with different effects on the speed of sound, an echo is created. Medical, and in this case, breast US, produces visual images based on echoes that occur at such interfaces (20).

As with mammography, the role of US in the evaluation of breast disease continues to evolve. Historically, US was used to differentiate the cystic versus solid nature of mammographically identified, nonpalpable breast lesions (Fig. 1.9). Even cysts as small as a few millimeters in size may be diagnosed under proper circumstances. If a cyst is demonstrated, then further mammographic workup may be avoided (21). Increasing quality of US equipment beginning in the early 1990s included availability of high-frequency and multifrequency linear array transducers and computer-enhanced imaging, all of which led to increased quality of breast US images (22,23). Improved imaging has allowed for better delineation of a number of US characteristics of breast lesions; this in turn facilitated their categorization into groups based on the increasing likelihood of benign versus malignant (24–26). The improved quality of US equipment has expanded indications for breast US to include evaluation of a questionably palpable mass on physical examination associated with a negative or nonspecific mammogram (27) (Figs. 1.10 A,B). US may be useful in evaluating dense breasts, especially in young women before mammographic age, and is the procedure of choice in those who are pregnant (28,29). Breast US may be useful in the postoperative period in evaluating a possible hematoma or seroma (Fig. 1.11). It may be helpful in evaluating patients with mastitis and may be useful in identifying an abscess that is difficult to visualize (30). Although MRI is generally considered the standard for evaluation of possible rupture of breast implants, US is extremely good at determining the presence of an implant rupture and/or leak. In addition to being far less expensive, it is more comfortable and convenient for the patient (31). As the quality of US continued to increase, it greatly

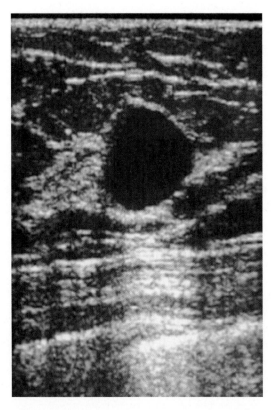

Figure 1.9 Diagnostic ultrasound of breast performed to evaluate a nonpalpable, nodular-appearing mass identified on mammogram and shown to be a simple cyst.

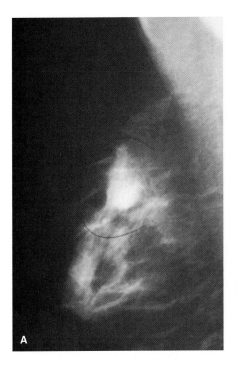
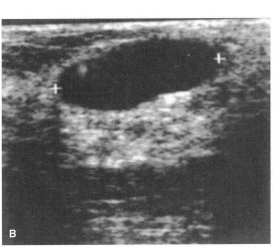

Figure 1.10 A. Left mediolateral view screening mammogram demonstrating a vaguely palpable nodular density (*circle*). **B.** Diagnostic ultrasound of breast demonstrating vaguely palpable and mammographically visualized mass lesion to be a simple cyst.

facilitated the use of US to guide interventional procedures of the breast for both biopsy and therapy (Figs. 1.12 A,B). US has been shown to be effective in guiding aspiration and biopsy of suspicious breast masses. It may also be used to localize those lesions identified to be atypical or suspicious on percutaneous biopsy. Potential advantages of such an approach include the placement of a guidewire into a breast lesion prior to performance of definitive excision. Placement by US allows for the wire to be placed in the

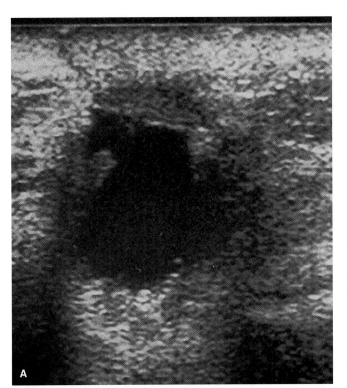
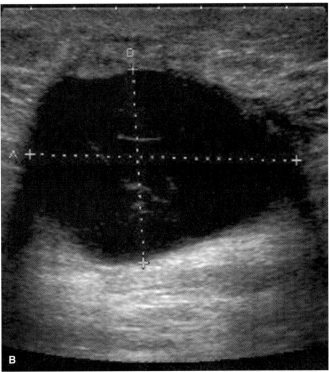

Figure 1.11 A. Multiechoic mass lesion in immediate postoperative period suggestive of a hematoma as compared with **(B)** an anechoic mass lesion with good through transmission consistent with a seroma.

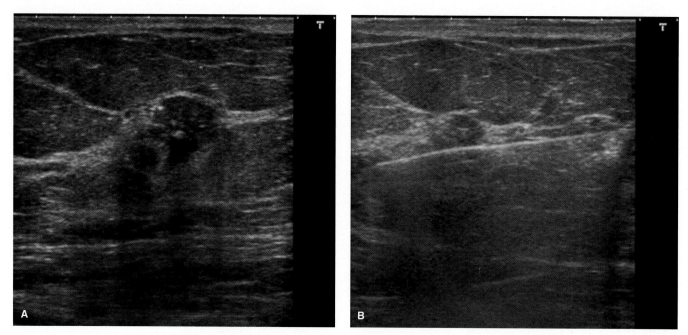

Figure 1.12 A. Diagnostic ultrasound demonstrating a suspicious breast mass characterized by multiechoic internal pattern with irregular margins and posterior shadowing. **B.** Ultrasound-guided core needle biopsy of breast mass demonstrated on Figure 11.2A and shown to be an infiltrating ductal carcinoma.

most direct route to the lesion. It is also convenient for the patient and avoids exposure to unnecessary radiation. Recent work has focused on the possible use of breast US in evaluation of the axilla; this may be valuable in preoperative staging and in the detection of recurrent disease.

Technique

When performing breast US, the patient is placed supine, with the ipsilateral hand over the head. A high-frequency transducer of at least 7 MHz and preferably 10 MHz is required. It is essential to scan the breast from the skin all the way down to the pectoralis musculature. A number of scanning methods have been described, including the transverse or sagittal sweep and the radial scan, also referred to as *ductal echography* (Figs. 1.13 A,B). The latter method, described by Teboul in 1988, follows the normal architecture of the breast lobes (32). With this technique, the transducer is swept over the breast, maintaining the nipple/areolar complex as the axis for the examination. This facilitates description of a lesions location and maintains the same orientation of anatomy regardless of quadrant. In most cases of breast US, a limited diagnostic study is performed on the basis of identification of a suspicious breast lesion. Between one-third and one-half of the breast is examined in an area defined by the mammogram. Once a lesion is identified, it must be viewed in at least two views, both the transverse and longitudinal views, in keeping with the standards of the American Institute of Ultrasound in Medicine. Adequate scanning of the nipple/areolar complex and retroareolar area requires placing the transducer on an angle adjacent to the nipple so as to avoid the strong posterior acoustic shadowing resulting from the dense connective tissue in this area (Fig. 1.14).

Normal/Abnormal Breast US

Normal structures evaluated in routine US evaluation of the breast include the skin, subcutaneous tissues, glandular tissue, underlying retromammary fat, pectoral muscles, and ribs. Upon completion of the breast portion of the examination and particularly in patients in whom malignancy is suspected, the axilla should be examined with attention to the possibility of abnormal lymph nodes. The skin appears as a homogeneous, hypoechoic zone between two hyperechoic layers. The subcutaneous fat appears as a

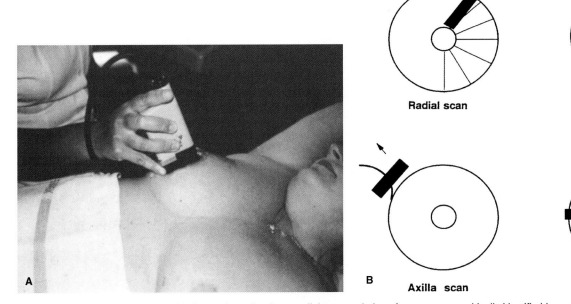

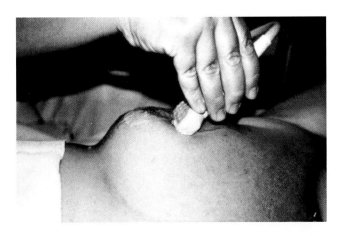

Figure 1.13 A. Diagnostic ultrasound being performed, using a radial scan technique for a mammographically identified breast mass and with patient supine and ipsilateral arm positioned above the patient's head. **B.** Graphical demonstration of multiple ultrasound scanning techniques including radial and transverse scans and axillary scan and tangential scan for evaluation of retroareolar area.

hypoechoic layer of variable depth just beneath the skin. The pectoral muscle appears as a hypoechoic zone, with interspersed hyperechoic ribs with strong posterior shadowing behind them. Glandular tissue has great variation in echogenicity, depending on the patient's age and menopausal status. Generally, lymph nodes are visible in the axilla only if they have pathologic changes within them (Fig. 1.15). Differentiation of the lymph nodes from vessels may be easily accomplished by simply noting the pulsatile nature of the vessels. When available, color flow Doppler imaging can be used to distinguish between them.

Smooth, well-defined margins in a breast lesion strongly support a lesion's benign nature, whereas even-jagged margins that may be indistinct indicate that a lesion is most likely malignant (Figs. 1.16 A,B). Solid breast nodules are most commonly hypoechoic although rarely they may be iso- or hyperechoic. Breast cancers are most often strongly hypoechoic and at times almost anechoic; they are generally heterogeneous. Despite that, degenerative fibroadenomas, complex cysts, and resolving abscesses may have a heterogeneous echo pattern (33). Benign lesions are more often homogeneous. Retrotumoral acoustic pattern may be useful; most benign breast lesions, particularly

Figure 1.14 Diagnostic ultrasound of the retroareolar area of the breast performed by placing the transducer on an angle adjacent to the nipple/areolar complex.

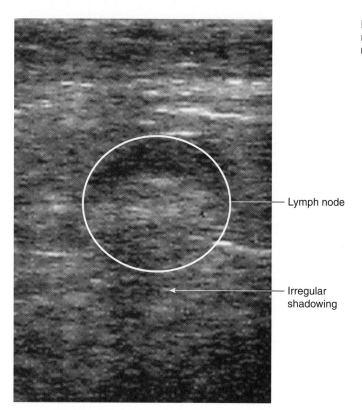

Lymph node

Irregular shadowing

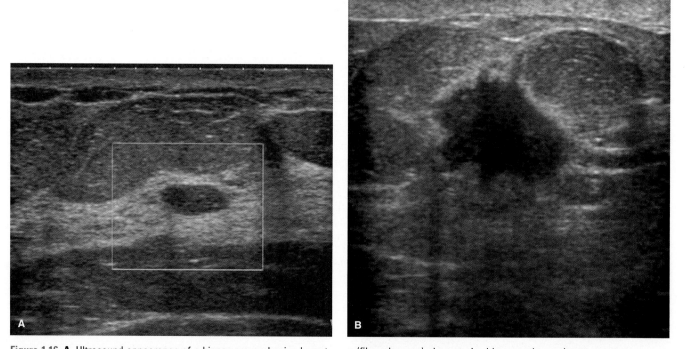

Figure 1.16 **A.** Ultrasound appearance of a biopsy-proven benign breast mass (fibroadenoma) characterized by smooth margins, homogeneous, hypoechoic interior, and a lateral:anteroposterior ratio greater than 1. **B.** Ultrasound appearance of a biopsy-proven malignant breast mass (infiltrating ductal carcinoma) characterized by irregular margins, multiechoic interior, asymmetric posterior shadowing, and a lateral:anteroposterior ratio less than 1.

simple cysts, will have good through transmission of sound waves, leading to posterior enhancement. The well-circumscribed, rounded nature of most benign lesions may lead to bilateral edge shadowing. Conversely, irregular posterior acoustic shadowing without previous trauma to the area is strongly suggestive of malignancy (34). Benign breast lesions can generally be compressed, whereas malignant lesions can not. Finally, a lesion's orientation may be useful in differentiation such that benign lesions frequently have a lateral:anteroposterior ratio greater than 1; benign lesions expand parallel to normal architecture, whereas malignant lesions do not respect normal tissues planes and tend to infiltrate. As such, malignant lesions often have a lateral:anteroposterior ratio less than 1.

Screening Breast US

There is considerable rationale to support the concept of screening breast US. Screening breast US visualization is actually improved with dense breast tissue. In addition to being well tolerated, it is inexpensive, involves no radiation, and may be conveniently performed in the clinician's office. A number of studies demonstrated that some breast cancers may be incidentally identified by screening breast US. This concept was supported by large studies that reported a 0.3% (and higher in "high-risk" patients) detection of incidental cancers (35,36). Recently, the ACR Imaging Network (ACRIN 6666) initiated a study aimed at better delineating the role of screening US. In this study, women with dense breast tissue in at least one quadrant were scanned; 2,637 have completed at least 12 months' follow-up. Forty patients were diagnosed with cancer: 8 suspicious on both US and mammogram, 12 on US alone, 12 on mammogram alone, and 8 on neither. The diagnostic yield for US plus mammogram versus mammogram alone was 11.8 versus 7.6/1,000, respectively; the diagnostic accuracy was 91% versus 78%, respectively. Unfortunately, the combined tests yielded a false-positive rate of 10.4% as compared with 4.4% for mammogram alone. These data added fuel to those already critical of screening breast US secondary to its high operator dependence, time-consuming nature, and increasing adoption of MRI. As such, numerous limitations persist to the routine adoption of screening US (37).

Axillary US

Lymph node status remains the single most important prognostic factor for patients with breast cancer. US of the axilla has been recommended as a standard component of the complete breast US examination and particularly for those in whom malignancy is suspected. Part of this is based on the high false-negative rate (30%–45%) associated with physical examination (38). US of the axilla may be useful in predicting the likelihood of malignancy; this prediction is based on the US appearance of lymph node size, shape, and contour. Axillary US is associated with a sensitivity of between 56% and 72% and a specificity of 70% to 90%. Unfortunately, the US signs of benignity and malignancy have sufficient overlap such that US-guided fine needle aspiration (FNA) has been recommended so as to increase the specificity of axillary US–based nodal staging (39). Holwitt et al. reviewed 311 breast cancer patients; 256 patients with clinically negative lymph nodes and 55 with clinically positive nodes. When combining US with US-guided FNA, they found a sensitivity of 71% and a specificity of 99%. This technique spared 29% of patients an additional axillary staging procedure.

Color Doppler Breast US

Color Doppler is an US technique which takes advantage of the Doppler effect, that is, US waves reflecting off moving blood cells are deflected (pitch is changed). This effect can be converted by computer enhancement to predict speed and direction of blood flow. Attempts to take advantage of this effect to quantify tumor vasculature and therefore predict the benign versus malignant nature of a lesion were initially thought to hold considerable promise (Fig. 1.17). However, more recent data showed color Doppler US to have an excessively high false-positive rate (40). Other reports have proposed that it may have a role in predicting prognosis; it has in fact been demonstrated to be an independent prognostic factor (41). It is unclear as yet whether color Doppler US may be used to predict response to chemotherapy.

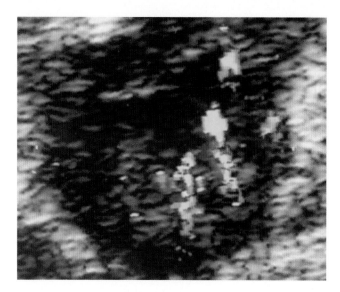

Figure 1.17 Ultrasound image of substantial color Doppler effect in a malignant breast lesion indicating its highly vascular nature.

Magnetic Resonance Imaging

Technique and Indications for Breast MRI

Although mammogram and now US have remained at the forefront of standard breast imaging, one approach, contrast-enhanced MRI, has also shown substantial progress and is frequently being touted for a number of routine breast-related indications. MRI technique images the very small (several particles/million) number of excess spins of protons (e.g., hydrogen nuclei) in a magnetized field. For breast MRI, the breast is scanned in a dedicated breast MRI device before and after the injection of a contrast agent (gadolinium DTPA); of note, what is imaged is the increased relaxation properties of the protons rather than the gadolinium itself. The precontrast images are then "subtracted" from the postcontrast images. Malignant masses are characterized by rapid initial contrast enhancement with a rapid washout in the delayed phase. Areas that have increased blood flow appear as bright spots on a dark background (Fig. 1.18). Breast MRI utilizes

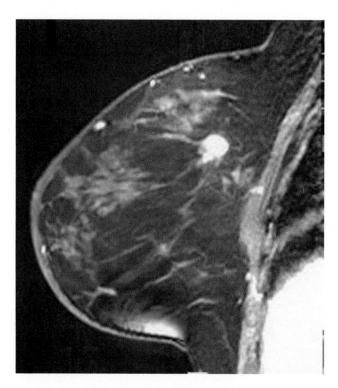

Figure 1.18 Contrast-enhanced magnetic resonance image demonstrating an approximately 1 cm spiculated bright-appearing mass on a dark background, consistent with a malignant breast lesion.

the increased uptake of gadolinium as a means to predict increased vascularity and therefore an increased likelihood of malignancy.

Breast MRI is recognized as a highly sensitive study; in fact, the sensitivity is reported to be substantially higher than that of either mammography or US. Moreover, while initially associated with a substantial number of false positives, specificity has improved secondary to improved practice guidelines that combine both structural and kinetic information; specificity rates greater than 80% are now being reported regularly. Nonetheless, MRI remains extremely expensive and relatively inconvenient for the patient. As a result, it has not been recommended as a routine screening study of the breast for the general population (42,43). However, because of its excellent sensitivity, the role of breast MRI has been considered for a number of subgroups. These circumstances continue to be reviewed but generally accepted indications for breast MRI now include the following:

- Screening for early disease in patients at high risk for breast cancer,
- In the evaluation of patients presenting with positive axillary lymph nodes but with disease that is otherwise occult on standard breast imaging, and
- As a means to evaluate the response to neoadjuvant chemotherapy.

Other indications being considered but for which there is still considerable debate include

- Patients diagnosed as having multifocal or multicentric disease,
- Patients with positive margins after lumpectomy, and
- Patients who recur after radiation therapy.

Efficacy of Breast MRI

Several large trials have looked at MRI as a screening tool for women at high risk for breast cancer; particularly women known or suspected to have mutations of BRCA1 or 2 (Fig. 1.19). The rationale for early identification of cancer in such patients is based on the high rate of interval cancers in such individuals with annual mammography alone. Bleicher and Morrow (44) reviewed five nonrandomized trials comparing MRI with mammography in high-risk women. These trials involved only those women who had at least a lifetime risk of developing breast cancer of 15%. Unfortunately, these studies were quite heterogeneous, with BRCA mutation carriers varying between 8% and 100%. The sensitivity of MRI for breast cancer detection ranged from 77% to 100% and was substantially higher than mammography (sensitivity from 25% to 40%). Three of these studies also demonstrated US to have a similarly low sensitivity similar to mammogram in

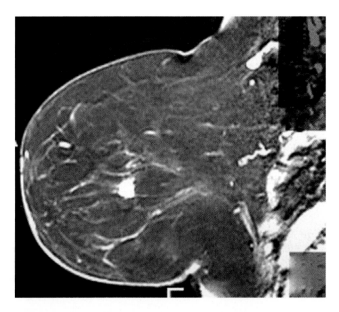

Figure 1.19 Suspicious area (bright-appearing mass) demonstrated on contrast-enhanced magnetic resonance imaging otherwise occult on other imaging studies in a patient with positive axillary adenopathy.

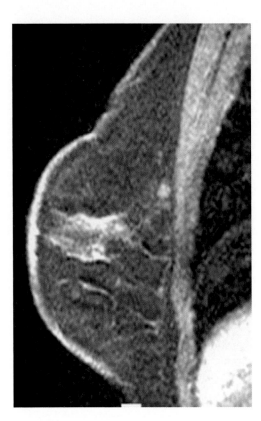

Figure 1.20 Large spiculated mass with rapid uptake and rapid washout of contrast on magnetic resonance imaging, consistent with a malignant lesion. Also noted is a small nodule in the low axilla and demonstrating rapid uptake found on biopsy to contain metastatic disease.

this patient population (45–47). In all studies reviewed, the specificity of MRI was lower than that of mammography. This lower specificity with MRI led to a substantially higher callback rate for additional studies as compared with mammography (11% vs. 4%, respectively) and a higher biopsy rate (3% vs. 1%, respectively) (48). Although no reduction in mortality has been reported secondary to MRI screening in high-risk women, the higher detection rate, and particularly at an earlier stage, has prompted the American Cancer Society to recommend annual MRI in the following cases:

- Women proven to be mutation carriers,
- Untested first-degree relatives of carriers, and
- Women with a lifetime risk for breast cancer of 20% or greater.

Breast MRI has been recommended in women presenting with a positive axilla and with negative physical, mammographic, and US examination of the breast (Fig. 1.20). In such circumstances, MRI may be expected to identify a primary lesion in at least 60% of cases. False positives may occur in up to 30% of patients, but false negatives are rare. In those cases where MRI is able to identify the primary, it becomes appropriate to offer patients the option of breast conservation therapy as an alternative to mastectomy (49).

MRI has been shown to offer an accurate estimate of the presence of residual disease in patients who have received neoadjuvant chemotherapy for locally advanced breast cancer (Fig. 1.21). Such an assessment is important to determine the extent of surgical resection required after such therapy (50). MRI was shown to be more accurate in determining the presence of residual disease compared with mammography (51). It has also been shown to be more accurate in determining the size of residual tumor compared with either physical examination or US.

However, MRI does have limitations in its ability to detect small residual foci. In a report by Sardanelli, serial sectioning was performed on mastectomy specimens and correlated with MRI findings. MRI was noted to miss 21% of multifocal/multicentric disease; the mean diameter of missed lesions was 5 mm. As such, MRI should not be viewed as a means to avoid definitive excision but rather as a tool to help guide what that excision should entail.

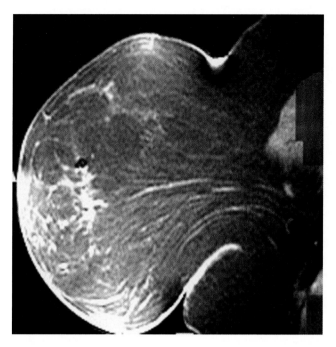

Figure 1.21 Diffuse stippled area of enhancement on contrast-enhanced magnetic resonance imaging demonstrating residual disease in a patient receiving neoadjuvant chemotherapy for biopsy-proven locally advanced breast cancer.

MRI has been suggested as a means to help guide definitive surgical resection in all women diagnosed with breast cancer. It has been proposed to assist in the evaluation of patients found to have multifocal or multicentric disease associated with the primary and in those circumstances where positive margins are identified after an initial excision (Figs. 1.22 A,B). Such recommendations are based on a number of studies demonstrating that MRI can identify additional tumor foci in a substantial number (e.g., 16%–37%) of cases (52). In those reports utilizing MRI to help guide surgical therapy, the impact of information gleaned from the study was such that a wider excision than initially planned and a higher amount of mastectomies resulted. MRI resulted

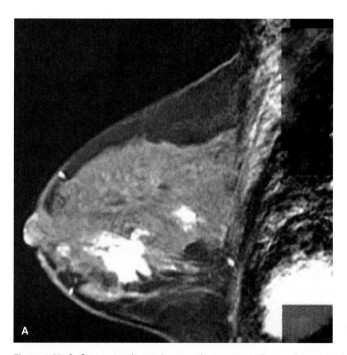

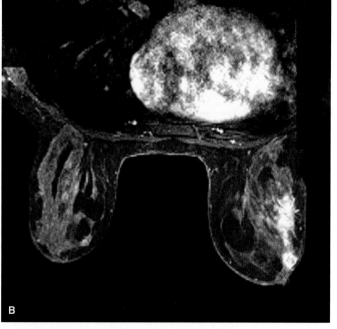

Figure 1.22 A. Contrast-enhanced magnetic resonance image demonstrating one large and two additional smaller lesions suspicious for malignancy. **B.** Coronal view magnetic resonance image of patient from Figure 22A demonstrating diffuse multifocal enhancement in left lateral breast.

in treatment changes in 20% to 55% of cases reviewed by Berg et al. (53). The concern, however, is that it is unclear as to whether such identification and treatment modification has any clinical benefit to the patient and that it may in fact result in more radical surgical intervention (i.e., mastectomy) than is necessary. Bleicher and Morrow (44) note that multifocal/multicentric carcinoma occurring beyond that resected in many lumpectomy specimens has long been recognized by serial sectioning of mastectomy specimens. Classic studies by Holland et al. (54) demonstrated that the cancer was limited to the primary site in less than 40% of cases and was within 2 cm of the primary in only 20% additional. Despite this, long-term follow-up would suggest that these areas are controlled by radiotherapy and systemic therapy. As a result, recent systematic review and meta-analysis by Houssami et al. (55) concluded that although MRI is able to identify additional disease as compared with clinical evaluation and standard imaging in a significant amount of women with breast cancer, randomized trials are necessary to determine the clinical value gleaned from this information.

The follow-up for patients after breast conservation therapy includes physical examination and mammography. Recently, MRI has been suggested as a possible means to detect recurrence at an earlier time. Although the ability for MRI to detect residual disease is well documented, it is unclear whether the same holds true for recurrent disease. Moreover, from a biological standpoint, it is not evident that such "early" identification would have any clinical significance. Since most recurrences are treated with mastectomy and the majority of patients are found to have operable disease, it is not likely that an earlier detection of local disease would have an impact on outcome.

Nonstandard (Investigational) Breast Imaging Techniques

Positron Emission Tomography/Mammography

Technique

Positron emission tomography (PET) is based on a unique chemical process involving the collision between an electron and a positron arising from a positron-emitting isotope that produces two photons and that can be detected by a PET scanner. Many such events occur at varying angles, necessitating multiple detectors surrounding the patient's entire body; these are then incorporated into a tomographic image by the computer.

On the basis of its favorable chemical characteristics, (18F) fluorodeoxyglucose (FDG) is the most commonly used isotope although other isotopes are being evaluated. The half-life of FDG is approximately 110 minutes. FDG uptake in tissues reflects the rate of trapping phosphorylated FDG and, therefore, is indicative of the rate of glycolysis. Uptake of FDG is increased in most malignant tissues as well as in areas of inflammation such as trauma, infection, and granulomatous disease.

PET scans require some patient preparation to optimize the image acquisition; this includes the patient having a normal blood glucose level with a period of fasting to occur prior to the study. Moreover, although patients should be adequately hydrated, no intravenous fluids containing glucose should be administered for at least 4 to 6 hours prior to the scan.

To adequately compare uptake given the variability between studies, a semiquantitative method is used to assess tracer uptake; this is measured as a standard uptake value (SUV). Initially performed as independent studies, in recent years, PET and computed tomography (CT) have been integrated into one study, thereby facilitating correlation of both functional and anatomic information. Despite this, limitations related to background and tissue attenuation result in the maximal resolution of whole-body PET being approximately 1 cm. As a result, it is not surprising that despite being specific for cancers of the breast, PET has limited resolution for small breast lesions and a rather low sensitivity (56–58).

Indications

The role of PET in imaging of the breast and axilla for breast cancer is ill defined. A recent review by the National Comprehensive Cancer Network task force on PET/CT scanning in cancer concluded that PET scan was not indicated for

- Detecting or screening of primary breast cancer;
- Staging of the primary tumor, axilla, or metastatic disease in patients with clinically early-stage disease; and
- Posttreatment disease surveillance (59).

However, a number of areas have been suggested to hold promise for PET in breast cancer. These include locoregional staging for locally advanced disease, as a means to monitor response to neoadjuvant chemotherapy, and for treatment response in metastatic disease.

Although PET was initially suggested as a possible means of evaluating the axilla in patients diagnosed with breast cancer, it has excessively low sensitivity as compared with techniques such as sentinel lymph node biopsy (SLNB) to justify its routine use as such. In a study by Wahl et al. (60) of 360 patients with newly diagnosed breast cancer who underwent PET scans to evaluate the axilla, they reported a sensitivity of 61% and specificity of 80% in detecting axillary lymph node involvement. These authors found that those cases where there was a false negative tended to be associated with fewer and smaller lymph nodes. In a large study by Veronesi et al. (61) of patients with breast cancer and clinically negative axillae, FDG PET was compared with SLNB. Although specificity was higher with PET, the low sensitivity (37%) was such that it was recommended that PET not be used to stage early breast cancer (61). Although evidently not able to replace SLNB, PET has also been proposed as a means to evaluate patients with high risk for positive axilla to avoid SLNB and go directly to axillary dissection; this suggestion must be taken in consideration of alternative techniques such as US-guided FNA of axillary adenopathy that require only minimal intervention and accomplish the same task and with increased reliability (Fig. 1.23).

Several studies have suggested that PET may be useful in evaluating not only the response of breast cancer to systemic therapy but also as a predictor for survival. Tumor cell metabolic activity may be inferred with PET by measuring both perfusion via ^{15}O water and tumor glucose utilization via FDG (62,63). Dunnwald et al. (64) used serial quantitative PET tumor blood flow and metabolism as in vivo measurements to predict patient outcome. They demonstrated that persistent or increased blood flow or

Figure 1.23 Positron emission tomography demonstrating a hypermetabolic mass (standard uptake value = 11) in right axilla consistent with malignant adenopathy.

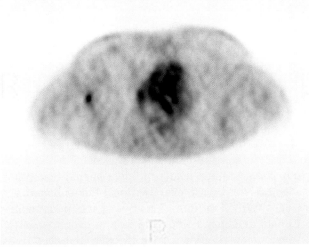

FDG transport after chemotherapy administration predicted for increased recurrence and decreased overall survival (64). These authors also demonstrated that tumor blood flow and high glucose utilization predicted for more chemoresistant tumors (65). Schwarz-Dose et al. (66) demonstrated that the level of FDG uptake at baseline and after each cycle of chemotherapy predicted for treatment response. Work is also ongoing to determine whether a decrease in SUV on PET may be able to distinguish complete versus partial response after neoadjuvant chemotherapy (67). Such information would be useful to determine indications for surgical resection and timing.

Positron Emission Mammography

Given the associated technical limitations, whole-body PET is poorly able to image the breast; therefore, it has not been viewed as appropriate for use in detecting or screening for primary cancer. Part of this difficulty in resolution is related to the normally dense nature of breast tissue that results in considerable background noise, but it is also related to the whole-body equipment requirement for multiple detectors placed some distance from the patient to detect photon emissions. In an attempt to improve sensitivity for breast examination, positron emission mammography, or PEM, uses small breast-specific detector heads oriented parallel to one another and adjacent to the anterior and posterior surface of the breast. This results in a significantly increased percentage of photons being detected as compared with whole-body scans and substantially improves spatial resolution of the breast (68). In a study by Levine et al. (69), sensitivity was 86% and specificity was 91%. Despite such enhancements, this technique is still limited by difficulty with anatomic specificity; it is hoped that this may be aided substantially by careful correlation with other studies such as mammogram, US, CT, or MRI.

Scintimammography

Technique and Indications

Technetium 99m (99mTc) sestamibi was approved in 1990 for clinical use as a perfusion agent for the detection of coronary artery disease. It was noticed to also be taken up by breast tissue. The mechanism for uptake is unclear, although it is thought to be related to mitochondrial activity. In 1987, Muller used for the first time 99mTc sestamibi to evaluate tumors (70). Shortly thereafter, Khalkhali et al. (71) investigated the use of 99mTc sestamibi for the detection of breast cancer (71). Part of the appeal of this technique in the breast is its apparent independence from breast tissue density (72). Although studies reported a specificity ranging from approximately 70% yo 100% for 99mTc sestamibi detection of breast cancer, the overall sensitivity was only approximately 75% and even less for lesions less than 1 cm in diameter (73–76). Khalkhali et al. reported on the usefulness of scintimammography to diagnose axillary lymph node metastasis in 15 patients with known breast carcinoma. These patients had scintimammography prior to axillary node dissection in the anterior upright position, and sensitivity and specificity were 60% and 90%, respectively. However, a large study by Massardo et al. (77) of standard scintimammography prior to 150 axillary dissections in 149 patients demonstrated sensitivity of only 28%, with specificity of 92%. Therefore, standard scintimammography is not recommended for routine evaluation of the axilla in patients with breast cancer.

Breast-Specific Detectors

It is believed that the principle factor limiting the sensitivity of scintimammography is related to limits in detector technology. Akin to the limits of photon detectors associated with whole-body PET, the relatively large gamma detectors used for whole-body nuclear scans are poorly applied to breast scanning, leading to poor spatial resolution. Evolution of dedicated gamma detectors for breast examination offer substantially enhanced resolution and, therefore, sensitivity. Preliminary results of scintimammography with a breast-specific gamma camera demonstrated an increase in overall sensitivity for breast cancer detection. In lesions smaller than 1 cm in size, the sensitivity increased from less than 50% with a traditional gamma camera to nearly 70% when a high-resolution breast-specific gamma camera was used (78). Utilization of such breast-dedicated detectors has been referred to as *molecular breast imaging* (MBI) by Hruska et al. (79) to distinguish it from conventional scintimammography.

MBI attributes its enhanced results to increased proximity of detectors to the breast, use of two detectors rather than one, and optimized collimation to increase counts per pixel in the images. Moreover, patients are placed in the same position as mammography, facilitating comparison. In an ongoing screening study of MBI, 650 women have been examined to date. Of these, nine cancers have been diagnosed; five detected by MBI, one by mammogram, two by both, and one by neither. It has been suggested by the authors that since MBI accuracy is independent of breast density, it may serve as a valuable adjunct in this patient population. Furthermore, these authors and others suggest that MBI detects cancers that are occult to mammography (80). What is as yet unclear is the ability of MBI to detect microcalcifications. As such, despite its evident improvement over conventional scintimammography, MBI also remains an adjunct to mammography rather than its replacement.

References

1. Ferrini R, Malur S, Wurdinger S, et al. Comparison of written reports of mammography, sonography and magnetic resonance mammography for preoperative evaluation of breast lesions, with special emphasis on magnetic resonance mammography. *Breast Cancer Res.* 2001;3:55–60.
2. Pisano E, Gatsonis C, Hendrick E, et al. Diagnostic performance of digital versus film mammography for breast cancer screening. *N Engl J M.* 2005;353:1773–1783.
3. Singletary SA. Imaging breast cancer; new answers for old problems. *General Surgery News.* 2007;34(3).
4. Gershon-Cohen J, Strickler A. Roentgenologic examination of the normal breast; its evaluation in demonstrating early neoplastic changes. *Am J Roentgenol Radium Ther.* 1938;40:189–201.
5. Gershon-Cohen J, Forman M. Mammography of cancer. *Bull N Y Acad Med.* 1964;40:674–689.
6. Egan RL. Fifty-three cases of carcinoma of the breast, occult until mammography. *Am J Roentgenol Radium Ther.* 1962;88:1095–1011.
7. Egan RL. Mammography: report on 2,000 studies. *Surgery.* 1963;53:291–302.
8. Kalisher L, Schaffer DL. Xeromammography in early detection of breast cancer. *JAMA.* 1975;234:60–63.
9. Sickles EA. Xeromammography versus screen-film mammography—pros and cons of the two techniques. *West J Med.* 1981;134:273–274.
10. Miller AB, Baines CJ, To T, et al. Canadian National Breast Screening Study, I: breast cancer detection and death rates among women ages 40–49 years. *Can Med Assoc J.* 1992;147:1459–1498.
11. Nystrom L, Rutqvist I, Wall S, et al. Breast cancer screening with mammography: overview of Swedish randomized trials. *Lancet.* 1993;341:973–978.
12. Gotzche PC, Nielsen M. Screening for breast cancer with mammography. *Cochrane Database Syst Rev.* 2006:4:CD001877.doi:10.1002/1451858.
13. Armstrong K, Moye E, Williams S, et al. Screening mammography in women 40–49 years of age: a systematic review for the American College of Physicians. *Ann Intern Med.* 2007;146:516–526.
14. Humphrey LL, Helfand M, Chan BK, et al. Breast cancer screening: a summary of the evidence for the U.S. Preventive Services Task Force. *Ann Intern Med.* 2002;137:347–360.
15. Qaseem A, Snow V, Sherif K, et al. Screening mammography for women 40 to 49 years of age: a clinical practice guideline: American College of Physicians. *Ann Intern Med.* 2007;146:511–515.
16. Smith RA, Cokkinides V, Eyre HJ. American Cancer Society guidelines for the early detection of cancer, 2006. *CA Cancer J Clin.* 2006;56:11–25.
17. ACOG Practice Bulletin. Clinical management guidelines for obstetrician-gynecologists: breast cancer screening. *Obstet Gynecol.* 2003;101:821–831.
18. Ringash J. Preventive health care, 2001 update: screening mammography among women aged 40–49 years at average risk of breast cancer. *Can Med Assoc J.* 2001;164:469–476.
19. U.S. Preventive Services Task Force. Screening for breast cancer: recommendations and rationale. *Ann Intern Med.* 2002;137:344–346.
20. Staren ED. Physics and principles of breast ultrasound. *Am Surg.* 1996;62:103–107.
21. Staren ED, Fine RE. Breast ultrasound. *Prob Gen Surg.* 1997;14:46–53.
22. Dempsey PJ. Breast sonography: historical perspective, clinical application, and image interpretation. *Ultrasound Q.* 1988;6:69–90.
23. McSweeney MB, Murphy CH. Whole breast sonography. *Radiol Clin North Am.* 1985;23:157–167.
24. Jackson VP. The role of ultrasound in breast imaging. *Radiology.* 1990;177:305–311.
25. Jackson VP, Rothschild PA, Kreipke DL, et al. The spectrum of sonographic findings of fibroadenoma of the breast. *Invest Radiol.* 1986;21:34–40.
26. Leucht W. *Teaching Atlas of Breast Ultrasound.* New York, NY: Thieme Medical Publishers, 1992.
27. Staren ED, O'Neill TP. Breast ultrasound. *Surg Clin North Am.* 1998;78:219–235.
28. Jackson VP, Hendrick RE, Feit SA, et al. Imaging of the radiographically dense breast. *Radiology.* 1993;188:297.
29. Hackeloer BJ, Duda V, Lauth G. *Ultrasound Mammography.* New York, NY: Springer-Verlag, 1989.
30. Karstrup S, Nolsoe C, Braeband K, et al. Ultrasound-guided percutaneous drainage of breast abscess. *Acta Radiol.* 1990;30:157–159.
31. Levine RA, Collins TL. Definitive diagnosis of breast implant rupture by ultrasonography. *Plast Reconstr Surg.* 1991;87:1126–1128.
32. Teboul M. A new concept in breast investigation: echo-histological acino-ductal 13 analysis or analytic echography. *Biomed Pharmacother.* 1988;42:289.
33. Staren ED. Ultrasound-guided biopsy of non-palpable breast masses by surgeons. *Ann Surg Oncol.* 1996;3:476–482.
34. Mendelsohn EB. Evaluation of the postoperative breast. *Radiol Clin North Am.* 1992;30:107.
35. Gordon PB, Goldenberg SL. Malignant breast masses detected only by US: a retrospective review. *Cancer.* 1995;76:626–630.
36. Kolb TM, Lichy J, Newhouse JH. Occult cancer in women with dense breasts: detection with screening US—diagnostic yield and tumor characteristics. *Radiology.* 1998;207:191–199.
37. Kopans DB. Breast sonographic screening is not ready for prime time. *Am J Roentgenol.* 2003;181:1426–1428.

38. BonnemaJ, VanGeel An, Ooijen BV et al. Ultrasound guided aspiration biopsy for detection of nonpalpable axillary node metastases in breast cancer patients: new diagnostic method. *World J Surg.* 1997;21:270–274.

39. Holwitt DM, Swatske ME, Gillanders WE, et al. The combination of axillary ultrasound and ultrasound-guided biopsy is an accurate predictor of axillary stage in clinically node-negative breast cancer patients. *Am J Surg.* 2008;196:477–482.

40. Lee SK, Lee T, Lee KR, et al. Evaluation of breast tumors with color Doppler imaging: a comparison with image-directed Doppler ultrasound. *J Clin Ultrasound.* 1995;23:367–373.

41. Waterman D, Madjar H, Sauerbrei W, et al. Assessment of breast cancer vascularisation by Doppler ultrasound as a prognostic factor of survival. *Oncol Rep.* 2004;11:905–910.

42. Kriege M, Brekelmans CTM, Boetes C, et al. Efficacy of MRI and mammography for breast cancer screening in women with a familial or genetic predisposition. *N Engl J Med.* 2004;351: 427–437.

43. Lehman CD, Blume JD, Weatherall P, et al. Screening women at high risk for breast cancer with mammography and MRI. *Cancer.* 2005;102:1898–1905.

44. Bleicher RJ, Morrow M. MRI and breast cancer: role in detection, diagnosis, and staging. *Oncology.* 2007;21:1521–1533.

45. Kuhl CK, Schrading S, Leutner CC, et al. Mammography, breast ultrasound, and magnetic resonance imaging for surveillance of women at high familial risk for breast cancer. *J Clin Oncol.* 2005;23:8469–8476.

46. Warner E, Plewes DB, Hill KA, et al. Surveillance of BRCA1 and BRCA2 mutation carriers with magnetic resonance imaging, ultrasound, mammography, and clinical breast examination. *JAMA.* 2004;292:1317–1325.

47. Lehman DC, Issacs C, Schnall MD, et al. Cancer yield of mammography, MR, and US in high-risk women: prospective multi-institution breast cancer screening study. *Radiology.* 2007;244: 381–388.

48. Saslow D, Boetes D, Burke W, et al. American Cancer Society guidelines for breast screening with MRI as an adjunct to mammography. *CA Cancer J Clin.* 2007;57:75–89.

49. Buchanan CL, Morris EA, Dorn PL, et al. Utility of breast magnetic resonance imaging in patients with occult primary breast cancer. *Ann Surg Oncol.* 2005;12:1045–1053.

50. Segara D, Krop IE, Garber JE, et al. Does MRI predict pathologic tumor response in women with breast cancer undergoing preoperative chemotherapy? *J Surg Oncol.* 2007;96:474–480.

51. Esserman L, Hyltom N, Yassa L, et al. Utility of magnetic resonance imaging in the management of breast cancer: evidence for improved preoperative staging. *J Clin Oncol.* 1999;17:110–119.

52. Van Goethem M, Tjalma W, Schelfout I, et al. Magnetic resonance imaging in breast cancer. *Eur J Surg Oncol.* 2006;32: 901–910.

53. Berg WA, Gutierrrez L, NessAiver MS, et al. Diagnostic accuracy of mammography, clinical examination, US, and MR imaging in preoperative assessment of breast cancer. *Radiology.* 2004; 233:830–849.

54. Holland R, Veling SH, Mravunac M, et al. Histologic multifocality of Tis, T1-2 breast carcinomas: implications for clinical trials of breast-conserving surgery. *Cancer.* 1985;56:979–990.

55. Houssami N, Ciatto S, Macaskill P, et al. Accuracy and surgical impact of magnetic resonance imaging in breast cancer staging: systematic review and meta-analysis in detection of multifocal and multicentric cancer. *J Clin Oncol.* 2008;26:3248–3258.

56. Tse NY, Hoh CK, Hawkins RA, et al. The application of positron emission tomographic imaging with fluorodeoxyglucose to the evaluation of breast disease. *Ann Surg.* 1992;216:27–34.

57. Gorres GW, Steinert HC, von Schulthess GK. PET and functional anatomic fusion imaging in lung and breast cancers. *Cancer J.* 2004;10:251–261.

58. Frangioni JV. New technologies for human cancer imaging. *J Clin Oncol.* 2008;26:4012–4021.

59. Podoloff DA, Advanti RH, Alfred C, et al. NCCN Task Force report: positron emission tomography (PET)/computed tomography (CT) scanning in cancer. *J Natl Compr Canc Netw.* 2007;5: S1–S22.

60. Wahl RI, Siegel BA, Coleman RE, et al. Prospective multicenter study of axillary nodal staging by positron emission tomography in breast cancer: a report of the staging breast cancer with PET Study Group. *J Clin Oncol.* 2004;22:277–285.

61. Veronesi U, De Cicco C, Phillips N. A comparative study on the value of FDG-PET and sentinel node biopsy to identify occult axillary metastases. *Ann Oncol.* 2007;18:473–478.

62. Smith IC, Welch AE, Hutcheon AW, et al. Positron emission tomography using fluorodeoxyglucose to predict the pathologic response of breast cancer to primary chemotherapy. *J Clin Oncol.* 2000;18:1676–1688.

63. Schelling M, Avril N, Nahrig J, et al. Positron emission tomography using fluorodeoxyglucose for monitoring chemotherapy in breast cancer. *J Clin Oncol.* 2000;18:1689–1695.

64. Dunnwald LK, Gralow JR, Ellis GK, et al. Tumor metabolism and blood flow changes by positron emission tomography: relation to survival in patients treated with neoadjuvant chemotherapy for locally advanced breast cancer. *J Clin Oncol.* 2008;26: 4449–4457.

65. Mankoff DA, Dunnwald LK, Gralow JR, et al. Changes in blood flow and metabolism in locally advanced breast cancer treated with neoadjuvant chemotherapy. *J Nucl Med.* 2003;44: 1806–1814.

66. Schwarz-Dose J, Untch M, Tiling R, et al. Monitoring primary systemic therapy of large and locally advanced breast cancer by sequential positron emission tomography imaging with [18F] fluorodeoxyglucose. *J Clin Oncol.* 2009;27:535–541.

67. Kim SJ, Kim SK, Lee ES, et al. Predictive value of FDG PET for pathological response of breast cancer to neoadjuvant chemotherapy. *Ann Oncol.* 2004;15:1352–1357.

68. Hofmann M. From scintimammography and metabolic imaging to receptor targeted PET—new principles of breast cancer detection. *Phys Med.* 2006;21:11.

69. Levine EA, Freimanis RI, Perrier NC, et al. Positron emission mammography: initial clinical results. *Ann Surg Oncol.* 2003; 10:86–91.

70. Muller ST, Guth-Tougeides B, Creutzig H. Imaging of malignant tumors with Tc-99 MIBI SPECT. *J Nucl Med.* 1987;28(suppl): P562.

71. Khalkhali I, Cutrone J, Mena I, et al. Technitium-99m-sestamibi scintimammography of breast lesions: clinical and pathological follow-up. *J Nucl Med.* 1995;36:1784–1789.

72. Khalkhali I, Baurn JK, Villanueva-Meyer J, et al. 99mTc-sestamibi breast imaging for the examination of patients with dense and fatty breasts: multicenter study. *Radiology.* 2002;222: 149–155.

73. Brem RF, Rapelyea JA, Zismann G, et al. Occult breast cancer: scintimammography with high-resolution breast-specific gamma camera in women at high risk for breast cancer. *Radiology.* 2005; 237:274–280.

74. Khalkhali I, Vargas HI. The role of nuclear medicine in breast cancer detection: functional breast imaging. *Radiol Clin North Am.* 2001;39:1053–1068.

75. Khalkhali I, Villanueva-Meyer J, Edell SL, et al. Diagnostic accuracy of 99mTc-sestamibi breast imaging: multicenter trial results. *J Nucl Med.* 2000;41:1973–1979.

76. Khalkhali I, Cutrone J, Mena I, et al. Technitium-99m-sestamibi scintimammography of breast lesions: clinical and pathological follow-up. *J Nucl Med.* 1995;36:1784–1789.

77. Massardo T, Alonso O, Llamas-Ollier A, et al. Planar Tc99m-sestamibi scintimammography should be considered cautiously in the axillary evaluation of breast cancer protocols: results of an international multicenter trial. *BMC Nucl Med.* 2005;5:4.

78. Brem RF, Rapelyea JA, Zismann G, et al. Occult breast cancer: scintimammography with high-resolution breast-specific gamma camera in women at high risk for breast cancer. *Radiology.* 2005;237:274–280.

79. Hruska CB, Boughey JC, Phillips SW, et al. Molecular breast imaging: a review of the Mayo Clinic experience. *Am J Surg.* 2008;196:470–476.

80. Coover LR, Caravaglia G, Kuhn P. Scintimammography with dedicated breast camera detects and localizes occult carcinoma. *J Nucl Med.* 2004;45:553–558.

2 Drainage of Breast Cysts and Abscesses

Amy C. Degnim

Breast Cysts

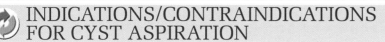

INDICATIONS/CONTRAINDICATIONS FOR CYST ASPIRATION

Breast cysts are common, both as identifiable symptomatic lesions and as asymptomatic findings during screening or diagnostic breast imaging. Prior to the widespread use and availability of ultrasound, most cysts were diagnosed and treated simultaneously with fine needle aspiration. In the current era, management of breast cysts is determined by their imaging appearance and symptoms. A symptomatic breast cyst classically presents as a smooth, well-circumscribed, mobile, soft-to-firm lump; tenderness is variable and is based on the degree of fluid tension within the cyst. Cysts that present as palpable breast lesions should be evaluated with ultrasound prior to intervention, if at all possible. This is a feasible goal, given common availability of good-quality portable ultrasound units and increasing numbers of surgeons trained in basic ultrasound. Diagnostic mammography is also standard in the imaging evaluation of new palpable lesions in women 35 years and older.

The breast is a glandular organ that serves the purpose of postpartum lactation. The normal anatomy comprises 15 to 20 lobar structures that are supported in fibrofatty stromal tissue. The lobar glandular elements are connected via microscopic ducts that converge in the central breast under the areola and exit through the nipple (Fig. 2.1A). In the subareolar location, the ducts dilate as lactiferous sinuses that act as small reservoirs of milk in the lactating state. Breast cysts can occur anywhere in the breast but most commonly are found within the parenchyma of the breast outside the nipple/areolar location (Fig. 2.1B).

Ultrasound is the primary diagnostic modality for diagnosis of breast cysts, with high sensitivity at discriminating fluid versus solid lesions. By ultrasound, normal breast tissue demonstrates some heterogeneity in echogenicity of the parenchyma but does not show discrete abnormalities (Fig. 2.2). When evaluating cysts sonographically, the location, size, borders, and internal echogenicity should be noted and recorded in detail to facilitate future comparison. The ultrasonographic criteria for diagnosis of a simple cyst are well established, such that asymptomatic simple cysts do not require aspiration. These strict

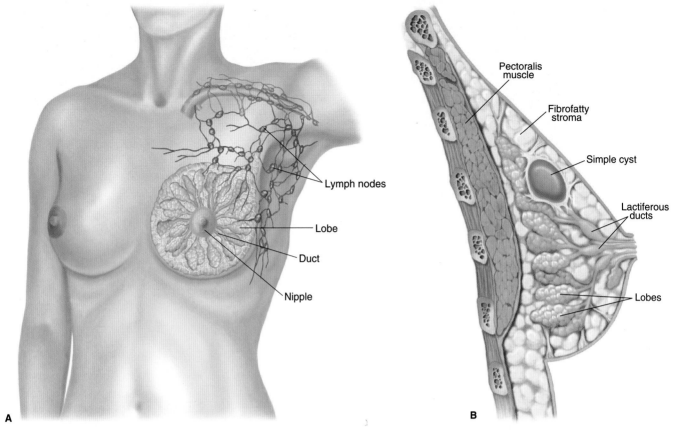

A   **B**

Figure 2.1 Normal breast anatomy.

sonographic features are anechoic (containing no echoes), sharply circumscribed margins, posterior acoustic enhancement, and refractive (edge) shadows (Fig. 2.3A). Simple cysts that meet these criteria do not require aspiration unless painful or worrisome to the patient. Some overlap exists with features and terminology of complex cysts and complex masses, but any solid component of a lesion in the breast should undergo tissue biopsy. Complex cysts are those that truly are cysts but do not meet the strict sonographic criteria for simple cysts (Fig. 2.3B). When ultrasound shows internal echoes, ill-defined margins, or wall thickening, the lesion should be described as a complex mass despite the presence of some cystic features (Fig. 2.3C). Complex cysts should undergo aspiration, and complex masses should be treated as solid masses and undergo core needle biopsy. In summary, cysts with indications for aspiration are simple cysts that are symptomatic, and complex cysts that do not meet strict sonographic criteria for simple cysts.

Figure 2.2 Normal breast ultrasound.

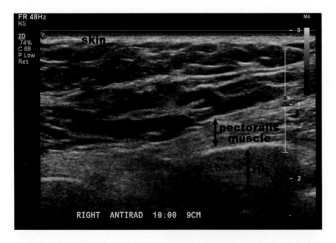

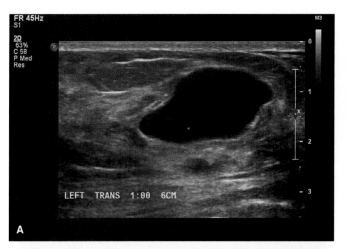

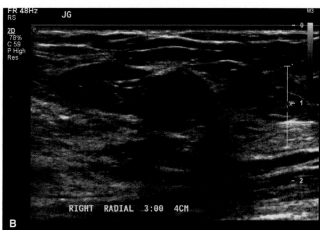

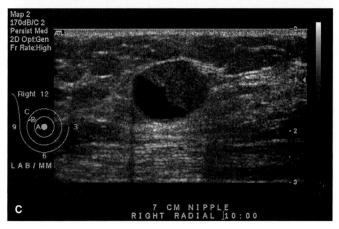

Figure 2.3 Cyst ultrasound: (**A**) simple cyst, (**B**) complex cyst, and (**C**) complex mass.

 PREOPERATIVE PLANNING

Percutaneous aspiration of a cyst can be performed either in freehand fashion or with ultrasound guidance. Ultrasound guidance is strongly preferred for several reasons: (1) it will help to achieve maximal drainage and (2) it will evaluate for any residual mass after aspiration that may be present but not palpable once the bulk of fluid is removed. It is not necessary to discontinue aspirin or anticoagulants such as warfarin for a fine needle aspiration. As with all procedures, informed consent should be obtained via discussion with the patient. All materials should be assembled and ready, including skin prep solution, sterile drape and gloves, 21-gauge needle, 5- or 10-mL syringe, and a plastic strip bandage. After skin prep and drape, the needle should be attached to the syringe and the plunger worked to ensure it is moving freely. If ultrasound is not available, a freehand technique may be used.

PROCEDURAL TECHNIQUES

Freehand Technique of Cyst Aspiration

For this approach, the lesion is stabilized between the thumb and the fingers of the non-dominant hand (Fig. 2.4A). The syringe is grasped with the dominant hand across the palm with the needle end of the syringe extending between the thumb and the forefinger, such that the fourth finger and the fifth finger can withdraw the plunger, enabling the operator to direct the needle and apply suction simultaneously (Fig. 2.4B). Local anesthetic can be applied in a skin wheal but is not necessary. Needle entry site is

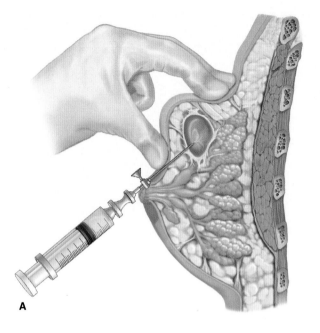

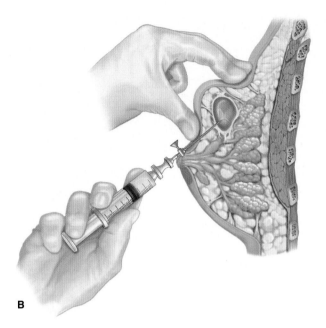

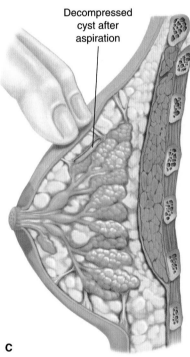

Decompressed
cyst after
aspiration

Figure 2.4 Freehand aspiration of palpable cyst: (**A**) Stabilize palpable cyst between the thumb and the forefinger of nondominant hand; (**B**) hold needle and syringe across palm of dominant hand, applying traction on plunger with fourth finger; and (**C**) collapsed cyst after aspiration.

planned such that the needle tract will be parallel to the chest wall in order to avoid pneumothorax. After skin prep, the needle is placed under the skin and negative pressure is applied to the syringe. The needle is advanced directly into the lesion, maintaining negative pressure in the syringe. The cyst is aspirated until there is no residual palpable mass (Fig. 2.4C). Aspirated fluid that is nonbloody may be simply discarded. If the aspirate is bloody or gelatinous, postaspiration imaging and tissue biopsy are indicated. Cytologic evaluation of bloody aspirate fluid is obtained in some practices, but this practice is not routinely recommended, as false-negative cytology is common among inexperienced samplers and pathologists not specially trained in cytology. Should a residual mass be palpable after cyst aspiration, repeat imaging is required to evaluate whether there is persistent cystic fluid that was not adequately drained or whether there is a residual solid component to the palpable mass that requires tissue biopsy.

Ultrasound-guided Percutaneous Aspiration of a Breast Cyst

Ultrasound-guided percutaneous aspiration of a breast cyst is performed according to standard techniques for image-guided breast biopsy. As in freehand aspiration, a 21-gauge needle and a 5- or 10-mL syringe are used. The lesion is visualized optimally with ultrasound and stabilized under the transducer with the nondominant hand (Fig. 2.5A,D). After antiseptic skin prep, the needle is advanced at a 45-degree angle in line with the long axis of the ultrasound transducer into the field of view and into the center of the cyst (Fig. 2.5B,E). All fluid is aspirated until the cyst completely disappears (Fig. 2.5C,F). As in freehand aspiration, any lesions with bloody aspirate or residual mass–like features require core needle diagnostic biopsy.

 PEARLS AND PITFALLS

Having all necessary materials available and ready facilitates a smooth procedure. It is also helpful to have an assistant available to converse with the patient and provide reassurance during the procedure; in addition, this reduces interruption of the procedure if an additional syringe or other supply is needed. Always be aware of the depth of the target lesion within the breast and the position of the needle tip in order to avoid pneumothorax as a possible complication. If frank blood is encountered in an aspiration, withdraw the needle and hold direct pressure over the site for at least 5 minutes. The procedure should be aborted and reattempted another day, once any hematoma has resolved.

 POSTPROCEDURE MANAGEMENT

For palpable/symptomatic simple cysts, a follow-up visit in 4 to 6 weeks is recommended to identify early recurrence of the cyst, although the value of this practice has been recently questioned. If the cyst recurs within this short period of time, then surgical excision is recommended. If the cyst is not palpable and initial diagnostic imaging was negative other than the cyst, then the patient is recommended to return to routine breast cancer screening guidelines. Simple cysts that are detected incidentally do not require any specific follow-up, and routine screening guidelines may be resumed.

 COMPLICATIONS

There are very few complications of cyst aspiration. Bruising, hematoma, and infection can occur rarely, and the risk of pneumothorax is remote.

 RESULTS

Ultrasound is the preferred diagnostic evaluation for suspected cystic lesions, and diagnostic mammography should also be performed for women aged 30 to 35 years and older. Simple cysts that are asymptomatic do not require aspiration, which is indicated for symptomatic simple cysts and complex cystic lesions. Most aspirated cysts do not recur rapidly, with only approximately 10% clinically apparent at 6- to 8-week follow-up visit. Ultrasound guidance is recommended for aspiration and allows immediate determination of the therapeutic benefit of the procedure as well as determination of any residual mass lesion and thus which patient should undergo core needle biopsy, since up to 25% of complex cysts and 50% to 60% of cystic masses harbor cancer.

Part II: Breast Biopsy

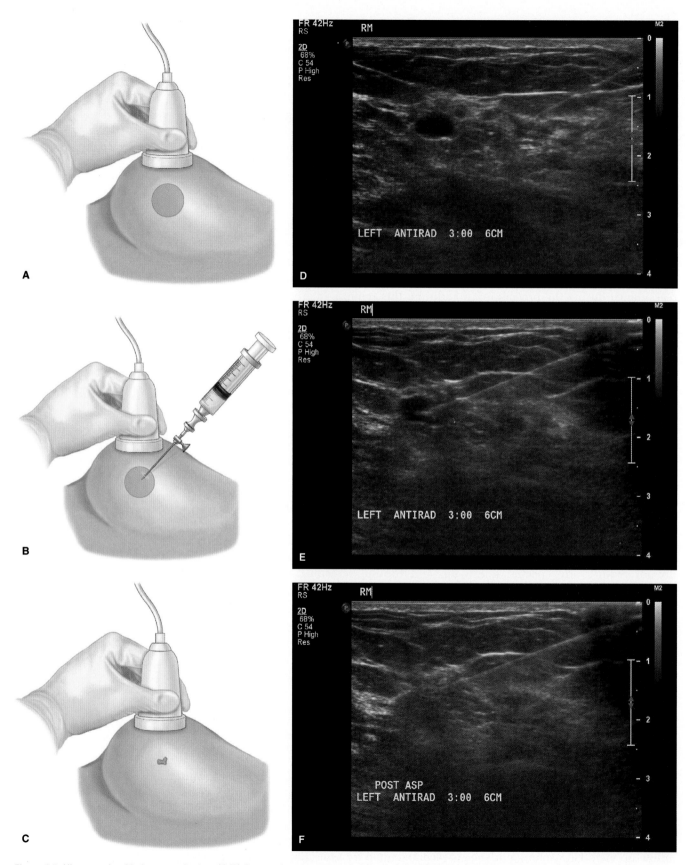

Figure 2.5 Ultrasound-guided cyst aspiration: (**A/D**) Center ultrasound transducer over cyst, (**B/E**) direct needle along long axis of transducer over the cyst, and (**C/F**) collapsed cyst after aspiration.

TABLE 2.1	Features of Lactational and Nonlactational Abscesses	
	Lactational	**Nonlactational**
Etiology	Untreated infectious mastitis	Squamous metaplasia of central nipple duct lining with keratin plugging, duct ectasia, and periductal inflammation
Age	Childbearing years (third decade of life)	Any age
Microorganism	*Staphylococcus aureus*	Aerobes and/or anaerobes *Staphylococcus aureus* *Staphylococcus epidermidis* *Bacteroides* *Streptococci* *Enterococci*
Relapse	Rare	Common without excision of nipple ducts
Location	Segmental area of peripheral parenchyma	Subareolar location

Breast Abscesses

Breast abscesses are generally categorized as one of two types: lactational abscesses and nonlactational abscesses (alternate terminology is puerperal and nonpuerperal abscesses). These two different types of breast abscesses have different profiles in terms of etiology, location, microbiology, and relapse patterns (Table 2.1; Fig. 2.6A,B). Nonlactational breast abscesses can occur at virtually any age, whereas lactational abscesses are most common in the third decade of life as would be expected around the childbearing years. Because of differences in their nature and treatment, these two entities will be discussed separately.

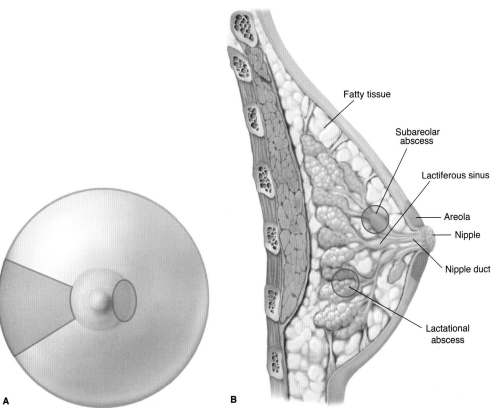

Figure 2.6 Abscess locations: (**A**) frontal diagram and (**B**) sagittal diagram.

Fatty tissue

Subareolar abscess

Lactiferous sinus

Areola

Nipple

Nipple duct

Lactational abscess

A

B

Lactational Abscesses

INDICATIONS/CONTRAINDICATIONS FOR DRAINAGE

By definition, lactational abscesses are associated with lactation in the puerperium. Specifically, this includes abscesses occurring during pregnancy, lactation, or within the first 3 months after cessation of lactation. Inspissated secretions and stasis of the breast milk with its intrinsic sugar content provide the ideal bacterial culture medium, and infection can progress rapidly. The responsible organism is almost always *Staphylococcus aureus*, attributable to the skin flora of the breast and also present in the oral flora of the suckling infant. Usually, lactational abscesses are preceded by lactational mastitis, characterized by fever, malaise, and exquisite tenderness (with or without overlying erythema) in a segmental area of the breast gland. Occasionally, systemic sepsis can be evident. Prompt treatment with antibiotics is paramount to prevent progression to abscess—oral antibiotics if the patient is stable and intravenous if septic. Dicloxacillin for 14 days is the recommended regimen. Rest, increased fluid intake, and more frequent suckling of the infant are additional important components of treatment to help clear the ductal obstruction. Diagnostic ultrasound should be obtained if there is any suspicion of abscess at presentation or if rapid clinical improvement does not occur with antibiotic therapy. If mastitis progresses to lactational abscess, then drainage is indicated.

For unifocal or multifocal abscesses in a stable patient, percutaneous aspiration should be attempted. Abscesses smaller than 3 cm in diameter can be simply aspirated, whereas larger abscesses can be approached either with aspiration or with percutaneous catheter drainage. Ultrasound guidance should be used in order to achieve maximal drainage of pus from the abscess, and the aspirate should be sent for culture with microbial sensitivities to tailor antimicrobial treatment. Although the responsible organism is usually *Staph aureus*, resistant strains are increasing in the community and non-*Staphylococcal* species can be identified on occasion. Dicloxacillin is safe for the suckling infant, but if another antibiotic is chosen because of an unusual or resistant bacteria, safety for the infant should be addressed since the medication and/or metabolites are routinely transmitted via the breast milk. Antibiotics are prescribed as mentioned earlier, and the patient returns for repeat ultrasound and reaspiration every other day until no fluid remains in the cavity. For larger abscesses, a small percutaneous closed suction drain can be placed as an alternative approach to serial aspiration. Any of the following constitutes failure of nonoperative treatment and is an indication for surgical drainage:

- worsening systemic illness despite aspiration and antibiotics,
- abscess cavity does not progressively diminish in size, or
- local progression evidenced by skin necrosis or other changes.

Other indications for initial operative drainage are very large abscess size, complicated and extensive pattern of infected fluid collections throughout the breast, and inability to obtain adequate drainage of infected material with a percutaneous approach.

There is no contraindication to drainage of an abscess. Abscesses require drainage, either percutaneously or surgically.

PREOPERATIVE PLANNING

When a patient presents with typical features of early lactational mastitis with duration of symptoms less than 48 hours, antibiotics and additional supportive measures as mentioned earlier are recommended. If the patient does not improve within 36 hours, then breast ultrasound is indicated to look for a fluid collection defining the presence of an abscess. If the patient's initial presentation includes any signs concerning for abscess (indications that the infection is fluctuant or pointing), then breast ultrasound should be performed at the first evaluation (Fig. 2.7A,B). Mammography will not be possible at

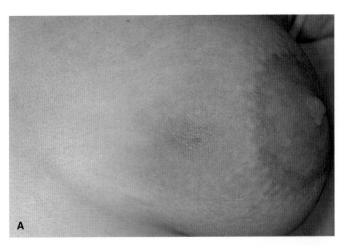

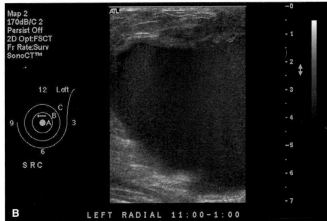

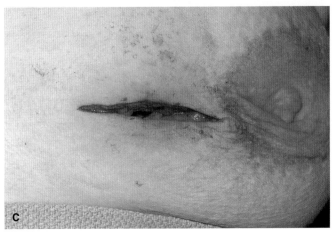

Figure 2.7 A 24-year-old woman with lactational mastitis treated for 1 month with antibiotics. **A.** Despite some improvement, focal pain and erythema persisted. **B.** Ultrasound showed a fluid collection underlying the site of erythema, connected with a larger fluid collection occupying the entire subareolar space, and having an estimated size greater than 10 cm. Because of large size and chronicity of symptoms, decision was made for surgical drainage. **C.** A radially oriented incision was made in the medial breast, 160 mL of pus was drained, abscess wall was debrided, and tissue sent for biopsy, which was benign.

initial presentation in affected patients due to exquisite tenderness. In cases of documented lactational abscess, consultation with a lactation consultant is appropriate preoperatively to help manage ongoing lactation postoperatively and to ensure proper lactation techniques to help correct problems that could predispose the contralateral breast similarly to mastitis and abscess. Cessation of lactation is not necessary. If the patient wishes to stop nursing, gradual rather than immediate cessation of lactation is preferred because of the ensuing engorgement that occurs with abrupt cessation of lactation, magnifying postoperative pain and possibly increasing the risk of milk fistula. If the infectious process is severe with extensive tissue necrosis, consultation with a plastic surgeon is advisable to help plan the surgical approach and optimize the cosmetic result.

SURGERY

Surgical Technique

For operative drainage of a lactational or peripheral breast abscess, an incision is placed transversely over the abscess, if possible (Fig. 2.7C). In the medial and lateral breast, this will be a radially oriented incision, whereas in the upper and lower central breast, this will constitute a transverse (antiradial) incision. The incision needs to be long enough that the resulting abscess cavity can be packed easily and the skin will not heal over before the depth of the wound has contracted. The incision is deepened into the abscess cavity, and intraoperative cultures are obtained, with care to provide the culture specimen in the correct medium/container to allow both aerobic and anaerobic cultures. All pus is drained and necrotic tissue is debrided. Although coincidental carcinoma in an abscess cavity is rare, biopsy of the abscess cavity is reasonable for cases

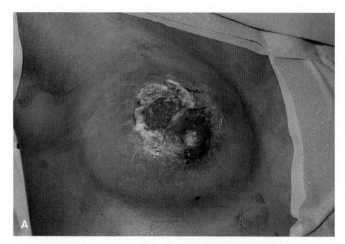

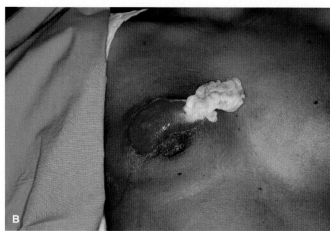

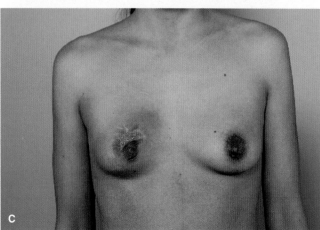

Figure 2.8 A 28-year-old lactating female who developed erythema and tenderness of the right breast 2 weeks postpartum. Lactation was discontinued and the process worsened. One week later, she underwent superficial incision and drainage in the emergency department. Four days later, she presented with worsening infection. **A.** Physical examination showed an enlarged inflamed breast with an open ulcerated wound, tissue necrosis, and a fluctuant area at 1 to 2 o'clock. Ultrasound showed complex fluid collections in both upper quadrants and a third fluid collection in the deep upper inner quadrant. At operation, necrotic skin was debrided, unroofing the medial abscess cavity. Pus extended throughout the central breast and into the retromammary space, and tissue biopsy was benign. Dressing changes were performed in the operating room at 24 and 48 hours at which time a wound vac was placed. **B.** The wound granulated well by 2 weeks and showed dramatic contraction and healing by 4 weeks (**C**).

that proceed to open drainage as long as this can be performed without compromising the cosmetic result because of excess tissue removal. Any necrotic overlying skin is debrided, and the wound is explored for loculations and tracts to ensure complete drainage (Fig. 2.8A–C). Vigorous irrigation and meticulous hemostasis are performed, and the wound is packed loosely with saline moistened gauze.

🔄 PEARLS AND PITFALLS

Lactational abscess can be locally destructive of normal tissues, so it is necessary to adequately debride necrotic tissue. Alternatively, do not remove extra healthy tissue; it is not necessary to excise back to normal-appearing tissue, as this will increase the tissue defect without any wound-healing benefit. If the tissue defect is large (greater than approximately 20% of the breast volume), it is advisable to have a plastic surgeon evaluate the wound early on to help with managing the long-term cosmetic result. Even large abscess cavities will usually heal with a good cosmetic result by secondary intention (Fig. 2.8A–C). Although excision of a small abscess and primary closure is tempting to avoid dressing changes, primary closure is contraindicated.

→ POSTOPERATIVE MANAGEMENT

The open wound is packed with saline-moistened gauze three times a day, reducing to twice a day once the wound has a bed of clean granulation tissue. Antibiotic treatment is continued for 2 weeks postoperatively. Additional supportive care with ongoing lactation is also recommended as mentioned earlier. Clinical signs of acute inflammation should resolve within a week; if not, repeat ultrasound should be performed to look for any undrained fluid collections. Once healed by secondary intention, recurrence of a lactational abscess is rare. All patients should undergo diagnostic mammogram after resolution of the breast abscess to establish a baseline mammogram.

 ## COMPLICATIONS

Significant breast deformity is unlikely but may occur, especially after open drainage and healing of larger abscesses by secondary intention. Plastic surgery consultation can be considered in the elective setting once the infection has resolved. Recurrent abscess can result from inadequate operative drainage or premature closure of the skin before healing of the deep tissues, which may be due to an incision that is too small or due to inadequate wound care. Milk fistula is a rare complication of open drainage in the lactating breast. This is characterized by milk that drains directly from an open surgical wound in the lactating breast. Classically, the milk drains during feedings and remains dry in between feedings. Wound management is indicated to protect the skin, and moist dressings should be maintained in the subcutaneous tissue. Usually, the tissues will granulate, with spontaneous resolution of the milk drainage within 4 to 6 weeks. If a milk fistula persists beyond 6 to 8 weeks, then cessation of lactation from the involved breast is indicated.

 ## RESULTS

Greater than 90% of lactational abscesses can be successfully treated without surgery, with a treatment plan of antibiotics and repeat percutaneous aspiration every other day until resolution of the abscess fluid. Lactational abscesses that require surgical drainage uniformly resolve with proper treatment, and cosmetic compromise is uncommon.

 ## CONCLUSIONS

Lactational abscesses result from inadequately treated lactational mastitis. These abscesses generally occur away from the nipple areolar complex but can be rapidly progressive. The usual microorganism is *Staph aureus*, but cultures and sensitivities should be obtained. Serial percutaneous aspiration is preferred for small abscesses in a stable patient. For larger abscesses, percutaneous catheter drainage can be successful. For those that fail percutaneous drainage or progress despite aspiration, operative drainage is indicated. Tissue biopsy of the abscess cavity is recommended for those cases that proceed to open drainage. Diagnostic mammography and ultrasound should be performed 3 months after resolution of the abscess to rule out any residual mass or findings suspicious for malignancy.

Nonlactational (Subareolar) Abscesses

 ## INDICATIONS/CONTRAINDICATIONS FOR INTERVENTION

Nonlactational abscesses occur almost exclusively in the subareolar/periareolar location. Nonlactational abscesses that occur in the periphery of the breast should be treated similar to lactational abscesses with two primary differences: (1) broad-spectrum antimicrobial therapy is needed and (2) biopsy of the abscess cavity is strongly suggested to rule out cancer at the time of open drainage. The most common type of nonlactational abscess occurs in the subareolar location and is a late manifestation of the "mammary duct–associated inflammatory disease syndrome" (MDAIDS), a term coined by Meguid et al. Subareolar abscesses result from keratin plugging of the major mammary

Figure 2.9 Photomicrograph of keratin plugging in an excised nipple crease and associated obstructed lactiferous duct in patient with chronic subareolar abscess. (From Li S, Grant CS, Degnim A, Donohue J. Surgical management of recurrent subareolar breast abscesses: Mayo Clinic experience. *Am J Surg.* 2006;192: 528–529, with permission.)

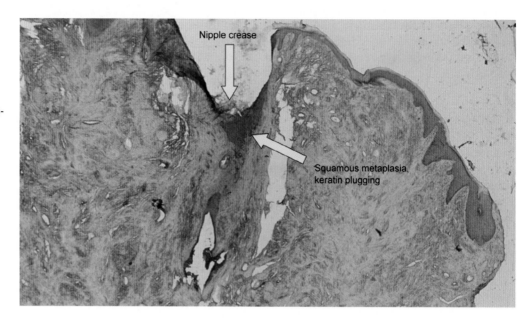

ducts in the nipple (Fig. 2.9), with superinfection of obstructed secretions. These abscesses are strongly associated with a smoking history, with greater than 70% of affected patients being active smokers. If subareolar abscesses are untreated, they will spontaneously drain (usually at the vermilion border of the areola) and progress to chronic fistula. Treatment is based upon the stage of the inflammatory process.

Early Abscess

For early abscess (Fig. 2.10A) consisting of an indurated subareolar mass without fluid collection on ultrasound, a 2-week course of antibiotic therapy should be prescribed. Antibiotic treatment must provide coverage for *Staphylococcal* species as well as for anaerobes. The most common organisms isolated are *Staph aureus* and *Staph epidermidis*, but other reported isolates include *Streptococcus, Corynebacterium, Bacteroides, Peptostreptococcus, Propionobacterium,* and *Candida albicans* (which occurs in HIV patients). In the absence of culture results, suggested empiric regimens are minocycline and levofloxacin (Levaquin) or cephalexin and metronidazole. The patient should be seen weekly to assess improvement or sooner for progression of symptoms. Some authors recommend elective excision, whereas others recommend reserving operation for cases that recur. If there is any visible associated abnormality of the nipple (retraction, inversion, or a central crease), the likelihood of abscess recurrence is high, and the patient should be counseled regarding the option for elective excision of the abscess site and involved central nipple duct(s).

Mature Abscess

In patients with mature abscess (Fig. 2.10B) that is fluctuant, serial percutaneous aspiration and bacterial culture are recommended as in initial percutaneous treatment of lactational abscesses. If the abscess is pointing with near necrosis of the skin at the areolar edge, then incision and drainage under local anesthesia will facilitate drainage and provide material for bacterial culture, with prompt symptomatic relief for the patient. The draining tract should be packed with a gauze wick until healed. Combined antibiotic therapy is recommended as for early abscess, tailoring treatment to culture results. Once the acute inflammation has resolved (usually 2–4 weeks), elective excision of the abscess cavity and central nipple duct is recommended. If the abscess is very small, has no fistula, and resolves with a single aspiration and antibiotic therapy, then operation can be omitted, but subareolar abscesses recur commonly without excision of the abscess cavity and associated obstructed nipple duct(s).

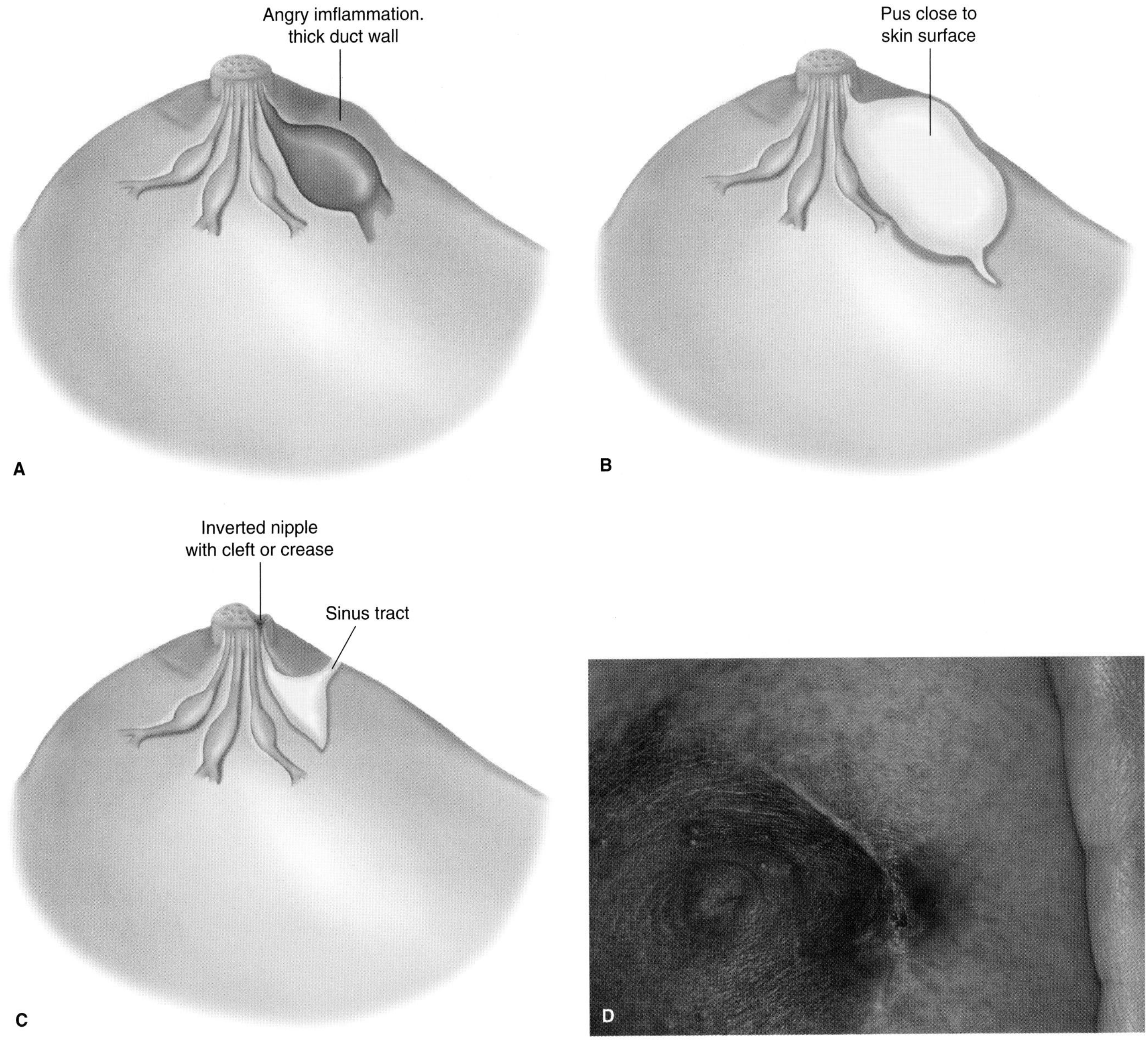

Figure 2.10 Subareolar abscess: (**A**) early, (**B**) mature, (**C**) chronic with fistula, (**D**) with periareolar fistula.

Chronic Abscess with Fistula

Once a chronic infection (Fig. 2.10C,D) is established in the subareolar space with a draining fistula, operative treatment is necessary for resolution of the infectious process. For the rare patient who presents with multiple fistulae resection of the entire nipple areolar complex may be necessary, and preoperative consultation with a plastic surgeon is advised.

PREOPERATIVE PLANNING

During preoperative physical examination, a detailed inspection of the nipple surface is recommended, looking for nipple inversion, retraction, a nipple crease, or other surface nipple abnormality that may cause obstruction. The nipple stalk should also be rolled between the thumb and the forefinger to identify any masses or enlarged/thickened ducts, as well as discharge of pus from the nipple surface. In the setting of acute inflammation, ultrasound should be obtained to define whether an abscess is present (Fig. 2.11). Diagnostic mammogram should be obtained in a few weeks when the acute inflamma-

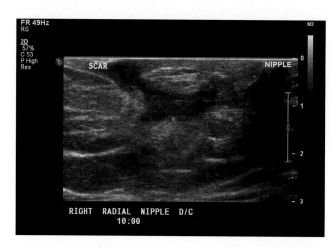

SCAR   NIPPLE

RIGHT RADIAL NIPPLE D/C
10:00

Figure 2.11 Ultrasound of subareolar abscess cavity extending from nipple to fistula.

tion has receded and the patient is able to tolerate the imaging. These imaging studies should focus particular attention to the subareolar and periareolar region. No benefit has been demonstrated for preoperative fistulogram. Diagnostic imaging studies should be performed prior to definitive operation.

The patient should be counseled regarding the possibilities of altered cosmesis and decreased nipple sensation after operation. If the patient is of childbearing age, she should also be informed of possible difficulty with future lactation due to disruption of the central nipple ducts. The patient should be treated pre- and postoperatively with broad-spectrum antibiotics (as described above) that continue for 10 to 14 days postoperatively.

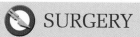 SURGERY

Surgical Technique

General anesthesia is recommended for surgical treatment of subareolar abscess. Definitive operation consists of excision of the abscess cavity, fistula(e) if present, and affected central nipple duct(s). Following sterile prep and drape, the nipple should be compressed to identify the location of any ducts with purulent discharge. If no fistulous tract was ever associated with the abscess, a periareolar incision is elected. The inferior areolar border is cosmetically preferred to an incision at the superior areolar edge (Fig. 2.12A). Dissection

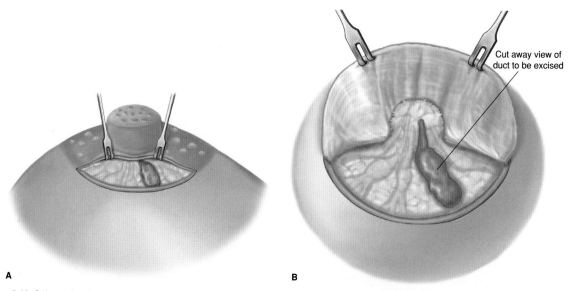

Cut away view of duct to be excised

A   B

Figure 2.12 Subareolar duct excision technique. **A**. Incise skin at inferior areolar edge and elevate areolar skin flap dissecting toward central ducts. **B**. Identify enlarged/diseased duct and excise in entirety including plugged duct of nipple dermis.

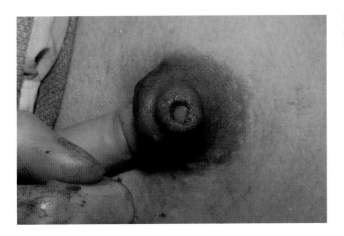

Figure 2.13 Excision of central nipple dermis to completely remove superficial portion of plugged duct(s).

proceeds in the subcutaneous plane toward the central nipple ducts. The involved area can be identified either by its abnormal central duct or by the residual inflammatory tissue changes. The residual inflammation of the abscess is localized with palpation and excised en bloc with the associated diseased duct (microdochectomy), which is usually visibly enlarged and extends to the nipple (Fig. 2.12B). In postmenopausal women, excision of the entire major central duct bundle (mammodochectomy) is appropriate for treatment as well as for prevention of future subareolar abscess. If there is an associated nipple retraction or obvious nipple crease, a small ellipse of skin at the apex of the nipple is excised for complete removal of the duct and its keratinous plug (Fig. 2.13).

In cases of abscess with fistula, the fistulous tract must also be excised with the abscess cavity and associated central nipple duct(s) (Fig. 2.14A,B). Incision planning is primarily determined by the location of the fistula opening. Regarding incisions, various approaches have been reported with success and good cosmetic outcomes, including radial and periareolar incisions. Generally, transversely oriented incisions are favored, such that radial incisions work well for fistulae located in medial and lateral positions whereas supra-areolar and infra-areolar incisions work well for fistulae in those locations. The accomplished breast surgeon should be aware of various incision options so that the selected incision is tailored to the patient on the basis of the fistula location and the size and shape of the breast and nipple–areolar complex.

The essential elements of excision are (1) a small ellipse of skin around the fistula opening, (2) the abscess cavity, and (3) the central nipple skin and associated duct leading to the abscess cavity (Fig. 2.15). When possible, en bloc resection of these elements is optimal, but treatment can be successful even with excision of elements separately.

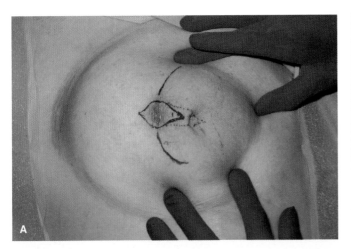
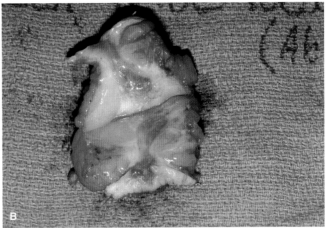

Figure 2.14 Chronic subareolar abscess with fistula and marked nipple retraction. **A.** Radial incision for chronic subareolar abscess with fistula. **B.** Cross-sectional appearance of chronic abscess cavity and fistula tract.

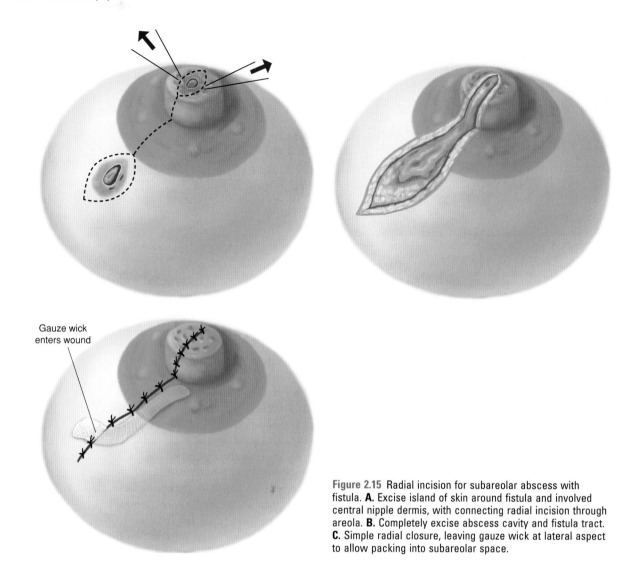

Figure 2.15 Radial incision for subareolar abscess with fistula. **A.** Excise island of skin around fistula and involved central nipple dermis, with connecting radial incision through areola. **B.** Completely excise abscess cavity and fistula tract. **C.** Simple radial closure, leaving gauze wick at lateral aspect to allow packing into subareolar space.

Gauze wick enters wound

After skin incision, dissection proceeds in the subcutaneous plane toward the central nipple ducts. The entire inflammatory mass is excised back to healthy tissue, and the involved duct(s) are excised with a small ellipse of associated nipple dermis. The specimen is oriented and sent for definitive pathologic review (Fig. 2.14B). If pus is encountered in the dissection or if prior cultures were negative, a small portion of excised tissue can be sent for culture.

The central subareolar parenchymal tissue defect must be approximated in order to provide support for the nipple–areolar complex and prevent recurrent nipple retraction with the normal contraction of healing. Depending on the size of the parenchymal defect and the nature and laxity of the patient's tissue, this can be performed by approximating the parenchyma with interrupted 3-0 Vicryl (Ethicon, Inc., Cincinatti, OH) in a transverse or pursestring approach (Fig. 2.16). For larger defects, a small rotational advancement flap of nearby parenchyma can be performed. If a radial incision is made from the nipple and extends past the areolar edge, then the base of the nipple is approximated with a single buried interrupted absorbable suture in the deep dermis and the vermilion border of the areola is similarly sutured. Consideration should be given to placing a pursestring stitch or Z-stitch in the deep dermis of the nipple base to reestablish normal nipple projection, if needed (Fig. 2.17), anticipating some degree of contraction with the healing process that could lead to flattening of the nipple. The nipple dermis is approximated with fine interrupted nonabsorbable sutures. The remainder of the incision is partially closed with interrupted nylon sutures, leaving a 7- to 10-mm space to place and exteriorize an iodoform gauze wick packed into the central depth of

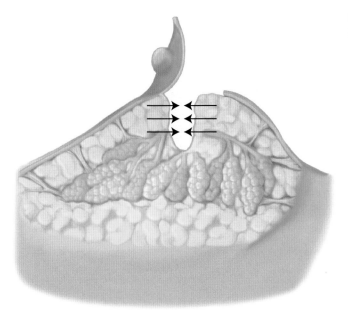

Figure 2.16 Closure of subareolar parenchymal defect.

the wound (lateral to the areolar closure if a radial incision is used) (Fig. 2.18A–D). Antibiotic ointment is placed on the nipple, and a nonadhesive sterile transparent occlusive dressing is placed to prevent catching and pulling of the sutures.

PEARLS AND PITFALLS

A key to success in the management of subareolar abscess is to excise the involved central nipple duct(s) up through the dermis of the nipple in order to reduce future recurrence. Performing a complete closure of the incision is debatable for cases of chronic recurrent subareolar abscess. Even though the abscess cavity has been excised, the wound bed is still contaminated. Partial closure of the wound encourages the skin edges to heal in a cosmetically favorable way, and placing a narrow gauze wick and proceeding with dressing changes via this open portion of the wound allow adequate drainage and healing by secondary intention.

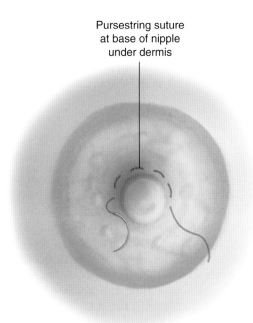

Pursestring suture at base of nipple under dermis

Figure 2.17 Absorbable pursestring suture placed at base of nipple/deep aspect of dermis to reestablish normal nipple projection.

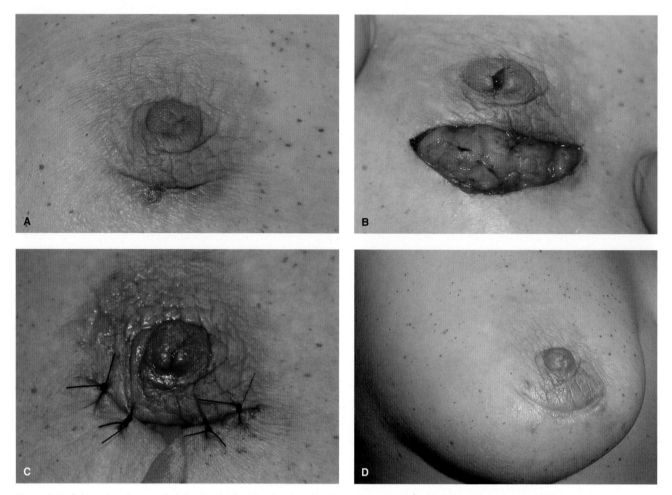

Figure 2.18 Subareolar abscess. **A.** Infra-areolar incision for chronic subareolar abscess with fistula. **B.** Appearance after resection of fistula tract and central nipple ducts via small ellipse of nipple skin. **C.** Gauze wick is exteriorized for packing. **D.** Postoperative result. (From Li S, Grant CS, Degnim A, Donohue J. Surgical management of recurrent subareolar breast abscesses: Mayo Clinic experience. *Am J Surg.* 2006;192:528–529, with permission.)

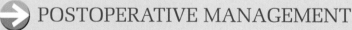

POSTOPERATIVE MANAGEMENT

If a gauze wick is placed (Fig. 2.18C), this packing is removed the day after surgery, and the patient is taught to change the dressing daily. Alternately, the wound can be cleansed daily with cotton swabs dipped in hydrogen peroxide, taking care to probe the wound to its depth. Complete healing usually requires 3 to 4 weeks. Oral antibiotics are continued for 10 to 14 days postoperatively.

COMPLICATIONS

The primary complication of operation for subareolar abscess is recurrence of the abscess. Rates of recurrence are proven to be linked to resection of involved obstructed nipple ducts, with 80% to 90% risk of recurrence without resection of the central nipple duct skin compared with 10% to 28% with resection of this nipple tissue. Poor cosmesis of the nipple–areolar complex can occur if there is skin necrosis, if the subareolar pillar is not reconstructed, or if excessive contraction associated with the healing process occurs. Necrosis of the nipple and areolar skin is primarily a theoretical concern since this has not been described in the major series of operative cases reported in the literature. Decreased nipple sensation and difficulty with lactation are expected sequelae, although also not quantified in the literature.

RESULTS

Over one-half of initial subareolar abscesses can be treated successfully with percutaneous aspiration and antibiotics, and success is better for those aspirated with ultrasound guidance probably due to more complete drainage. Surgical treatment should be considered for abscesses that recur or do not resolve with a percutaneous approach. For patients presenting with a history of multiply recurrent subareolar abscess or with fistula, surgical excision is necessary, and the success of this approach highly depends on excising the affected duct within the nipple. With excision of the associated diseased nipple duct, recurrence is uncommon (on the order of 10%–20% in most published series). Without excision of the nipple duct, reported recurrence rates are 40% to 80%. Partial closure leaving a gauze wick is a safer approach than primary closure, although primary closure has been performed with very low infection rates as long as there is no frank pus at surgery and the involved nipple duct is also excised. More than 80% of patients are happy with the cosmetic outcome. For those who are not, plastic surgery consultation should be obtained.

CONCLUSIONS

In summary, nonlactational abscesses occur primarily in the subareolar location and are associated with keratinous plugging of nipple ducts. Aerobic and anaerobic microorganisms can be involved. Early inflammation may be treated successfully with oral antibiotics. If the process progresses to abscess with fluid collection, it should be drained either percutaneously or surgically with simultaneous antibiotic therapy. Diagnostic breast imaging should be obtained once the acute inflammation recedes and before definitive operation. Patients with subareolar abscess are likely to develop recurrent infection without definitive surgical treatment, and those who have a draining fistula mandate operation for adequate treatment. At the time of surgery, the abscess cavity, associated nipple ducts and nipple skin, and any draining fistulous tract need to be excised in order to maximally reduce abscess recurrence.

Suggested Readings

Berg WA, Campassi CI, Loffe OB. Cystic lesions of the breast: sonographic-pathologic correlation. *Radiology.* 2003;227:183–191.

Berna-Serna JD, Madrigal M, Berna-Serna JD. Percutaneous management of breast abscesses. An experience of 39 cases. *Ultrasound Med Biol.* 2004;30:1–6.

Bhate RD, Chakravorty A, Ebbs SR. Management of breast cysts revisited. *Int J Clin Pract.* 2007; 61:195–199.

Chang Y-W, Kwon KH, Goo DE, et al. Sonographic differentiation of benign and malignant cystic lesions of the breast. *J Ultrasound Med.* 2007;26:47–53.

Christensen AF, Al-Suliman N, Nielsen KR, et al. Ultrasound-guided drainage of breast abscesses: results in 151 patients. *Br J Radiol.* 2005;78:186–188.

Gordon PB. Image-directed fine needle aspiration biopsy in nonpalpable breast lesions. *Clin Lab Med.* 2005;25:655–678.

Hamed H, Coady A, Chaudhary MA, Fentiman IS. Follow-up of patients with aspirated breast cysts is necessary. *Arch Surg.* 1989; 124:253–255.

Hook GW, Ikeda DM. Treatment of breast abscesses with US-guided percutaneous needle drainage without indwelling catheter placement. *Radiology.* 1999;213:579–582.

Lannin DR. Twenty-two year experience with recurring subareolar abscess and lactiferous duct fistula treated by a single breast surgeon. *Am J Surg.* 2004;188:407–410.

Li S, Grant CS, Degnim A, Donohue J. Surgical management of recurrent subareolar breast abscesses: Mayo Clinic experience. *Am J Surg.* 2006;192:528–529.

Meguid MM, Oler A, Numann PJ, Khan S. Pathogenesis-based treatment of recurring subareolar breast abscesses. *Surgery.* 1995;118:775–782.

Pinkney TD, Raman S, Piramanayagam B, Corder AP. The results of structured diagnostic pathway to minimise the chance of breast cancer misdiagnosis. *EJSO Eur J Surg Oncol.* 2007;33:551–555.

Scott BG, Silberfein EJ, Pham HQ, et al. Rate of malignancies in breast abscesses and argument for ultrasound drainage. *Am J Surg.* 2006;192:869–872.

Venta LA, Kim JP, Pelloski CE, Morrow M. Management of complex breast cysts. *AJR Am J Roentgenol.* 1999;173:1331–1336.

Versluijs-Ossewaarde FNL, Roumen RMH, Goris RJA. Subareolar abreast abscesses: characteristics and results of surgical treatment. *Breast J.* 2005;11:179–182.

Part II: Breast Biopsy

3 Ultrasound-guided Breast Percutaneous Needle Biopsy

Richard E. Fine

The number of biopsies required for diagnosis of image-detected abnormalities has increased with the continued promotion of screening for the early detection of breast cancer. In fact, each year in the United States, women undergo approximately 1.8 million breast biopsies. As confirmed by the 2005 International Consensus Conference II on diagnosis and treatment of image-detected breast cancer, minimally invasive image-guided percutaneous breast biopsy should be the first-line intervention for both palpable and nonpalpable image-detected abnormalities. Being less invasive and more cost-effective, image-guided percutaneous breast biopsy has essentially eliminated the need for open surgical biopsy for diagnosis, without sacrificing accuracy. Patients diagnosed with breast cancer by image-guided percutaneous biopsy may then proceed to definitive surgical management or be monitored with appropriate imaging and clinical follow-up if their pathology is benign.

Many of the early concerns about instituting an image-guided breast biopsy program such as patient acceptance (sampling rather than excision), accuracy (false-negative rate), overutilization (maintenance of proper indications), and qualifications (performed by radiologists or surgeons) have been resolved. The vast majority of patients with breast cancers and benign breast lesions will have their diagnosis made accurately with percutaneous image-guided needle biopsy, with many of these with ultrasound guidance.

INDICATIONS/CONTRAINDICATIONS

Almost any patient with an indeterminate, image-detected lesion, palpable or nonpalpable, should undergo a minimally invasive image-guided percutaneous biopsy. The modalities for image guidance include ultrasound, stereotactic, or magnetic resonance imaging (MRI) guidance. These abnormalities fall into the following categories established by the ACR (American College of Radiology) BI-RADS (Breast Imaging Reporting and Data System) lexicon:

- BI-RADS 5—highly suspicious abnormalities; biopsy provides a histology diagnosis for preoperative patient consultation

■ BI-RADS 4—indeterminate abnormalities; require biopsy and may avoid a trip to the operating room for an abnormality with perhaps only a 20% risk of malignancy
■ BI-RADS 3—(probably benign, 2%–4% risk of malignancy); abnormalities identified in a patient with a strong family history, difficult clinical and imaging examination, or a patient with a high level of anxiety.

The choice of image guidance is dependent on the modality of detection, the lesion type, and the tissue density of the breast parenchyma. The most common indication for ultrasound-guided percutaneous biopsy is the indeterminate or suspicious, ultrasound-visible, solid mass. However, some solid masses are better visualized on mammography because of a large fatty replaced breast parenchyma in which stereotactic guidance would be preferable. The usual approach for the patient with mammogram-detected microcalcifications without a mass is with stereotactic-guided percutaneous needle biopsy. However, rarely, with the advent of high-end, high-resolution ultrasound equipment, a prominent cluster of indeterminate calcifications can be biopsied with ultrasound guidance. Performing a second-look, directed ultrasound on a patient with an MRI-detected enhancing mass lesion will identify a lesion amenable to ultrasound guidance approximately 60% of the time. The advantage of ultrasound guidance over other imaging modalities includes patient comfort, lying supine (as opposed to prone with neck extension on the stereotactic table), and availability of ultrasound as an office-based procedure minimizing costs and scheduling delays.

The presence of a nonpalpable, solid mass is an indication for an ultrasound-guided needle core biopsy to obtain a histology diagnosis. It is also appropriate to utilize ultrasound guidance for the solid, palpable mass according to the American Society of Breast Surgeons Position Statement on Image-guided Percutaneous Biopsy of Palpable Breast Lesions (January 29, 2001). Without the adjunct of image guidance, the surgeon would be unable to confirm the proper penetration of the core needle through the lesion or the alignment of the tissue-sampling portion of a vacuum-assisted or rotating core device, leading to false-negative results.

The surgeon should categorize these abnormalities on the basis of their risk of malignancy. Smooth, well-defined margins suggest that a lesion is benign, whereas irregular, indistinct margins suggest malignancy. Heterogeneous internal echo pattern implies malignancy, whereas benign lesions usually display homogeneity. Posterior enhancement represents transmission of sound through the lesion related to lesion homogeneity and causes a brighter echo pattern behind the lesion, which is usually benign. The heterogeneous nature of many cancers will cause haphazard sound refraction, which leads to irregular shadowing. However, bilateral edge shadows are consistent with a smooth-walled benign lesion. Finally, benign lesions tend to be wider than they are tall (width greater than anterior–posterior diameter). In contrast, cancers tend to disrupt the adjacent normal tissue planes and appear taller than they are wide. Familiarity of these characteristics will help the surgeon anticipate the diagnosis. Any discordance between the image analysis and the pathology results would require excision of the lesion.

Unless the surgeon's assessment of the lesion finds all characteristics falling strictly in the benign category, they would categorize the lesion as indeterminate and some type of intervention is required. A smooth, well-circumscribed, anechoic lesion with bilateral edge shadowing and posterior enhancement representing a simple cyst, which is also asymptomatic, would require no intervention. For the small (less than 1 cm) solid, hypoechoic lesion with smooth margins, a homogeneous internal echo pattern and ellipsoid shape, ultrasound-guided needle biopsy can confirm a benign diagnosis, but a surgeon with experience in ultrasound interpretation and pathologic correlation may choose to monitor the lesion, especially with a highly compliant patient (Fig. 3.1A, and 3.1B).

"Indeterminate-risk" lesions often have heterogeneous interiors, indistinct yet smooth margins, and they may have a lateral/anterior–posterior dimension ratio greater than 1. If a surgeon cannot characterize a lesion as a simple cyst, aspiration to distinguish a complex cyst from a solid mass is required. A lesion with a mixed internal echo

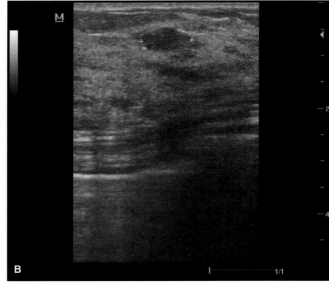

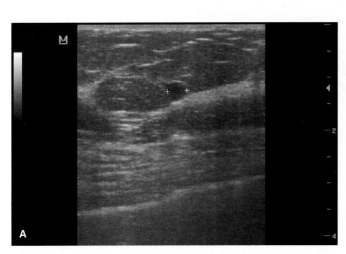

Figure 3.1 With experience in ultrasound interpretation and pathologic correlation, a surgeon may choose short-term follow-up ultrasound as opposed to biopsy for a small, benign appearing lesion **(A)**. Once a solid lesion is larger than 1 cm, the risk of occult malignancy rises and intervention may be required **(B)**.

pattern and posterior enhancement suggests the presence of fluid versus a solid lesion and an aspiration may be preferable prior to a core biopsy (Fig. 3.2). Chapter 2 addresses the details of cyst aspiration. Another indeterminate lesion requiring intervention is the cystic appearing abnormality with a mural or solid-appearing component. Only resolution of a complex cyst or a specific benign diagnosis on percutaneous needle biopsy will avoid surgical excision (Fig. 3.3).

Higher risk of malignancy requires a pathology diagnosis. For the more suspicious, high-risk lesions with jagged edges, nonhomogeneous internal echo patterns and irregular shadowing, the malignant diagnosis obtained with ultrasound-guided biopsy in a cost-effective, efficient manner in the office setting, facilitates planning of the definitive management (Fig. 3.4).

Ultrasound-guided percutaneous biopsy of highly suspicious (BI-RADS 5) lesions is optimal for planning the management of malignant lesions. Confirmation of the

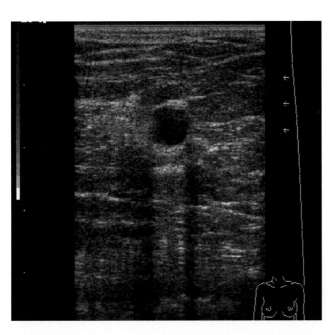

Figure 3.2 This lesion exhibits a mixed internal echo pattern and posterior enhancement, and although thought to be a solid lesion, it may prove to be a complex cyst on aspiration attempt.

Part II: Breast Biopsy

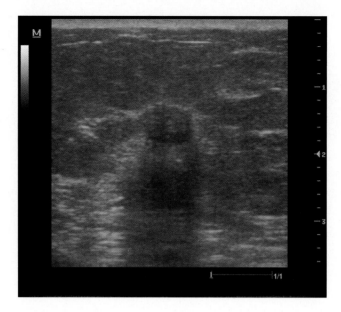

Figure 3.3 This lesion has both benign and indeterminate characteristics. The lesion is smooth but has a heterogeneous internal echo pattern and questionable shadowing.

histology eliminates an initial operating room procedure for diagnosis or a return to the operating room for contaminated resection margins. Encountering positive margins is twice as frequent at definitive surgery if not preceded by an image-guided percutaneous biopsy to confirm the malignant diagnosis. Patients who may be candidates for neoadjuvant or preoperative chemotherapy will ideally be diagnosed with image-directed percutaneous biopsy. The needle core biopsy tissue provides many of the ancillary markers required for appropriate management (estrogen/progesterone receptors and Her-2 neu).

The most common indication for an ultrasound-guided percutaneous biopsy is the indeterminate solid mass (BI-RADS 4), where approximately 80% will have a benign diagnosis. The previous standard for diagnosis of image-detected abnormalities with open surgical biopsy had several disadvantages including

- anesthesia requirements often resulting in time loss from work not only for the patient but also for the provider of needed transportation;
- the separate, time-consuming trip to the radiology suite for lesion localization, adding to the discomfort and emotional stress;

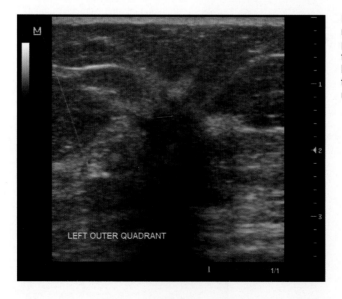

Figure 3.4 With irregular, indistinct margins; heterogeneous internal pattern; posterior shadowing and in this case an anterior–posterior to lateral dimension ratio greater than 1; this lesion should be malignant unless biopsy proves otherwise.

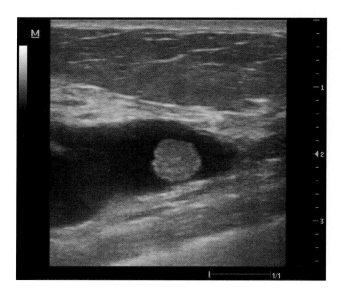

Figure 3.5 Dilated, subareolar duct with an intraductal solid lesion suggestive of an intraductal papilloma.

▓ larger incisions/scars, including scars within the parenchyma, leading to alterations on future mammograms; and

▓ potentially deforming surgery to remove a benign lesion that did not require removal.

If the benign pathology diagnosed with ultrasound-guided percutaneous biopsy fully explains the imaged findings, the surgeon need not remove the lesion, whether palpable or nonpalpable. The patient must also be comfortable with the reassurance of a benign diagnosis without removal of the suspect lesion. An image-guided percutaneous biopsy would be inadvisable for the patient who desires complete removal of the lesion, especially when it is palpable. The surgeon should avoid a percutaneous image-guided biopsy if surgical excision of a target lesion were part of the definitive management because the suspected pathology result would not be acceptable without excision. An example would be subareolar lesions with or without associated nipple discharge that are suspicious for papillary lesions where the pathologist requires intact histology architecture to eliminate atypia or papillary carcinoma (Fig. 3.5).

Ultrasound-guided percutaneous excision is an alternative to open surgical excision for those patients who desire the removal of their lesions, especially when palpable, despite being well informed. The surgeon may accomplish percutaneous excision with either one of the vacuum-assisted biopsy (VAB) devices or one of the devices capable of removing a large, single intact core of tissue. The procedure may be both therapeutic and diagnostic in a single setting. Percutaneous management of benign lesions has several benefits. In addition to the previously discussed disadvantages of the surgical approach, the patient avoids the physical and emotional trauma and added cost. Further indications for percutaneous excision with ultrasound guidance include but are not limited to the following:

▓ Nonoperative potential therapy for benign lesions
▓ Remove image evidence and or palpability of the lesion
  ▓ Clinically apparent fibroadenomas in younger patients
  ▓ Palpable lipoma causing location-related discomfort (inframammary fold)
▓ Nonoperative potential therapy for malignant lesions;
▓ Highly suspicious masses or densities
  ▓ Lesions ≤1.5 cm with large intact sampling devices

PREOPERATIVE PLANNING

The initial step, prior to ultrasound-guided breast biopsy, is to take an appropriate history, which includes an assessment of risk factors for breast cancer, and perform a clinical breast examination. A knowledge of anticoagulant medications can prevent

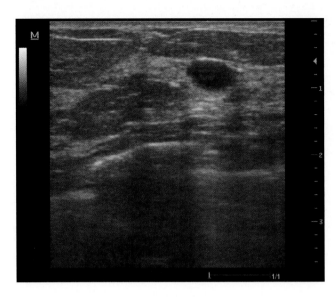

Figure 3.6 The posterior enhancement seen with this presumed solid, benign-appearing lesion suggests the possibility of complex cystic fluid that may be aspirated before attempting a core biopsy.

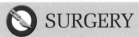

bleeding complications, including significant hematomas. A significant risk profile might lead the surgeon to perform an image-guided percutaneous biopsy on a lesion of low malignant potential (BI-RADS 3). The physician responsible for performing the biopsy should perform a clinical breast examination, confirming correlation between any suspicious palpable mass detected and the image-detected abnormality. The physician should also reevaluate the diagnostic ultrasound examination in complement to additional imaging available such as mammogram or MRI. Careful evaluation of the diagnostic ultrasound performed at an outside institution may suggest lesion characteristics, such as posterior enhancement, that allows the physician to attempt a cyst aspiration and eliminate the unnecessary wasting of an expensive disposable biopsy tool for a presumed solid lesion (Fig. 3.6).

The surgeon should outline the details of the benefits and risks of an ultrasound-guided percutaneous breast biopsy and have the patient sign an appropriate consent. Specific to the image-guided percutaneous procedures, the physician should emphasize to the patient that this is diagnostic procedure and that further intervention, including surgical excision may be necessary, depending on the concordance between the pathology and the impression of the ultrasound. It is important that the patient understands that unless the surgeon specifically plans a percutaneous excision, the mass may remain on future imaging and continue to be palpable. With ultrasound-guided percutaneous excision, it should be pointed out that a small percentage of lesions either will not be successfully removed in their entirety or will again be visualized on the follow-up imaging studies.

SURGERY

Positioning

The success of an ultrasound-guided percutaneous biopsy begins with proper positioning of the patient, physician, and equipment. The physician may place a pillow under the shoulder, with the ipsilateral arm raised to optimize the patient's supine position. This allows the breast to disperse more evenly on the chest wall, eliminating some of the thickness of the breast parenchyma. In addition, the lateral decubitus patient position provides the surgeon with access to deeper or posterior lesions by keeping the biopsy device parallel with the pectoral muscle. Placement of the equipment in the procedure room enhances the physician's visualization and comfort. By placing the ultrasound unit on the opposite side of the patient, the physician prevents turning his/her head away from the biopsy field to see the ultrasound monitor, further adding to the comfort. The physician's best visualization of the advancing biopsy device is along a

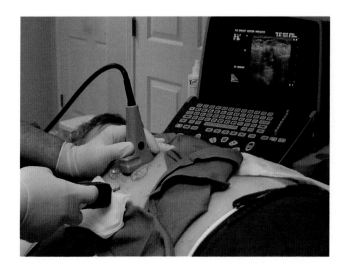

Figure 3.7 Alignment of physician, intervention device, and ultrasound equipment for optimal approach.

straight line of sight between the physician's vision, the physician's arm, down the length of the biopsy device, along the long axis of the ultrasound transducer, and up to the ultrasound monitor (Fig. 3.7).

Optimizing the Ultrasound Image and Scanning Technique

The ability to perform a successful ultrasound-guided percutaneous breast biopsy is also dependent on the ultrasound image quality and the physician's ultrasound scanning skill. The appropriate overall gain and time-gain-compensation slope should provide a uniform grayscale throughout the image. An improper overall gain setting may alter the appearance of the internal echo pattern and limit the ability to distinguish solid from cystic lesions. To achieve the optimal lateral resolution, the physician must align the focal zone with the target lesion. This will better illustrate the retrotumoral characteristics such as posterior enhancement (Fig. 3.8A–C). Once properly visualized, the physician compares the target lesion with the original ultrasound images and then documented, labeled, and measured.

The physician performing the biopsy should be facile with two basic scanning techniques that are crucial for identifying the area of greatest lesion diameter and positioning the lesion on the ultrasound monitor to limit the skin to lesion distance. Movement of the transducer in a motion perpendicular to the long axis of the transducer allows the scanner to visualize the lesion from end to end and find the widest portion of the lesion. Sliding the transducer in the direction parallel with the long axis will change the position of the lesion on the ultrasound monitor (Fig. 3.9A and 3.9B). To avoid veering off the edge of the lesion, the physician should position the ultrasound transducer so that the greatest diameter of the lesion is within the ultrasound plane, preventing missing the lesion with the needle core biopsy device. By correctly positioning the lesion on the ultrasound monitor, the physician will traverse the least amount of breast tissue with the biopsy device.

Biopsy Devices

The physician performing the ultrasound-guided percutaneous biopsy must decide on the proper device or instrument that best accomplishes the goal of the procedure. The most common objective of any image-guided biopsy procedure is of course to obtain a

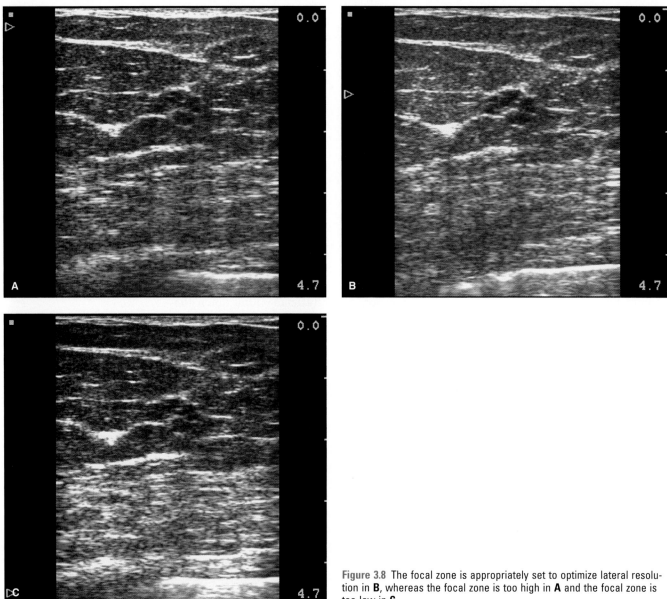

Figure 3.8 The focal zone is appropriately set to optimize lateral resolution in **B**, whereas the focal zone is too high in **A** and the focal zone is too low in **C**.

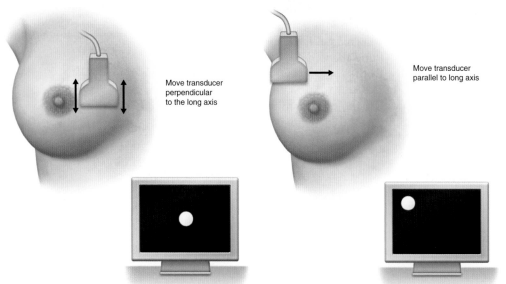

Move transducer perpendicular to the long axis

Move transducer parallel to long axis

Figure 3.9 Movement of the ultrasound transducer perpendicular to its long axis (painting) will allow the physician to determine the lesion's greatest diameter (**A**). The position of the lesion on the side of the monitor closest to where the biopsy device enters the skin is adjusted by moving the transducer along its long axis (skiing) (**B**).

A

B

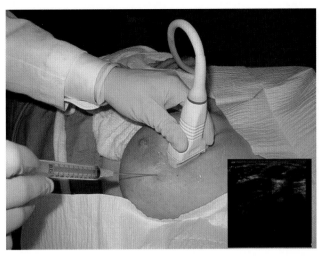

Figure 3.10 An ultrasound-guided fine-needle aspiration of an intra-mammary lymph node with an inset illustrating the visualization of the needle within the lesion.

benign or malignant diagnosis but the patient's desire or clinical presentation may influence the physician. The tools for specimen acquisition have evolved from fine-needle aspiration (FNA), automated Tru-cut (ATC) core needle, vacuum-assisted core biopsy devices to large-core, intact sample instruments, providing either "sampling" capability, adequate for most lesions or "removal" (by percutaneous excisional biopsy) capability for selected lesions. The surgeon must select the most appropriate instrumentation and biopsy type for each case.

Despite the criticism related to the degree of insufficient sampling and the need for expert cytopathology, FNA biopsy is a quick, inexpensive technique to delineate benign from malignant solid breast masses. Unfortunately, even with specialized experience and expertise, FNA yields inferior false-negative diagnosis rates for primary breast cancer compared to those obtained with core biopsy. However, ultrasound-guided FNA is ideally suited to evaluate lesions in areas where more invasive biopsy devices may be difficult, dangerous, such as the axilla, or adjacent to a breast implant. The diagnosis of lymph node metastasis by FNA can assist with pre-operative staging in consideration of neo-adjuvant chemotherapy or eliminate sentinel lymph node biopsy by confirming positive cytology in clinically suspicious lymph nodes (Fig. 3.10).

The use of ATC needle core biopsy (Fig. 3.11) eliminates the problems with FNA such as insufficient sampling and the inability to provide the histological type and grade of a diagnosed cancer. The 14-G spring-loaded core biopsy needle has been the most common device for ultrasound-guided percutaneous biopsy device of solid lesions at most centers since the mid-1990s and remains the most commonly used type for ultrasound-guided core "sampling," especially for the larger, easily targeted suspicious masses requiring only diagnosis. Spring-loaded core biopsy is adequate in most circumstances (Fig. 3.12A and 3.12B).

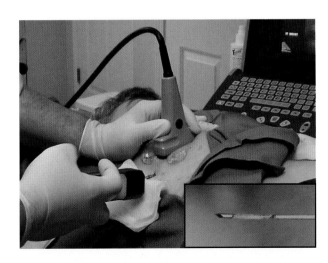

Figure 3.11 A 14-G, 20-mm core of tissue can provide a specific benign diagnosis and can distinguish between invasive and in situ carcinomas.

Part II: Breast Biopsy

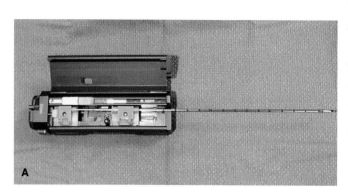

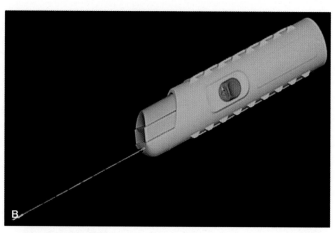

Figure 3.12 The spring-loaded automated Tru-cut devices are available as a nondisposable handpiece utilizing disposable core needle inserts **(A)** or as a single-piece disposable handheld biopsy tool **(B)**.

Despite accurate histology with spring-loaded core needles, specimens that are more substantial, obtained with the larger, vacuum-assisted/rotational core devices, offer advantages. Reduction in discordant pathology results with imaging and decreased upgrades in diagnosis (from atypical hyperplasia to cancer or from ductal carcinoma in situ [DCIS] to invasive cancer) is achieved with more tissue obtained at image-guided core biopsy. Accurate biological characterization of the individual breast cancer, including hormone receptor status, genomic profile, and protein expression, obtained with initial tissue-sampling is the result of optimal tissue fixation and preservation and in selected cases of neoadjuvant treatment provides needed information to guide therapy.

Vacuum-assisted and rotational core technology (Fig. 3.13) available with ultrasound guidance allow tissue acquisition with either multiple insertions of the device or a single device insertion allowing multiple tissue samples or a single large intact core sample. Understanding similarities and differences in available technology enables the surgeon to select the most appropriate device and application. In addition, the choice of device depends on the desired result of either "sampling" for diagnosis, with the advantages of larger core size/volume, or percutaneous excision of selected solid masses.

Development of the first directional VAB device, Mammotome Breast Biopsy System (Ethicon Endo-Surgery, Inc., Cincinnati, Ohio), satisfied the requirement of increasing the size of the core sample and the contiguous nature of the sampling as a proposed solution to the diagnosis upgrading issue (atypia to cancer) seen with stereotactic biopsy of microcalcifications. The improved accuracy with the directional VAB device significantly lowered the upgrading of diagnosis compared with spring-loaded needle core biopsy technology.

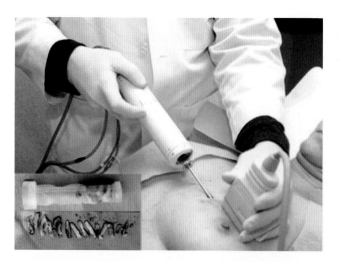

Figure 3.13 Vacuum-assisted biopsy technology allows multiple tissue samples with a single-device insertion. The tissue samples are larger and may improve diagnostic accuracy and/or allow potential removal of image evidence of the lesion (*insert*).

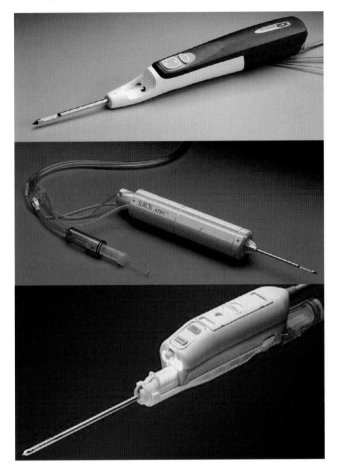

Figure 3.14 Ultrasound-guided vacuum-assisted biopsy devices: *top*—Mammotome EX, Ethicon Endosurgery, Cincinnati, Ohio; *middle*—ATEC, Hologic, Bedford, Massachusetts; *bottom*—EnCor, SenoRx, Irvine, California.

Part II: Breast Biopsy

Two additional directional, side-cutting VAB devices offer the same advantages as the Mammotome. The Automated Tissue Excision and Collection (ATEC) Breast Biopsy and Excision System (Hologic, Inc., Bedford, Massachusetts), pneumatically driven and lightweight, obtains cores faster than the Mammotome but collects them in a closed chamber. The EnCor (SenoRx, Inc., Aliso Viejo, California) offers 10-G and 7-G (the largest gauge currently available in this category) versions. In addition, all three devices are available in handheld versions for ultrasound-guided procedures and in versions that are compatible with MRI-guided biopsy (Fig. 3.14).

The directional, side-cutting VAB devices (Mammotome, the ATEC, and the EnCor) remove multiple tissue samples with a single insertion of the device into the breast—a significant advancement in technology. The vacuum applied to the side-cutting sampling portion of the device eliminates the pinpoint accuracy required with spring-loaded biopsy needles by pulling the lesion toward the sampling chamber. With the ability of the VAB sampling to be directional, the surgeon can overcome small targeting deviations by directing the biopsy aperture, rotating it toward the lesion. This directional capability with the ultrasound-guided VAB devices is helpful in also dealing successfully with deep target lesions because the physician positions the device below the lesion and directs the sampling superiorly, away from the chest wall or an implant. Manually inserting the device without having to utilize a "firing" mechanism could help deal with the deep lesion, avoiding the risks of penetrating the pectoral muscle or implant. Compared with samples obtained with the 14-G spring-loaded needle core device, the samples obtained are considerably larger.

Other currently available devices designed to remove larger core samples, utilizing either vacuum or rotating cutter, include EnCor 360 (formerly the SenoCor 360; SenoRx), Celero spring-loaded handheld breast biopsy devices (Hologic, Inc., Bedford, Massachusetts), and Vacora Breast Biopsy System (Bard Biopsy Systems, Tempe,

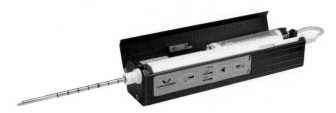

Figure 3.15 Vacora Breast Biopsy System, Bard Biopsy Systems, Tempe, Arizona.

Arizona) (Fig. 3.15). These devices require less capital expense than the Mammotome, ATEC, or EnCor while providing the diagnostic advantage of being able to capture larger tissue specimens. They require reinsertion for each core sample and do not generally provide percutaneous excisional capability. An additional larger core device utilizing a rotating cutter, the Flash (Rubicor Medical, Redwood City, California) (Fig. 3.16), provides a single-insertion, multisample device in a self-contained disposable unit employing a closed collection chamber and requires no capital cost.

The indications for ultrasound-guided VAB or rotational cutter devices are similar to those for needle core biopsy including any indeterminate, ultrasound-visible, palpable or nonpalpable solid masses. If the physician were interested in percutaneous excision, single-insertion, multisample VAB devices or large intact sampling devices would be required. Both of these device categories have successfully demonstrated their ability to remove image evidence and especially palpability of probably benign solid masses.

With an expected benign diagnosis, devices that permit the percutaneous multicore excision of even larger lesions are ideal when the patient wants it removed entirely. The Mammotome, ATEC, and EnCor are capable of removing all imaged evidence or palpability of a lesion (percutaneous excisional biopsy), such as a benign fibroadenoma. Devices that remove a very large single-core specimen are most suitable when pathologic examination of the entire intact lesion is desirable.

Large single-core devices, designed to remove an intact, single block of tissue include the Intact Breast Biopsy System (Intact Medical Corporation, Natick, Massachusetts) and the Halo Breast Biopsy Device (Rubicor Medical, Inc., Redwood City, California) (Figs. 3.7, 3.17A, and 3.17B). The main advantage of these devices is that they make it possible to excise a single larger sample of intact tissue than with the other VAB devices described earlier. This capability provides maximal diagnostic certainty and may prove particularly helpful in removing challenging lesions such as radial scar, lesions with associated atypia (atypical ductal hyperplasia [ADH], atypical lobular hyperplasia [ALH]), and lesions with pathologic diagnoses that are difficult without the entire lesion (papilloma, nodular adenosis, phyllodes tumor). Now that devices such as the Intact and Halo are available, surgeons and their patients have another option over surgical excision in selected cases. In such cases, these newer image-guided approaches are superior because of the precise targeting and preservation of tissue and the cost saving obtained by avoiding operating room charges.

Technique

A sterile or clean field is prepared. This technique is physician preference. There are disposable povidone/iodine (Betadine) swabs available, which can be used in combination with disposable sterile towels and individual packets of sterile ultrasound gel (Fig. 3.18). Others have chosen to use Betadine gel for both the antiseptic and the acoustic coupling. Alternative antiseptic solutions such as Hibiclens are available to

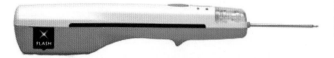

Figure 3.16 Flash single-insertion multisample core needle device, Rubicor Medical, Redwood City, California.

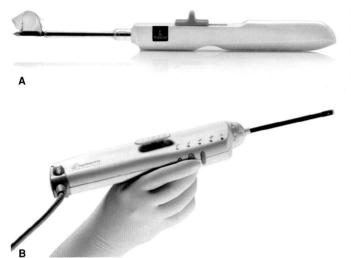

Figure 3.17 **A.** Halo large, single core breast biopsy device, Rubicor Medical, Redwood City, California. **B.** BLES large, single core breast biopsy device, Intact Medical, Natick, Massachusetts.

those with an iodine allergy. A sterile ultrasound transducer cover is optional. If utilized, it is necessary to place ultrasound gel inside the cover for acoustic coupling between the transducer and the cover. Appropriate antiseptic solutions are, however, a minimum requirement. The physician then identifies the target lesion, positioning the ultrasound transducer to demonstrate the lesion's greatest diameter and minimizing the skin to lesion distance.

With positioning and imaging optimized and the target lesion location in the breast reestablished, physicians the ultrasound transducer, with its long axis oriented in a direct line between themselves and the ultrasound monitor. The approach of the biopsy device toward the target lesion will be along the long axis of the transducer. The decision of the position of the entry site and the distance of the entry site from the transducer edge is dependent on the type of biopsy device and the depth of the lesion. Devices that require positioning beneath the lesion and those lesions that are deeper in the breast may require an entry site further away from the transducer edge to maintain a biopsy needle/device approach that parallels the skin and pectoral muscle. This allows better visualization of the approaching biopsy device and therefore improves accuracy and safety (Fig. 3.19).

Adequate local anesthesia is achieved by injecting at the proposed skin entry site and then into the deeper breast parenchyma under direct ultrasound visualization. The advantage of real-time imaging with ultrasound allows the physician to use greater volumes of local anesthetic for patient comfort and at the same time preventing creating any "pseudo" lesions or fluid collections that could interfere with visualization of the

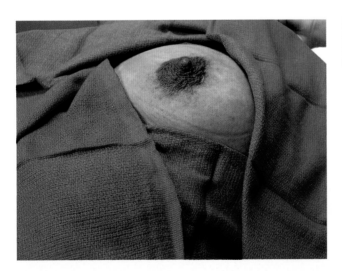

Figure 3.18 The field has been prepped with a disposable povidone/iodine swab in combination with disposable sterile towels.

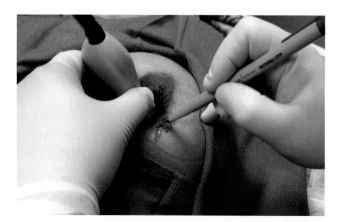

Figure 3.19 The physician marks the device entrance site based on the type of device and the depth of the lesion on ultrasound.

target lesion and accurate targeting. Injection along the pathway of the device to the target lesion and then creating a field block around the lesion is desirable (Fig. 3.20). The physician can accomplish this technique by injecting anterior and posterior to the lesion and then directing the needle superior and inferior to the lesion. Anesthetizing the breast parenchyma on the far side of the lesion, where the tip of a spring-loaded device may end its excursion, adds to patient comfort. The ability to direct the placement of local anesthesia can also be valuable in moving a superficial lesion away from the skin or lifting a deep posterior lesion off the underlying pectoral muscle or augmentation implant capsule. This can be especially important when utilizing a biopsy device that requires placement under the target.

The size of the skin incision made with a disposable 11-blade scalpel is a function of biopsy device but usually is between 2 and 6 mm. Once inserted through the skin incision, the physician must guide the biopsy device along the long axis of the transducer, maintaining the needle in the 1- to 1.5-mm thickness scan plane, constantly keeping the advancing needle tip in view on the ultrasound image (Fig. 3.21). By propping the patient with a pillow laterally and by gently pushing the far end of the transducer into the breast, keeping the device parallel to the sole of the ultrasound transducer allowing better visualization of the advancing device tip, possibly even demonstrating a comet tail artifact, further confirms the biopsy device position for intervention (Fig. 3.22).

Advancement of a forward cutting or coring device, such as the ATC device, toward the target lesion under direct ultrasound visualization continues until the needle tip abuts against the lesion. With the ATC device, as well as other forward cutting/coring

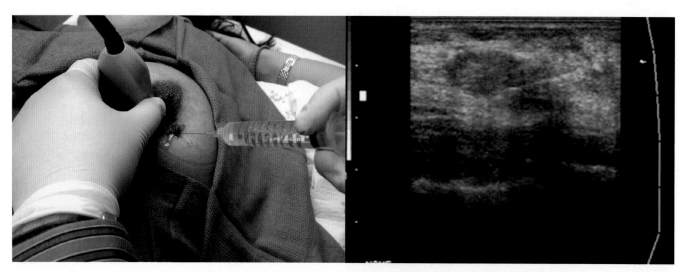

Figure 3.20 Ultrasound allows real-time visualization of the local anesthetic injection, allowing a complete field block without limiting the visibility of the lesion. The lesion can be moved away from the skin and/or chest wall by appropriate placement of local anesthetic.

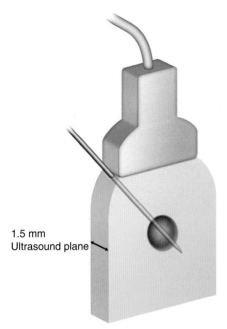

Figure 3.21 The biopsy needle is guided along the long axis of the ultrasound transducer and must be maintained within the narrow (1.5 mm) ultrasound plane.

1.5 mm
Ultrasound plane

devices, lesion sampling occurs with piercing by the sampling portion of the device. Before withdrawing the device to acquire the tissue sample, the physician should perform a confirmation scan. By scanning the ultrasound transducer in a motion perpendicular to its long axis, toward the superior end of the lesion, and then back past the portion of the lesion containing the biopsy needle toward the inferior end of the lesion, it can be ensured that the needle is in the lesion (Fig. 3.23). The goal is to see a portion of the lesion without a biopsy needle on either side of the scan plane containing the needle. Seeing the lesion on both sides of the device confirms that the device is inside the lesion and rules out the "image averaging" artifact that can occur when the device is immediately adjacent to the lesion (Fig. 3.24). Finally, the surgeon can obtain further confirmation by turning the transducer perpendicular to the device and imaging a cross section of the device within the lesion. With this orientation, the device appears as a small bright dot within the mass. Acquisition of the tissue sample follows the confirmation scan. Rolling the tissue off the needle trough onto a moistened telfa pad or rinsing it off in a container of saline solution is the physician preference. The multiple insertion devices requiring withdrawal from the breast for each tissue sample obtained prepared (cocked)

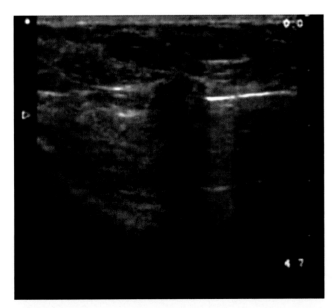

Figure 3.22 With proper positioning of the patient and tilting the ultrasound transducer, the needle remains parallel to the transducer face, allowing better visualization of the advancing needle tip.

Part II: Breast Biopsy

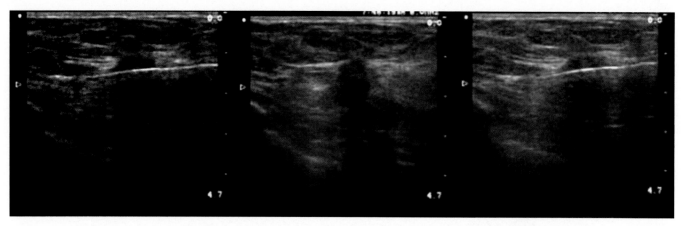

Figure 3.23 A confirmation scan is performed by moving the ultrasound transducer perpendicular to its long access from one end of the lesion to the other. By visualizing the needle within the lesion and then lesion without needle at either end of the confirmation scan confirms that the biopsy needle and tissue obtained can come from nowhere else but the lesion.

for additional sampling is reinserted into the breast through the same incision. It is important to adjust the biopsy needle tip toward different portions of the lesion to acquire adequate samples and avoid a sampling error and a resulting discordant diagnosis.

Positioning of either a side-cutting, VAB device or a radiofrequency loop device designed for acquiring a large, single, intact sample is beneath the target lesion for sampling. The first steps of the procedure are the same with a few exceptions including (1) positioning the patient in a more pronounced lateral decubitus position (especially for deeper lesions) to allow the device to remain parallel to the pectoral muscle and be guided beneath the lesion; (2) the use of larger amounts of local anesthetic both for comfort and to use the local anesthetic to lift a more posterior positioned lesion off the chest wall, to allow the device between the muscle and the lesion; and (3) the need for a slightly larger incision (usually 4–10 mm) depending on the gauge of the VAB device or the size of the lesion that will be extracted from the breast through the incision in a single intact specimen. Positioned beneath the lesion, rotating the ultrasound transducer 90 degrees confirms the proper alignment of the lesion with the sampling portion of the device by being able to see the circular artifact of the device directly below the center of the lesion (Fig. 3.25).

The goal of the ultrasound-guided percutaneous biopsy helps determine the amount of sampling for any of the devices chosen. For purely diagnostic purposes, especially confirmation of a suspicious lesion as malignant, approximately five good-quality cores

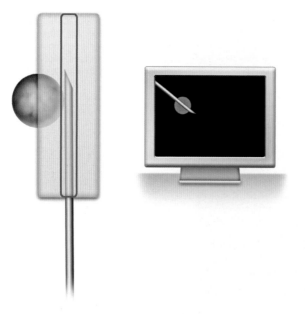

Figure 3.24 The confirmation scan helps avoid image averaging, where a needle misses but is up against the lesion and therefore is seen in the same ultrasound plane as the lesion, causing the physician to be falsely reassured that the biopsy needle has successfully penetrated the lesion.

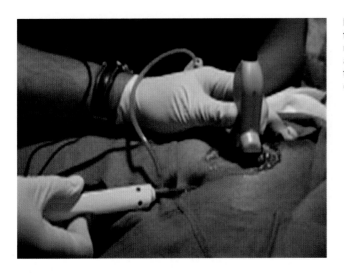

Figure 3.25 Ninety-degree rotation of transverse imaging is performed when utilizing either a vacuum assisted or a large intact sample biopsy device to confirm the position of the device centered underneath the lesion.

should be obtained. If the purpose of the procedure is to remove the image evidence of a solid mass that has a greater likelihood of being benign (i.e., fibroadenoma), a VAB device may require a much greater number of core samples. The gauge of the device may also influence the number of cores needed.

With the VAB device appropriately positioned, excision of the lesion proceeds in multiple cores, beginning at the deepest aspect and moving superficially with rotation of the sampling aperture superiorly and inferiorly. The Halo large intact loop device has a radiofrequency-activated cutting loop that is brought out lateral (3 o'clock position) and circumferentially rotated over the top of the lesion, followed by loop closure that completes the excision with the lesion contained within a small attached sampling bag. The physician withdraws the device from the breast, maintaining loop closure (Figs. 3.26 and 3.27).

Localizing marker placement before ending the procedure is common with percutaneous image-guided biopsy and is influenced by the purpose for the marker and the prospective next step in management. Deployment of a simple metallic marker in the center of a malignancy of a highly suspicious target lesion after a biopsy to confirm

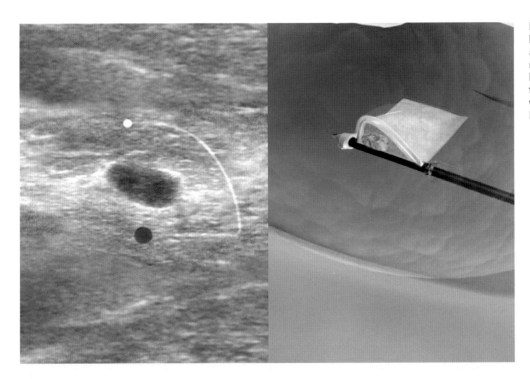

Figure 3.26 The Halo large intact loop device has a radiofrequency-activated cutting loop, which is rotated circumferentially, and with loop closure completes the percutaneous excision of the lesion within a small attached sampling bag.

Part II: Breast Biopsy

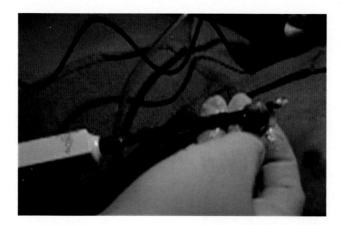

Figure 3.27 After the device is removed from the breast, the radiofrequency loop is reexpanded and the physician removes the lesion from the bag. The physician sometimes, as in this case, is able to palpate the entire fibroadenoma that has been excised.

malignancy will help identify the lesion location after the patient undergoes neoadjuvant treatment. The technique of guiding the marker applicator through the biopsy incision along the long axis of the transducer follows the similar ultrasound-guidance principles associated with performing the biopsy (Fig. 3.28). Removal of the image evidence of a lesion with a VAB device or as a larger single intact sample core or if a small lesion is difficult to visualize after removal of multiple cores requires markers with ultrasound visibility characteristics. These markers serve two purposes. If the lesion requires surgical intervention for cancer or for discordance between the pathology and the radiographic interpretation: the ultrasound-visible markers allow the surgeon to eliminate a preoperative trip for their patient to radiology for wire localization and allow them to perform their own intraoperative ultrasound localization for definitive surgery (Fig. 3.29A and 3.29B). If the ultrasound-guided percutaneous biopsy diagnosis is benign, the metallic portion of the marker remaining allows for future orientation and evaluation of the ultrasound biopsy site on mammogram. Others do not routinely utilize specialized ultrasound visible localization markers and rely instead on the routinely ultrasound visibility of the residual VAB or large intact device cavity and associated small hematoma for intraoperative localization.

PEARLS AND PITFALLS

Regardless of the imaging modality, the most significant error in image-guided breast biopsy is of course missing or inadequately sampling the lesion and providing the patient a false sense of security, with a benign diagnosis. Careful evaluation of the diagnostic ultrasound performed at an outside institution is essential for determining the

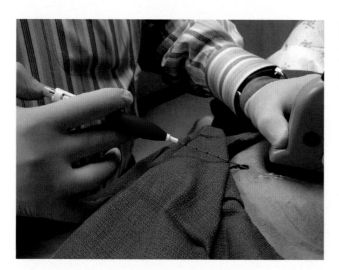

Figure 3.28 The placement of a localization marker may be accomplished by guiding the applicator along the long axis of the transducer by using the same principles as described for ultrasound-guided intervention.

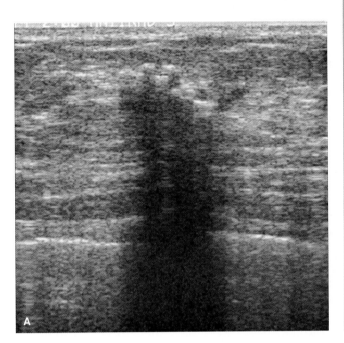

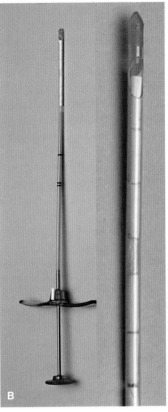

Figure 3.29 **A.** The localization marker with ultrasound visible pellets allows surgeons to perform their own intraoperative localization with ultrasound when needed. **B.** Ex-vivo clipand device.

Part II: Breast Biopsy

appropriate indication for biopsy, the correct image-guidance and the optimal biopsy device. For example, any suggestion of posterior enhancement or other characteristics of a possible complex cyst should first lead to an attempt at aspiration, eliminating the unnecessary wasting of an expensive disposable biopsy tool for a lesion that may actually turn out not to be solid.

Too much local anesthetic injected into the breast parenchyma carries the risk of the inability to visualize a smaller target lesion. In addition, the injection of too much local anesthetic in one area can create a false lesion that mimics a cyst. This can be especially frustrating when the target lesion is partially cystic. Physicians inject adequate local anesthetic under ultrasound guidance. However, if they have altered lesion visibility, they may wait for some of the local anesthetic to be reabsorbed before proceeding. Attempting to perform the biopsy without optimal visualization of the lesion could only result in an inadequate sampling of the lesion and a diagnosis that may falsely reassure the patient.

Also, among the potential problems is the inability to confirm the position of the advancing biopsy device. The key to visualizing the advancing tip of any device resides in both maintaining alignment of the device with the ultrasound scan plane and keeping the advancing device as parallel with the face of the ultrasound transducer as possible. To achieve parallel with the transducer, regardless of the lesion depth will require positioning the patient in a lateral decubitus with a pillow behind the shoulder. In addition, the physician gently tilts the far end of the ultrasound transducer into the breast away from the advancing device.

Failure to confirm with ultrasound imaging that the biopsy device tip or its sampling area is aligned correctly with the lesion will lead to inadequate biopsy of the lesion and potentially falsely reassuring a patient of a benign diagnosis. To avoid missing significant portions of the lesion with ultrasound-guided needle core biopsy, by the forward movement of the inner and outer cannula, the needle tip is brought just to the front edge of the lesion and does not penetrate into the lesion before firing.

When performing a needle core biopsy, it is crucial to know whether the needle has penetrated the lesion, and the physician must perform a confirmation scan to avoid image averaging, an artifact created by the overlap of the narrow ultrasound scan plane with the needle just at the edge of the lesion (Fig. 3.23). The physician may view the ultrasound image and interpret it as a successful biopsy but the needle has not actually penetrated the lesion. By moving the ultrasound transducer perpendicular to its long axis, the lesion can be visualized from one end through its middle to the other end of the lesion. It is necessary to see a portion of the lesion without the needle, on either side of the lesion with the needle. This will confirm the needle is in the lesion. The physician can also rotate the ultrasound transducer 90 degrees to visualize a cross section of the needle within the lesion. The most common error made by surgeons who are gaining skill in ultrasound device guidance is failure to line up the device with the transducer. Small alignment deviations result in failure to visualize the tip of the device and to be able to anticipate the trajectory of the advancing tip. Frequent direct visual checks of device–transducer alignment will help to prevent this dangerous situation. Further alignment is required if the full length of the device is not well seen.

The physician paying careful attention to the technical aspect of the procedure can enhance the success of ultrasound-guided VAB or large intact-sample biopsy. Patient positioning (lateral decubitus), injection of local anesthetic posterior to the lesion for a lifting effect, and torquing down of the biopsy device handle as the probe approaches the underside of the lesion all serve to provide a shallow angle of insertion and easier access underneath the lesion, especially when the lesion is deep within the breast parenchyma.

When the VAB or large-intact Halo biopsy device is in position, to ensure an adequate sampling requires a confirmation scan to assess the relationship of the device and the lesion. If not positioned beneath the breast target lesion, the artifact created by the device would eliminate visualization of any portion of the lesion below the biopsy probe. The surgeon may also use this cross section scan to confirm the position of a biopsy device beneath the target lesion. One advantage of the directional capability of the VAB devices is the ability to rotate the sampling aperture toward the direction of lesion deviation. Physicians must utilize the technique of scanning perpendicular to the long-axis of the transducer to determine the direction they should rotate the sample chamber and then scanning back again to visualize the forward movement of the cutter across the sample opening.

Occasionally, the physician encounters a patient with multiple imaging abnormalities (diffuse cystic mastopathy), but there is only one specific lesion requiring a pathology diagnosis. If there is any doubt that the lesion biopsied with ultrasound guidance is the same as that seen on mammogram, the physician may perform a postprocedure mammogram to confirm the marker placement and alignment with the mammogram abnormality (Fig. 3.30).

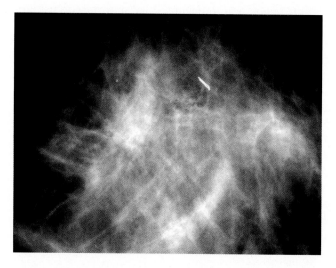

Figure 3.30 All localization markers contain a permanent metallic component, allowing for either mammographic localization or monitoring the biopsy site on future mammograms.

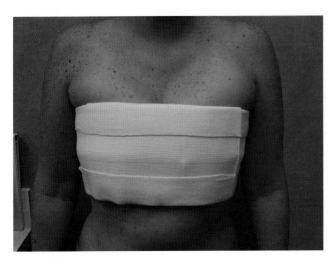

Figure 3.31 A supportive wrap is utilized to help reduce the incidence of bleeding and postprocedure hematoma, especially with vacuum-assisted and large intact procedures. This GentleWrap (Gentle Med Solutions, Marietta, Georgia) is an elastic, compressive wrap, with front Velcro closure that allows patients to adjust and rewrap themselves without assistance.

 POSTOPERATIVE MANAGEMENT

The physician terminates the procedure when adequate sampling of the target lesion has occurred. Either the physician or the assistant applies manual compression for hemostasis. If medical assistants have this responsibility, they should be instructed in the importance of applying pressure not only at the needle entrance site but also along the tract and especially at the site of the lesion or resultant cavity from lesion removal. This usually requires 5 minutes of uninterrupted compression. Steri-strips or Derma-bond are used to reapproximate the incision with Tegaderm (preferably with a telfa island) for dressing. The need for further pressure dressing with gauze and compression tape is dependent on the amount of intra- and postprocedure bleeding observed. Utilizing a supportive pressure wrap may be advisable for a cavity associated with lesion removal from either a VAB or a large intact sample device (Fig. 3.31).

Prior to transport to the pathology laboratory, the assistant transfers the tissue sample(s) into formalin. Time documentation of sample placement in formalin helps confirm proper fixation of the samples to ensure accuracy of ancillary studies performed for malignancy and is a more frequently requirement by many laboratories.

Patients are instructed in home wound care instructions and told when to call for the pathology results. Whether all patients who undergo an ultrasound percutaneous needle biopsy require a short-term postprocedure visit is physician choice but regardless, tracking mechanisms for pathology notification and follow-up imaging studies is essential. Office-based ultrasound-guided percutaneous biopsy has a zero-day global period for AMA CPT coding; and therefore, postprocedure visits are allowed and may be charged as an established patient visit. Regardless of whether this visit occurs, the patient must have appropriate follow-up imaging in 4 to 6 months.

Lack of concordance between breast imaging findings and the histopathology report is the most significant requirement for surgical excision after an ultrasound-guided percutaneous biopsy despite a benign diagnosis. To avoid excision, the surgeon must be satisfied that the findings reported by the pathologist fully explain those on mammography, ultrasound, and physical examination. The physician must review each pathology diagnosis, preferably with the pathologist, to eliminate a false-negative result. Having access to a multidisciplinary imaging/pathology conference is ideal for any image-guided biopsy program.

 COMPLICATIONS

During the course of any image-guided breast biopsy procedure, bleeding can occur. An excessive amount of intraprocedural bleeding can potentially interfere with sampling and, as a result, an accurate biopsy. During the ultrasound-imaging phase of the procedure, it should be determined whether there are vessels near the lesion, which may be in the pathway of the biopsy device, to be avoided.

The most common adverse event associated with percutaneous image-guided biopsy is bruising and small hematoma formation. The incidence of significant hematoma reported is 2% to 8%. The size of the hematoma of course will contribute to the level of pain and discomfort experienced by the patient. Manual compression is the mainstay for achieving hemostasis in image-guided breast biopsy and preventing hematomas. It is important to instruct medical assistants and radiology personnel applying pressure across the biopsy track created by the device. The larger biopsy cavity resulting from removal of the image evidence of the lesion with a VAB or large intact sample device creates a greater risk of bleeding and hematoma. Application of manual pressure and a pressure dressing to the site of the lesion and not only at the incision is crucial. The injection of additional local anesthesia with 1:100,000 epinephrine can be helpful. Utilizing a chest wrap influences prevention of a hematoma. Conservative management with ice and pressure wraps is sufficient. It is extremely rare for bleeding or hematoma to result in surgical intervention.

Pneumothorax, hemothorax, and biopsy of pectoral muscle (with associated increased bleeding and pain) are among the potential problems associated with the inability to confirm the position of the advancing biopsy device. The physician must maintain alignment of the device with the ultrasound scan plane and keep the advancing device as parallel with the face of the ultrasound transducer as possible to prevent these injuries. Local anesthesia can also be injected under direct ultrasound visualization and by directing the needle beneath the lesion; it can be raised off or away from the pectoral muscle. Another way to avoid inadvertent pneumothorax is to use a nonfiring device. The VAB the large intact sample devices are positioned below a lesion without a spring-loaded "firing" mechanism and the acquisition of tissue is directed superiorly.

RESULTS

FNA biopsy is successful in delineating benign from malignant solid breast masses. Fornage and colleagues evaluated 355 breast masses with ultrasound-guided FNA biopsy and demonstrated a sensitivity of 97% and a specificity of 91%. Gordon et al. confirmed the diagnosis of malignancy with ultrasound-guided FNA in 213 of 225 cases, yielding a 95% sensitivity and a specificity of 92%. Six of 12 of false-negative cases in this series were lobular carcinoma. Lobular carcinoma does not shed cells well at aspiration and therefore limits the usefulness of FNA in these cases.

FNA has several potential pitfalls. This includes insufficient sampling, as high as 38% in some series, with sensitivity ranging between 68% and 93% and specificity between 88% and 100%. Cytology rarely provides a specific benign diagnosis and cannot distinguish between invasive and in situ carcinoma.

ATC core needle biopsy has a lower false-negative rate compared with FNA. The standard use of the 14-G needle essentially eliminated the issue of insufficient sampling. Staren et al. reduced the initial false-negative rate obtained with ultrasound-guided FNA from 20% to 3.6% by using ultrasound-guided 14-G core biopsy in 210 patients with nonpalpable mammogram-detected lesions. There were no false positives. There were no cancers detected in a median follow-up of 18 months in the patients with a benign diagnosis.

The lower rate of insufficient sampling and increased sensitivity without increased complications has led to a minimum size of 14 G as a standard. Lieberman et al. studied the number of cores needed to make an accurate diagnosis dependent on presentation. In this study, 145 lesions were biopsied: 92 were nodular densities and 53 were microcalcifications. Five cores with a 14-G ATC needle yielded a diagnosis in 99% of biopsies for breast masses. Five cores yielded a diagnosis in only 87% of the microcalcification cases, and more than six cores yielded a diagnosis in 92% of the cases. Because studies of needle core biopsy for microcalcifications demonstrated upgrading to carcinoma from (48%–52%) atypical hyperplasia identified on stereotactic core biopsy, atypical hyperplasia diagnosed at stereotactic core biopsy became an indication for open biopsy. The larger core samples obtained with VAB and rotational core devices afford more extensive pathologic and biologic analyses than the 14-G spring-loaded needle simply in collecting more tissue for the pathologist's review. Comparison of multiple devices have shown that the use of vacuum-assisted larger-gauge devices reduces the upgrade rate from ADH on core biopsy to DCIS or infiltrating carcinoma (IC), or from DCIS to IC, on excision. Another clear advantage is improved pretreatment characterization (receptor status, genomic and proteomic analysis) of breast lesions obtained in the case of locally advanced breast cancers destined for preoperative chemotherapy.

Except when the surgeon wishes to remove the lesion as an intact specimen, the Mammotome, ATEC, and EnCor combine the features ideal for allowing maximal tissue removal through the smallest possible incision. The Mammotome is the well-established standard for image-guided percutaneous tissue excision, providing significant data regarding its use in the diagnostic setting along with improved clinical outcomes. Researchers have reported clinical trial outcomes of procedures performed with the goal of removing the lesion.

A multiinstitutional investigation evaluated outcomes after lesion removal with ultrasound-guided 11-G and 8-G Mammotome excision of palpable masses below 15 mm and 15 to 30 mm, respectively. Biopsies performed in 127 patients with the 8-G probe and the 11-G probe in 89 patients demonstrated 98% of the lesions remained nonpalpable at 6-month follow-up, including 73% with no ultrasound-visible abnormality at the biopsy site. Complications were mild and anticipated. Most patients (98%) were satisfied with incision appearance; 92% of patients said they would recommend the procedure to others.

The main advantage of devices designed to remove a single large block of tissue—the Intact and the Halo—is that they make it possible to excise a single larger sample of intact tissue than with the other VAB devices described earlier. However, there are limited data available, supporting the use of these devices with the goal of complete removal of imaged evidence of the lesion. More information is available concerning lesion removal in series whose primary goal was accurate diagnosis. Small, successful pilot studies have demonstrated the value of the Intact device for definitive removal of lesions containing atypical ductal hyperplasia and small cancers.

Fine and Staren demonstrated a favorable comparison with VAB devices in the successes of complete removal of fibroadenomas with the Rubicor Halo large intact-sample device. Of the 100 patients selected for the procedure, the indications included palpable mass (ultrasound visible) in 77, abnormal mammogram in 13, and abnormal ultrasound in 10. Ultrasound guided the procedure in 82 patients, and stereotactic guidance was used in 18 patients. At 4- to 6-month follow-up, 72 of 78 (92%) patients evaluated demonstrated no physical or imaging evidence of residual fibroadenoma.

Atypical ductal and lobular hyperplasia require excision to eliminate the possibility of missing associated malignancy. An alternative to open surgical excision is the removal of these lesions as an intact specimen with a large intact-sample device. The Intact Percutaneous Excision Trial (I-PET; Intact Medical) design includes blinded pathology and radiologic review to determine prediction of outcome on open excision. Upgrade rates from ADH to cancer approached zero with percutaneous excisional biopsy in a retrospective series of patients who underwent ultrasound-guided percutaneous biopsies. If studies such as I-PET should define reproducible clinical and pathologic criteria, confirmation of pathologic removal may save patients and their surgeons an unnecessary trip to the operating room.

CONCLUSIONS

Minimally invasive image-guided percutaneous breast biopsy should be the first-line intervention for image-detected abnormalities. The vast majority of patients with breast cancers and benign breast lesions will have their diagnosis made accurately with percutaneous image-guided needle biopsy, with many of these with ultrasound guidance. The advantage of ultrasound guidance over other imaging modalities includes patient comfort, lying supine (as opposed to prone with neck extension on the stereotactic table), and availability of ultrasound as an office-based procedure minimizing costs and scheduling delays.

The presence of a palpable or nonpalpable solid mass is the most common indication for an ultrasound-guided needle core biopsy to obtain a histology diagnosis. It is optimal for planning the management of malignant lesions. If the benign pathology diagnosed with ultrasound-guided percutaneous biopsy fully explains the imaged findings, the surgeon need not remove the lesion if the patient is comfortable with the reassurance of a benign diagnosis, without removal of the suspect lesion. Ultrasound-guided percutaneous excision is an alternative to open surgical excision for those patients who desire the removal of their lesions, especially when palpable, despite being well informed.

The tools for specimen acquisition have evolved from FNA, ATC core needle, vacuum-assisted core biopsy devices to large-core, intact sample instruments, providing either "sampling" capability, adequate for most lesions, or "removal" (by percutaneous excisional biopsy) capability for selected lesions. The surgeon must select the most appropriate instrumentation and biopsy type for each case.

The most significant error in image-guided breast biopsy is of course missing or inadequately sampling the lesion and providing the patient a false sense of security, with a benign diagnosis. The physician paying careful attention to the technical aspect of the procedure can enhance the success of ultrasound-guided percutaneous biopsy and eliminate the difficulties in correctly advancing the device and positioning it for appropriate sampling or excision.

Lack of concordance between breast imaging findings and the histopathology report is the most significant requirement for surgical excision after an ultrasound-guided percutaneous biopsy despite a benign diagnosis. To avoid excision, the surgeon must be satisfied that the findings reported by the pathologist fully explain those on mammography, ultrasound, and physical examination. The physician must review each pathology diagnosis, preferably with the pathologist, to eliminate a false-negative result. Having access to a multidisciplinary imaging/pathology conference is ideal for any image-guided biopsy program.

Suggested Readings

Fine RE, Staren ED. Percutaneous radiofrequency-assisted excision of fibroadenomas. *Am J Surg.* 2006;192:545–547.

Fine RE, Staren ED. Updates in breast ultrasound. *Surg Clin N Am.* 2004;84:1001–1034, v–vi.

Fine RE, Whitworth PW, Kim JA, et al. Low-risk palpable breast masses removed using a vacuum-assisted hand-held device. *Am J Surg.* 2003;186:362–367.

Killebrew LK, Oneson RH. Comparison of the diagnostic accuracy of a vacuum-assisted percutaneous intact specimen sampling device to a vacuum-assisted core needle sampling device for breast biopsy: initial experience. *Breast J.* 2006;12(4):302–308.

Philpotts LE, Hooley RJ, Lee CH. Comparison of automated versus vacuum-assisted biopsy methods for sonographically guided core biopsy of the breast. *AJR Am J Roentgenol.* 2003;180: 347–351.

Rao R, Lilley L, Andrews V, et al. Axillary staging by percutaneous biopsy: sensitivity of fine-needle aspiration versus core needle biopsy. *Ann Surg Oncol.* 2009;16:1170–1175.

Silverstein MJ, Lagios MD, Recht A, et al. Image-detected breast cancer: state of the art diagnosis and treatment. *J Am Coll Surg.* 2005;201(4):586–597.

Sperber F, Blank A, Mester U, et al. Diagnosis and treatment of breast fibroadenomas by ultrasound-guided vacuum-assisted biopsy. *Arch Surg.* 2003;138:796–800.

4 Stereotactically Guided Breast Percutaneous Needle Biopsy

Arthur G. Lerner

Introduction

History of Stereotactic Breast Biopsies

Stereotactic breast biopsies were first discussed in 1977 (1). Dr. Kambiz Dowlatshahi, a surgeon at Rush Presbyterian Medical College in Chicago, Illinois, brought the first prone stereotactic table to the United States in the mid-1980s. After learning this technology at the Karolinska Institute in Germany, Dr. Dowlatshahi performed the first stereotactic breast biopsy in 1987 (2) (Fig. 4.1). Since that time, there have been many significant changes in the stereotactic technology and in the biopsy techniques and devices employed during these interventions.

Initially, the prone stereotactic technology was an analog imaging system. The determination of the location of the image abnormality was accomplished using a digitizer. By placing marks on the mammogram films with a T square, measurements were taken and the co-ordinates of the lesion were determined and entered into the system by hand, using a set of micrometer dials. Today, the system is completely digital, and the determination of the co-ordinates of the mammographic abnormality is made electronically from the digital images. This work is done at the imaging console (Fig. 4.2). The data points are entered into the system electronically without having to manually place the co-ordinates into the table's database.

Another significant improvement in the biopsy methodology has been the evolution of the biopsy devices (3,4). In the early 1990s, spring-loaded core needles were developed to replace the fine needle aspiration (FNA) technique. The early core needle devices were 16 to 18 gauge, and eventually 14-gauge devices became the standard (Fig. 4.3). Large core, rotating cutter, vacuum-assisted biopsy devices have replaced the spring-loaded 14-gauge core needles (Figs. 4.4–4.9). Radiofrequency devices are also in use and have the potential to remove the entire imaging abnormality in a single intact specimen (Figs. 4.10 and 4.11). These new tools represent a significant change in biopsy devices from the original FNA technology first employed on the stereotactic table. The

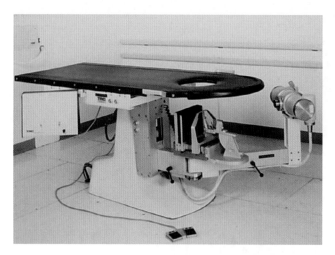

Figure 4.1 The first stereotactic biopsy in the United States was performed by Dr. Kambiz Dowlatshahi in 1987 on this table. Dr. Dowlatshahi brought this table from Germany where he learned the technology. (Photograph reprinted with the permission of Dr. Dowlatshahi.)

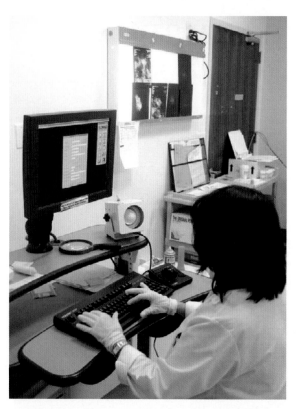

Figure 4.2 Computer station for image viewing, targeting of the lesion, and transmission of the data electronically to the table.

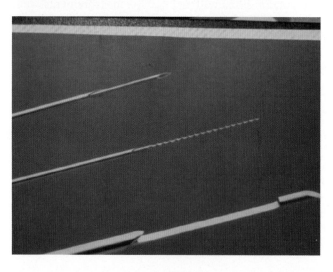

Figure 4.3 Tissue sampling was initially performed with a fine needle aspiration cytology technique. (Photograph reprinted with the permission of Dr. Kambiz Dowlatshahi.)

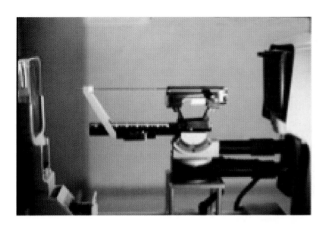

Figure 4.4 The first early spring-loaded core needles used on the prone stereotactic table.

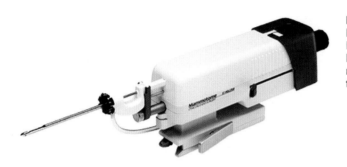

Figure 4.5 The first vacuum-assisted biopsy device was manufactured by Biopysis. This product was eventually bought by Ethicon Endo-Surgery and manufactured and sold as Mammotome.

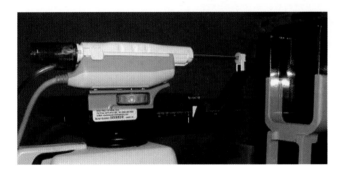

Figure 4.6 Encore vacuum-assisted biopsy device by SenoRx.

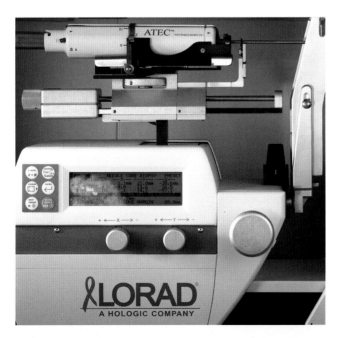

Figure 4.7 The ATEC vacuum-assisted biopsy device manufactured by Suros, Inc.

Part II: Breast Biopsy

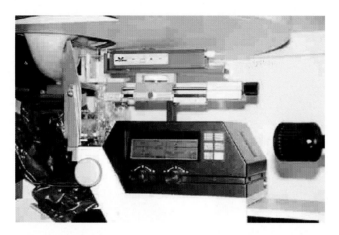

Figure 4.8 Vacuum-assisted multiple insertion biopsy device manufactured by Bard Inc.

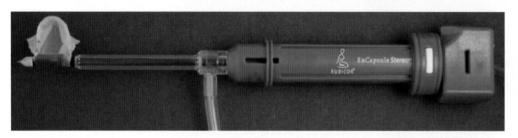

Figure 4.9 Large core biopsy needle from Site Select. This rotating cutter needle cores a single large sample to include the targeted lesion.

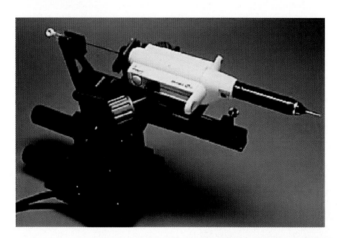

Figure 4.10 Radiofrequency biopsy needle manufactured by Rubicor. It has a loop and a bag that is deployed and rotated around the target. The loop is energized and cuts the tissue, which is captured in the bag and extracted from the breast.

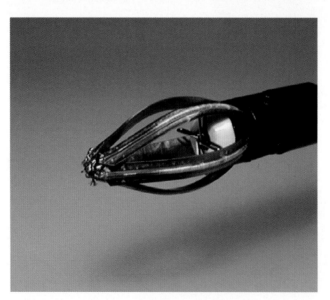

Figure 4.11 In Tact, a radiofrequency device that has an energized basket at the tip of the device that surrounds the target when deployed. The energized basket arms cut the tissue, and once the tissue is secured in the basket, the device is removed from the breast with a single sample of tissue that includes the targeted lesion.

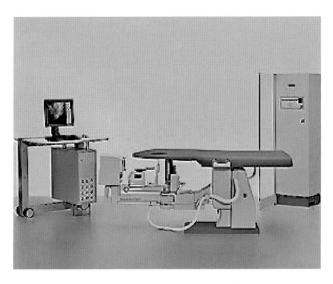

Figure 4.12 The original Fischer Mammotest system with the table, workstation, and x-ray generator. This is a unidirectional table. The patient is always facing the same way once in the prone position on the table. The C arm rotates through a 270-degree arc, allowing all approaches to the breast except a caudal to cranial approach.

result has been a decrease in the nondiagnostic and false-negative biopsies as a result of the larger samples these devices provide for pathologic analysis.

Presently, almost all diagnostic breast biopsies can be accomplished with a needle rather than with a knife (5).

The Technology

There are two different targeting systems employed in the stereotactic technology (6,7). The table originally developed by Fischer Imaging of Denver Co. (Fig. 4.12) utilizes a polar co-ordinating system, where the co-ordinates of the indexed mammographic lesion are defined by the distances from a fixed point and angular distances from a reference line. The horizontal and vertical co-ordinates are expressed in degrees, while the depth to the center of the lesion is given in millimeters.

On the Lorad Multicare table (Fig. 4.13), a Cartesian co-ordinating system is used. Here, distances are determined from a reference point, where the horizontal, vertical, and depth axes intersect at right angles and define the target. Utilizing this system, all co-ordinates are given in millimeters.

A third prone table technology made by Giotto, in use at this time mainly in Europe, also utilizes a Cartesian targeting system, incorporated into a mammography unit with patient positioning on a prone table.

There are numerous "add-on" or upright systems, where a targeting and biopsy technology is added to an existing mammography unit, and the targeting and biopsy are done with the patient either upright or lying on her side (Fig. 4.14). These add-on systems allow the mammography unit to be used for screening or diagnostic mammography when biopsies are not being performed. This differs from the prone systems, which are only for stereotactic procedures and not applicable to standard mammography.

The advantages of the prone tables are the ability to biopsy the lesion in the breast from multiple approaches, where on the upright systems the approaches are somewhat limited.

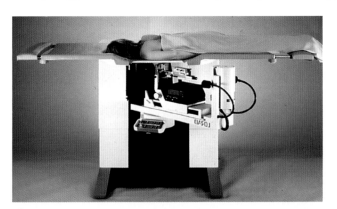

Figure 4.13 The Lorad Multicare prone stereotactic table. This is a bidirectional table. The patient can be positioned in either direction, allowing any approach to either breast.

Part II: Breast Biopsy

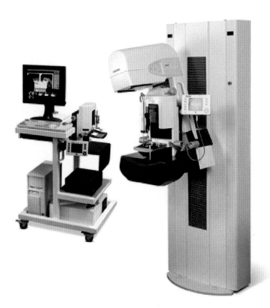

Figure 4.14 A Lorad upright or add on system. Photograph provided by Lorad.

There are more patient issues reported with the "add-on" systems, particularly vasovagal reactions. These upright systems do, however, allow access to lesions close to the chest without needing exaggerated positioning that may be necessary on the prone tables.

 ## INDICATIONS/CONTRAINDICATIONS

Any mammographic abnormality classified as Breast Imaging-Reporting and Data System (BI-RADS) 4 or 5 should be considered for a stereotactic biopsy, unless the lesion is visible on ultrasound. In that case, an ultrasound-guided needle biopsy should be performed instead of a stereotactic biopsy.

The most common indication for a stereotactic breast biopsy is a cluster of indeterminate microcalcifications (8). Asymmetric densities and architectural distortions, frequently not imaged with breast ultrasound, may also prompt a stereotactic biopsy. The mammographic abnormality seen in only one mammographic view may possibly be biopsied stereotactically.

Breast thickness in compression is the first requirement for a safe successful stereotactic biopsy. As a stereotactic program begins, a compression thickness of the breast during mammography of 28 mm should be the minimum thickness for a stereotactic biopsy. With experience, a woman with a compression thickness of as little as 20 mm may still be a candidate for a stereotactic biopsy.

The prone tables have a weight restriction of 300 lb. Patients must be able to accept the prone position without moving for the duration of the procedure, which may last from 20 minutes to 1 hour. The ability to lie on a hard uncomfortable table without moving may be an issue for patients with musculoskeletal problems, chronic obstructive pulmonary disease (COPD), or extreme anxiety.

The position of the abnormality in the breast is an important consideration. Difficult lesions to biopsy with stereotaxis are superficial lesions, lesions close to the chest wall, and lesions in the axillary tail of the breast. However, with experience, most abnormalities can be safely biopsied with utilizing stereotaxis. Initially, these difficult lesions may challenge the learning curve of the surgeon and the radiology technologist.

 ## PREOPERATIVE PLANNING

Preparing the Patient for a Stereotactic Biopsy

The patient should be made aware of the position she will be asked to assume during the procedure. Local anesthesia will be utilized and the procedure should be painless.

If pain is experienced, additional local anesthesia can be administered. She should be told that a metallic clip would be placed at the biopsy site in case a surgical excision is required as a result of the core needle pathology. This clip will remain in the breast for life unless the diagnosis requires a surgical excision at which time the clip will be removed. The patient should be made aware of the significant frequency with which ecchymosis may develop, which will dissipate with time. The patient should also be told that rarely the procedure must be cancelled for unexpected technical reasons. It is further suggested that the common diagnoses found on pathology be discussed, including those that will require a subsequent surgical resection. Lastly, the patient should be made aware of an approximately 2% incidence of a discordant biopsy requiring another biopsy, possibly performed with a needle localization and surgical excision.

SURGERY (THE PROCEDURE)

Setting up a Stereotactic Biopsy Room

If biopsies will be done with add-on, upright unit, an existing mammography room will be used. If there is a choice of rooms, utilize the largest room possible since a stretcher may be needed if the patient is to be placed on her side for a lateral or medial approach.

If a prone table is to be used, a room large enough to accommodate the table and the computer workstation, as well as additional room for supplies, should be utilized. A view box should also be installed close to the workstation, and a bright light and magnifying glass should be available. Two low rolling stools are needed for the physician and technologist to sit on under the raised stereotactic table. Adequate storage for supplies is also required. Dimmers on the overhead lights are recommended to allow adequate ambient lighting for the procedure, but a reduced level of light for image interpretation. A changing area for patients should be close to or within the stereotactic room.

Some method for obtaining a specimen radiograph to be certain the imaging abnormality has been sampled is a requirement. Cores can be radiographed with a mammography unit, a dedicated specimen imaging system such as a Faxitron (Fig. 4.20), or a digital image of the cores taken using the table's imaging system.

The Biopsy

The first step in the sequence of a stereotactic biopsy begins with the determination of how the patient should be positioned on the table. The Lorad Multicare table is a bidirectional table, where the patient can be positioned with her head at either end of the table, allowing any approach to the breast. The original Fischer table is unidirectional, and this allows any approach except caudal to cranial. Determining how the lesion will be approached is required before the patient can be placed on the stereotactic table.

Other factors that must be considered to determine the approach to the breast include the following:

1. The location of the lesion in the breast.
2. The shortest distance from skin to lesion.
3. The mammographic views, on which the abnormality is most clearly evident.

Whichever table is selected for use, the positioning must result in the lesion index visualized in the 0-degree scout view in the center third of the 5-cm square window through which the images are obtained and the biopsy is to be performed.

For each digital image obtained, the ability of the physician to maximize the image quality using the digital imaging functions of the system is available in the software of both table technologies. Brightness and contrast (window leveling), magnification, inverting the images, and filtering the images are techniques available. It should be realized that using these digital imaging manipulations to compensate for a poorly exposed image would result in a loss of image sensitivity. Re-exposing an under- or overexposed image is always superior to attempting to improve upon a poor-quality image.

A 0-degree scout is obtained first, and the indexed lesion must be clearly identified. It is common to have to reposition the patient's breast several times before the lesion is properly positioned on the scout image in the center one-third of the front compression paddle window. Once the lesion is identified on the scout image, a stereotactic pair of images is obtained. Each stereotactic image is offset 15 degrees from the scout. Therefore, the stereotactic pair of images is 30 degrees apart.

It is on the stereotactic pair of images that the targeting to obtain the co-ordinates of the lesion is performed. In the unusual event that the lesion is identified on only the scout and one of the two stereotactic images, the targeting can be accomplished utilizing the scout and one of the stereo pair. Since this targeting utilizes images with only 15 degrees between them, the sensitivity of the targeting is reduced. It is therefore recommended that all efforts should be made to visualize the lesion on both stereotactic images before attempting to target the lesion using what Fischer originally called "target on scout."

Icons are then placed over the target on both stereo images. The principle of parallax shift is employed to determine the depth of the lesion in the breast. On the Lorad table the depth is determined from the reference point, which is located on the front compression paddle. On the polar technology employed by the Fischer table, the depth of the lesion is determined from the back of the breast to the lesion.

The horizontal and vertical axes are automatically displayed in millimeters in the Cartesian system, and in degrees on the polar table, and appear on the computer screen. Once these co-ordinates are displayed, the stroke margin is determined.

Stroke margin refers to the distance from the "fired" tip of the biopsy needle to the back of the breast (Fig. 4.15). An adequate stroke margin, at least 4 mm, must be available for a safe biopsy. A negative stroke margin will result in the needle, when fired, striking the back breast support, first going through the unanesthetized skin of the back of the breast. This is a completely avoidable complication. If a negative stoke margin is calculated, the safest next step is to reposition the patient and try a different approach to the lesion until a positive stroke margin is obtained.

On the polar tables, the stroke margin is displayed automatically on the computer screen. For those working on a Cartesian table, a simple calculation must be made at

Figure 4.15 Stroke margin, the distance from the tip of the fired biopsy device to the back breast support.

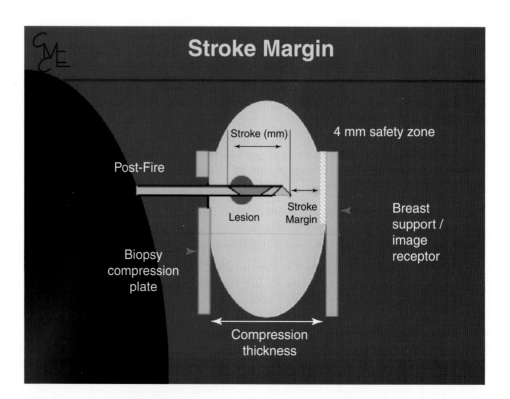

this time to avoid violating the requirement of an adequate stroke margin. Depending on the needle being utilized, the compression thickness of the breast is noted. Most commonly, 5 mm is added to the calculated depth of the lesion. If that total is equal to or less than the compression thickness of the breast, a positive stroke margin exists and the procedure may continue safely. It should be noted that this difference between the compression thickness and the sum of the depth plus 5 mm is not the actual stroke margin, but just a number within the range of a positive stroke margin. If the approach chosen results in a positive stroke margin, the procedure can continue safely.

On the Fischer table, the biopsy needle to be used is selected from a series of needle icons displayed on the computer screen. On the Lorad table, the needle chosen must be "zeroed." This process brings the needle tip to the reference point in the front compression paddle. This process is necessary each time a new patient is biopsied.

Once the lesion is targeted, a positive stroke margin is determined, the co-ordinates are transmitted electronically from the computer to the table. It is suggested that confirmation of the electronic transfer of the data be obtained by comparing the coordinates on the computer screen and the numbers that appear on the table data.

A topical antiseptic solution is placed on the skin, and local anesthesia is administered. A skin wheal is created for the insertion of the needle into the breast. It is important not to use local anesthesia with epinephrine in the skin. A skin ulcer may develop when the local anesthesia includes dilute epinephrine. The biopsy site is then anesthetized. Epinephrine may be utilized in the breast tissue if there are no contraindications.

On both tables, the biopsy device is held on the stage, which moves upon command to aim the needle at the target. On the Fischer table, the needle is aimed at an upward angle, whereas on the Lorad table, the needle is always parallel to the table. The physician must manually advance the needle to the proper depth.

Many of the needles have a "pull back," which is a distance the tip of the needle must be pulled back from the calculated depth in order to have the needle's sampling through the lesion. If the needle is position to the calculated depth, the sampling area may be too deep.

The vacuum-assisted needles are all "fired" or advanced forward. Most commonly, this is done in the breast tissue, but some prefer to fire the needle outside the breast and place it into the breast in that fired position. If the needle is to be fired in the breast, it is advanced to the "prefire" position and a stereotactic pair of images is obtained (Fig. 4.16). In the case where the needle is fired outside of the breast, it is positioned according to the determined co-ordinates.

Prefire images and postfire images are always taken to determine the relative position of the needle to the lesion. "Snow plowing" or lesion movement is common with needle insertion, and it is crucial to determine which way and how far from the needle the lesion has moved (Figs. 4.17 and 4.18).

Once fired in the breast, or if fired ex vivo and then inserted into the parenchyma, the exact relationship of the target to the needle must be determined so that the biopsy sequence can be planned. The vacuum needles are capable of being rotated through

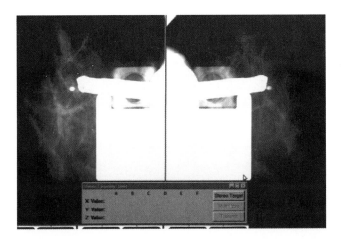

Figure 4.16 A prefire stereotactic pair of images. The target, a calcification, can be seen in both images almost equidistant from the tip of the needle. This alignment should be observed before a device is fired in the breast.

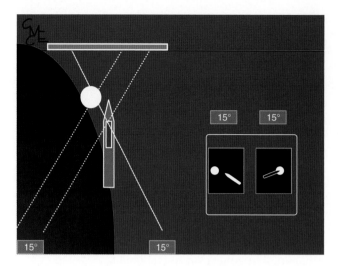

Figure 4.17 When a target moves away from the biopsy needle either during needle insertion or with needle firing the direction, the lesion moves must be appreciated to determine if there must be repositioning of or retargeting to obtain new co-ordinates for the target. Here the target has moved to the right of the needle. The stereotactic images represented here are created by the x-ray energy superimposing the needle over the lesion on the +15-degree image. On the −15-degree image, the needle tip and target are separated as the x-ray energy strikes the back image receptor.

360 degrees along their long axis. If the target has moved to the 6-o'clock position relative to the needle, the needle's sampling area may be rotated to that position for the initial samples (Fig. 4.19).

Usually, the number of samples taken depends on the size of the biopsy tool and the nature of the lesion being biopsied. For solid lesions, five to six cores usually provide adequate tissue for the pathologist. When sampling microcalcifications, 6 cores with an 8- to 9-gauge device and 12 cores with an 11-gauge device should allow for an accurate diagnosis.

At the end of the sampling sequence, an image of the cores must be obtained to be certain that tissue with microcalcifications has been sampled (Fig. 4.20). This specimen image can be obtained with a mammography machine, a Faxitron (a dedicated specimen imaging system), or a digital image, performed by placing the cores in the compression plate window after the patient is out of compression. Once the decision that enough cores have been obtained, a marker clip is usually placed through the biopsy tool at the biopsy site. A marker can be avoided if there is enough of the lesion remaining to be a target for a needle localization should the diagnosis require surgical intervention.

Before releasing the breast from compression, images should be taken to be certain the clip was deployed. If possible, a two-view mammogram is helpful to be certain that there has not been a malplacement of the clip.

Pressure should be held on the biopsy site. Once oozing has stopped, the small incision can be closed with a Steri-Strip. A pressure dressing is also used by many physicians. This can be accomplished with a circumferential ace bandage or by using a Gentle Wrap bandage (Fig. 4.21).

A two-view mammogram is recommended postbiopsy if a marker or clip has been placed, and when asymmetric densities are biopsied to make certain that the correct density has been sampled. If a mammography unit is not in proximity to the stereotactic

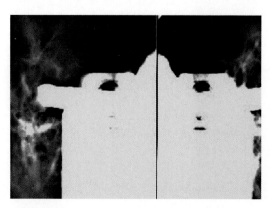

Figure 4.18 A stereotactic pair of images demonstrating the target has moved to the right of the needle tip during its insertion.

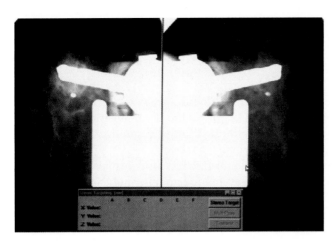

Figure 4.19 Stereotactic postfire images demonstrating the lesion has moved to the 6-o'clock position relative to the needle. The amount of movement may have the target too far from the needle to be captured in a core. The needle should be repositioned before attempting sampling. The distance from the needle to the target can be measured on the images. It is suggested that when a distance of 4 mm or greater is found, retargeting before sampling is recommended.

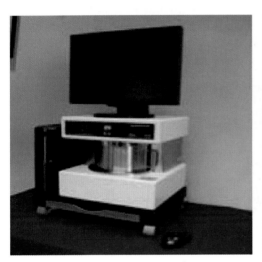 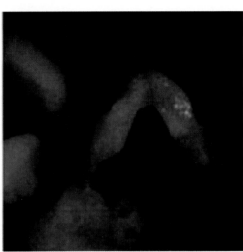

Figure 4.20 A digital specimen x-ray system on the left by Faxitron-Ray, LLC. On the right, the cluster of microcalcifications can be seen in a single core.

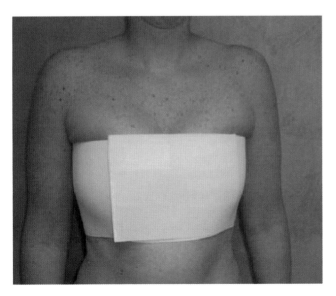

Figure 4.21 Gentle Wrap, a self-adhering pressure wrap distributed by Rubicor, Inc. This wrap allows an ice pack to be inserted between the layers to reduce postbiopsy swelling and ecchymosis.

Part II: Breast Biopsy

room, the patient should be referred for the indexed breast postprocedure mammogram as soon after the biopsy as practical.

Processing the Cores

For microcalcification cases, place the cores with calcium into one specimen bottle. A second specimen container can be used for the cores without calcifications. This tells the pathologist which cores are potentially the most diagnostic should there be issues with identifying the microcalcifications on permanent section.

Analysis of estrogen receptor/progestin receptor (ER/PR) on cores is a reliable technology. Cores fix very well, and fixation is a key to an accurate analysis. Human epidermal growth factor receptor 2 (HER2) analysis on cores is more problematic. If an immunohistochemical (IHC) assay is employed for HER2 overexpression, and the results for overexpression are negative, this suggests a reliable result. If however, HER2 is overexpressed with IHC analysis performed on cores, consider repeating the analysis on the surgical specimen. If there is no residual pathologic tissue in the surgical specimen, HER2 analysis of the core should be repeated with fluorescent in situ hybridization (FISH) (9).

Interpreting the Results of the Biopsy

Upon completion of the pathologic analysis of the cores, a determination of the adequacy of the biopsy must be made.

▪ Did the pathology answer the questions raised on the mammogram?
▪ Was the biopsy concordant or discordant?

There should not be a discordance rate higher than 2% to 3% in any series of biopsies. That analysis is the responsibility of the physician performing the biopsy. Once it is determined that the biopsy was concordant, a decision must be made if there is a need to examine a larger volume of tissue. For atypia or the lobular neoplasias, surgical excision to provide the pathologist with more tissue volume will ensure a reduction in sampling error (9,10).

If atypia is confirmed histologically, either ductal or lobular, surgical excision of the biopsy site is suggested with an expected incidence of upgrading the diagnosis with additional pathologic examination of the larger tissue sample. Other lesions that require consideration for excision following a stereotactic needle biopsy include a radial sclerosing lesion (radial scar) that is larger than 6 mm or an intraductal papilloma with residual papilloma still in the breast. Fibroadenomas admixed with stromal cellularity have approximately a 17% incidence of upgrading to a phyllodes tumor and should be excised. The lobular neoplasias, which do not have a reliable imaging marker, with the exception of pleomorphic lobular carcinoma in situ (LCIS), should also be excised (11).

It is important to discuss with the pathologist their expectations for an upgrading of any lesion of concern, that is, columnar cell change with atypia should be excised because of the incidence of invasive tubular carcinomas associated with columnar cell change with atypia.

 ## COMPLICATIONS

Common to all invasive procedures, bleeding and infection are the most common postbiopsy complications. Bleeding can be minimized with compression postbiopsy for 5 to 10 minutes. An additional option is placement of a pressure dressing either with an ace bandage or with a Gentle Wrap bandage. Patients should be warned that postbiopsy ecchymosis is not uncommon. Infection is rare and in most centers prophylactic antibiotics are not necessary.

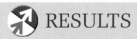

RESULTS

In an active biopsy program, the discordant rate should not be higher than 2%. A discordant biopsy should not be an issue as long as the discordant biopsy is recognized and additional tissue sampling is planned. Cancer should not be missed as long as the surgeon works closely with the pathologist and breast imager to assess the adequacy of the biopsy (12).

CONCLUSIONS

Image-guided needle biopsies should replace excisional biopsies for the diagnosis of breast lesions whenever possible. For nonpalpable mammographic abnormalities, a stereotactic biopsy should be the first consideration. Unless there are special circumstances, (e.g., small breast or the inability of the patient to lie prone without moving), a minimally invasive stereotactic needle biopsy is advisable and should be recommended. This approach compared to a surgical biopsy will save health care dollars. Approximately, 80% of patients with BI-RADS 4 and 5 abnormalities can avoid operation. A stereotactic approach allows less scaring, less morbidity, and elicits fewer complications without sacrifice of diagnostic accuracy.

References

1. Bolmgren J, Jacobson B, Nordenstrom B. Stereotaxic instrument for the needle biopsy of the mamma. *AJR Am J Roentgenol.* 1977;129:121–125.
2. Dowlatshahi K, Jokich PM, Schmidt R, et al. Cytologic diagnosis of occult breast lesions using stereotaxic needle aspiration. *Arch Surg.* 1987;122:1343–1346.
3. Elvecrog EL, Lechner MC, Nelson MT. Nonpalpable breast lesions: correlation of stereotactic large-core needle biopsy and surgical results. *Radiology.* 1993;188(2):453–455.
4. Parker, SH, Lovin JD, Jobe WE, et al. Nonpalpable breast lesions: stereotactic automated large core biopsies. *Radiology.* 1991;180(2):403–407.
5. International Breast Cancer Consensus Conference. Image-detected breast cancer: state of the art diagnosis and treatment. International Breast Cancer Consensus Conference. *J Am Coll Surg.* 2001;193:297–302.
6. Parker SH, Jobe WE, eds. *Percutaneous Breast Needle Biopsy.* New York, NY: Churchill Livingstone; 1993.
7. Fajardo LL, Pizzutello RJ, Willison KM, eds. *A Comprehensive Approach To Stereotactic Breast Biopsy.* Cambridge, MA: Blackwell Science; 1996.
8. Dershaw DD, Liberman L. Stereotactic breast biopsy: indications and results. *Oncology (Williston Park).* 1998;12(6):907–916.
9. Park SY, Kim KS, Lee TG, et al. The accuracy of preoperative core biopsy in determining histologic grade, hormone receptors, and human epidermal growth factor receptor 2 status in invasive breast cancer. *Am J Surg.* 2009;197(2):266–269.
10. Rosen PP, Hoda SA, eds. *Breast Pathology: Diagnosis by Needle Core Biopsy.* Philadelphia, PA: Lippincott Williams & Wilkins; 2005.
11. Liberman L. Clinical management issues in percutaneous core breast biopsy. *Radiol Clin North Am.* 2000;28(4):791–807.
12. Jackman RJ, MarzJoni TA Jr, Rosenberg J. False negative diagnosis at stereotactic vacuum-assisted needle breast biopsy: long-term follow-up of 1,280 lesions and review of the literature. *AJR Am J Roentgenol.* 2000;192(2):741–751.

Part II: Breast Biopsy

5 Breast Ductoscopy

William C. Dooley

Introduction

Interest in breast endoscopy came from Oriental investigators in the early 1990s where bloody nipple discharge was a more common presentation of breast cancer (1–3). The early techniques using a single microfiber scope without ductal distension were successful in navigating only the first 1 to 3 cm of the ducts and fraught with technical problems such as scope breakage and poor image quality. In spite of these barriers, there has been increasing use of this technology in Japan and more widespread acceptance as the technology of scope design improved (4–12).

Dooley and others recently tested a new method of obtaining a rich cytologic specimen from the ducts of high-risk women (13–15). This method is known as ductal lavage. The success of this procedure was that it detected severe cytologic and malignant atypia in clinically and radiographically normal breasts. Reproducibly, the same breast duct could be cannulated and severely atypical cytology obtained. The problem arose in identifying the lesion within the breast, which was the source for the atypia. New American multifiber microendoscopes were applied to solve this problem in an initial series of patients with abnormal cytology to identify the lesions (16). Success of that series led to wider application of the imaging technology and eventual adoption of this imaging modality to help guide during all nonmastectomy breast surgeries where fluid could be elicited from the nipple to identify the duct connecting to the lesion for which surgery was being performed. Initial reports have demonstrated the findings in certain subpopulations early in the use of this technology (17–19). With experience the technology has improved, and operator results have also improved. This series reviews the entire experience with this relatively new technology, the learning curve, and the effect of improved intra-operative visualization afforded to the operative surgeon technically on nonmastectomy breast surgery.

INDICATIONS/CONTRAINDICATIONS

Mammary ductoscopy is a surgical tool that allows identification of intraductal intraluminal growths and mapping of the branching patterns of the mammary ductal systems in vivo. Most successful breast endoscopists use submillimeter scopes and distend the ductal system in some way. The most obvious indication is naturally one of diagnostic and therapeutic direction of excisional biopsy for bloody or pathologic nipple discharge. Papillomas account for a large percentage of these underlying lesions for this indication. Many of these papillomas will be present in the first 20 mm of the breast duct and can be easily identified for removal. The technology of completely removing these large central papillomas from within the limitations of a submillimeter ductoscope is evolving. Simple transillumination of the skin in the central breast can easily direct a minimal-access approach to removing these lesions. Deeper proliferative lesions causing pathologic nipple discharge are much more likely to reveal premalignant or frankly malignant changes. These lesions are almost always found within the larger ductal branches. This raises the important question of were these branches larger before the lesions arose or did they just dilate since the lesions were making fluid. Since these worrisome lesions are in the most dilated ductal branches, scoping down the largest ducts usually finds the most suspicious pathology.

Ductoscopy can be used in other ways as an adjunct to a planned surgical breast resection. Here ductoscopy allows mapping of the involved ductal tree and identification of intraluminal growths down to about 1/100 mm. This resolution is far below that of external imaging techniques such as mammography, ultrasound, and magnetic resonance imaging. Unfortunately, there is a large visual overlap in the appearance of some malignant/premalignant and benign lesions. Transscope biopsy techniques are still in their infancy, so until these are available, all intraluminal growths must be assumed to be proliferative and therefore potentially important to sample or excise. In the case of ductal carcinoma in situ or T1 breast cancers, about 60% have very small fields or zones of surrounding proliferation. The remaining 40% however seem to have a field defect within the ductal tree, leading to widespread proliferative changes at several stages of development. It is these cases that give rise to the extensive intraductal component, and multifocality or multicentricity seen in pathologic mapping of breast cancers and as secondary cancers in magnetic resonance imaging and advanced imaging cases.

Ductoscopy of a fluid-producing duct in the same quadrant of a known breast cancer will reveal a direct connection to the cancer in more than 85% of the cases and allow the surgeon to determine the presence or absence of associated proliferative changes. By mapping out these changes, using skin transillumination, the surgeon can then resect an entire ductal tree or perform a subsegment resection to incorporate the allied proliferative disease. My prospective but nonrandomized series has shown a dramatic fall in positive margin rates at initial resection (arguably because of larger resections when associated with proliferative disease) and a dramatic reduction in the local failure rate of traditional breast conservation. As more surgeons become facile with breast endoscopy, hopefully, these results can be proven even more conclusively in a prospective randomized multicenter trial.

PREOPERATIVE PLANNING

The most important aspect of successful breast endoscopy is being able to reliably identify the correct duct and repeatedly be able to get fluid from it for successful cannulation in the operating room (OR). First, you need to develop the skill of expression of nipple fluid during your clinical exams. The La Leche League has an excellent video primer on expression of milk during lactation. The techniques it explains in detail are excellent for expressing the microliters of ductal fluid in nonlactating women with underlying proliferative breast disease. Most series report high expression of nipple fluid using such techniques in those with strong breast cancer history or high Gail model risk. A brief description of the technique is as follows: begin with careful gentle dekeratinization of the nipple papilla using a mild facial exfoliant. Next, the breast is lubricated away from the nipple with a thin moisturizing cream. The breast is then kneaded in a centripetal fashion from the edges toward the nipple as shown in Figure 5.1. Then, the dilated lactiferous sinuses in the retroareolar space are individually compressed to express milk or fluid as shown in Figure 5.2.

Next is repeatedly being able to find the offending duct between your clinic exam and the OR. You can draw a clock face on the areola and take a picture. Cannulating

Figure 5.1 Centripetal breast massage.

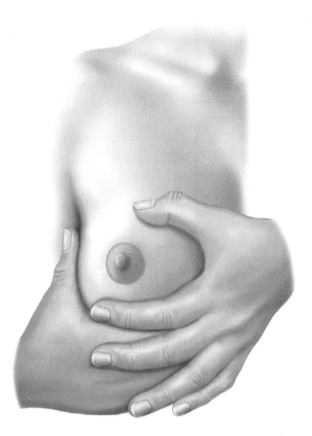

Figure 5.2 Compression of lactiferous sinuses.

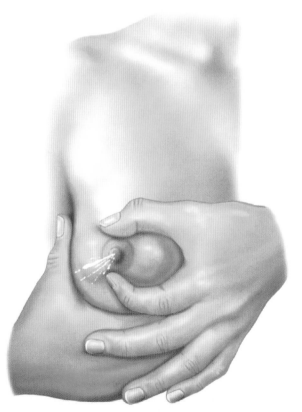

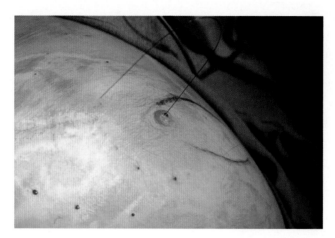

Figure 5.3 Nipple cannulated with prolene suture.

the duct with a soft suture such as a 2-0 prolene can further assist in correct duct identification (Fig. 5.3). With a little practice, using a grid much as in the child's game Battleship with letters on the x axis and numbers on the y axis, you can code position on the nipple and be able to find the ducts without the added picture step (Fig. 5.4). Remember, for the ducts to produce fluid, the patient will need to be well hydrated. To some extent, consumption of methyl xanthines such as caffeinated drinks will stimulate some additional ductal secretion and assist you. Clearly, being NPO (nothing by mouth) for 12 hours prior to surgery can make fluid more difficult to elicit from the nipple. I encourage women to "superhydrate for at least a couple of days before." Giving intravenous fluids liberally on the day of surgery and keeping the nipple warm prior to attempts to elicit fluid are important.

Third is being sure that keratinous debris and crusty dried secretions do not limit your ability to find the duct of interest. I have found using some minimally abrasive facial exfoliant and a 4″ × 4″ gauze pad the most expeditious way to scrub off the plateau of the nipple papilla for this purpose.

Finally is the massage in the OR prior to prepping the patient. Using the La Leche techniques and hand lotion, the breast is kneaded from chest wall toward nipple to push deep pockets of fluid into the lactiferous sinuses behind the nipple. After prepping, simple radial compression of the sinuses allows easy identification of the ducts producing fluid (Fig. 5.2).

SURGERY

Anatomy

What has been written about the anatomy of the ducts and the nipple is very confusing. This can best be summarized by noting that nipple cross-sections usually reveal 18 to 25 ducts but lactational studies looking at the orifices that actually produce milk show only

LEFT

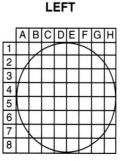

RIGHT

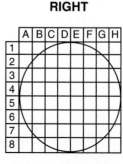

Figure 5.4 Grid for labeling ductal orifice location.

8 to 12 ductal orifices. Most now believe that many of the ducts seen on histology are truncated and short ducts that never really develop into formal lactiferous ducts with branching glands. These truncated ducts usually end around the areolar edge and may be associated with the relatively common periareolar abscess etiology. The larger ducts can branch widely and into differing quadrants. This is perhaps best seen on wax injections of the ductal trees. Usually, the ducts arising from the outer one-third of the nipple papilla branch widely and cover large areas. The more centrally located ducts have a branching pattern making a teardrop-like system directly back from the nipple.

Ductal Identification

Cannulate the fluid-producing duct—in case of pathologic discharge, use a 2-0 prolene cut to a gentle taper; for breast cancer cases, the orifice will be smaller and produce much less fluid. In these cases, inject 1% isosulfan blue (Lymphazurine) and local anesthetic in the region around the tumor first to be better able to select the correct low-volume duct. Cannulate with the 2-0 prolene if possible or more rigid introducers such as the smallest lacrimal duct dilators or stents when needed. Then, progressively dilate in Seldinger fashion using 24 G and 22 G angiocaths. With each size angiocath, inject 1 cc to 5 cc of local anesthetic into the duct for distension or alternatively, small lacrimal dilators can be used gently (Fig. 5.5).

Ductoscopy—Diagnostic

The scope sheath is introduced in Seldinger fashion with the hollow introducer being removed and replaced by the scope. It is important to have the scope well focused and white balanced before introduction into the breast ducts. The duct can then be distended by saline or local anesthetic while preventing leakage by compressing the nipple papilla against the scope with the thumb and the index finger. The scope is advanced as distension is obtained. Distraction of the nipple outward and gentle motion

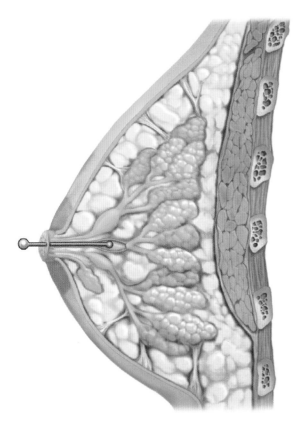

Figure 5.5 Dilation of nipple papilla.

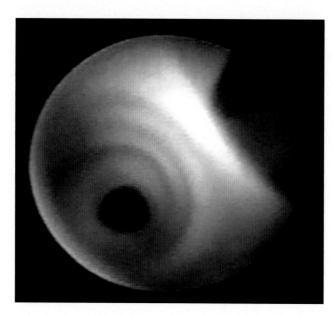

Figure 5.6 Branch point as seen on endoscopy.

of the underlying breast mound back and forth can be used to negotiate the varying branches. The scope sheaths all come with markings to help keep track of depth. When you come to multiple branches, the largest diameter branch usually takes you to the most proliferative lesion (Fig. 5.6).

To find the position of the scope tip if an abnormality is seen that needs excisional biopsy, turn off all the overhead lights in the OR and use the transilluminate from the scope tip to identify your site for biopsy (Fig. 5.7). The scopes can all be readily seen with ultrasound so that minimal-access biopsy devices can be used for same lesions near the scope tip using percutaneous ultrasound-directed techniques.

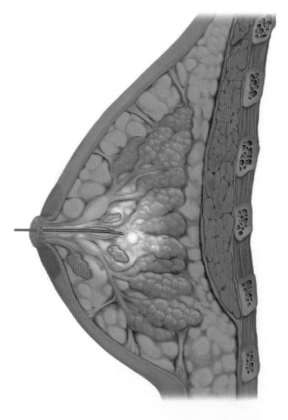

Figure 5.7 Transillumination to see position in breast.

Ductoscopy—Therapeutic

In the case of directing breast cancer procedures, remember that the volume of expressed fluid may be small and the ductal cannulation may be substantially more challenging. Do not perforate the ductal system or efforts to distend the ducts will fail. Be gentle and expect that distension may take longer.

The ductal orifice chosen should usually be within 100 to 110 degrees radially from the nipple papilla of the known lesion position in the breast. Always scope down largest branches first since these are more likely to connect to tumor. Once the obstructing tumor is found, mark position on the skin by transillumination. Work your way backward scoping each smaller branch and mark each site of intraductal luminal defects by transillumination on the breast surface.

Leave the scope at the most proximal extent of nipple-ward progression of intraluminal disease or replace it with a prolene suture. Design your excision of the subsegmental quadrant to include from scope tip to a pie-shaped wedge to the periphery of the breast from the known tumor. The width of this wedge is determined by the intraluminal disease foci you identified in side branches (Fig. 5.3 shows the region abnormally marked on the skin surface). Most resections can be easily adapted to one of the newer oncoplastic incisions to hide the resection defect.

 POSTOPERATIVE MANAGEMENT

These patients require no different care than that which is given after any surgical breast tissue excision. It is normal for bloody fluid to drain from the nipple for several days following ductoscopy. I encourage women to avoid tape on the sensitive breast skin and wear a feminine napkin strategically placed within a bra to catch the nipple fluid that may drain.

 PEARLS AND PITFALLS

Perforation of the lactiferous sinus in the immediate retroareolar space is common. There are no known or described complications reported. The most disturbing aspect is that it may limit your ability to find the distal segment of the duct to scope. As soon as a perforation is seen or suspected from soft-tissue infiltration in the retroareolar space, stop instilling any fluid through the scope. Careful circular motion of the scope will usually allow you to find the crescent-like collapsed distal duct. If you can manipulate the scope to engage this remnant, regular scoping with saline distension can resume after getting 10 to 15 mm down this segment.

Most patients will drain fluid from the nipple for 1 to 5 days after the procedure and this is normal.

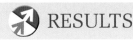 RESULTS

The earliest results from ductoscopy came in the early 1990s, when surgeons in Japan, where nipple discharge is a more common complaint among new breast cancer patients, began to experiment with endoscopes less than 2 mm in diameter (1). The initial effort was successful at identifying the cause of symptomatic bloody nipple discharge in a majority of patients. Unfortunately, the technology was cumbersome and expensive, which limited its early widespread use. Mammography has however been a poor tool for the diagnosis of breast cancer because of small breast size and high breast density in the Oriental population. Persistent efforts in the 1990s with ductoscopy in Japan, Korea, and Hong Kong began to show increasing success and developed a loyal following of surgical advocates as equipment improvements made this more practical (2–7).

The Oriental technique of breast endoscopy was to identify the ductal orifice draining blood, dilate the orifice, and introduce an optical fiber rigid scope with a chip camera mounted at a distance of about 6 inches. The fiber carried both the light and the image, and a very small working channel allowed air insufflation to distend the ducts (1,7,8). The air distension led to bubbles within a fluid-secreting duct, which then appeared as glistening reflective balls in the image. Clearly, this limited exposure until the duct was cleared of bubbles. Lesions seen were collapsed to the sidewall from the intraluminal air distension, but the bleeding source could usually be recognized easily and resection could be guided by transillumination through the skin. Further refinements of this technique have allowed cyst puncture and cystoscopy directly through the puncture tract (9–11).

American efforts to perform ductoscopy began with experimentation with much smaller and very flexible single-fiber scopes (12). These were even harder to direct and manipulate through the ductal system than their Oriental rigid counterparts. No working port was available and so active distension of the ductal system during endoscopy was not feasible. To achieve distension prescope distension of the duct with saline was needed, which afforded some increase in manipulation room.

While participating in the initial ductal lavage trial, I recognized the problem of identifying a single ductal orifice that could reliably multiply lavage for cancerous cells without any lesion being found clinically or radiographically (13,14). Aware of both the prior Oriental and American experiences with ductoscopy, Dooley et al. sought to find a semirigid submillimeter scope through which we could perform saline distension of the ductal tree. Further to avoid the torque issue of the camera at the end of a long lever arm, we wanted an optical fiber that was long and flexible enough to not interfere with driving the scope down the ducts. The Acuity 9-mm microendoscope fit these criteria, and we began a small pilot series to identify the cause of malignant and severe atypia from ductal lavage or nipple aspiration fluids. Quickly, it became apparent that the scope identified both the source of abnormal cells and bleeding from the intraluminal inspection (15,16). As cancer patients were examined more closely, it also became apparent that a small volume of fluid could be elicited from the duct connecting to the tumor in a majority of patients. Even where this fluid did not contain cytologically detectable cancer cells, fragments of cancer cell DNA could be identified and when endoscoped the cancerous lesion and proliferative disease around it could often be identified (17).

Expanding the use of breast endoscopy, first Dooley et al. used it to direct investigations and biopsies for bloody nipple discharge (18). These investigators found that the most proximal intraductal lesion was often not the source of the blood, and results suggested that multiple lesions are much more common than previous blind retroareolar duct excisions had suggested. Next, when fluid could be elicited from cancerous breasts, those ducts were endoscoped at the time of surgical lumpectomy (19). The majority of cancers were seen and the ductoscopy proved to be a very reliable way of both documenting the presence or absence of extensive intraductal carcinoma and directing complete resection at first attempt at lumpectomy. In a lumpectomy series, I was able to demonstrate that more than 40% of early-stage breast cancer patients had extensive intraductal proliferative changes. In these patients with this lobar distribution of proliferation around their cancer, lumpectomy was then fashioned to include the entire proliferative intraductal surface. This maneuver resulted in cutting the positive margin rate at initial lumpectomy attempt by more than 80%. Furthermore, it resulted in a four- to fivefold decrease over the next 5 to 8 years in the local hazard rate for recurrence in the conserved breast (16).

At present the clinical use of ductoscopy is limited because of steep learning curves to successfully cannulate, distend, and navigate the ductal branches. Furthermore, since the number of intraductal photographs with pathologic correlates is still small, the learning curve also includes building up your own personal repertoire of pathologic correlates. Equipment prices continue to fall and the technology is becoming more affordable as multiple manufacturers of submillimeter endoscopes worldwide are adapting their technologies to breast duct applications. A number of intraductal biopsy tools are beginning to appear to allow biopsy through these submillimeter scopes. Unfortunately, the specimen size is often less than 0.1 mm and would be more appropriately characterized as "chunky cytology" than a true histopathologic specimen. Pathologists will have to modify their approach to such specimens to try to give meaningful and precise answers with such small tissue samples.

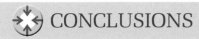 CONCLUSIONS

Ductoscopy can currently be used as an aid to identification of the root causes of pathologic nipple discharge. Its role in the management of early-stage breast cancer is evolving but clearly directs us toward the goal of anatomic resection of proliferative disease instead of the more traditional nonanatomic lumpectomy. Perhaps the greatest importance however of ductoscopy is the ready access to the ductal epithelium in vivo for research purposes. Just as the polyp model of colon cancer with its sequence of genetic alterations, the ability to visualize, and repeatedly sample and monitor chemoprevention efforts will direct us in unlocking the secrets of breast cancer carcinogenesis and prevention, development of molecular markers might even allow us to screen for the precancerous stages and prevent breast cancer instead of waiting till there is an invasive cancer in the majority of patients.

References

1. Okazaki A, Okazaki M, Asaishi K, et al. Fiberoptic ductoscopy of the breast: A new diagnostic procedure for nipple discharge. *Jpn J Clin Oncol.* 1991;21(3):188–193.
2. Okazaki A, Okazaki M, Hirata K, Tsumanuma T. Progress of ductoscopy of the breast [in Japanese]. *Nippon Geka Gakkai Zasshi.* 1996;97(5):357–362.
3. Okazaki A, Hirata K, Okazaki M, et al. Nipple discharge disorders: Current diagnostic management and the role of fiber ductoscopy. *Eur Radiol.* 1999;9(4):583–590.
4. Shen KW, Wu J, Lu JS, et al. Fiberoptic ductoscopy for patients with nipple discharge. *Cancer.* 2000:89(7):1512–1519.
5. Shao ZM, Liu Y, Nguyen M. The role of the breast ductal system in the diagnosis of cancer . *Oncol Rep.* 2001;8(1):153–156.
6. Matsunaga T, Ohta D, Misaka T, et al. Mammary ductoscopy for diagnosis and treatment of intraductal lesions of the breast. *Breast Cancer.* 2001;8(3):213–221.
7. Shen KW, Wu J, Lu JS, et al. Fiberoptic ductoscopy for breast cancer patients with nipple discharge. *Surg Endosc.* 2001; 15(11):1340–1345.
8. Yamamoto D, Shoji T, Kawanishi H, et al. A utility of ductography and fiberoptic ductoscopy for patients with nipple discharge. *Breast Cancer Res Treat.* 2001;70(2):103–108.
9. Yamamoto D, Ueda S, Senzaki H, et al. New diagnostic approach to intracystic lesions of the breast by fiberoptic ductoscopy. *Anticancer Res.* 2001;21(6A):4113–4116.
10. Makita M, Akiyama F, Gomi N, et al. Endoscopic classification of intraductal lesions and histologic diagnosis. *Breast Cancer.* 2002;9(3):220–225.
11. Tamaki Y, Miyoshi Y, Noguchi S. Application of endoscopic surgery for breast cancer treatment [in Japanese]. *Nippon Geka Gakkai Zasshi.* 2002;103(11):835–838.
12. Love SM, Barsky SH. Breast-duct endoscopy to study stages of cancerous breast disease. *Lancet.* 1996;348(9033):997–999.
13. Dooley WC, Ljung B-M, Veronesi U, et al. Ductal lavage for detection of cellular atypia in women at high risk for breast cancer. *J Natl Can Inst.* 2001;93(21):1624–1632.
14. Khan SA, Baird C, Staradub VL, Morrow M. Ductal lavage and ductoscopy: the opportunities and the limitations. *Clin Breast Cancer.* 2002;3(3):185–191; discussion 192–195.
15. Dietz JR, Crowe JP, Grundfest S, et al. Directed duct excision by using mammary ductoscopy in patients with pathologic nipple discharge. *Surgery.* 2002;132(4):582–587; discussion 587–588.
16. Dooley WC. Routine operative breast endoscopy during lumpectomy. *Ann Surg Oncol.* 2003;10(1):38–42.
17. Evon E, Dooley WC, Umbricht CB, et al. Detection of breast cancer cells in ductal lavage fluid by methation-specific PCR. *Lancet.* 2001;357:1335–1446.
18. Dooley WC. Routine operative breast endoscopy for bloody nipple discharge. *Ann Surg Oncol.* 2002;9(9):920–923.
19. Dooley WC. Ductal lavage, nipple aspiration, and ductoscopy for breast cancer diagnosis. *Curr Oncol Rep.* 2003;5(1):63–65.

Part II: Breast Biopsy

6 Excisional Breast Biopsy of Palpable Lesions

Stephen R. Grobmyer, Juan C. Cendan, and Edward M. Copeland, III

 INDICATIONS/CONTRAINDICATIONS

Clinical physical examination of the breast and breast self-examination are tools currently utilized in the detection of breast cancer. These modalities should be used in conjunction with annual mammographic examinations for the detection of breast cancer.

A wide spectrum of benign, potentially malignant, and malignant lesions of the breast may present as a palpable nodule or lump in the breast. When patients present with a new palpable lesion or a new lesion is detected on physical examination by a health care provider, further characterization of the lesion is warranted. Many but not all palpable lesions are detectable and assessable on breast imaging studies. When imaging studies suggest the possibility of a malignant breast lesion, image-guided percutaneous biopsy (fine needle aspiration, ultrasound-guided core, stereotactic, or magnetic resonance imaging [MRI]–guided core) is preferred to achieve a pathologic diagnosis in most patients. This approach allows detailed multidisciplinary treatment planning for patients who have breast cancer and potentially limits the number of operative interventions ultimately required.

At present, we perform excisional biopsy of palpable breast lesions to the following five indications:

1. Palpable lesions that cannot be detected on breast imaging studies
2. Discordance between percutaneous biopsy results and imaging studies
3. Lesions strongly suspected to be consistent with fibroadenomas in younger women
4. Lesions in an unfavorable position for percutaneous biopsy (near chest wall or near an implant)
5. Patients with a bleeding diathesis in whom percutaneous biopsy may be associated with high risk of postprocedural bleeding

 PREOPERATIVE PLANNING

The assessment of patients with palpable breast lesions should begin with a detailed history and physical examination. Particular attention should be given to personal breast health history (including prior breast biopsies and prior breast operations), other cancer

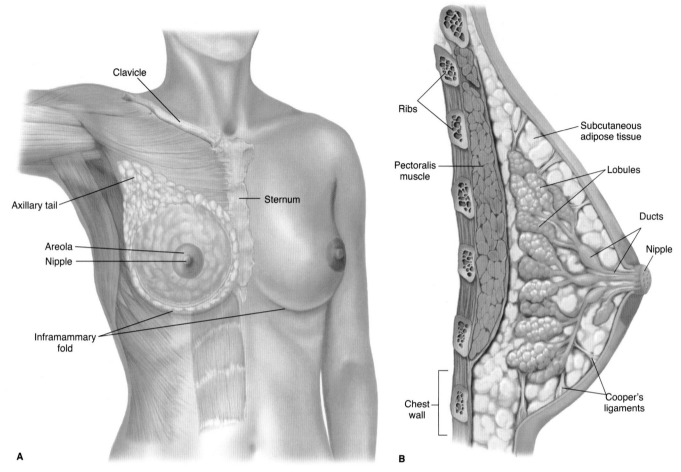

Figure 6.1 A. and **B.** Normal breast anatomy. Anterior view (**A**) and lateral view (**B**).

history, family cancer history, and other risks factors for breast cancer. Information regarding the details of a palpable lesion includes size, rate of change in size, location in the breast, texture, method of detection (patient or other health care provider), and associated symptoms (e.g., skin changes, nipple discharge, nipple inversion, pain, tenderness). These details can provide important clinical clues regarding the etiology of a mass or nodule. The presentation of a new dominant lump in the breast of a female in her 20s, which is smooth, round, and mobile, suggests a fibroadenoma. In contrast, a firm palpable mass in the breast of a postmenopausal woman with associated overlying skin changes suggests a malignant process, either with or without a familial history of breast carcinoma.

Physical examination of the breast should be performed and carefully documented. We prefer to perform breast examination with patients in both the sitting and lying positions. Mass size, texture, location, mobility, and tenderness should be recorded. Particular attention should also be given to associated findings including adenopathy (axillary or supraclavicular), nipple inversion, and nipple discharge. Normal breast anatomy is demonstrated in Figure 6.1A and B. Clinical features suggesting malignancy are shown in Table 6.1.

TABLE 6.1	Clinical Features of Palpable Breast Lesions That Suggest Malignancy
History	**Physical Examination**
Rapid growth	Firm
Not mobile	Fixed
Large	Irregular borders
	Associated adenopathy (axillary or supraclavicular)
	Other breast changes involving skin or nipple

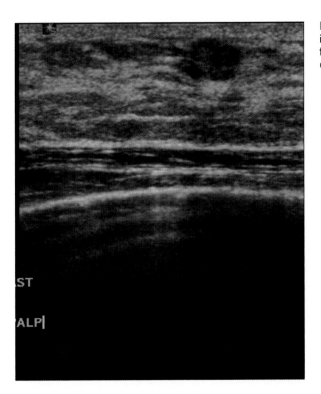

Figure 6.2 Breast ultrasound demonstrating a hypoechoic mass consistent with fibroadenoma. Fibroadenomas are typically wider than tall as shown.

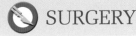

Part II: Breast Biopsy

It can be difficult in some patients, particularly those with dense or fibrocystic breast tissue, to discriminate on clinical examination between normal breast changes and breast lesions that warrant further attention. Significant clinical experience is required in judging the clinical need for biopsy in these situations.

Radiographic imaging is generally indicated in the initial investigation of breast lumps or masses. The work-up should be tailored to the specifics of a given patient's clinical presentation. This often includes a mammogram and ultrasound of the breast. Mammography is an important component of the evaluation but can be technically limited in younger patients and for lesions located in the upper medial breast. The recent addition of digital mammography to the radiologist armamentarium has somewhat eliminated the problem of dense breasts. Ultrasound is excellent for determining whether a palpable breast lump is cystic or solid and used alone may suffice for young patients who present with typical features of fibroadenoma (Fig. 6.2). Magnetic resonance imaging is not generally recommended for the evaluation of palpable breast lumps or masses.

Finally, patients with either an inherited or medically induced bleeding diathesis will need specific consideration. We prefer to work closely with the patient's hematologist in the case of inherited disorders in an effort to minimize the operative hemorrhage risk. Likewise, and quite commonly, co-ordination will require direct communication with the patient's other physicians, particularly cardiologists who may have initiated an anticoagulant in conjunction with placement of coronary stents. In these cases discontinuation of the anticoagulant prematurely may be of greater risk to the patient than that presented by the breast mass and a comprehensive plan must be agreed upon prior to surgery.

SURGERY

Before taking the patient to the operating room for biopsy, we mark the palpable abnormality with the patient awake with the patient in the supine position. This procedure helps ensure removal of the index lesion and reduces the chance of wrong site surgery. Practically, we have also found that small lesions may be somewhat obscured by infiltration of the local anesthetic agent, and marking the lesion prior to infiltration of the dermis is critical. On the day of operation, we also have available prior breast imaging studies and results of previous biopsies for review.

For operation, patients are generally placed supine on the operating room table. Excisional breast biopsy for palpable lesions can be performed under local anesthesia or general anesthesia. For patients with small or subtle palpable breast nodules, general anesthesia may be preferred in order to prevent the local anesthesia from obscuring the tactile properties of the lesion and complicating removal. For patients in whom general anesthesia is elected, our group generally prefers laryngeal mask airway to endotracheal intubation in selected patients. For local anesthesia during operation, a 1% lidocaine solution *without epinephrine* is utilized. We prefer local anesthetic without epinephrine, as the use of epinephrine may be associated with delayed postoperative bleeding and has been associated with sloughing of the skin at the incision margins. Bupivacaine (Marcaine) (0.25%) is administered toward the end of the operation to the operative site for prolonged local anesthesia.

An intravenous antibiotic (e.g., first-generation cephalosporin) is given within 30 minutes of the incision preoperatively. No postoperative doses of antibiotics are given. Sequential compression devices are placed on the calves to help reduce the risk of perioperative deep venous thrombosis. Chemoprophylaxis (e.g., subcutaneous heparin) against deep venous thrombosis is not utilized routinely in patients undergoing excisional breast biopsy for palpable lesions.

Technique 1: Excision of Fibroadenoma

Excision of lesions thought to be consistent with fibroadenoma makes up a large portion of excisional breast biopsies because of the frequency of this lesion, particularly in younger women. Considerations on the excision of fibroadenoma differ in subtle ways from the approach for palpable breast lesions not thought to be fibroadenoma. For patients in whom there is a strong clinical suspicion for a fibroadenoma, we prefer a periareolar incision when possible, as this approach may be associated with improved cosmetic outcomes in the postoperative period (Fig. 6.3). For lesions far from the central breast, this approach may not be technically possible. In these cases, we will utilize either an incision in the orientation of Langer's lines (Fig. 6.4) or a transverse incision (Fig. 6.5). As a general rule, skin incisions should not be made at great distances from the incident lesion. If the lesion proves to be malignant, all the normal tissues surrounding the tunnel through which the cancer exited must be considered contaminated with breast cancer cells.

The skin of the breast and surrounding areas are prepared in a sterile fashion. The incision is made with a scalpel (no. 15 blade) and deepened through the dermal layers with electrocautery (Figs. 6.6 and 6.7). For excisional breast biopsies, we prefer use of the guarded tip cautery (Fig. 6.7). Tissue flaps are then elevated using Metzenbaum scissors in all directions and particularly in the direction of the palpable lesion (Fig. 6.8A and B). These flaps allow greater exposure through smaller excision. The underlying breast parenchyma is divided with cautery or sharp dissection working in the direction of the palpable lesion. As the tissue is divided, the underlying tissue is exposed using fixed

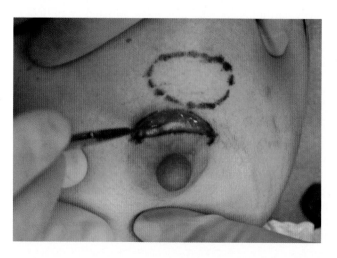

Figure 6.3 Periareolar incision in a patient with a fibroadenoma in the upper central left breast (inferior view). The dashed circle is the area of the palpable fibroadenoma.

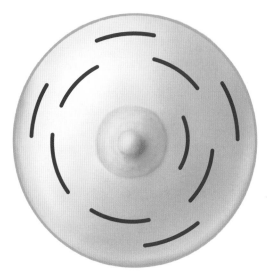

Figure 6.4 Incisions for excisional biopsies may be made in the orientation of Langer's lines, which are oriented around the breast.

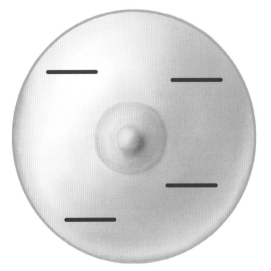

Figure 6.5 Incisions for excisional biopsies may be alternatively made in a transverse orientation.

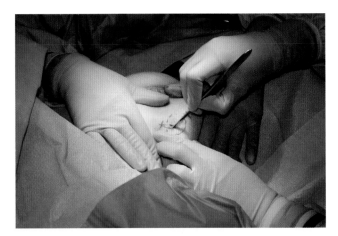

Figure 6.6 Skin incision is made with no. 15 blade scalpel. Retraction on the breast tissue facilitates incision.

Part II: Breast Biopsy

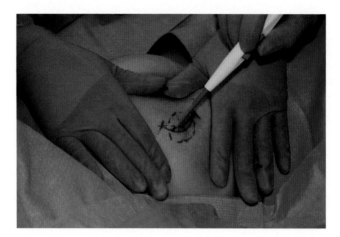

Figure 6.7 Skin incision is deepened through superficial tissue using electrocautery. We prefer guarded tip cautery, as shown, for excisional biopsy of palpable breast lesions.

angle retractors (Fig. 6.9). We prefer Eastman retractors for this exposure (Fig. 6.10), as they are very versatile and can be used for a variety of wound sizes. For a more superficial lesion, rake retractors may also be useful (Fig. 6.11). Dissection is carried down until the palpable lesion of interest is identified (Fig. 6.9). In the case of a fibroadenoma, only the mass needs to be removed. A silk stitch is then placed in the mass to provide the gentle retraction necessary to facilitate its removal (Fig. 6.12). Alternatively, an Adair tenaculum may be used to provide retraction (Fig. 6.13). Fibroadenomas are then removed using a combination of sharp and blunt dissection (Fig. 6.11). No attempt is made to remove a margin of normal breast tissue in conjunction with the fibroadenoma, as this does not improve outcomes and is associated with unnecessary cosmetic deformity. As fibroadenomas tend to push surrounding breast tissue when they grow, cavity closure following removal of fibroadenomas is not necessary. In fact, an attempt to remove a portion of normal tissue surrounding a large fibroadenoma is wrong since the normal tissue has been compressed by the enlarging fibroadenoma, and if normal tissue is removed, this compressed normal breast tissue is not available to expand to fill the excision cavity. Frozen section is not performed on lesions that are clinically consistent with fibroadenoma. Specimen radiograph is not necessary and is not performed on these lesions following removal. After removal of the lesion, we digitally inspect the biopsy cavity to confirm the absence of other suspicious lesions (Fig. 6.14). Hemostasis is controlled in the cavity using electrocautery. Local anesthesia without epinephrine is administered for long-acting pain control (Fig. 6.15). No drains are placed in the breast. The dermal layer is reapproximated using 3-0 absorbable sutures. The skin is closed with rapidly absorbing subcuticular sutures (Fig. 6.16). We prefer superficial wound closure without the use of buried stitches (Fig. 6.17), as this avoids "spitting" of knots in the postoperative

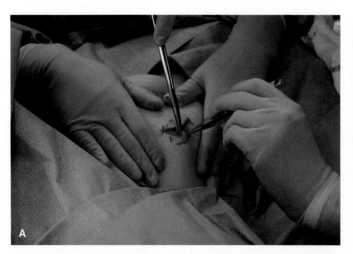

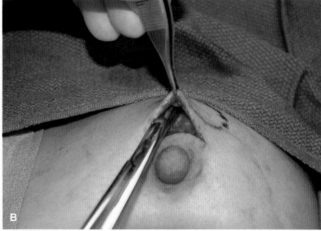

Figure 6.8 **A.** and **B.** Subcutaneous flaps are raised using Metzenbaum scissors in all directions to facilitate exposure.

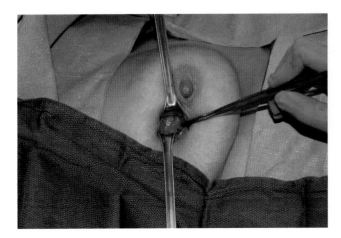

Figure 6.9 Breast tissue is separated using Eastman retractors as dissection is carried down to palpable lesion. The forceps are pointing to area of palpable abnormality in this patient.

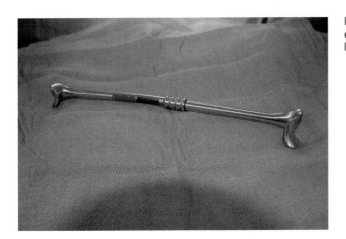

Figure 6.10 Eastman retractor used in excisional biopsy of palpable breast lesion.

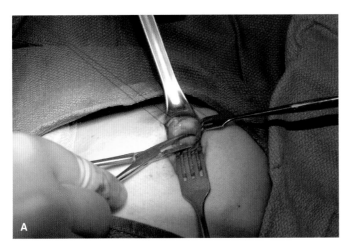
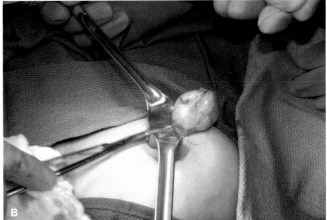

Figure 6.11 **A.** and **B.** Fibroadenomas may be removed with a combination of sharp and blunt dissection. Rake retractors are being used to facilitate exposure for the superficial portion of the excision.

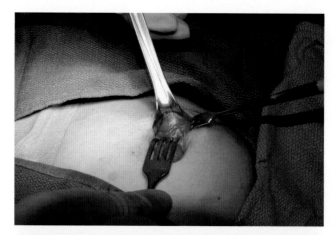

Figure 6.12 A figure-of-eight silk stitch has been placed in the palpable fibroadenoma to facilitate retraction and exposure.

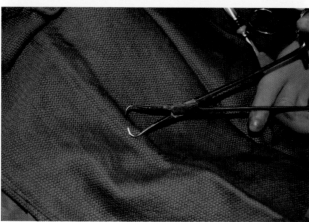

Figure 6.13 An Adair tenaculum may be used to grasp palpable lesions in an atraumatic fashion to facilitate excision of palpable breast lesions.

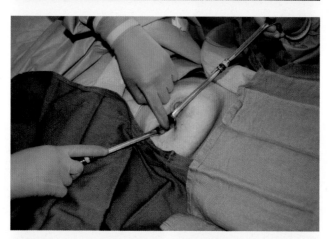

Figure 6.14 Following excision of a palpable breast lesion, the cavity should be inspected to exclude any additional suspicious lesions.

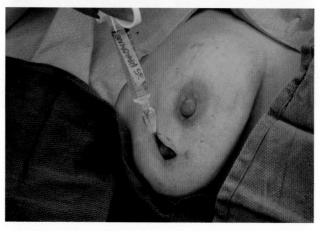

Figure 6.15 Administration of long-acting local anesthetic is performed prior to final wound closure.

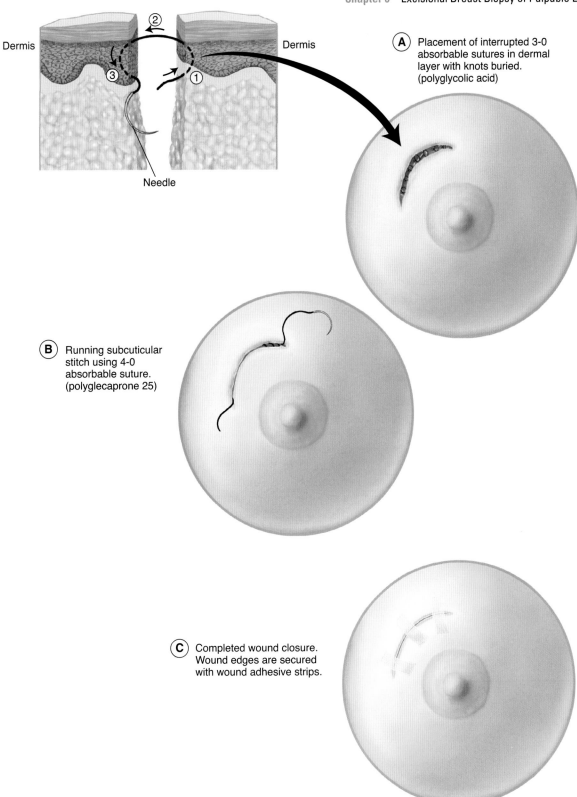

Dermis

Needle

Dermis

(A) Placement of interrupted 3-0 absorbable sutures in dermal layer with knots buried. (polyglycolic acid)

(B) Running subcuticular stitch using 4-0 absorbable suture. (polyglecaprone 25)

(C) Completed wound closure. Wound edges are secured with wound adhesive strips.

Part II: Breast Biopsy

Figure 6.16 Schematic of wound closure following excisional biopsy of palpable lesions. First, interrupted absorbable sutures are placed in the dermal layer with knots buried. Then, the skin is closed with a running subcuticular suture. No knots are used and ends are left to exit wound on each end. Finally, wound edges are secured with wound tapes as shown.

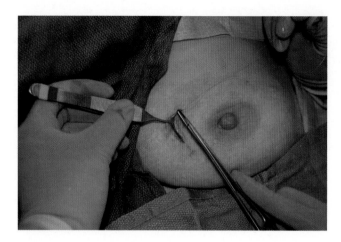

Figure 6.17 Subcuticular wound closure is achieved using rapidly absorbing suture. No knots are used on the corners of the closure as this prevents "spitting" of the knots in the postoperative period.

period. Wound edges and the free ends of the suture are secured with Steri-Strips following closure (Fig. 6.18). A surgical bra is then placed following the procedure, as it eliminates the need for tape on the breast and it provides support and gentle compression to the surgical site.

Technique 2: Excision of Palpable Breast Lesions Not Consistent with Fibroadenoma

Patient preparation and positioning is similar to that outlined in Technique 1. For these lesions with a greater chance of associated malignancy, we prefer incisions placed in close approximation to the lesions to avoid contamination of the surrounding normal breast tissue where tunneling is required to reach the lesion. Consideration should also be given to the need for inclusion of the skin incision in the mastectomy specimen where this operation is required (Fig. 6.19). Incision and exposure are similar to that performed in Technique 1. Once the lesion is identified by palpation, it can be grasped with an Adair tenaculum (Figs. 6.13 and 6.20) or secured with a traction suture. The lesion can then subsequently be excised using sharp or cautery dissection. Serial palpation is critical during biopsy of the lesions in order to accurately define the area of abnormality requiring excision. Once these lesions are removed, they should be oriented for pathologic evaluation (Fig. 6.21). Digital inspection of the biopsy cavity is important to ensure the absence of other suspicious areas (Fig. 6.14). Hemostasis is controlled with the electrocautery. Frozen section is obtained only in situations in which the result will alter immediate management as discussed with the patient preoperatively (such as proceeding directly to mastectomy if frozen section demonstrates invasive cancer). For these procedures, we prefer parenchymal closure, as parenchymal closure is associated with lower rates of infection and seroma formation. Parenchymal closure is done using interrupted absorbable sutures (Fig. 6.22). The remainder of the

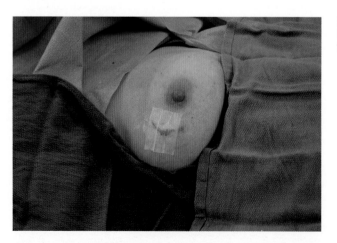

Figure 6.18 Steri-Strips are used to help secure wound edges and protect the wound following skin closure.

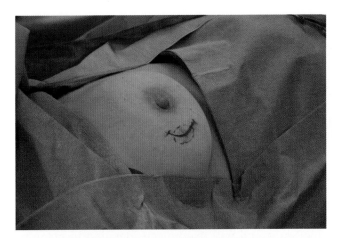

Figure 6.19 Planned incision in a patient with a palpable lesion of the lateral right breast (superior–lateral view). Dashed circle is the palpable abnormality not seen on imaging studies. The curved line is the planned incision.

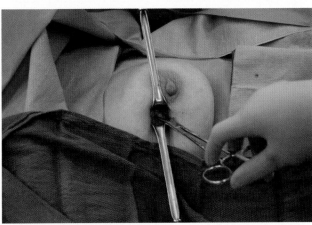

Figure 6.20 The palpable abnormality is grasped with an Adair tenaculum to facilitate exposure and excision.

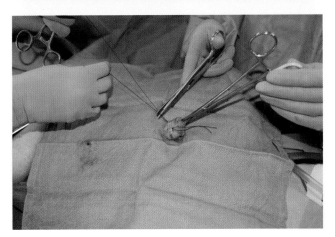

Figure 6.21 Following removal of palpable lesions of the breast, the specimen is oriented for pathologic evaluation. We place a short suture on the superior margin and a long suture on the lateral margin.

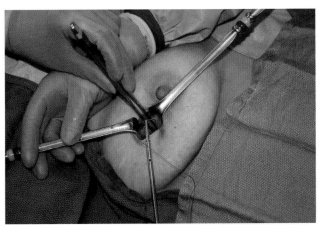

Figure 6.22 Closure of the deep tissue is performed using absorbable sutures.

closure and wound management are similar to that performed in Technique 1 discussed earlier (Fig. 6.16).

Special Considerations on Excisional Biopsy of Palpable Breast Lesions

There are several clinical settings in which special consideration should be given to excisional biopsy of palpable lesions.

Lymphoma

In patients in whom lymphoma of the breast is suspected, specimens should be sent to pathology fresh and sterile to allow analysis by flow cytometry—it cannot be placed in formalin. This may pose a problem for operations being performed in outpatient surgical units separate from the pathology suite and will require consideration in planning for the transport of the tissue.

Granulomatous Mastitis

In patients with a breast mass that is thought possibly to be consistent with granulomatous mastitis, specimens should be sent for culture and gram stain in addition to routine histologic analysis.

Pseudoangiomatous Stromal Hyperplasia

Patients with pseudoangiomatous stromal hyperplasia (PASH) may present with a dominant large mass of the breast. Following percutaneous biopsy, surgical biopsy may be advised to confirm the diagnosis, in patients with symptoms, enlarging lesions, or those classified as BI-RADS 4 or 5. For other select patients, incisional biopsy may be preferable to excisional biopsy to avoid potential cosmetic deformity associated with complete excisional biopsy.

Phyllodes Tumor

Rarely, lesions that are excised as fibroadenomas are found to be phyllodes tumors. In this situation, re-excision is required of the surrounding breast tissue to reduce the rate of recurrence. This re-excision should be done as soon as possible to allow recognition of the original biopsy cavity (remembering that excision of normal breast tissue is not recommended for fibroadenomas regardless of size).

 ## POSTOPERATIVE MANAGEMENT

We encourage patients to keep an ice pack on the surgical area after biopsy for 48 hours to reduce postprocedural swelling. Oral pain medication is prescribed. Usually narcotics are not necessary. Patients are allowed to take shower beginning 48 hours following the operative procedure.

Patients are seen for a follow-up visit in the clinic 7 to 14 days following the operation. The wound is inspected (Fig. 6.23) and the final pathology report is reviewed with the patient. Other treatment planning is discussed as indicated. In general, we recommend follow-up imaging of the operated breast 6 months following the procedure to document postprocedural changes.

 ## COMPLICATIONS

Potential complications in the patient undergoing excisional biopsy of palpable lesions of the breast include infection, seroma formation, hematoma formation, and Mondor disease.

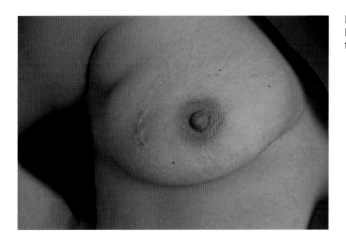

Figure 6.23 Appearance of a properly healing breast incision on postoperative day 10.

Breast infection in the postoperative period may range from mild cellulitis to abscess formation. In patients suspected of having an infection, ultrasound can be helpful in distinguishing abscesses from cellulitis of the breast. Cellulitis may be treated with oral antibiotics; however, in cases where cellulitis fails to respond to oral antibiotics, intravenous antibiotics may be warranted. Abscesses of the breast following excisional biopsy, requires incision and drainage.

Seroma formation occurs commonly in the course of recovery following excisional biopsy of the breast. We typically reserve percutaneous aspiration for symptomatic patients.

Low volume hematomas following breast excisional biopsy may be managed using symptom-directed strategies typically resulting in resolution. Larger hematomas may require surgical evacuation of the clot.

Mondor disease (thrombosis of the thoracoepigastric vein) can occur after excisional breast biopsy. Mondor disease presents as a palpable cord between the breast and the abdominal wall. Conservative management is warranted, as this condition typically is self-limited.

A special circumstance is the postoperative management of a patient who requires a breast biopsy while still lactating. Milk fistulization through the biopsy incision is an expected result and must be discussed in detail with the patient, especially if she insists on breast-feeding following biopsy if the lesion is benign. These typically resolve following cessation of breast-feeding.

✺ CONCLUSIONS

A thorough understanding of the evaluation and work-up of palpable breast lesions is essential for the breast surgeon. With the widespread availability of percutaneous biopsy technology, excisional biopsy of the breast for palpable lesions should be reserved for specific clinical situations that we have outlined in this chapter. An understanding of the current surgical strategies and the potential complications resulting from excisional breast biopsy for palpable lesions can reduce morbidity and optimize patient outcomes.

Suggested Readings

Chaney AW, Pollack A, McNeese MD, et al. Primary treatment of cystosarcoma phyllodes of the breast. *Cancer.* 2000;89:1502–1511.

Collins JC, Liao S, Wile AG. Surgical management of breast masses in pregnant women. *J Reprod Med.* 1995;40:785–788.

Foxcroft LM, Evans EB, Joshua HK, et al. Breast cancers invisible on mammography. *Aust N Z J Surg.* 2000;70:162–167.

Grady I, Gorsuch H, Wilburn-Bailey S. Long-term outcome of benign fibroadenomas treated by ultrasound-guided percutaneous excision. *Breast J.* 2008;14:275–278.

Liberman L. Clinical management issues in percutaneous core breast biopsy. *Radiol Clin North Am.* 2000;38:791–807.

Park YM, Kim EK, Lee JH, et al. Palpable breast masses with probably benign morphology at sonography: can biopsy be deferred? *Acta Radiol.* 2008;49:1104–1111.

Pocock B, Taback B, Klein L, et al. Preoperative needle biopsy as a potential quality measure in breast cancer surgery. *Ann Surg Oncol.* 2009;16:1108–1111.

Vitug AF, Newman LA. Complications in breast surgery. *Surg Clin North Am.* 2007;87:431–451.

Wilson JP, Massoll N, Marshall J, et al. Idiopathic granulomatous mastitis: in search of a therapeutic paradigm. *Am Surg.* 2007;73: 798–802.

Part II: Breast Biopsy

7 Needle Localization Biopsy of Nonpalpable Breast Lesions

Virginia M. Herrmann

The increasing use of screening, and in particular digital mammography, ultrasound, and breast magnetic resonance imaging (MRI), has resulted in earlier detection of breast cancer (1,2). Screening mammography has improved significantly in the last two decades. This, coupled with emphasis on breast screening and guidelines recommending annual mammography for women 40 years of age and older, has contributed to the increased detection of small, nonpalpable lesions. The early detection of nonpalpable lesions led to the development of breast needle localization (BNL) to obtain a tissue diagnosis. Mammographic detection of lesions requiring BNL include a nonpalpable mass or density within, but distinct from normal breast parenchyma, architectural distortion, and clustered calcifications. These lesions are frequently discovered during screening mammography, and in most screening programs, approximately 15% of all lesions detected are malignant (3). The diagnosis of breast cancer at a very early stage has resulted in improved overall and disease-free survival for patients.

History and Rationale

The technique of BNL for nonpalpable lesions was first described by Dodd in 1966 (4,5). Nonpalpable lesions were localized by using a stiff needle placed near the lesion. This method was associated with several problems, including movement or dislodgement of the stiff needle during the period between its placement in radiology and transporting the patient to the operating room, movement of the needle during compression mammography, and movement or dislodgment of the needle during surgery. Inadequate tissue sampling was a frequent result.

Subsequent reports described the use of a combination of a needle and hooked wire with excellent accuracy and low biopsy failure rates. The wire was recommended to be placed within 1 mm of the lesion and secured within the breast tissue (6,7). In this method, the needle is removed, leaving the wire in place, with the wire hook placed within or immediately adjacent to the lesion. The hooked wire makes removal or dislodgment of the wire less likely than with a rigid needle.

BNL of suspicious nonpalpable lesions has been shown to be a reliable method for obtaining a diagnosis and has been the standard of care for the past several decades (8). The procedure can be performed by using local anesthesia and has been associated with a less than 2% chance of a missed lesion and a relatively low complication rate, similar to excisional biopsy of palpable lesions (9).

And while BNL of nonpalpable lesions is highly accurate, it can still be associated with some failures in obtaining the lesion seen on imaging. Whether the procedure was performed for diagnostic or therapeutic purposes, a review indicates the overall miss rate of this procedure is between 0% and 18% (mean 2.6%) and a cancer miss rate or false-negative BNL is 0% and 8% (mean 2.0%) (9–11).

BNL generally requires the patient undergo a separate procedure (wire or needle localization) in a separate department (radiology) from the operating room, where the lesion is removed. This technique is also associated with some morbidity and complications, to include pain and anxiety during needle placement, dislodgment of the needle or wire prior to operative removal, displacement of the wire when the breast is taken out of compression, and transecting the wire during surgery. The procedure requires significant anesthesia (e.g., monitored anesthesia care with intravenous sedation and local anesthetic, or general anesthetic) and has the potential for causing scar or distortion on subsequent mammography. Additional problems include excision of excess amount of tissue if the needle localization is not ideally centered in the lesion, resulting in possible cosmetic defect.

Historically, BNL performed as the primary procedure has been associated with the frequent need for a second operation if malignancy is found. When BNL was performed as the initial procedure and malignancy was found, the incidence of positive margins ranged from 55% to 83% (12,13).

With the development of stereotactic and MRI-guided biopsy techniques, the need for BNL of nonpalpable lesions has decreased. Stereotactic, ultrasound-guided, and MRI-guided biopsy have allowed the pathologic confirmation of benign lesions, obviating the need for surgery in many patients. Open excisional biopsy of many or most benign lesions is probably not necessary.

INDICATIONS/CONTRAINDICATIONS

Despite the advances in image-guided, minimally invasive biopsy for breast lesions, BNL continues to have an important role in the management of patients with nonpalpable breast lesions. Indications for this procedure include the following:

- Suspicious microcalcifications or solid lesions located too close to the chest wall to allow safe stereotactic core biopsy are generally considered for BNL. Ultrasound localization of lesions close to the chest wall is often a preferred and safer method of BNL (Fig. 7.1).
- Calcifications or papillary lesions in the immediate retroareolar area are often difficult to biopsy with image-guided technique and may be more amenable to BNL (Fig. 7.2).
- Atypical hyperplasia (ductal or lobular) found on core biopsy, and not associated with a palpable lesion, generally requires BNL because of the high incidence of ductal carcinoma in the associated tissue.
- Nonpalpable papillary lesions found on core biopsy should be excised with BNL to exclude papillary carcinoma.
- Radial scar, diagnosed either by mammogram or by core biopsy, should be totally excised by using BNL. These lesions, even if benign on core biopsy, are associated with a significant incidence of associated atypia or ductal carcinoma in situ (DCIS), necessitating complete excision (Fig. 7.3).
- BNL is the procedure of choice if breast conservation therapy is anticipated for patients with nonpalpable cancers and a prior core biopsy confirming malignancy (Figs. 7.4 and 7.5).

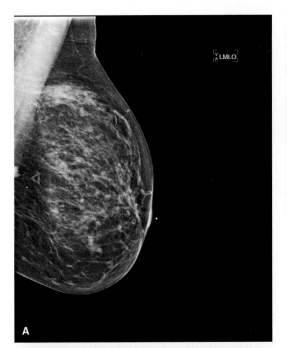

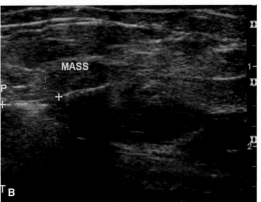

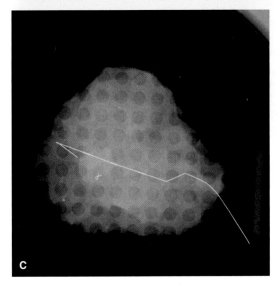

Figure 7.1 **A.** Lesion seen posteriorly near chest wall on mammogram. **B.** Lesion seen on ultrasound. **C.** Lesion successfully removed by using ultrasound localization.

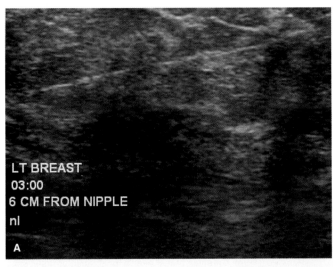

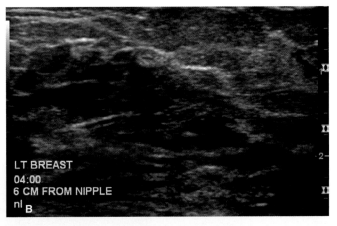

Figure 7.2 **A.** Papillary lesion on ultrasound at 3 o'clock position. **B.** Second papillary lesion seen on ultrasound at 4 o'clock position. **C.** Both papillary lesions localized by ultrasound. Mammogram taken for breast needle localization in operating room. (*continued*)

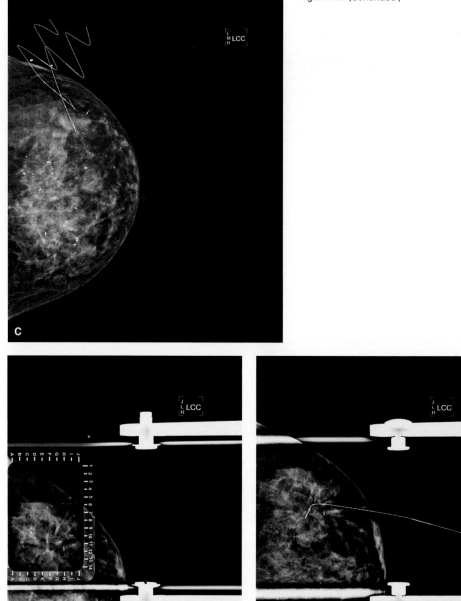

Figure 7.2 (*Continued*)

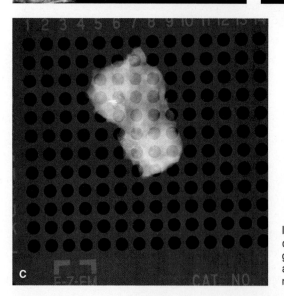

Figure 7.3 **A.** Radial scar on mammogram with clip from previous core biopsy. **B.** Mammographic breast needle localization of radial scar and clip. **C.** Specimen radiograph with clip and radial scar.

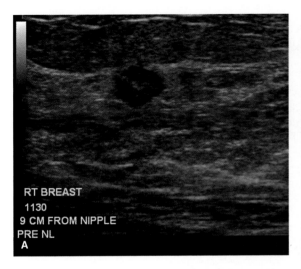

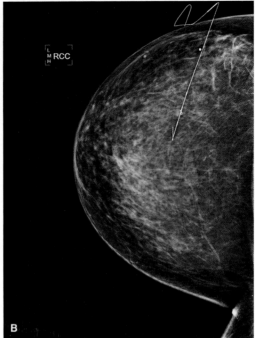

Figure 7.4 A. Pre–breast needle localization (BNL) of cancer seen on ultrasound. **B.** Mammogram of BNL showing small, nonpalpable cancer.

■ BNL is used to localize clip placement, or the "epicenter" of the tumor or tumor bed in patients treated with neoadjuvant chemotherapy. These patients ideally have had a clip or marker placed before commencing neoadjuvant chemotherapy, which localizes the area of cancer. Following treatment, the clip may be the only sign of the previously noted malignancy (Fig. 7.6).

Technical Considerations

Radiologists and surgeons have refined the technique of BNL to allow more accurate localization of breast lesions. The use of various needle or wire lengths allows access

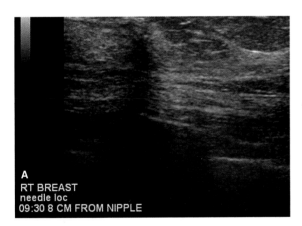

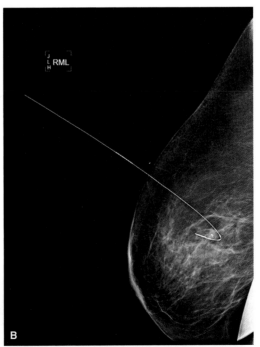

Figure 7.5 A. Small invasive tubular carcinoma on ultrasound. **B.** Mammographic breast needle localization of tubular invasive carcinoma.

Part II: Breast Biopsy

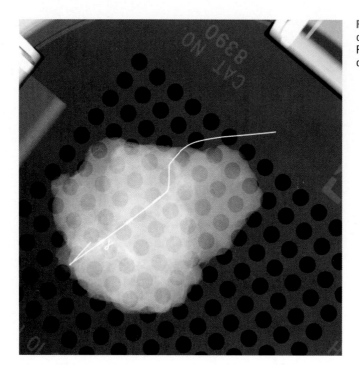

Figure 7.6 Specimen radiograph confirming clip in small tumor bed. Patient treated with neoadjuvant chemotherapy.

to lesions that may be deep in the breast or access to lesions in patients with large breast volume (Fig. 7.7). There are several needles used to localize lesions, most commonly, the Kopan needle, the Homer needle (J-wire), and the Hawkins retractable wire.

Image-guided BNL can be performed by using mammography, ultrasound, or MRI. The decision of which imaging modality to use for BNL is largely determined by the following:

- the type of lesion,
- how the lesion is best visualized, and
- available equipment and expertise in any given institution.

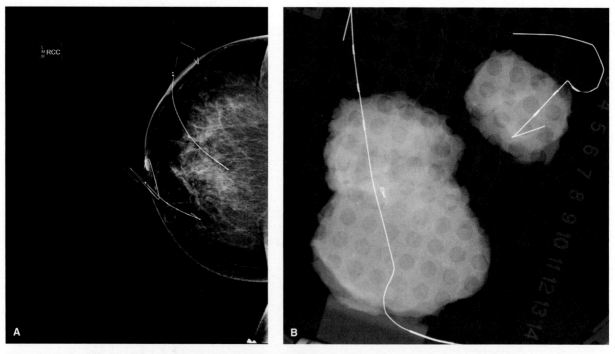

Figure 7.7 **A.** Two lesions localized with different lengths of wire. **B.** Specimen radiograph of each lesion with wire.

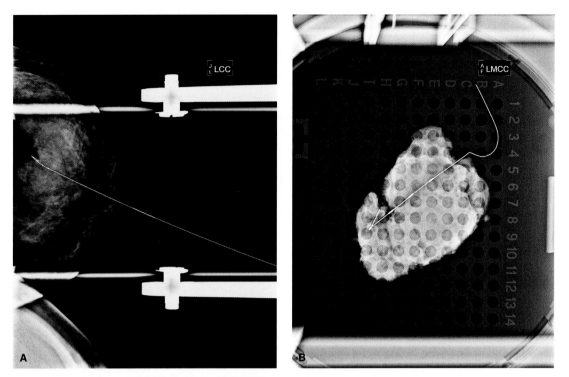

Figure 7.8 A. Breast needle localization of calcifications. **B.** Specimen radiograph confirming calcifications in specimen.

The decision of which modality to use is generally suggested by the radiologist, often with input from the surgeon.

Mammography

Breast microcalcifications are often best biopsied by using mammographic BNL (Fig. 7.8). A needle containing a wire is inserted into the breast. The needle is removed, and the wire hook "anchors" the wire in the breast lesion. A variable length of wire will extend beyond the skin. The wire tip should ideally be placed within the lesion or within 1 mm of the lesion and be well anchored in the breast tissue. Studies have indicated a failure rate of 2% to 4% if the wire is placed within 1 to 3 cm of the lesion (7). Generally, radiologists prefer to enter the skin parallel to the chest wall and approach the lesion from above (Fig. 7.9). A postlocalization mammogram is performed and should be available to the surgeon in the operating room as a visual guide to assess the depth of the lesion and

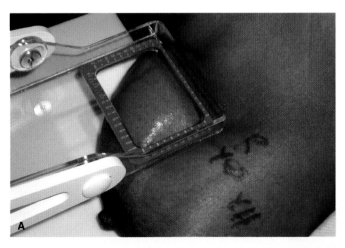
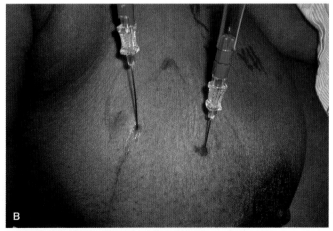

Figure 7.9 A. Lesion approached from above for breast needle localization (BNL). **B.** BNL completed with lesion approached from above.

needle, the proximity of the needle tip to the lesion, and the extent of the lesion. The increasing availability and use of digital mammography has expedited BNL. Recent data have demonstrated that full-field digital mammography is superior to screen–film mammography in the time needed for BNL (14). The time needed to position the patient and place the needle was shorter with digital mammography than screen–film mammography. In addition, digital mammography may provide superior image quality, reduced radiation exposure, and fewer delays as film processing is unnecessary.

Prior to BNL, the surgeon should review the radiographs with the radiologist to provide a clear understanding of the lesion(s) to be localized and the imaging method to be used for wire placement (e.g., ultrasound-, mammogram-, or MRI-guided biopsy).

Bracketed needle localization is particularly helpful in certain circumstances. Patients with extensive microcalcifications may not be ideal candidates for stereotactic core biopsy. More commonly, however, bracketed needle localization is used to identify the extent of calcifications in a patient with core biopsy-proven DCIS (Fig. 7.10). The

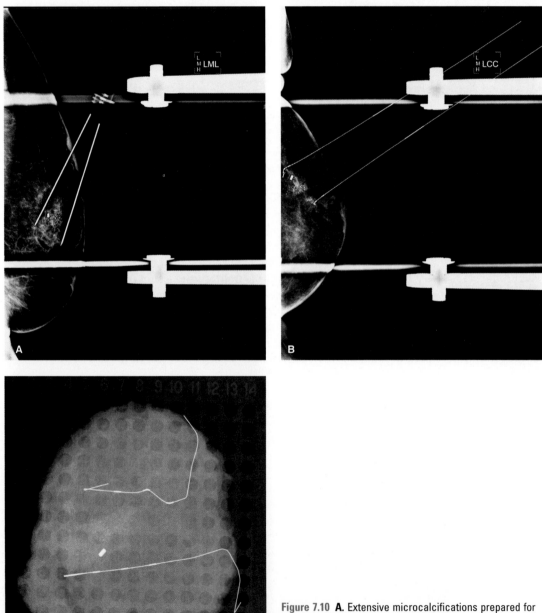

Figure 7.10 A. Extensive microcalcifications prepared for breast needle localization. **B.** Same patient with wires to bracket area of calcifications. **C.** Specimen radiograph showing successful removal of calcifications.

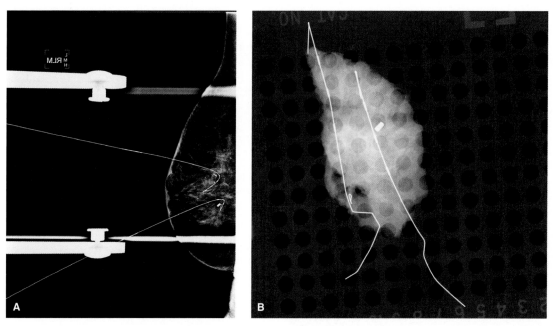

Figure 7.11 **A.** Two lesions (atypical ductal hyperplasia and invasive ductal cancer) previously diagnosed by core biopsy and clip placement. **B.** Same patient with both lesions removed on specimen radiograph.

extent of calcifications may underestimate the extent of DCIS; therefore, every attempt should be made to remove all of the suspicious calcifications with adequate margins. In bracketed needle localization, a wire is placed generally at the anterior and the posterior extent of calcifications. Two or more wires may be used to "bracket" the area of concern. Bracketed needle localization is also helpful to identify two or more lesions in the same quadrant (i.e., multifocal) lesions (Fig. 7.11). Two or more lesions can be removed through one incision. If the lesions are biopsy-proven or suspected to be malignant, both lesions can be removed along with the tissue between the two lesions and an adequate margin (Fig. 7.12).

Specimen radiography is strongly recommended following needle localization of suspicious breast lesions. The incidence of false-positive specimen radiographs may be as high as 7.8% and the false-negative rate as high as 55% (15). Hasselgren et al. (15) found that the incidence of missed lesions was 3.2%, and the incidence of incompletely excised lesions was 6.4%. The accuracy of needle localization has certainly improved with advances in mammography and the use of digital mammograms. Nevertheless, if there is any question whether or not the targeted lesion has been adequately resected, or if there is discordance between the initial mammogram, specimen radiograph and final pathology, a postoperative mammogram should be ordered (16).

Ultrasound-Guided Needle Localization

The increasing use of ultrasound of the breast has allowed identification of lesions, ultrasound-guided biopsy, and if necessary, needle localization using sonography. If a lesion is seen on both mammogram and ultrasound, ultrasound BNL is often easier for both the radiologist and patient and is better tolerated than mammographic BNL by patients (Fig. 7.13). If a lesion requires removal with excision and is accessible by ultrasound, a needle can be placed by using ultrasound guidance and secured at the skin level while the patient is transported to the operating room. Ultrasound needle localization is particularly useful for lesions that are seen better by ultrasound than by mammogram (e.g., small hypoechoic lesions in a mammographically dense breast) and for lesions in the immediate retroareolar area (e.g., papillary lesions requiring excisional biopsy). Calcifications are typically not easily identified by ultrasound and, therefore, are best excised with mammogram placement of the needle or wire.

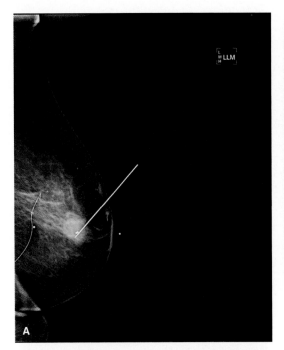

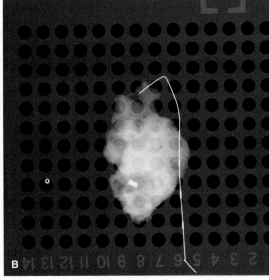

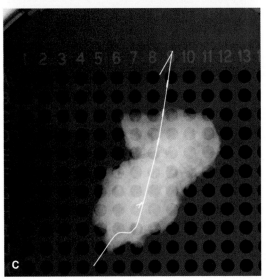

Figure 7.12 A. Two lesions (small invasive ductal cancer posteriorly and papillary lesion more anteriorly, diagnosed by core biopsy with clip placement. **B.** Papillary lesion with clip on specimen radiograph. **C.** Breast needle localization of small invasive cancer from double needle localization.

MRI-Guided Needle Localization

The past decade has witnessed a sharp increase in the use of MRI as a breast imaging modality. Breast MRI is more sensitive than mammography but has a lower specificity and a high false-positive rate. The positive predictive value of MRI-detected lesions is directly related to the lesion size. Biopsy is generally not necessary for lesions smaller than 5 mm as these lesions have been shown to have a low probability of being cancer (3%) (17). Lesions detected by MRI imaging but not seen on mammography or ultrasound may be amenable to MRI-guided core biopsy or MRI-guided needle localization and excisional biopsy (18–20). It may be difficult to confirm accurate or adequate removal of the MRI localized lesion, as the enhancement of the lesion diminishes with time and does not occur once the lesion has been removed. Specimen radiography has been shown to be a reliable method to confirm the removal of the targeted lesion and is a cost-effective alternative to repeated MRI scanning (21–23).

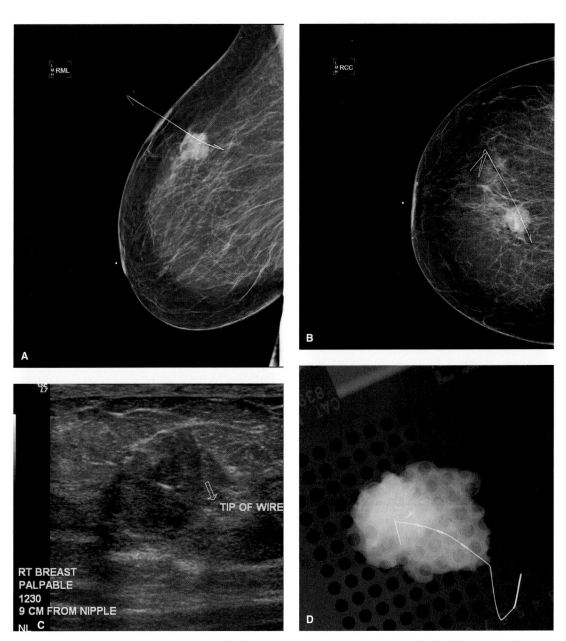

Figure 7.13 A. Lesion on medial lateral oblique (MLO) view of mammogram. Vaguely palpable. **B.** Lesion on cranial-caudal (CC) view of mammogram. **C.** Lesion localized by ultrasound. **D.** Specimen radiograph following ultrasound.

There are several technical challenges associated with dynamic MRI-guided wire localization. There is limited access to the patient with closed MR units, and the need to transfer the patient in and out of the MR scanner increases the time of the procedure. In addition, the insertion of the needle needs to be performed outside the magnet, and movement of either the breast tissue or needle is not necessarily detected during insertion and cannot be immediately corrected. Lesions located close to the chest wall, in the axillary tail of the breast, or close to implants may be difficult to localize with MR guidance. Real-time MRI, however, has distinct advantages over dynamic MRI (24). Real-time MRI-guided localization allows for correction of the needle during insertion and allows access to lesions close to the chest wall, axillary tail, or implants. It is associated with a satisfactory period for the procedure and is increasingly used as a modality to localize lesions not visualized on a mammogram or an ultrasound.

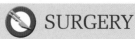 PREOPERATIVE PLANNING

Before performing BNL, surgeons and radiologists should discuss the procedure with the patient so that there is a clear understanding of the procedure, expected incision, and possible need for further surgery or reexcision. Surgeons often ask radiologists to leave the needle in place over the wire, as the needle is more easily palpable during surgery and facilitates accurate resection. Radiologists and/or staff will likely secure the wire in place with various methods, using a dressing, Steri-Strips, or other means to secure the wire, and avoid potential movement or dislodgement. BNL can be performed under either general or local anesthesia with intravenous sedation.

SURGERY

Relevant Anatomy

The first step in planning for the location of a partial mastectomy incision is to remember that the patient may have to proceed with mastectomy if margins are not clear; and therefore, placement of the partial mastectomy incision should be in close proximity to a potential future skin-sparing mastectomy incision. Curvilinear incisions following Langer lines are appropriate for upper hemisphere breast lesions, whereas a vertically placed 6 o'clock incision can be used for those lesions between 5 and 7 o'clock position (see Fig. 14.2). Some surgeons prefer circumareolar incisions to enhance cosmetic outcome. After incising the skin, it is optimal to dissect directly down to the lesion and avoid undermining thin skin flaps if possible. If a lesion is close to the skin and especially if retraction is present, a small portion of skin overlying the retraction may need to be excised. Skin removal creates a mastopexy effect and can contribute to slight asymmetry when compared with the contralateral breast. Excision of extensive skin should be avoided unless coupled with oncoplastic surgical techniques for a closure that addresses the contralateral breast as well.

Procedure

The patient's arm on the side of the lesion should be gently secured on an armboard at approximately 90 degrees to the body. The surgeon should remove the outer dressing or Steri-Strips securing the wire before the breast is prepped with surgical soap.

The entry site of the wire in the breast should not necessarily dictate the incision on the breast. The incision on the breast is dictated by the location of the breast lesion and cosmetic considerations. Many if not most breast lesions can be accessed through circumareolar incisions (Fig. 7.14).

Technical Considerations

■ Often, the wire enters the skin of the breast at some distance from the lesion and may not be near the areolar border (Fig. 7.15).

■ The surgeon may mark the anticipated skin incision and make an incision remote from the wire (Fig. 7.16).

■ A skin flap is then carefully created in the somewhat avascular fatty plane between the skin and breast tissue, using small skin hooks, until the wire is visualized in the breast (Fig. 7.17).

■ Using wire cutters, the wire is then cut several millimeters above the skin at its entry point, and the external portion is removed from the operative field (Fig. 7.18).

■ The skin flap is carefully carried beyond the wire so that the entire circumference of breast tissue can be easily visualized where the wire enters the breast tissue. The wire is gently grasped at its proximal end with a clamp, such as an Allis clamp, to include some of the surrounding breast tissue (Fig 7.19).

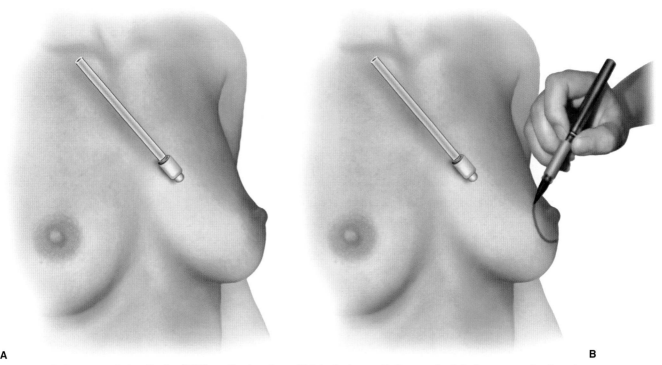

A   B

Figure 7.14 **A.** Breast needle localization (BNL) needle placed very high in the breast. **B.** Same patient's lesion was at wire tip and a circumareolar incision was drawn preoperatively and used to remove the lesion.

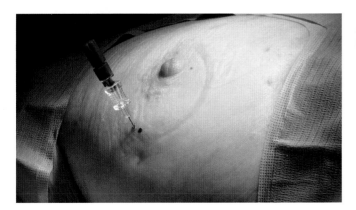

Figure 7.15 Wire enters the skin of the breast distant from the lesion.

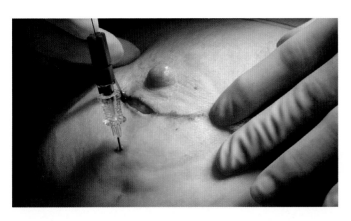

Figure 7.16 Surgeon marks incision site remote from wire.

Part II: Breast Biopsy

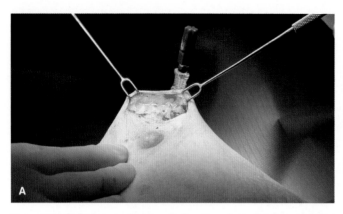
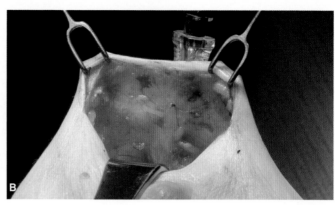

Figure 7.17 **A.** Periareolar incision. **B.** Creation of skin flap from periareolar incision to lesion site.

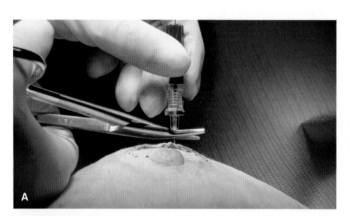
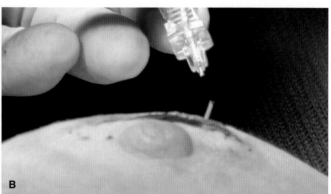

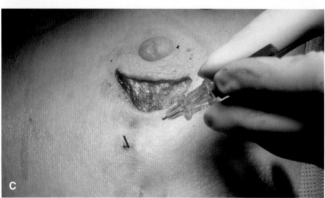

Figure 7.18 **A–C.** Using wire cutters, the wire is cut several millimeters above the skin at its entry point, and the external portion is removed from the operative field.

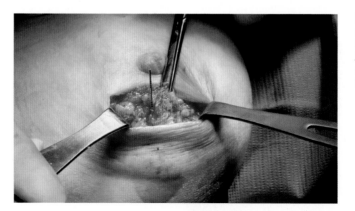

Figure 7.19 The cut end of the needle/wire is brought into the incision site and grasped with an Allis clamp to secure it to surrounding tissue to ensure en bloc resection.

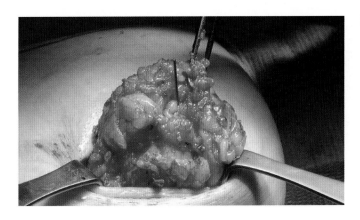

Figure 7.20 The tissue is removed as a cylinder or a rectangular portion of tissue around the wire.

- It is critically important for the surgeon to remove a cylinder or a rectangular portion of tissue around the wire. If the tissue is removed in a "triangular" fashion with the tissue toward the wire tip being the point of the triangle, the lesion may be missed or inadequately excised. Therefore, a trough is made around the wire at the superior, medial, inferior, and lateral sides of the wire by using either the scalpel or electrocautery (Fig. 7.20).
- Each trough is carefully carried down to below the wire tip or further if the lesion is distal to the wire tip. The entire "cylinder" of tissue is gradually brought upward (Fig. 7.21).
- The specimen should ideally be labeled with sutures or other suitable markers while it is in vivo to ensure accurate orientation (e.g., short suture for the superior margin, long suture for the lateral margin). At least two sutures or markers should be used for proper orientation and margin assessment (Fig. 7.22).
- The depth of the trough is determined by the depth of the needle, and the trough around the needle generally extends beyond the tip of the wire to allow adequate excision of the tissue at the wire tip, where the lesion is generally located.
- The specimen is then divided at its deep or posterior margin and removed from the operative field. The surgeon should aim to achieve a 1-cm margin around the lesion and should palpate the tissue before removing the specimen from the operative field (Fig 7.23).
- The specimen is carefully placed on a grid for imaging to confirm adequate excision of the lesion. The specimen should not be handled by the sutures marking the margins (Fig. 7.24).
- Hemostasis is of course meticulously achieved, and the wound can be infiltrated with local anesthetic (e.g., bupivacaine) for postoperative anesthesia.
- If the lesion excised is a known or suspected cancer, the surgeon may place several hemoclips in the surgical bed to mark the area for eventual radiotherapy (Fig. 7.25).

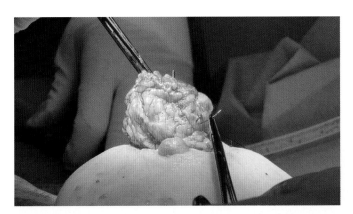

Figure 7.21 The entire "cylinder" of tissue is gradually brought upward.

Part II: Breast Biopsy

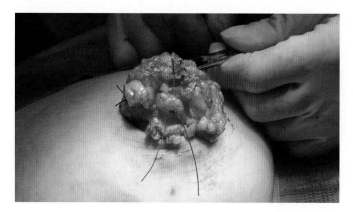

Figure 7.22 Specimen is labeled in vivo to ensure correct orientation. Short suture marks the superior margin and long suture marks the lateral margin.

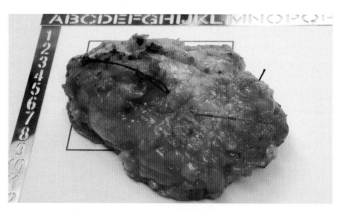

Figure 7.23 The specimen is then divided at its deep or posterior margin and removed from the operative field.

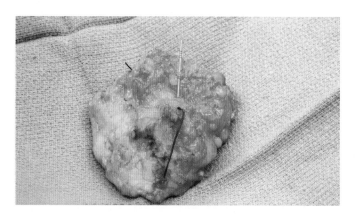

Figure 7.24 Specimen is oriented on a grid for specimen x-ray.

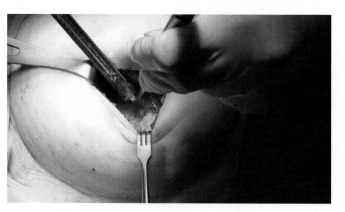

Figure 7.25 Hemoclips mark the surgical bed for radiotherapy.

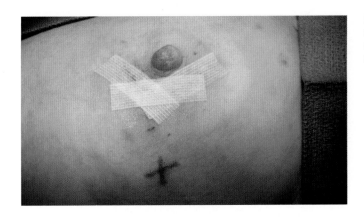

Figure 7.26 The circumareolar (or other) incision is closed with sutures and dressed with steristrips.

■ The circumareolar (or other) incision is then closed in usual fashion, allowing a satisfactory cosmetic result, even though the lesion was removed from this area (Fig. 7.26).

If the lesion is not accessible via a circumareolar incision, either due to the location of the lesion or due to the size of the areola compared with the breast size, then appropriate incisions should be made to allow access to the lesion with a satisfactory cosmetic result. Incisions may be made directly at the area of needle/wire insertion. The procedure is similar, in that a flap is created on either side of the wire, and a similar cylindrical specimen is removed. Lesions in the lower pole of the breast may be approached through an inframammary or a radial incision.

If the lesion is a suspected cancer, the surgeon should be mindful of the possible decision for mastectomy. The incision should be placed in such a manner to allow eventual skin-sparing mastectomy. Incisions along the Langer lines of the breast may be problematic if further surgery is indicated. Radial incisions are generally preferred, as these can then be incorporated in the mastectomy incision if needed.

PEARLS AND PITFALLS

There are several problems or pitfalls associated with needle localization of breast lesions. Some of these problems are of a pragmatic nature, whereas others are more technically challenging. Anticipation of potential problems or "pitfalls" will assist the surgeon in the care of patients with nonpalpable lesions.

Missed lesions on needle localization are of the more frustrating complications following BNL biopsy.

■ Pitfall: Missed lesions can be the result of a less than optimally placed needle or wire.
■ Pearl: Review of the needle localization mammogram or ultrasound with the radiologist, prior to the procedure, is extremely helpful. The discussion allows a detailed explanation of the approach used and the proximity of the lesion to the wire. This gives the surgeon valuable knowledge about the length of the wire within the breast and the extent of the lesion. More importantly, if the needle or wire is not ideally placed, the radiologist can guide the surgeon as to the distance between the wire tip or hook and the lesion, allowing for adequate resection.
■ Pitfall: More commonly, missed lesions are due to technical errors during the operative procedure (Fig. 7.27).
■ Pearl: The specimen excised should include an adequate (1 cm) amount of tissue around the targeted lesion to allow for satisfactory removal and margins. The surgeon should excise a cylinder or a rectangular area of tissue around the wire tip or around the targeted lesion. The more experience a surgeon has with needle localization, the more adequate is the excision, without removing excessive tissue.
■ Pitfall: Specimen radiographs may show removal of the targeted area but may not adequately demonstrate complete removal of the lesion, particularly if calcifications are the targeted lesion.

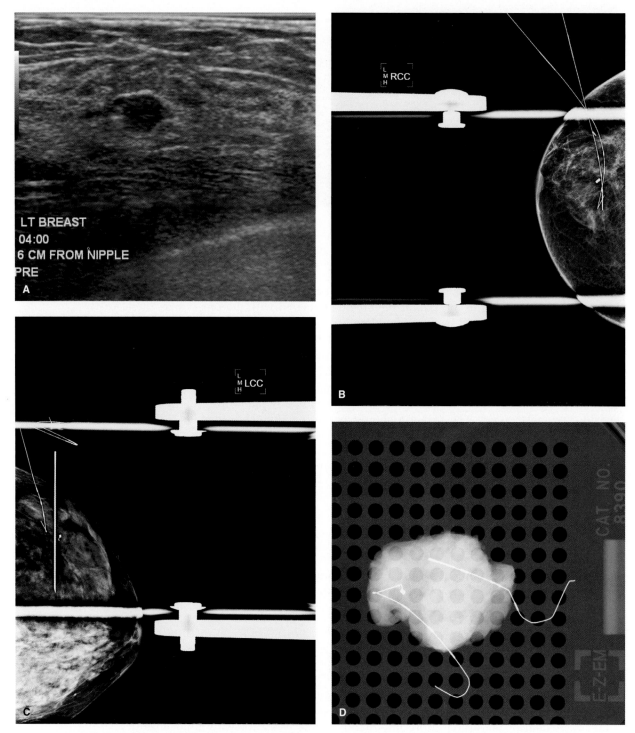

Figure 7.27 **A.** Lesion seen and targeted with ultrasound breast needle localization (BNL). **B.** Successful BNL of both clip and ductal carcinoma in situ. **C.** Lesion from ultrasound BNL in Figure 7.13A was not seen on specimen radiograph. Mammographic BNL was done. **D.** Successful mammographic BNL.

■ Pearl: Review of specimen radiographs is essential. If there is any question about removal of the targeted area, detailed review and discussion with the radiologist can be very helpful in assessing adequacy of excision. Surgeons should obtain a postexcision mammogram or ultrasound if there is any question about whether or not the lesion has been adequately or completely excised. BNL performed for DCIS with associated calcifications should be accompanied by a postexcision mammogram prior to radiotherapy to ensure all the suspicious calcifications have been removed.

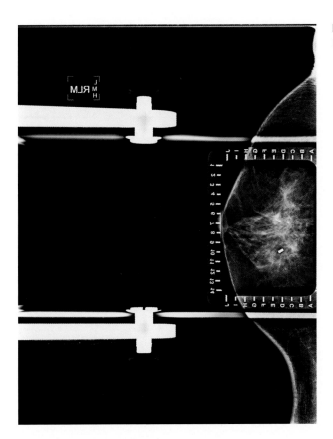

Figure 7.28 Inferior clip migration in a patient with ductal carcinoma in situ.

- Pitfall: Clip migration is possible following core biopsy and clip placement at the site of the lesion. This occurs with some frequency and, if not recognized preoperatively, is associated with needle localization of the clip and a potential of missing the lesion (Fig. 7.28).
- Pearl: Surgeons need to be aware if clip migration has occurred. If recognized, the lesion can still be successfully removed with needle localization. Again, careful review of the imaging with the radiologist preoperatively will allow recognition of clip migration. The radiologist may be able to target the lesion on the basis of other anatomic markers in the breast tissue. If so, the surgeon must review the preoperative needle localization images carefully with the radiologist to ensure the excisional biopsy is directed to the targeted lesion and not the clip.
- Pearl: Newer clip devices are available with a "cage" that helps prevent clip migration (Fig. 7.29).
- Pearl: A postbiopsy mammogram or ultrasound may be essential to confirm removal of a subtle lesion if clip migration has occurred (Fig. 7.30).
- Pitfall: Specimen radiographs will confirm the absence of the clip, even though the lesion has been successfully removed. Presumably, the clip used to localize the lesion during previous core biopsy has been lost. Intraoperative loss of clips placed during image-guided biopsy has been described in as many as 3.8% of patients undergoing BNL (25).
- Pearl: Surgeons need to be aware of clip loss that can occur intraoperatively. The failure to identify the clip in the specimen radiograph frequently leads to excision of additional specimens. Accurate clip placement and avoiding of excessive suctioning during the operative procedure can minimize clip loss. Careful evaluation of the specimen radiograph utilizing anatomic markers other than the clip, and communication between the radiologist and surgeon may help minimize removal of excessive breast tissue. Subsequent concordance between the targeted lesion pathology and breast imaging must be established. Postexcisional mammogram should be done if there is any question of discordance between the specimen pathology and imaging.
- Pitfall: The surgeon thinks the lesion has been removed, but subsequent imaging shows the lesion is still present.

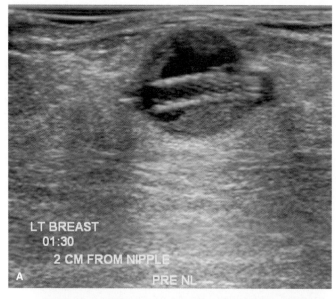

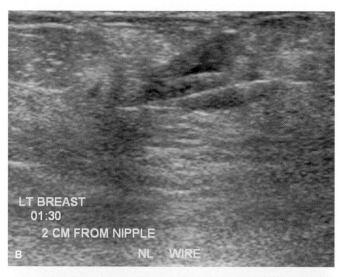

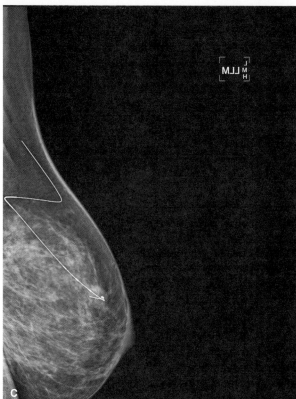

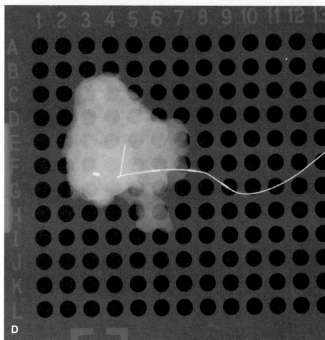

Figure 7.29 A. Papillary lesion seen on ultrasound. **B.** Clip placed in papillary lesion with a cage to prevent clip migration. **C.** BNL of clip with cage. **D.** Specimen radiograph confirming presence of clip and lesion.

- Pearl: This is a particularly untoward complication of BNL. Establishing concordance between the original imaging, core biopsy results, and subsequent needle localized specimen pathology is essential. If results are discordant, postoperative imaging should be done. Reexcision of the area may be needed to ensure adequate removal of the targeted lesion if there is discordance between the initial imaging or core biopsy results and the pathology on the excised specimen.
- Pitfall: The patient is transported to the operating room after needle localization. The dressing around the needle is removed and the wire is no longer in the breast, but is in the dressing.
- Pearl: The hook in the wire makes this an infrequent complication. Nevertheless, when it occurs, it is very troublesome, as it necessitates relocalization of the lesion. Securing

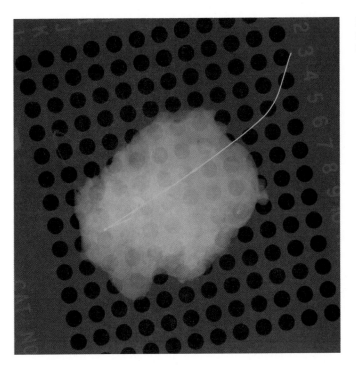

Figure 7.30 Specimen radiograph confirming clip, which had migrated, and lesion.

the needle or wire with Steri-Strips is helpful. Radiology technicians should be trained in the proper securing of the wire. The dressing around the wire should be removed only by the operating surgeon, or someone on the operating room team who has been carefully instructed as to removal of the surrounding dressing (Fig. 7.31).

- Pitfall: Failure to consider possible pathologic results may allow the surgeon to make an incision during BNL that allows easy access to the lesion but that complicates future surgery or limits choices if a mastectomy and reconstruction is needed.
- Pearl: Lesions that are potentially malignant should be excised through incisions that will allow easy reoperation or skin-sparing mastectomy should that be necessary.

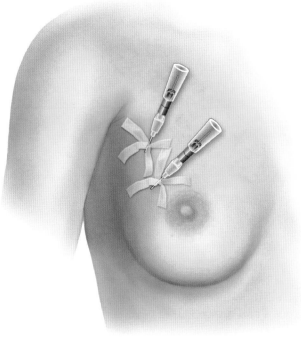

A

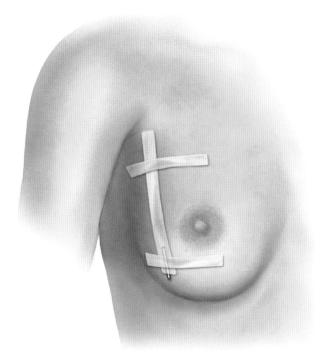

B

Figure 7.31 A. Needles secured prior to transport to operating room. **B.** Wire secured prior to transport to operating room.

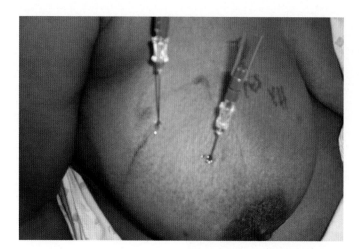

Figure 7.32 Bracketed breast needle localization. Circumareolar incision will allow removal of the suspicious area and still allow satisfactory incision if mastectomy is performed.

Circumareolar incisions are ideal; however, if a circumareolar incision is not easily done, a radial incision extending toward the areola generally allows for skin-sparing mastectomy with satisfactory cosmetic outcome.

■ Pearl: If the lesion to be excised is highly suspicious for cancer, or has been determined by prior core biopsy to be malignant, the incision in the breast should be made with the anticipation that the patient may require or desire subsequent mastectomy. Incisions ideally should be circumareolar but, if not, may be a radial incision, extending toward the areola, and one that would easily accommodate subsequent skin sparing mastectomy if necessary (Fig. 7.32).

■ Pitfall: Frequently, BNL procedures are regarded as easy, straightforward, and fairly routine. Preoperative discussion with patients may be brief. The procedure may be regarded by residents as simple and uncomplicated.

■ Pearl: The ideal BNL procedure will remove the targeted lesion, with an adequate, but not excessive, amount of surrounding tissue. The procedure necessitates a substantial understanding of breast imaging and the ability to appreciate three dimensions operatively while interpreting a two-dimension radiograph. The success of BNL in removing the targeted lesion, achieving satisfactory cosmetic outcome and expedient operative time, is directly related to the experience of the surgeon.

■ Pearl: Comprehensive communication with patients prior to the procedure is essential. Patients should understand the procedure will involve the coordination and cooperation of two departments and specialists (i.e., radiology and surgery). A discussion preoperatively of expected results (removal of the targeted lesion) and potential complications (missed lesion or need for post biopsy imaging) and possible need for reexcision for malignant lesions), will prepare the patient for these outcomes and establish trust between the patient and surgeon.

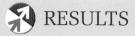 RESULTS

Surgeons in particular have sought alternatives to BNL because of the attendant difficulties described, scheduling issues, and the need for patients to be seen in two departments (e.g., radiology and the operating room). These include using intraoperative ultrasound (26–28) radioactive seed localization (29,30), and iatrogenically induced hematoma (28,31). More recently, a prospective randomized study evaluated cryo-assisted localization compared with needle wire localization for breast lesions visible by ultrasonography (32). A cryoprobe is introduced into the breast lesion by using ultrasound guidance in the operating room, and an ice ball is created. The ice ball is then resected.

When this technique is compared with BNL, the positive margin status is not statistically different; however, the volume of tissue removed is significantly less.

CONCLUSIONS

Although various procedures all have some utility, and each has some advantage over standard BNL, they have not replaced the need for well-done BNL.

References

1. Ernst M, Avenarius J, Schuur K, et al. Wire localization of nonpalpable breast lesions: out of date? *Breast*. 2002;11(5):408–413.
2. Cady B. Traditional and future management of nonpalpable breast cancer. *Am Surg*. 1997;63:55–58.
3. Al-Sobbhis, Helvie M, Pass H, et al. Extent of lumpectomy for breast cancer after diagnosis by stereotactic core versus wire localization biopsy. *Ann Surg Oncol*. 1999;6:330–335.
4. Dodd G, Fry K, Delany W. Pre-operative localization of occult carcinoma in the breast. In: Nealon TF, ed. *Management of the Patient with Cancer*. Philadelphia, PA: WB Saunders, 1966: 88–113.
5. Dodd G. Preoperative radiographic localization of non-palpable lesions. In: Gallagher HS, ed. *Early Breast Cancer Detection and Treatment*. New York, NY: John Wiley & Sons, 1975: 151–152.
6. Frank H, Hall F, Steer M. Pre-operative localization of nonpalpable breast lesions demonstrated by mammography. *N Engl J Med*. 1976;295:259–260.
7. Homer M, Pile-Spellman E. Needle localization of occult breast lesions with a curved-end retractable wire: technique and pitfalls. *Radiology*. 1986;161:546–548.
8. Liberman L, LaTrenta L, Dershaw D, et al. Impact of core biopsy on the surgical management of impalpable breast cancer. *Am J Roentgenol*. 1997;68:495–498.
9. Kaelin C, Smith T, Homer M, et al. Safety, accuracy, and diagnostic yield of needle localization biopsy of the breast performed using local anesthesia. *J Am Coll Surg*. 1995;179(3):267–272.
10. Jackman R, Marzoni F. Needle localized breast biopsy: why do we fail? *Radiology*. 1997;204:677–684.
11. Jackman R, Nowels K, Rodriguez-Soto J, et al. Stereotactic, automated, large-core needle biopsy of nonpalpable breast lesions: false negative and histologic underestimation rates after long-term follow-up. *Radiology*. 1999;210:799–805.
12. Whitten T, Wallace T, Bird R, et al. Image-guided core biopsy has advantages over localization biopsy for the diagnosis of non-palpable breast cancer. *Am Surg*. 1997;12:1072–1077.
13. Yim J, Barton P, Weber B, et al. Mammographically detected breast cancer: benefits of stereotactic core versus wire localization biopsy. *Ann Surg*. 1996;6:688–700.
14. Yang W, Whitman G, Johnson M, et al. Needle localization for excisional biopsy of breast lesions: comparison of effect of use of full-field digital versus screen-film mammographic guidance on procedure time. *Radiology*. 2004;231:277–281.
15. Hasselgren P, Hummel R, Georgian-Smith D, et al. Breast biopsy with needle localization: accuracy of specimen x-ray and management of missed lesions. *Surgery*. 1993;114(4):836–840.
16. Urist M, Bland K. Indications and techniques for biopsy. In: Bland K, Copeland E, eds. *The Breast: Comprehensive Management of Benign and Malignant Disorders*. 3rd ed. St. Louis, MO: Saunders, 2004: 787–801.
17. Liberman L, Mason G, Morris E, et al. Does size matter? Positive predictive value of MRI-detected breast lesions as a function of lesion size. *AJR Am J Roentgenol*. 2006;186:426–430.
18. Morris E, Liberman L, Dershaw d, et al. Preoperative MR imaging-guided needle localization of breast lesions. *AJR Am J Roentgenol*. 2002;178:1211–1220.
19. Prat X, Sittek H, Grosse A, et al. European quadricentric evaluation of a breast MR biopsy and localization device: technical improvements based on phase-I evaluation. *Eur Radiol*. 2002;12: 1720–1727.
20. Schneider E, Rohling K, Schnall M, et al. An apparatus for MR-guided breast lesion localization and core biopsy: design and preliminary results. *J Magn Reson Imaging*. 2001;14:243–253.
21. Erguvan-Dogan B, Whitman G, Nguyen V, et al. Specimen radiography in confirmation of MRI-guided needle localization and surgical excision of breast lesions. *AJR Am J Roentgenol*. 2006; 187:339–344.
22. Chagpar A, Yen T, Sahin A, et al. Intraoperative margin assessment reduces re-excision rates in patients with ductal carcinoma in situ treated with breast conserving surgery. *Am J Surg*. 2003;186:371–377.
23. McCormick J, Keleher A, Tikhomirov V, et al. Analysis of the use of specimen mammography in breast conservation therapy. *Am J Surg*. 2004;188:433–436.
24. Gossmann A, Bangard C, Warm M, et al. Real-time MR-guided wire localization of breast lesions by using an open 1.0-T imager: initial experience. *Radiology*. 2008;247:535–542.
25. Smith L, Rubio I, Henry-Tillman R, et al. Intra-operative ultrasound-guided breast biopsy. *Am J Surg*. 2000;180:419–423.
26. Rahusen F, Bremers A, Fabry J, et al. Ultrasound-guided lumpectomy of nonpalpable breast cancer versus wire guided resection: a randomized clinical trial. *Ann Surg Oncol*. 2002;9: 994–998.
27. Bennett I, Greenslade J, Chiam H. Intraoperative ultrasound guided excision of nonpalpable breast lesions. *World J Surg*. 2005;29:369–374.
28. Cox C, Furman B, Stowell N, et al. Radioactive seed localization breast biopsy and lumpectomy: can specimen radiographs be eliminated? *Ann Surg Oncol*. 2003;10:1039–1047.
29. Gray R, Salud C, Nguyen K, et al. Randomized prospective evaluation of a novel technique for biopsy or lumpectomy of nonpalpable breast lesions: radioactive seed versus wire localization. *Ann Surg Oncol*. 2001;8:711–715.
30. Smith L, Henry-Tillman R, Harms S, et al. Hematoma-directed ultrasound-guided breast biopsy. *Ann Surg*. 2001;233:669–675.
31. Tafra L, Fine R, Whitworth P, et al. Prospective randomized study comparing cryo-assisted and needle wire localization of ultrasound visible breast tumors. *Am J Surg*. 2006;192:462–470.
32. Calhoun K, Giuliano A, Brenner J. Intraoperative loss of core biopsy clips: clinical implications. *Am J Roentgenol*. 2008;190: 196–200.

Part II: Breast Biopsy

8 Intraoperative Ultrasound-Guided Excision of Nonpalpable Lesions

V. Suzanne Klimberg

Introduction

It has been little more than three decades since mammograms were first employed. Mammograms have contributed greatly to the decreased size at which breast cancer can be diagnosed. Initially nonpalpable lesions were removed by the surgeon's best estimate of where the mass or calcification was located in the breast from triangulation of the mammogram views. Large resections were usually needed often for benign lesions, targeted entities more frequently missed, and reoperations more often required when cancer was diagnosed. Needle localization breast biopsy (NLBB) (see Chapter 7) became the new standard in the 1980s for diagnosis and removal of nonpalpable lesions. Miss rates remain in the 5% to 9% range and vasovagal episodes seen in 10% to 20% percent of patients. Today, the consensus is that image-guided needle core biopsy prior to surgery is the standard of care and can determine whether open biopsy can be avoided (in up to 80% of cases) or whether cancer is present and more than just excision is needed.

In the last decade, surgeons have become very facile with ultrasound (US). As more than half of nonpalpable masses diagnosed on mammography can be seen with US, intraoperative-guided excisional biopsy became in vogue for lesions that needed complete removal. Unfortunately, this left an increasing number of patients diagnosed on mammography with calcifications. Stereotactic needle core biopsy was developed in the 1990s in order to minimally invasively biopsy microcalcifications and non–US-visualized masses. If after stereotactic biopsy further open excision was required, NLBB of the stereotactically placed clip has remained the standard to remove such lesions. Recently, hematoma-directed ultrasound-guided (HUG) excision has been described. This method utilizes intraoperative US to locate the hematoma left behind after image-guided core biopsy (mass or calcifications) and intraoperatively guide the excisional biopsy by line of sight.

INDICATIONS/CONTRAINDICATIONS

Indications for US-guided excisional breast biopsy (EBB) include those lesions described as indeterminate or suspicious on core biopsy including but not exclusive of atypical lobular or ductal hyperplasia, incompletely excised papillomas and papillomas associated with atypia whether completely excised or not, lobular carcinoma in situ, radial scar, and nonconcordance of imaging with the pathology. Occasionally, patients will present with a nonpalpable lesion that is almost certainly benign but is greater than 2 cm in size or is growing, painful, or recurring (e.g., a previously aspirated cyst) or simply because of patient preference or fear of needles.

Contraindications to intraoperative US-guided biopsy is simply poor or nonvisualization of the lesion after core biopsy. This may occur in patients if the image-guided core biopsy has been longer than 5 weeks. By this time significant resorption of the biopsy cavity hematoma would have occurred. Hematoma-directed ultrasound-guided biopsy may also not be useful if there is a massive hematoma after image-guided core biopsy, making the localization relatively nonspecific.

PREOPERATIVE PLANNING

Preoperative Core Biopsy and Diagnosis

Although some advocate the use of fine needle aspiration, a definitive diagnosis via core needle biopsy before performing EBB is preferred. All outside pathology should require rereview within the institution performing the EBB. A preoperative benign diagnosis (e.g., fibroadenoma) will permit some patients to forgo EBB. A preoperative diagnosis of cancer allows for a single definitive cancer operation in most cases compared with only 25% to 60% of patients in whom NLBB is used for diagnosis.

Ultrasound

A high-quality US is needed for intraoperative use and it should be tested prior to surgery and the settings appropriate to the patient's breast and transducer locked in. For intraoperative use, the small 15-MHz probe is ideal. The US should be placed on the opposite side of the table from where the surgeon will be standing for ease of visualization during the procedure. The US should be covered with a sterile clear drape such that the operator can adjust the machine with sterile technique during the procedure. Likewise, a sterile drape will be needed to cover the US transducer (Fig. 8.1).

Relevant Anatomy

Figure 8.2A demonstrates the intraductal nature of cysts, papilloma, atypia, and ductal carcinoma in situ (DCIS), with most cancers thought to arise from the terminal ductal

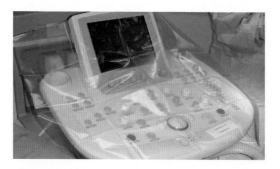

Figure 8.1 Draping of US into the field.

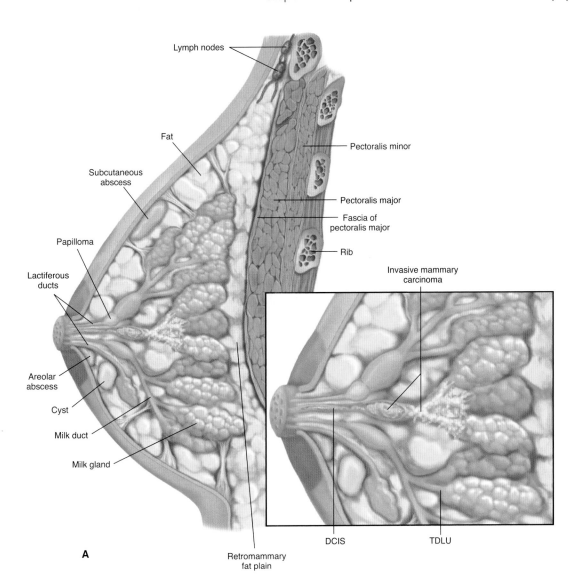

Lymph nodes

Fat

Subcutaneous abscess

Pectoralis minor

Pectoralis major

Fascia of pectoralis major

Rib

Papilloma

Invasive mammary carcinoma

Lactiferous ducts

Areolar abscess

Cyst

Milk duct

Milk gland

DCIS

TDLU

A

Retromammary fat plain

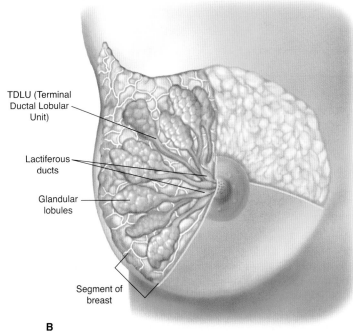

TDLU (Terminal Ductal Lobular Unit)

Lactiferous ducts

Glandular lobules

Segment of breast

B

Figure 8.2 A. Demonstrates anatomy of ducts and relationship to lesions. **B.** Demonstrates the radial nature of the ducts of the breast. DCIS, ductal carcinoma in situ; TDLU, terminal ductal lobular unit.

Figure 8.3 Cross-sectional anatomy of the breast.

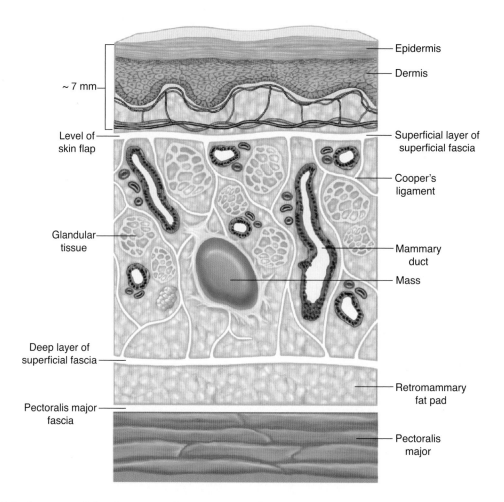

lobular unit of the breast, and Figure 8.2B demonstrates the radial nature of the segments of the breast.

Figure 8.3 demonstrates the important layers of the breast in cross-section. Retention of the subcutaneous layer just below the skin significantly contributes to the cosmesis after EBB. Likewise, preservation of the integrity of posteriorly located fascia covering the pectoralis major prevents the formation of tense seromas.

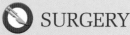 SURGERY

Surgical Technique

Anesthesia

Excision of breast lesions can be performed under local, with or without sedative, or general anesthesia, although some reports have suggested better margin clearance under general anesthesia. With a very cooperative patient, local anesthesia with a mixture of short- and long-acting anesthetic with epinephrine and mild sedation is easily doable.

Positioning

The patient is placed supine or in a lawn chair position, with the arm on the affected breast extended at a right angle such that the operator and the assistant can stand on either side of the arm board (Fig. 8.4). The patient should be at the very edge of the table so that the surgeon can stand in close proximity to the patient and not have to unduly lean over the table to operate (spares back strain). The US monitor is positioned on the opposite side of the table in direct line of sight of the surgeon. The arm does not need to be draped into the field but should be place on sufficient padding to relieve any pressure on the radial nerve at the elbow. After sterile prep, a biodrape can be used to retract and stabilize a large pendulous breast in an optimal position for EBB.

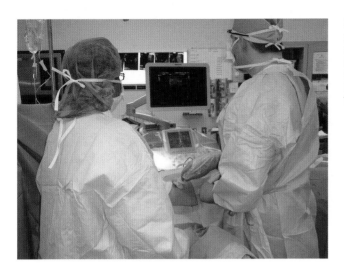

Figure 8.4 Demonstrates the proper position of the patient with surgeon and assistant above and below the arm and with the US machine directly across from the operator with the ultrasound probe sterilely draped into the field.

Intraoperative Localization

A 7.5-, 10-, or 15-MHz US transducer can be used to locate a nonpalpable mass or the residual hematoma from an image-guided biopsy of a nonpalpable mass or calcifications (Fig. 8.5A–D). A purple pen is used to outline the mass located by the US probe and determine the best position for the incision.

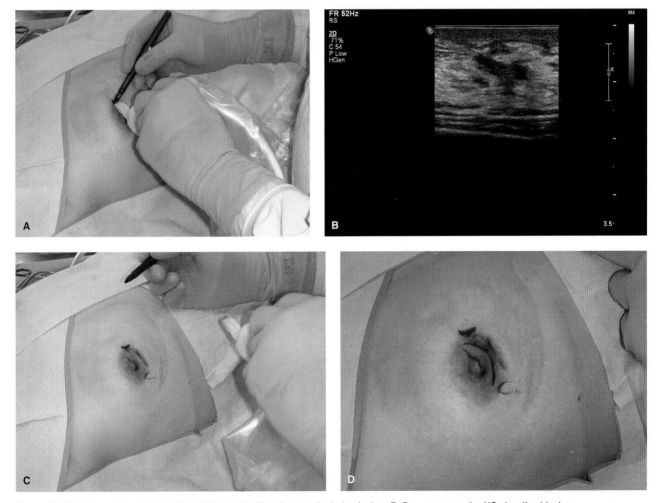

Figure 8.5 **A.** Demonstrates the position of the probe directly over the index lesion. **B.** Demonstrates the US-visualized lesion. **C.** Demonstrates the resultant marking for ultrasound localization. **D.** Demonstrates placement of the incision.

Part II: Breast Biopsy

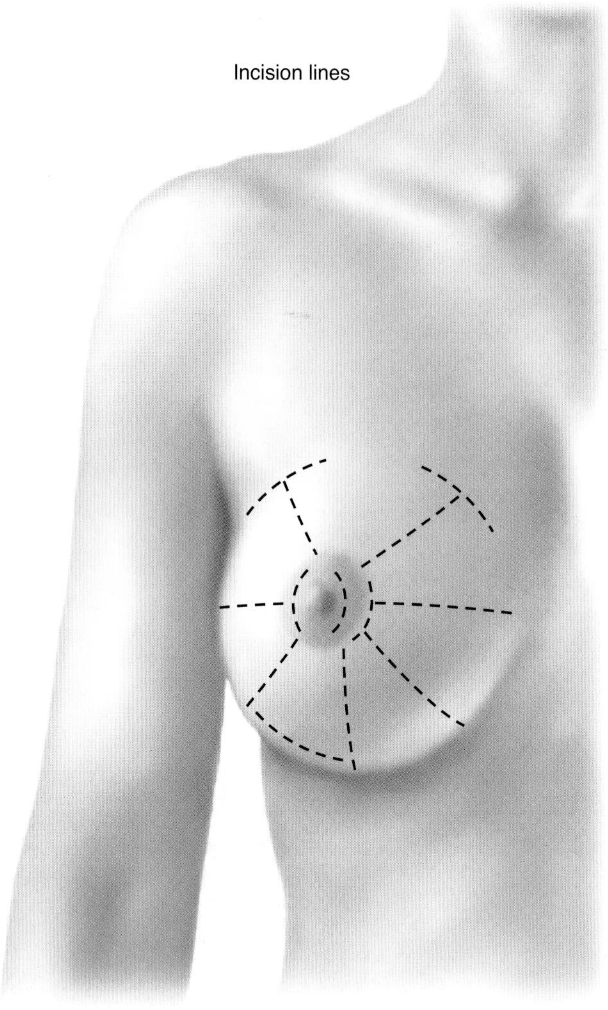

Figure 8.6 Demonstrates possible breast incisions.

Incision lines

Incision

Incisions along Langer's lines usually provide the best cosmesis in the upper quadrants of the breast (Fig. 8.6). Because radial incisions prevent distortion of the nipple downward in the lower pole of the breast, some surgeons prefer radial incisions altogether because of the radial nature of the growth of breast cancer (Fig. 8.2B). For benign lesions, some advocate a periareolar incision with tunneling to the lesion to prevent obvious scarring. An intra-areolar incision gives the least visible scar because of the already uneven surface of the areola. The patient should be warned of possible areolar hypesthesia when using such scars. In any case, when deciding on placement and orientation of the EBB scar, the possibility of a later mastectomy should be entertained and the scar placed in skin that would be subsequently taken.

The incision is marked directly over the lesion and the skin incised with a number 10 or 15 scalpel (Fig. 8.7A–C).

The edge of the dermis is then freed on each edge of the incision to facilitate retractor placement and closure of the dermis (Figs. 8.8A and B).

Margin Estimation

The surgeon can then place the US transducer into the wound (Fig. 8.9).

The surgeon should use the US transducer to aim for a 1-cm margin around the hematoma or mass as determined by line-of-sight guidance (Fig. 8.10) and to also judge the depth of the dissection.

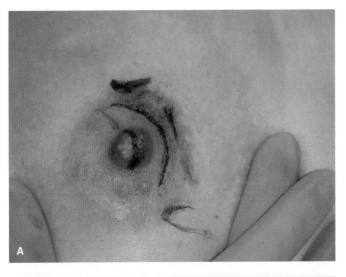

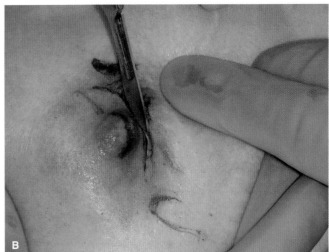

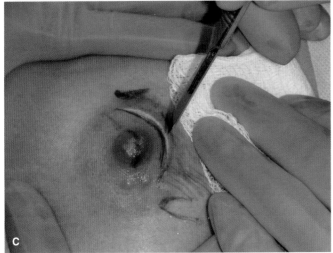

Figure 8.7 **A–C.** Demonstrate initial incision of skin.

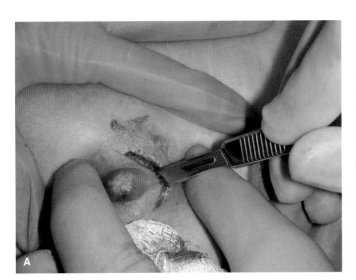

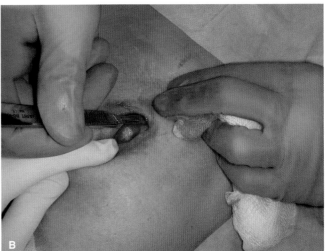

Figure 8.8 **A.** and **B.** Demonstrate freeing of the dermis at biopsy sight for optimal closure.

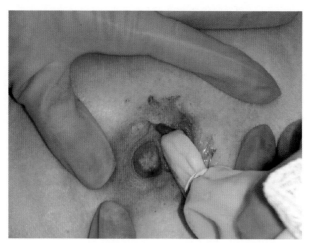

Figure 8.9 Introduction of the 15-mm US probe into the wound.

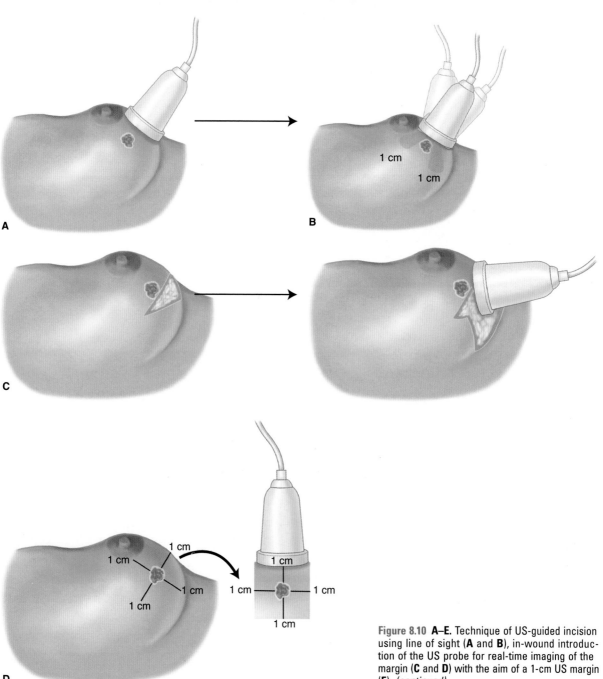

1 cm

1 cm

A

B

C

1 cm

1 cm

1 cm

1 cm

1 cm

1 cm

1 cm

1 cm

D

Figure 8.10 A–E. Technique of US-guided incision using line of sight (**A** and **B**), in-wound introduction of the US probe for real-time imaging of the margin (**C** and **D**) with the aim of a 1-cm US margin (**E**). *(continued)*

Figure 8.10 *(Continued)*

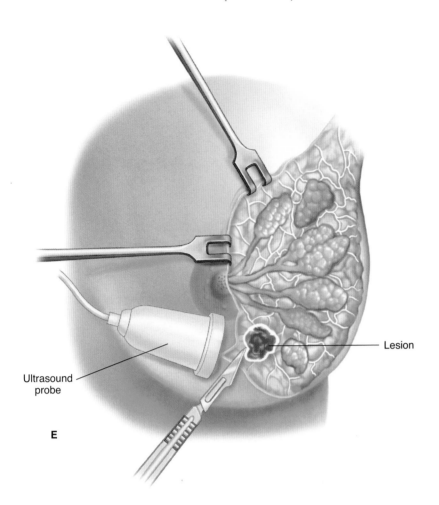

Ultrasound
probe

Lesion

E

Excision

The surgeon cuts each border in a stepwise fashion. For example, as demonstrated in Figure 8.11, the superior border (Fig. 8.11A) is incised first, then the inferior border (Fig. 8.11B), followed by the medial border (Fig. 8.11C), and finally the lateral border (Fig. 8.11D). In this way, the removed lesion is near square and can more easily be oriented for the pathologist. Once this has been done, the scalpel is turned almost flat with the chest wall, and the posterior depth of the lesion is rolled out of the wound (Fig. 8.11E and F). The US probe is brought in and out of the wound throughout the procedure to ensure that the lesion is centered within the EBB and adequate depth around the lesion (posterior margin) has been obtained.

Specimen Imaging

The removed lesion is then set on a sterile towel and inspected for obvious abnormality and breech of the lesion. A specimen US is then performed by either wetting the specimen with water or alternatively submersing the EBB specimen in a bowl of water (Fig. 8.12A and B). Avoid the use of gel especially if cytology is to be performed. Specimen US determines that the lesion has been removed by comparison to the original specimen as in Figure 8.12B, which shows that the hematoma is within the excised specimen. Also, as in this case of excision for cancer diagnosed by stereotactic core biopsy, the US determines that an adequate amount of tissue around the index lesion has been removed. In this way, any re-excision can be directed specifically to the close margin(s) (e.g., lateral). Specimen mammography should be performed to document removal of the clip (in this case not visible by US) and removal of any additional calcifications (Fig. 8.12C).

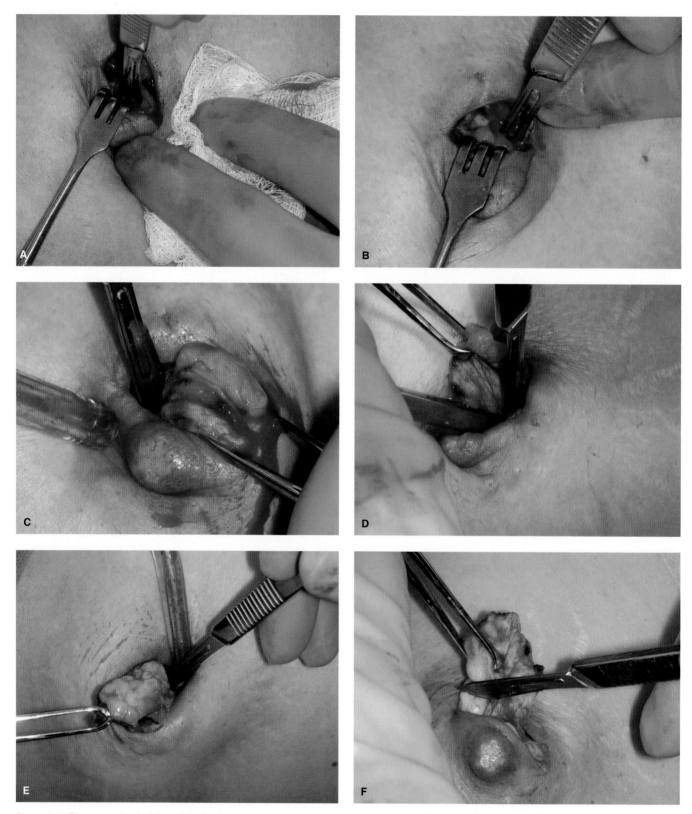

Figure 8.11 Demonstrating incision of the borders around the lesion: superior (**A**), inferior (**B**), medial (**C**), lateral (**D**), and posterior (**E** and **F**).

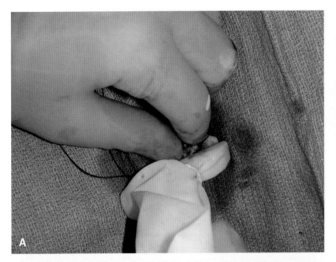

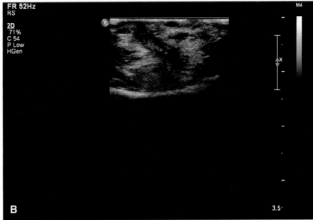

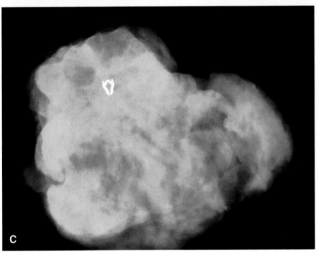

Figure 8.12 On-table specimen US (**A**) and US image of lesion within the specimen (**B**), specimen radiograph to document removal of the clip (**C**).

Part II: Breast Biopsy

Pathological Marking

The excised specimen should be marked in at least two different directions. This can be done with special markers sewn to the specimen, hemoclips, any of the marketed kits, or simply by putting a short stitch superiorly and a long stitch laterally (Fig. 8.13). Consistently marking in the same way every time causes less uncertainty when pathology tries to orient the usually very globular specimen.

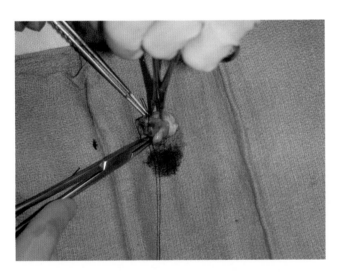

Figure 8.13 Specimen marking for pathological orientation.

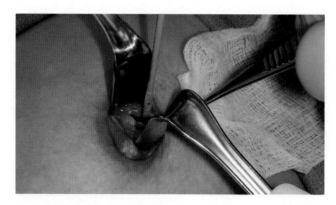

Figure 8.14 Hemostasis with electro-cautery.

Palpation of Cavity

Ultrasound and palpation of the cavity ensures that the lesion was removed and that nothing has been left behind. Any additional lesions not preoperatively appreciated can be removed at this time.

Cavity Irrigation

The wound is then irrigated with the solution of choice: saline, water, or a dilute mixture of water and hydrogen peroxide. The main objective is to remove most of the loose fat and debris, as well as any introduced bacteria.

Hemostasis

Hemostasis is extremely important in the very vascular breast to avoid lateral complications of a hematoma and infection. Electrocautery is usually sufficient (Fig. 8.14). Occasionally, a stick tie is necessary, but hemoclips should be avoided.

Pain Block

At our institution, the antibiotic is mixed with the anesthetic (a mix of short- and long-acting anesthesia) as a low-cost solution that gives high antibiotic levels in the wound at the time of closure, facilitates hemostasis, and aids in postoperative pain control (Fig. 8.15).

Closure

Cosmesis is a function of the presence and depth of subcutaneous tissue and not obliterating the EBB cavity. A drain is unnecessary and may also adversely affect cosmesis.

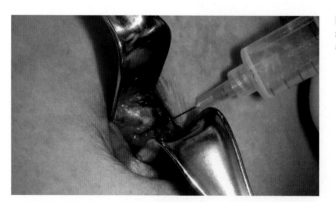

Figure 8.15 Pain block with a mix of short- and long-acting anesthetics and antibiotic.

Figure 8.16 Sagittal depiction of closure of biopsy cavity.

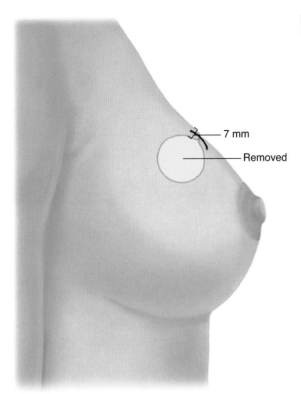

7 mm

Removed

A 7-mm thickness of subcutaneous tissue just below the skin should be reapproximated in case cancer is found, because this is the necessary thickness for partial breast irradiation (Fig. 8.16).

A 3.0 running or interrupted absorbable buried stitch is sufficient to close the dermis (Fig. 8.17A–D).

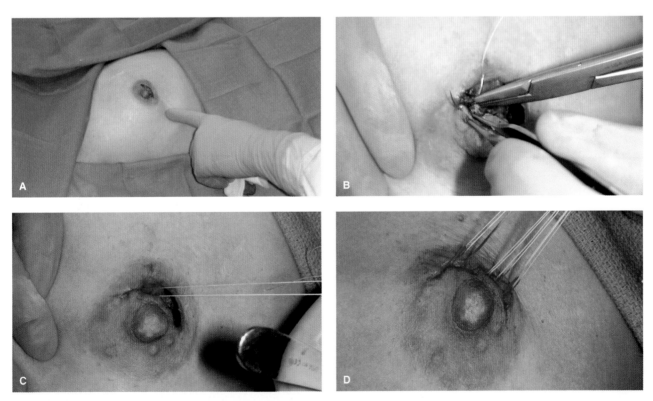

Figure 8.17 A–D. Closure of dermis with buried interrupted sutures.

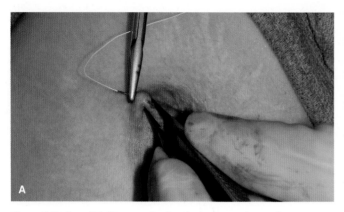
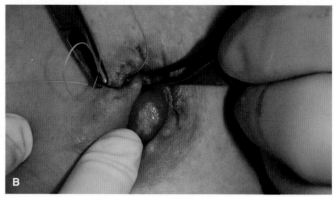

Figure 8.18 **A.** and **B.** Closure of subcuticular layer of wound.

A 4.0 absorbable suture is used to close the skin. As this stitch is mainly for cosmesis, knots are not necessary. The needle pierces the skin and is brought into the wound at the corner (Fig. 8.18A) and the a running subcuticular continued (Fig. 8.18B) and the stitch similarly exits the wound without tying in the opposing corner of the wound again without tying it.

Dressing

Closure of the wound with skin glue is sufficient and allows the patient to shower immediately after surgery (Fig. 8.19).

PEARLS AND PITFALLS

Make sure patients are off vitamin E, herbal remedies, and aspirin for 7 to 10 days and nonsteroidal anti-inflammatories for 3 days preoperatively, to avoid unnecessary bleeding. The surgery using HUG biopsy should proceed on average within 5 weeks to take maximum advantage of a hematoma postcore biopsy, as over time the hematomas will resorb.

Placing the patient in a comfortable position on the table (lawn chair position) with adequate padding under the arm and the wrist can avoid unnecessary pain of the arm, shoulder, and back in the postoperative period.

Sitting a patient with pendulous breast upright (at least 45 degrees) during surgery can often help with the decision of where and in what orientation to place the incision and optimizing the ultimate cosmetic result.

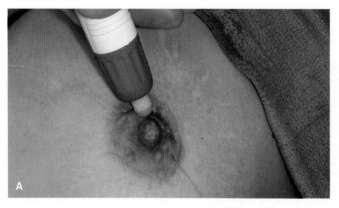
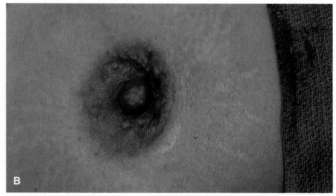

Figure 8.19 **A.** and **B.** Dressing of wound with skin glue.

Do not make thin skin flaps, as this will result in a poor cosmetic outcome.

Use the US to determine the depth and extent of the lesion. If the lesion is less than or equal to 1 cm from the skin, take skin over the lesion to avoid a positive anterior margin should the lesion be a cancer. Use the US to also determine the deep and horizontal margins of the lesion or hematoma by placing the transducer into the wound. Despite this sophisticated method, simple palpation and inspection of the removed specimen as well as of the wound cavity can often help determine the location of a missed lesion.

In addition to the use of US to document the removal of a lesion or postbiopsy hematoma, specimen radiograph also documents the removal of the marking clip and of any additional calcifications. Two-view specimen mammography is ideal to determine the location of the lesion within the specimen.

If the excision cavity continues to ooze, do not leave a drain but simply obliterate the dead space. Drains do not drain blood well.

Avoid knots at the corners of the wound when placing a subcuticular stitch, as these usually spit postoperatively.

Steri-Strips and wound bandages are unnecessary and a hindrance to the patient taking a shower. Wound glue is sufficient and allows complete visualization of the wound. Steri-Strips placed in right angles to the scar or on tension can often create a more unsightly scar than the surgery.

POSTOPERATIVE MANAGEMENT

Meticulous attention to hemostasis and use of a local pain block and skin glue instead of a dressing greatly simplify postoperative management. A sports bra instead of a pressure dressing may be used. The patient may or may not need pain medicine or may simply take over the counter medication for pain. A shower may be taken immediately.

COMPLICATIONS

Risk of complications has not been increased with US-guided EBB over that of NLBB or excision of palpable lesions. Potential complications include infection (abscess or cellulitis), hematomas, and bulging seromas. Cellulitis can usually be managed with antibiotics that cover the typical *Staphylococcus* in your institution. In a cellulitis that does not quickly resolve, an abscess should be suspected and either percutaneously drained if small or immediate open drainage if larger than a few centimeters in size or loculated.

Hematomas that take up more than one-third of the breast or are expanded require a trip back to the operating room to remove the hematoma and potential to eradicate the source of bleeding.

Seromas postoperatively are not necessarily a complication. Seromas can prevent unsightly dimpling of the biopsy cavity. A bulging seroma often requires drainage that can lead to secondary infection. Bulging seromas can be avoided by thick skin flaps and by closure of any defects made in the pectoralis fascia prior to closure.

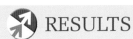 RESULTS

There is no doubt that intraoperative US-guided excision of nonpalpable lesions is a more comfortable procedure than NLBB for the patient with benign or malignant disease. Most mass-like lesions seen on mammogram can be localized by US for biopsy and then removal. Those lesions that are not initially US visualized or in the patient with calcifications require a preoperative stereotactic core biopsy for diagnosis. After core biopsy, almost all patients will have a hematoma at the core sight that can be visualized and removed by US for up to 5 weeks postoperation. Clips should be left after core biopsy, but these have been shown to be displaced by 1 cm more than half the time and displaced more than 2 cm 22% of the time. A recent comparison between NLBB and HUG biopsy demonstrated significantly less positive margins with HUG biopsy.

✦ CONCLUSIONS

Ultrasound-guided biopsy of nonpalpable lesion should be reserved for the specific clinical indications outlined above. The initial step in the work-up of any lesion should be a percutaneous core biopsy. The surgeon performing breast surgery must be facile with breast US for patient comfort and for optimizing patient outcome.

Suggested Readings

Schwartz GF, Veronesi U, Clough KB, et al. Consensus conference on breast conservation. *J Am Coll Surg*. 2006;203:198–207.

Silverstein M et al. Consensus conference of image-detected lesions. *JACS*. 2009.

Special Report: Consensus Conference III. Image-detected breast cancer: State-of-the-art diagnosis and treatment. *J Am Coll Surg*. 2009; Oct 209(4):504–520.

Thompson M, Henry-Tillman R, Margulies A, et al. Hematoma-directed ultrasound-guided (HUG) breast lumpectomy. *Ann Surg Oncol*. 2007;14(1):148–156.

Thompson M, Klimberg VS. Use of ultrasound in breast surgery [review]. *Surg Clin North Am*. 2007;87(2):469–484.

9 Breast Surgery after Radioactive Seed Localization

Richard J. Gray and Barbara A. Pockaj

INDICATIONS/CONTRAINDICATIONS

The goal of breast conserving therapy is to remove the lesion with the minimum tissue volume necessary to ensure negative margins, a low recurrence risk, and a good cosmetic result. More than two-thirds of breast cancers are nonpalpable, as are an even greater proportion of undiagnosed breast lesions. These nonpalpable lesions require radiologic localization for surgical treatment or biopsy. The standard procedure for excision of nonpalpable breast lesions is wire localization (WL). There are several disadvantages with the standard WL technique that include the following:

- Wire skin entry site may be far away from the tumor resulting in more difficulty planning the incision site and excess normal tissue being excised.
- Margins of excision have been reported to be positive, requiring a second operation for reexcision up to 50% of the time [1,2].
- Wire can be displaced during postlocalization mammogram and transfer to the operating room.
- Wire must be placed on the same day of surgery, resulting in logistical challenges for radiology and operative suites that may result in more inpatient stays due to operations occurring late in the day.

Radioactive seed localization (RSL) overcomes many of these disadvantages. The technique utilizes a 4.5 mm by 0.8 mm titanium seed labeled with ^{125}I (usual dose 0.100–0.150 mCi) (Fig. 9.1). The same radioactive seed is used for prostate brachytherapy. The radioactive seed is placed percutaneously, using radiologic guidance in a manner similar to that used for wire placement. Intraoperative localization is performed using a gamma counter set to detect ^{125}I. Several studies have demonstrated the safety, feasibility, and effectiveness of RSL, including a demonstration of virtually no radiation exposure to staff. Patients also benefit by as much as a 52% reduction in the rate of positive margins [3].

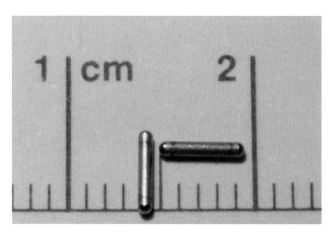

Figure 9.1 Radioactive seed.

PREOPERATIVE PLANNING

The first step in preoperative planning for RSL is ensuring an appropriate program is in place. RSL requires that the institution have a medical license issued by the Nuclear Regulatory Commission or an agreement state, as is the case for any institution using radioactive materials for any purpose. In addition, an authorized nuclear medicine physician or radiation oncologist must agree to oversee the safe use of radioactive seeds and develop systems for ensuring each seed is safely handled and returned to nuclear storage for decay after use. One must also clarify billing issues: the same Current Procedural Terminology (CPT) code is used for the operative procedure, but the CPT code for the radiologic placement of the radioactive seed must be clarified with payers. Current CPT codes to be considered include 19499, 19290, A4641, 77032, and 76942.

Radiologic placement of radioactive seeds is done with largely the same techniques as for WL. Seeds may be inserted up to 5 days before the operation, although 1 day prior to the operation is most common to allow concurrent injection of radiocolloid for sentinel lymph node (SLN) mapping. After assembling the necessary items (Fig. 9.2), the target(s) is confirmed with ultrasound or mammography and the approach determined. Unlike WL, in RSL, the radiologist may use the best available approach for accurate seed placement without concern for the skin entry site complicating the operative approach for the surgeon. Using reverse-spring tweezers, a sterile seed is loaded into an 18-G spinal needle, the tip of which has been occluded with bone wax. After providing adequate local anesthesia, the needle is advanced to the target under imaging

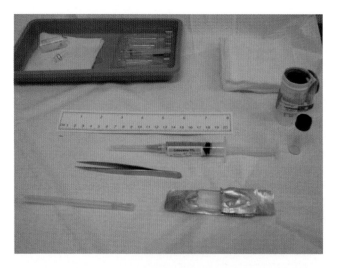

Figure 9.2 Equipment for radiologic placement of radioactive seed. (Photo courtesy of Michelle McDonough, MD.)

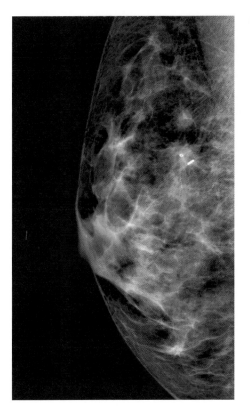

Figure 9.3 Postlocalization mammogram with radioactive seed and adjacent clip.

guidance and the seed deployed by advancing a stylet through the needle. A postlocalization mammogram confirms positioning of the seed (Fig. 9.3).

There are several potential RSL pitfalls of which the radiologist must be aware of.

■ The stylet must be placed part way into the spinal needle or additional bone wax placed into the needle hub during the localization to ensure the seed does not slide back out through the hub as the angle of the needle is manipulated.
■ The diameters of 18-G spinal needles and of the radioactive seeds can slightly vary, so one must ensure the seed passes through the needle adequately before beginning localization.
■ One must ensure the stylet passes through the bone wax for the seed to deploy, so note how far into the spinal needle the stylet fits before beginning each localization procedure.

Multiple radioactive seeds can be placed to localize multiple lesions or bracket a large lesion. Orienting these seeds to separate on a radial plane rather than in the anterior-to-posterior dimension allows the surgeon to more easily detect the seeds as separate gamma sources at the skin level. Having the ability to separately detect these signals allows surgeon to more precisely plan incision and dissection.

No patient or staff shielding is necessary, nor are patient warnings or precautions necessary when the patient leaves the radiology suite. A single ^{125}I seed provides little radiation exposure. The radiation dose at 15 cm from each low-dose seed is less than one-tenth the radiation exposure from a plane flight.

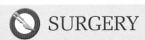 SURGERY

Steps of the Procedure

Excision of a nonpalpable breast lesion by using RSL requires only a gamma probe such as those used for SLN biopsy. The ^{125}I seed can be detected as a separate source from the ^{99}Tc colloid used for SLN mapping. The steps for the RSL surgical excision are as follows:

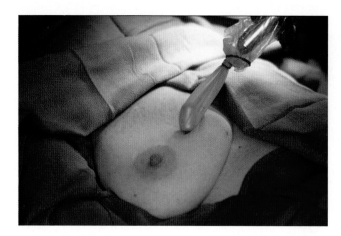

Figure 9.4 Using the gamma probe to detect the skin site with highest ^{125}I gamma activity.

- Set the gamma counter to detect ^{125}I. The setting for a SLN biopsy procedure is ^{99}Tc. It is critical that the gamma counter is changed for the RSL as the surgeon can be misled to think the ^{99}Tc injection site is the position of the radioactive seed. Some low-level gamma activity can be detected at the ^{99}Tc injection site even when the gamma probe is properly set to ^{125}I due to Compton scatter, so the surgeon must remain vigilant to find the highest gamma counts.
- After the patient is prepped and draped, the point of highest radioactivity is localized on the breast (Fig. 9.4). The skin incision is made over the point of highest radioactivity.
- After the incision is made, reevaluate the site of highest radioactivity and begin performing the lumpectomy dissection. Use the gamma counter to continuously reorient to the position of the seed (Fig. 9.5). Generally, a count of 40,000 to 45,000 approximates a 2 cm margin from the radioactive seed, resulting in a 1 cm gross margin. This is an estimate and will vary with the dose of ^{125}I in each radioactive seed and will vary on the basis of gamma probe sensitivity settings.
  - When performing the lumpectomy, care should be taken to not crush the breast specimen tightly with a surgical instrument because this may dislodge the seed.

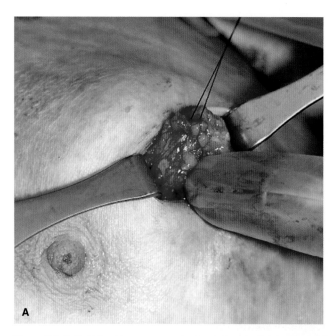

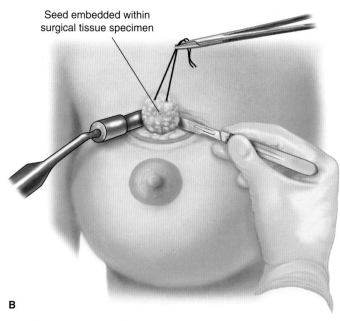

Seed embedded within surgical tissue specimen

Figure 9.5 A-B. Using the gamma probe to reorient to the position of the radioactive seed during dissection.

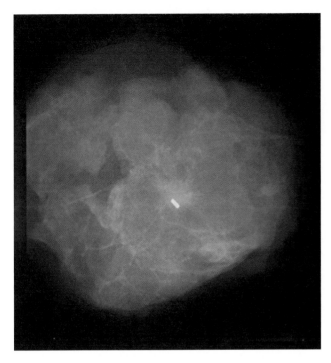
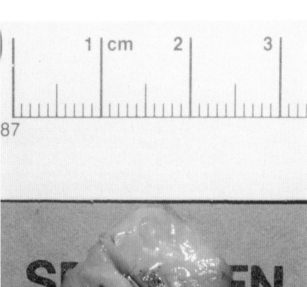
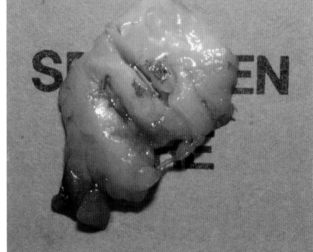

Figure 9.6 Specimen radiograph with radioactive seed and gross specimen.

Part II: Breast Biopsy

If traction on the breast specimen is desired, a suture can be placed for this purpose and then used for specimen orientation after the excision is completed.

- Care must also be taken to ensure the seed is not cut, although cutting a seed is extraordinarily difficult.
- After the specimen is excised and marked for orientation, the surgeon must ensure that ^{125}I gamma activity is within the specimen and that there is no ^{125}I radioactivity in the lumpectomy cavity.
- A specimen radiograph is obtained to document the retrieval of the seed and targeted lesion (Fig. 9.6).
- The lumpectomy cavity is closed in the standard manner.
- The pathologist inks the specimen as per institutional protocol and then sections the specimen to retrieve the seed and place it within a lead-lined container for transport to the nuclear medicine or radiation oncology suite for decay (4). If the seed is difficult to locate within the specimen, a gamma probe is used for direction.

PEARLS AND PITFALLS

- To ensure adequate margins, be sure to aim the gamma probe directly at the portion of the specimen containing the seed rather than obliquely or at another portion of the specimen during dissection.
- Be sure to check gamma signals in the specimen and wound to ensure the seed has been removed. This is particularly important when using two or more bracketing seeds.
- Use the counts from the gamma probe to estimate the adequacy of the margins in the excised specimen. Counts greater than 55,000 generally indicate the need for a reexcision of that margin.

■ Identifying and retrieving the seed from the specimen is easier if it is able to be sectioned perpendicular to the long axis of the seed.
■ The seed is small enough to be suctioned into a standard Yankauer suction device, so care must be taken to not dissect into the seed and dislodge it and to not suction the seed into the suction tubing or canister should this occur.

 POSTOPERATIVE MANAGEMENT

The postoperative management of patients undergoing RSL is the same as for patients undergoing WL. Appropriate oral analgesics are administered as needed. No specific additional breast imaging is required in the immediate postoperative period.

 COMPLICATIONS

The surgical complications are identical to those that occur after lumpectomy with WL. Specific issues related to this procedure are focused on the radioactive seed. The loss of a radioactive seed, inability to account for a deployed radioactive seed, and transection of a seed are radiation safety emergencies. Fortunately, there have been no reported cases of a radiation safety emergency while using RSL. In a study of 383 patients from three institutions, there were only two adverse events (5). One episode of seed migration 1 cm or larger occurred after radiologic placement. The migration was thought to be within a core biopsy hematoma, and the seed and lesion were nonetheless successfully retrieved. One seed was displaced after the specimen was removed. Documenting seed retrieval in the operating suite with gamma probe examination of the specimen is critical. Should there be no ^{125}I radioactivity within the breast specimen, a search for the radioactive seed must be performed. Places to search include the lumpectomy cavity (seed dislodged during dissection), on the drapes and sponges, and in suction tubing or suction canister.

 RESULTS

A summary of the reported series are shown in Table 9.1 (3,5–7). A large study randomized patients between RSL and WL (3). The overall time for the procedure and subjective ease of the procedure (rated by the radiologist, surgeon, and patient) were not different between the two techniques. The volume of tissue excised was less for the patients who underwent RSL, but it was not statically significant (RSL 55.7 mL vs. WL 73.5 mL, $p = 0.52$). The incidence of positive margins on the first specimen excised was significantly lower in the RSL group (26%) than in the WL group (57%, $p = 0.02$).

Two subsequent case series were performed (5,6). Both demonstrated the ability to retrieve the lesion and the radioactive seed in all cases. One study compared 200 consecutive lumpectomy patients (6). The first 100 underwent WL, and the second 100

TABLE 9.1	Published Radioactive Seed Studies								
Study	Randomized	Wire (*N*)	Intra-Op margin +	Final margin +	Seed (*N*)	Intra-Op margin +	Final margin +	*p* value	SLN identified
Gray, 2001 (3)	Yes	26	57%	NA	35	26%	NA	0.02	97%
Cox, 2003 (5)	No (case series)	NA	NA	NA	64	41%	27%	NA	NA
Gray, 2004 (6)	No (sequential case series)	99	46%	24%	100	24%	10%	0.01	100%
Hughes, 2008 (7)	No (comparison to historical controls)	99	46%	25%	383	27%	8%	<0.001	100%

underwent RSL. All WL procedures were performed on the day of surgery, whereas 68% of RSL patients had their localization procedure performed the day before. Of note, those patients who had their radioactive seed placed the day before also had their radiocolloid injection for the SLN biopsy performed the day before. Bracketing of lesions was used in 6% of the WL group and 7% of the RSL group. The incidence of positive margins was significantly reduced with RSL (10% vs. 24% for WL, $p = 0.01$). Patients were asked to rate their pain and convenience for both procedures. Pain was not different between the two procedures, but those patients who underwent RSL the day before surgery rated their convenience significantly higher than those who underwent same-day localization ($p < 0.01$).

Last, a three-site validation of RSL was performed (7). The first 99 patients underwent WL and served as controls, and the next 383 patients were treated with RSL. Again, there was a significant reduction in positive margins using RSL (8% vs. 25% for WL, $p < 0.001$). Convenience was again rated higher by patients undergoing RSL ($p = 0.02$) with no difference in pain.

CONCLUSIONS

RSL has been shown to be safe and accurate for the excision of nonpalpable breast lesions. The advantages to this procedure include the following:

- The rate of positive margins is reduced by 50% or more.
- Radiologist can place the radioactive seed percutaneously by using any approach.
- The radioactive seed may be placed up to 5 days before surgery, thus uncoupling radiology and operative schedules.
- No displacement by imaging or patient transportation.
- Precise skin incision.
- Reorientation from any angle during surgery.
- Improved patient convenience.

The difference between a standard WL procedure and the RSL procedure revolves around radiation safety and the Nuclear Regulatory Commission policies. With attention to radiation safety details, this intuitive procedure is safely adopted with enthusiasm by radiologists, surgeons, and patients and provides superior outcomes.

References

1. Wong MH, Windle I, Rose A, et al. Predictors of surgical margin status in breast-conserving surgery within a breast screening program. *Ann Surg Oncol.* 2008;15:2542–2549.
2. Velanovich V, Lewis FR, Nathanson SD, et al. Comparison of mammographically guided biopsy techniques. *Ann Surg.* 1999; 229:525–530.
3. Gray RJ, Salud C, Nguyen K, et al. Randomized prospective evaluation of a novel technique for biopsy or lumpectomy of nonpalpable breast lesions: radioactive seed versus wire localization. *Ann Surg Oncol.* 2001;8:711–715.
4. Pavlecek W, Walton HA, Karsteadt PJ, et al. Radiation safety with use of I-125 seeds for localization of nonpalpable breast lesions. *Acad Radiol.* 2006;13:909–915.
5. Cox CE, Furman B, Stowell N, et al. Radioactive seed localization breast biopsy and lumpectomy: can specimen radiographs be eliminated? *Ann Surg Oncol.* 2003;10:1039–1047.
6. Gray RJ, Pockaj BA, Karstaedt PJ, et al. Radioactive seed localization of nonpalpable breast lesions is better than wire localization. *Am J Surg.* 2004;188:377–380.
7. Hughes JH, Mason MC, Gray RJ, et al. A multi-site validation trial of radioactive seed localization as an alternative to wire localization. *Breast J.* 2008;14:153–157.

Part II: Breast Biopsy

10 Axillary Sentinel Lymph Node Biopsy

Julie A. Margenthaler

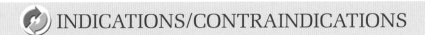

INDICATIONS/CONTRAINDICATIONS

Historical Considerations

The method and role of axillary staging for breast cancer has been in evolution since the 1960s. Historically, the prognostic information derived from axillary lymph node dissection was viewed so important to the overall patient management that clinically and pathologically uninvolved lymph nodes were removed for staging and treatment planning, though the therapeutic benefit was questionable. There has been a long-standing interest in the pathways of metastasis, with special emphasis placed on the draining regional lymphatics. The sentinel node concept was an elegant hypothesis founded on the principle that the lymphatic vessels draining a specific primary tumor travel to the first, or a finite group of several, "sentinel," lymph nodes in the respective regional lymphatic basin before disseminating to the remaining nonsentinel lymph nodes (1). Researchers at the John Wayne Cancer Institute (2,3) first demonstrated the sentinel node hypothesis in an animal model and subsequently validated it in a group of patients with melanoma. Following the success of intraoperative lymphatic mapping for melanoma, the technique of sentinel lymph node biopsy was quickly adapted to early-stage breast cancer (1).

Indications

The presence of metastatic disease in the axillary lymph nodes is considered the single most important prognostic factor for patients with breast cancer, whereby patients have a poorer prognosis with increasing numbers of metastatic lymph nodes (4). Sentinel lymph node biopsy has emerged as the standard method of axillary staging in breast cancer patients with clinically negative axillas (1,5–7). The goal of sentinel lymph node biopsy is to minimize morbidity while maintaining high sensitivity and a low false-negative rate, such that axillary staging is similar to the standard provided by axillary lymph node dissection pathology. Early experience with the procedure revealed a wide variation in reported rates of successful mapping and accuracy. However, training and quality control programs were initiated which have resulted in a large number of surgeons capable of performing sentinel lymph node biopsy in a standardized fashion with a high degree of pathologic accuracy (7). The National Surgical Adjuvant Breast and Bowel Project (NSABP) B-32 trial was primarily designed to demonstrate whether sentinel lymph node biopsy resulted in a mortality difference or differences in regional control compared to those patients undergoing axillary lymph node dissection. No significant differences were observed. In addition, the NSABP B-32 data were secondarily evaluated to demonstrate whether sentinel lymph node biopsy could achieve the same diagnostic accuracy as the gold standard, axillary lymph node dissection, while significantly decreasing morbidity (7). In more than 5,600 patients enrolled in NSABP B-32, the sentinel lymph node(s) were identified successfully in 97.2% of patients, with an overall accuracy of 97.1% (95% confidence interval [CI], 96.5 to 97.8) and a false-negative rate of 9.7% (95% CI, 7.6 to 11.9). The negative predictive value was 96.1% (95% CI, 95.2 to 97.0) (7).

Contraindications

Absolute and relative contraindications for the use of sentinel lymph node biopsy have been proposed, including prior mastectomy, prior axillary surgery or previous sentinel lymph node biopsy, palpable lymphadenopathy, prior excisional breast biopsy, T3 and T4 tumors, male breast cancer, neoadjuvant chemotherapy, and multicentric/multifocal breast cancers. However, as surgeon experience with sentinel lymph node biopsy has progressed, the previously described contraindications for sentinel lymph node biopsy have been successfully challenged. T4 and inflammatory breast cancer remain contraindications.

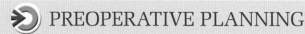

⟩ PREOPERATIVE PLANNING

Imaging

Prior to definitive surgical axillary staging, axillary ultrasound may be used to visualize the axillary lymph nodes. At our institution, this has become the standard for all newly diagnosed breast cancer patients with clinically negative axillae. Multiple reports in the literature suggest that axillary ultrasound is a potentially valuable technique for identifying axillary metastases (8). Axillary ultrasound permits the visualization of lymph node size, shape, contour, and changes in cortical morphology and texture that appear to be associated with the presence of axillary metastases (Figs. 10.1 and 10.2). However, sonographic signs of metastatic disease sometimes overlap with those of benign reactive changes, limiting the ability of this modality alone to accurately stage the axilla. The addition of fine needle aspiration biopsy has been shown to increase the specificity of nodal staging (9). If the patient is confirmed to have axillary nodal metastases by

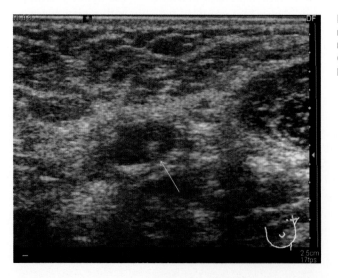

Figure 10.1 Axillary ultrasound of a normal-appearing lymph node. The node has a smooth, homogenous cortex with a centrally located, preserved fatty hilum (*arrow*).

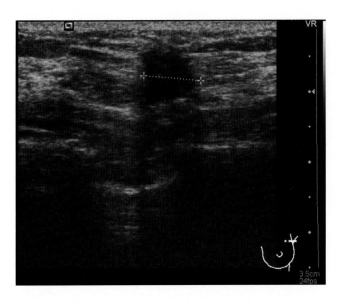

Figure 10.2 Axillary ultrasound of a suspicious-appearing lymph node. The node has a rounded appearance with an eccentrically thickened, heterogenous cortex and effacement of the fatty hilum.

cytopathology, full axillary lymph node dissection is recommended. However, if the axillary lymph nodes are morphologically normal or if the cytopathology is negative or nondiagnostic, sentinel lymph node biopsy should be performed.

Lymphoscintigraphy

Mapping and identification of the sentinel lymph node can be accomplished using radioactive colloid injection with or without lymphoscintigraphy and/or vital blue dye injection. For most surgeons who utilize radioactive colloid injection, the injection is performed by the nuclear medicine specialists at the institution prior to the planned surgical procedure. The recommended guidelines include an injection of approximately 0.5 mCi of 0.2-μm-filtered technetium sulfur colloid. This injection has traditionally been performed approximately 1 to 2 hours prior to the sentinel lymph node biopsy procedure. However, the method of injection varies widely. Options for site of injection include peritumoral versus subareolar and options for method of injection include intraparenchymal versus intradermal. A recent prospective randomized trial was performed to compare these modalities. Patients were randomized to receive radiocolloid injection by an intradermal route (placed in the skin overlying palpable tumors or in the same quadrant near the nipple areolar border for nonpalpable tumors), an intraparenchymal route (administered in a peritumoral fashion), or a subareolar route (at the upper, outer edge of the areolar complex directed medially 5 mm below the complex). Figures 10.3 to 10.5 depict the described injection methods. Intraoperative identification rates were 90% or more for all methods (100% for intradermal, 95% for subareolar, and 90% for intraparenchymal), further supporting the notion that sentinel lymph node biopsy is a robust technique regardless of the site and/or method of injection (10). However, the mean time to first localization on lymphoscintigram was 8 ± 14 minutes for intradermal injection, 53 ± 49 minutes for intraparenchymal injection, and 22 ± 29 minutes for subareolar injection (10). On the basis of these results, we have adopted the intradermal method of injection at our institution. Anecdotally, this has been very successful, and we now require our patients to present to the nuclear medicine department approximately 45 minutes prior to their surgical procedure, rather than 2 hours which was our previous practice with intraparenchymal injections.

Recently, Thompson et al. (11) reported their experience with intraoperative subareolar injection of radioactive sulfur colloid by the operating surgeon. They found that this was a safe, effective, and equally reliable method of identification of the sentinel lymph nodes. Further, intraoperative injection of the colloid avoided the patient pain, vasovagal events, operative delays, and costs associated with preoperative injections. One potential disadvantage of the intraoperative method of injection is the lack of access to lymphoscintigraphy. This may be important if the surgeon typically relies on the

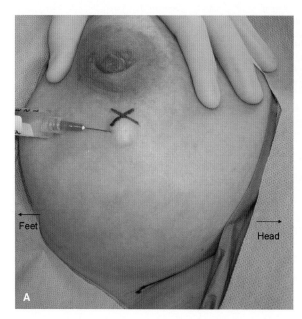

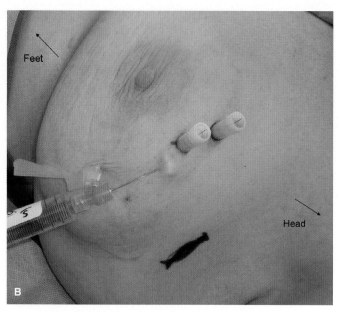

Figure 10.3 Radiocolloid injection using an intradermal injection method in a patient with a palpable breast cancer (**A**) or a nonpalpable breast cancer (**B**). In the case of patients with palpable breast cancers ("X" marks the palpable tumor), the injection is administered in a peritumoral location. In the case of patients with nonpalpable breast cancers, the injection is administered in nonpigmented skin in a location adjacent to but not involving the pigmented areolar skin in the same radial "o'clock" position in which the breast cancer is located. In both cases, an attempt is made to create a visible, raised, dermal skin wheal.

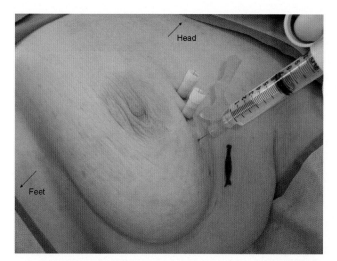

Figure 10.4 Radiocolloid injection using an intraparenchymal, peritumoral injection method. For patients with nonpalpable breast cancer, the injection is performed using imaging guidance or is directed along the pathway of the wire localization (as shown in the figure).

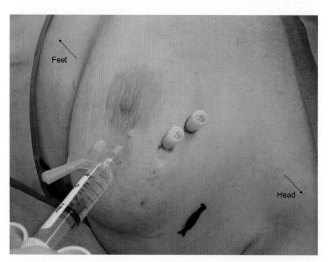

Figure 10.5 Radiocolloid injection using a subareolar injection method. The injection is performed by placing the needle at the upper, outer edge of the nipple areolar complex (at 10 o'clock for the right breast and at 2 o'clock for the left breast) and directing the tip medially toward the nipple and deep to (approximately 5 mm below) the central portion of the areolar complex. The injection is performed in the subdermal subcutaneous tissue plane.

lymphoscintigram for information regarding number of localized nodes, position of localized nodes in the axillary space, and presence of internal mammary sentinel lymph nodes.

Vital Blue Dye

The injection of a vital blue dye can be used alone or in conjunction with radioactive colloid injection for sentinel lymph node mapping. The vital blue dye is universally injected intraoperatively and will be discussed further in the technique section. However, options also exist for the type and method of blue dye injection planned. The issues of the site of blue dye injection are similar to those for radioactive colloid injection. Peritumoral or subareolar injections may be employed, though many surgeons have adopted subareolar and periareolar injections because of their simplicity and convenience. Further results of previous studies have validated the efficacy of subareolar and periareolar injections, supporting the hypothesis that the lymphatic drainage of the entire breast is to the same few sentinel lymph nodes (12).

The two available vital blue dyes for injection and sentinel lymph node localization are isosulfan blue dye and methylene blue dye. Isosulfan blue is a triphenylmethane-based dye and is one of the rosaniline dyes. It was the first blue dye of its class to be approved for use in lymphangiography by the Food and Drug Administration under the trade name Lymphazurin 1% (US Surgical Corp, Norwalk, Connecticut). Typically, 5 mL of Lymphazurin 1% is used for injection. Although isosulfan blue dye remains a popular choice of dye for sentinel lymph node localization, the rate of allergic reactions to the dye has also increased (13). This is likely related to the fact that this class of blue dyes is also used in many cosmetics, paper, and textile supplies, and patients may become sensitized from prior exposure. Patients with allergies to sulfa drugs are not significantly more likely to sustain an allergic reaction, and, therefore, sulfa allergy is not an absolute contraindication for the use of isosulfan blue dye. The rate of allergic and anaphylactic reactions to isosulfan blue dye is reported to be 1% to 3%, and the reactions may range from blue hives (Fig. 10.6) to serious anaphylaxis with hypotension and angioedema (14). I have personally witnessed two such cases of anaphylaxis in my patients, whereby both had marked swelling of the eyelids and lips and a severe hypotension approximately 20 to 30 minutes following the injection. Both were treated with epinephrine, fluid resuscitation, diphenhydramine, and methylprednisolone. Both were able to be extubated at the completion of the procedure and were discharged the following day without any long-term sequelae.

Methylene blue dye represents an alternative to isosulfan blue dye for sentinel lymph node localization. Recent reports suggest that methylene blue dye is efficacious with a similar sentinel lymph node identification rate (15). Methylene blue dye is also more cost-effective than isosulfan blue dye (at our institution, methylene blue dye is approximately 10% of the cost of isosulfan blue dye). Further, there have been no reports of anaphylaxis with the use of methylene blue dye. One disadvantage of methylene blue dye is that it can cause skin necrosis if injected intradermally; therefore,

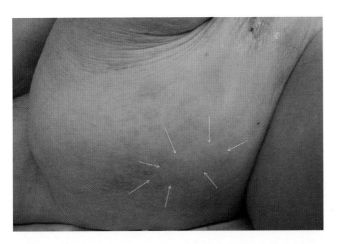

Figure 10.6 An example of a blue hive following injection of isosulfan blue dye for sentinel lymph node mapping (*yellow arrows* mark the circumference of the blue hive).

parenchymal injection is recommended. When using methylene blue dye, it is also helpful to dilute the dye to further reduce the risk of local inflammatory response and skin necrosis. At our institution, 1 mL of methylene blue dye is mixed with 4 mL of injectable normal saline, and the entire 5 mL solution is used for injection.

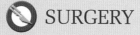 SURGERY

Relevant Anatomy

Mastery of the anatomy of the axilla is critical to perform an adequate sentinel lymph node dissection with minimal morbidity. The axillary space is defined by the axillary vein superiorly, the serratus anterior muscle medially, and the latissimus dorsi muscle laterally.

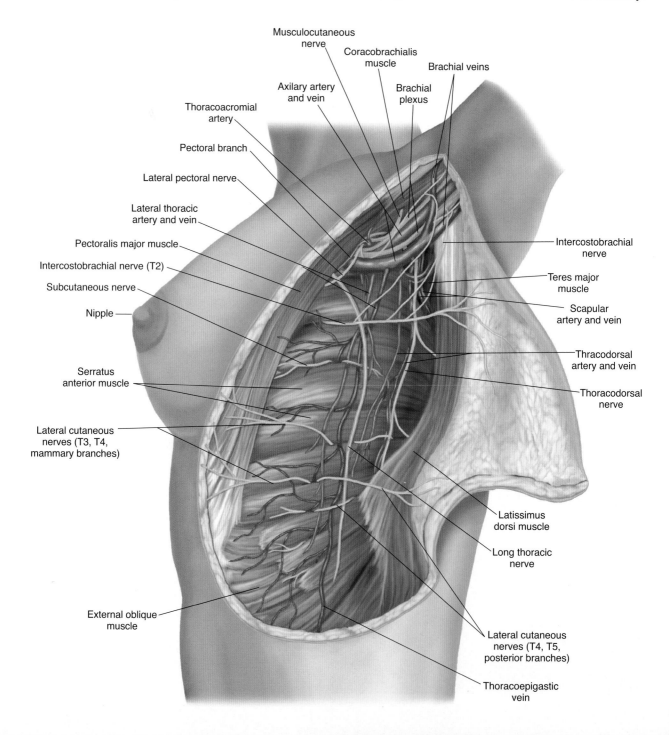

There is no specific bony or muscle landmark to indicate the inferior border. The clavipectoral fascia encloses the pectoralis minor muscle and the axillary fat pad. In order to identify the sentinel lymph nodes, it is necessary to open the clavipectoral fascia to expose the underlying fat pad. Once the axillary fat pad is exposed, the blue and/or radioactive lymphatics are identified and followed to the sentinel lymph nodes as described below. The major motor nerves of the axilla include the long thoracic nerve of Bell, which runs parallel to the chest wall and innervates the serratus anterior muscle and the thoracodorsal nerve, which mark the deep aspect of the axillary space and innervate the latissimus dorsi muscle. The major boundaries and motor nerves of the axillary space may not be visualized during sentinel lymph node biopsy, as they are during full axillary lymph node dissection. However, the intercostobrachial nerves are frequently encountered. These sensory nerves traverse the axilla to supply the skin on the medial and posterior arm, axilla, and posterior axillary line. The intercostobrachial nerves exit the fascia of the chest wall at the second and third intercostal spaces. Injury to the intercostobrachial nerves can be avoided by carefully dissecting the sentinel lymph nodes without wide excision of surrounding axillary fat as described below.

Preparation

On the day of surgery, the "correct" breast and axilla are confirmed and marked. The patient's medical history is reviewed in the holding area, with particular attention paid to allergies to drugs that may be used during and after surgery. The patient is then brought to the operating theater and placed supine on the operating table.

Positioning

Patients are positioned such that their arms are placed on arm boards at 90 degrees abduction from the chest wall. We prefer general anesthesia at our institution, though regional or local anesthesia may be utilized, depending on patient and surgeon preference. The operating room and equipment are arranged to facilitate the surgical procedure. As the surgeon, I prefer to stand on the side of the affected breast to be operated upon, with my first assistant positioned on the same side above the arm board. The gamma probe device and ultrasound machine (if applicable) are placed on the opposite side of the operating table, which allows a straight, unobstructed view of the machines and images (Figs. 10.7 and 10.8).

Technique

Once the patient has been prepped and draped in the standard surgical fashion, the vital blue dye, if used, is injected. I prefer a periareolar or subareolar injection site in

Part III: Lymph Node Mapping and Dissection

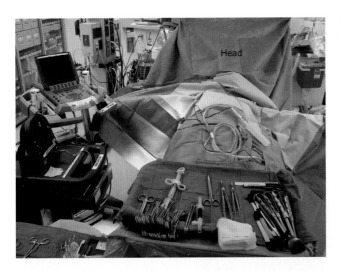

Figure 10.7 Positioning of patient and equipment in the operating room.

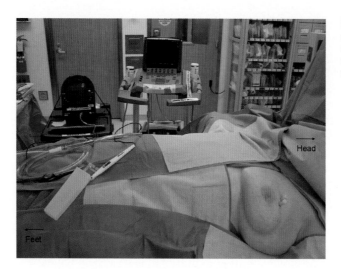

Figure 10.8 View of the patient and equipment from the standpoint of the operating surgeon who is standing on the patient's ipsilateral side (respective to the cancer) below the arm.

the same quadrant as the known cancer as shown in Figure 10.9. If the patient has had a prior excision of the cancer and only a cavity is in place, it is important to inject the blue dye outside of the cavity and lateral (toward the axilla) to the cavity. A 5-minute breast massage is then performed. A curvilinear incision is planned approximately 1 to 2 cm below the edge of the axillary hairline from the edge of the pectoralis major muscle laterally (Fig. 10.10). If a radioactive colloid injection was used pre- or intraoperatively, the navigator probe can be used to help localize the site of maximum tracer uptake for surgical incision planning (Fig. 10.11).

An incision is made with a scalpel and carried down through the dermis with electrocautery. Blue and/or "hot" lymphatics may be encountered just below the dermis if intradermal injections were utilized. However, the lymphatic channels of interest are located below the clavipectoral fascia. The subcutaneous tissue is divided and the clavipectoral fascia is identified (Fig. 10.12) and incised. Once the clavipectoral fascia is opened, the true axillary fat pad is revealed and a search for the blue and/or "hot" lymphatics may commence. Because I use a dual injection technique, I prefer to search for the blue lymphatic initially and use the navigator probe secondarily. Once the axillary space has been entered, the blue lymphatic is typically easily visible (Fig. 10.13). Without transecting the blue lymphatic, blunt dissection is used to carefully follow the lymphatic down onto the surface of the blue node (Fig. 10.14). At this point, the navigator probe is placed on the node and a count is taken. The node is then carefully excised from the surrounding tissues using electrocautery. By lifting the lymph node up into the surgical space and staying right on the node/fatty tissue interface, injury to surrounding structures can be avoided; very little surrounding fatty tissue is excised with the sentinel lymph node with this technique (Fig. 10.15). I have also found it help-

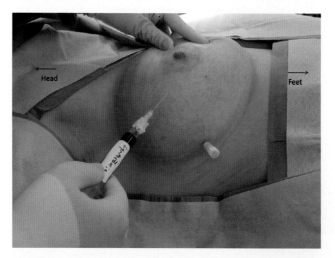

Figure 10.9 Periareolar injection of vital blue dye in the same quadrant as the needle localized cancer (in this case, 5 mL Lymphazurin 1% was utilized).

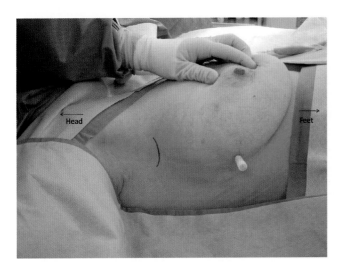

Figure 10.10 An incision is planned approximately 1 to 2 cm below the edge of the axillary hairline near the lateral edge of the pectoralis major muscle.

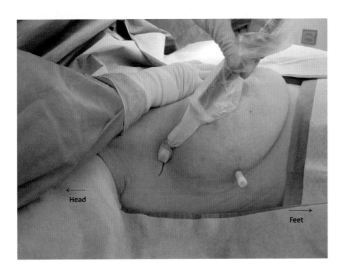

Figure 10.11 The navigator probe can identify the site of maximum tracer uptake to aid in surgical incision planning.

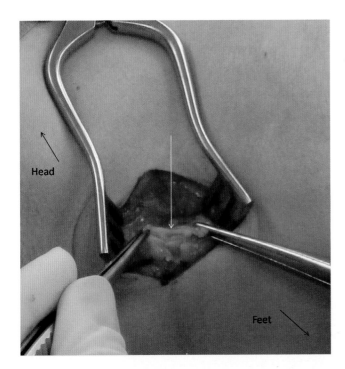

Figure 10.12 Identification and division of the clavipectoral fascia (*arrow*) represents entry to the true axillary fat pad.

Part III: Lymph Node Mapping and Dissection

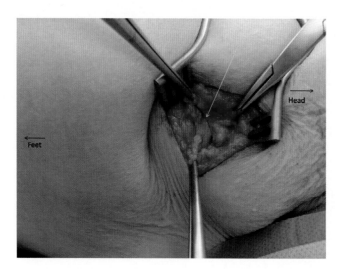

Figure 10.13 Identification of the blue lymphatic (*arrow*).

ful to clip or tie the blue and/or "hot" lymphatic to potentially decrease spillage of radioactive colloid into the axillary space and to help prevent future seroma formation. In cases where only radioactive colloid is used without the addition of vital blue dye, the procedure is similar, though the navigator probe is used to guide the dissection. When a "hot" spot is identified, the probe is angled to identify the point of maximum intensity; this is referred to as the "line-of-sight" method and it represents the angle in which the dissection continues until the lymph node is identified.

This process is continued until all sentinel lymph nodes are identified. The definition of a sentinel lymph node is a node that is either blue, "hot," and/or palpable. The blue lymphatic must be followed back to the point where it exits the breast and down into the axillary space to ensure complete identification of all blue nodes. Once all of the blue sentinel nodes have been identified, place the navigator probe in the space and perform a count. If the background count of the axilla is 10% or less of the most "hot" sentinel lymph node removed, I consider all blue and "hot" sentinel lymph nodes to be sufficiently harvested. The final step is to perform a palpation of the space to ensure that there are no abnormally palpable sentinel lymph nodes. This is a very important final step as it is possible for a sentinel lymph node to be obstructed and replaced by malignancy, thereby preventing the uptake of blue dye and/or radioactive colloid.

The space is then carefully inspected and hemostasis is achieved. The space is irrigated with sterile saline. The clavipectoral fascia is reapproximated with a single interrupted 3-0 Vicryl stitch (Fig. 10.16). The deep dermal layer is reapproximated with interrupted 3-0 Vicryl stitches and the skin is reapproximated with a running subcuticular stitch using a 4-0 Monocryl. Dermabond dressing is applied (Fig. 10.17).

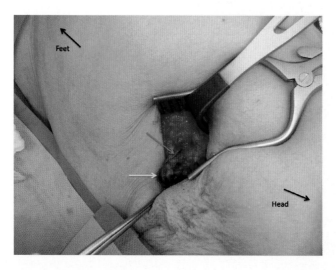

Figure 10.14 The blue lymphatic (*green arrow)* is followed down onto the surface of the blue sentinel lymph node (*yellow arrow*).

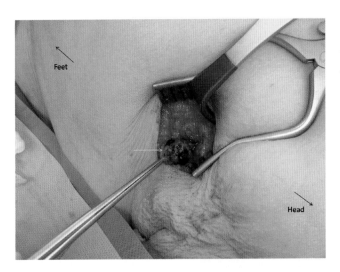

Figure 10.15 The blue sentinel lymph node (*arrow*) is elevated into the space and electrocautery is used to excise the node from the surrounding tissues.

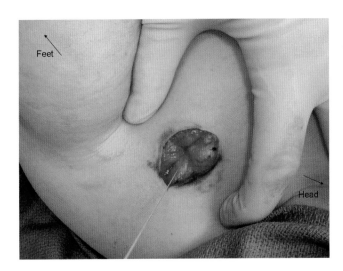

Figure 10.16 A single 3-0 Vicryl stitch is placed in the clavipectoral fascia to reapproximate and close the dead space.

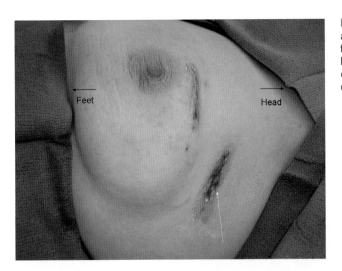

Figure 10.17 Final surgical appearance of the axillary incision (*arrow*) following closure of the deep dermal layer with 3-0 Vicryl, a running subcuticular with 4-0 Monocryl, and dermabond dressing application.

Part III: Lymph Node Mapping and Dissection

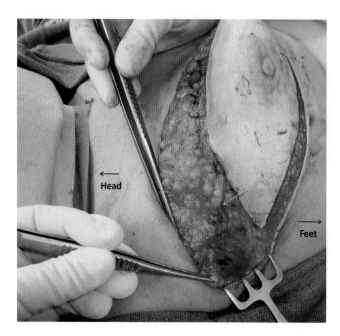

Figure 10.18 During mastectomy, as the lateral flap is being created, the blue (and/or "hot") lymphatic (*arrow*) can be located exiting the breast at the lateral edge of the pectoralis major muscle.

The technique described is universally employed for patients who are undergoing breast-conserving therapy. For patients who are undergoing mastectomy for treatment of their primary breast tumor, the sentinel lymph node biopsy can still be performed through an axillary counter-incision as described above. However, my preference is to perform the sentinel lymph node biopsy through the mastectomy incision. This is also a viable option for patients undergoing skin-sparing procedures. The injections and localization are performed in a similar fashion. The blue and/or "hot" lymphatic can be identified as the lateral flap is created at the edge of the pectoralis major muscle. Alternatively, the breast can be removed and the sentinel lymph node biopsy performed through the cavity. In either case, the clavipectoral fascia is divided along the lateral edge of the pectoralis major muscle, which facilitates identification of the lymphatic (Fig. 10.18). The lymphatic is then followed down to the sentinel lymph nodes (Fig. 10.19) and the procedure continues as described previously.

 COMPLICATIONS

Although sentinel lymph node biopsy is clearly less invasive than axillary lymph node dissection, sentinel lymph node biopsy is not without morbidity and anesthetic risk. The risk of allergic reaction and anaphylaxis to vital blue dye injection has been

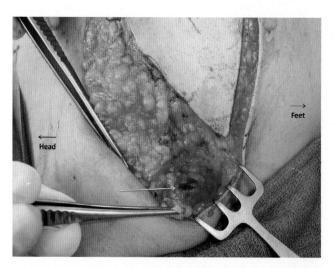

Figure 10.19 The sentinel lymph node (*arrow*) is identified during the mastectomy.

previously discussed. A recent randomized, prospective trial of sentinel lymph node biopsy versus axillary lymph node dissection confirms that complications of sentinel lymph node biopsy include seroma formation, lymphedema, sensory nerve injury, and limitation in range of motion (16). In addition, sentinel lymph node biopsy is often performed as a staged procedure, requiring that breast cancer patients undergo two or more operations for definitive staging and treatment of the axilla. Such patients include those who have node-positive disease by sentinel lymph node biopsy and require completion axillary lymph node dissection, those who undergo axillary staging prior to breast reconstruction, and those undergoing neoadjuvant chemotherapy. These clinical scenarios may represent up to 40% to 50% of patients treated for breast cancer. Future randomized studies devoted to the development of validated intraoperative assessment of sentinel nodal status and the use and timing of sentinel lymph node biopsy in patients receiving neoadjuvant therapy may help reduce the need for staged procedures.

Although the above complications can occur following sentinel lymph node biopsy, the morbidity and outcomes from sentinel lymph node biopsy are superior to axillary lymph node dissection. Analysis of the Axillary Lymphatic Mapping Against Nodal Axillary Clearance (ALMANAC) trial demonstrated that the relative risks of any lymphedema and sensory loss for patients undergoing sentinel lymph node biopsy compared with those patients undergoing standard axillary lymph node dissection were 0.37 (95% CI, 0.23 to 0.60; absolute rates 5% vs. 13%) and 0.37 (95% CI, 0.27 to 0.50; absolute rates 11% vs. 31%) at 12 months, respectively (17). Drain usage, length of hospital stay, and time to resumption of normal activities after surgery were statistically significantly lower in the sentinel lymph node biopsy group, and axillary operative time was reduced (17). Overall patient-recorded quality of life and arm functioning scores were statistically significantly better in the sentinel lymph node biopsy group throughout (17).

POSTOPERATIVE MANAGEMENT

Surgical Follow-up

Patients are seen in the surgical clinic at 10 to 14 days following the sentinel lymph node biopsy. Prior to this visit, restrictions include avoidance of submersion of the incision in water and limitation in lifting to less than 20 lb. Otherwise, we encourage our patients to resume their normal activities. At the postoperative visit, the incision is inspected to ensure proper healing and lack of seroma formation. If a significant seroma is present and is symptomatic, it can be percutaneously aspirated. Intercostobrachial nerve function is also assessed. If wound healing is uneventful, patients are encouraged to gradually increase their level of activity and range of motion. It is extremely rare for patients to have protracted difficulty with function; physical therapy can be initiated if the patient fails to return to full function within 6 weeks.

Pathological Interpretation

Final pathology results are reviewed carefully by the surgeon and with the patient. The increasing use of immunohistochemical staining and molecular biology techniques has led to an ability to detect extremely small metastatic lesions in axillary sentinel lymph nodes. Sentinel node metastasis is described as (1) macrometastasis (tumor deposit >2.0 mm), (2) micrometastasis (tumor deposit >0.2 to 2.0 mm), (3) isolated tumor cells (tumor clusters <0.2 mm), and (4) molecular positive only (reverse-transcriptase polymerase chain reaction). Although these potential findings have now been incorporated in the latest edition of the *American Joint Commission (AJCC) on Cancer Staging Manual* (17), the management and clinical importance of these lesions remain unclear. The current American Society of Clinical Oncology guidelines recommend routine axillary

Part III: Lymph Node Mapping and Dissection

lymph node dissection for patients with a macro- or micrometastasis on histopathologic examination (18). The clinical significance of isolated tumor cells and molecular metastasis is not known; therefore, no specific recommendations were made (18). The use of nomograms to predict the presence of nonsentinel lymph node metastases, such as the Memorial Sloan-Kettering Cancer Center nomogram (19), may aid in surgeons' decision making for individual patients with these findings. The current practice at our institution is to perform completion axillary lymph node dissection for patients with macro- and micrometastases and for patients with isolated tumor cells that are considered high risk for nonsentinel lymph node metastases (by nomogram and multidisciplinary tumor board discussion) (20).

RESULTS

Previous studies have validated the accuracy of sentinel lymph node biopsy. In NSABP B-32, the overall accuracy of sentinel lymph node biopsy compared with the gold standard of axillary lymph node dissection was 97.1% (95% CI, 96.5 to 97.8) with a false-negative rate of 9.7% (95% CI, 7.6 to 11.9) and a negative predictive value of 96.1% (95% CI, 95.2 to 97.0) (7). Veronesi et al. (21) demonstrated an overall accuracy for sentinel lymph node biopsy of 96.9%, a sensitivity of 91.2%, a specificity of 100%, and a false-negative rate of 8.8% in patients with T1 primary breast cancers. Giuliano et al. (22) reported their prospective results of sentinel lymph node biopsy in women with T1/T2 primary breast cancers who underwent only completion axillary lymph node dissection if the sentinel lymph node was positive for metastatic cells. They reported a 99% sentinel lymph node identification rate, and no locoregional recurrences were reported at 39 months' follow-up. Similar results have been observed in nonrandomized studies.

PEARLS AND PITFALLS

The false-negative rate for sentinel lymph node biopsy is likely related to injection methods, lymphatic physiology, aberrant lymphatic patterns, tumor-replaced nodes that do not readily take up blue dye or radiocolloid, and surgeon experience. Techniques to aid the surgeon who is beginning their experience with sentinel lymph node biopsy include (1) dual identification with blue dye and radiocolloid, (2) subareolar or periareolar injection techniques, (3) lateral (toward the axilla) pericavity injection for patients undergoing previous excisional biopsy, and (4) thorough palpation of the axillary fat pad following removal of blue and/or "hot" nodes. Using these techniques, many centers have demonstrated false-negative rates that have dropped to less than 5%.

CONCLUSIONS

Evaluation of the axilla by sentinel lymph node biopsy is an accurate, less invasive alternative to axillary lymph node dissection, and it has become the standard of care in patients with clinically node-negative breast cancer. Few contraindications exist for its use in early-stage breast cancer. Overall identification rates, accuracy, and negative predictive value vary little, regardless of the site, method, or type of injection used.

Acknowledgment

The author thanks her assistant, Circe W. Diggs, for her secretarial and administrative assistance in preparing this chapter.

References

1. Krag D, Weaver D, Ashikaga T, et al. The sentinel node in breast cancer: a multicenter validation study. *N Engl J Med.* 1998;339: 941–946.
2. Wong J, Cagle L, Morton D. Lymphatic drainage of the skin to a sentinel lymph node in a feline model. *Ann Surg.* 1991;214: 637–643.
3. Habal N, Giuliano AE, Morton DL. The use of sentinel lymphadenectomy to identify candidates for postoperative adjuvant therapy of melanoma and breast cáncer. *Semin Oncol.* 2001;28: 41–47.
4. Carter CL, Allen C, Henson DE. Relation of tumor size, lymph node status, and survival in 24,740 breast cancer cases. *Cancer.* 1989;63:181–187.
5. Veronesi U, Paganelli G, Viale G, et al. Sentinel lymph node biopsy and axillary dissection in breast cancer: results in a large series. *J Natl Cancer Inst.* 1999;91:368–373.
6. McMasters KM, Tuttle TM, Carlson DJ, et al. Sentinel lymph node biopsy for breast cancer: a suitable alternative to routine axillary dissection in multi-institutional practice when optimal technique is used. *J Clin Oncol.* 2000;18:2560–2566.
7. Krag DN, Anderson SJ, Julian TB, et al. Technical outcomes of sentinel lymph node resection and conventional axillary lymph node dissection in patients with clinically node negative breast cancer: results from the NSABP B-32 randomized phase III trial. *Lancet.* 2007;8:881–888.
8. Deurloo EE, Tanis PJ, Gilhuijs KG, et al. Reduction in the number of sentinel lymph node procedures by preoperative ultrasonography of the axilla in breast cancer. *Eur J Cancer.* 2003;39: 1068–1073.
9. Krishnamurthy SN, Sneige DG, Bedi BS, et al. Role of ultrasound-guided fine-needle aspiration of indeterminate and suspicious axillary lymph nodes in the initial staging of breast carcinoma. *Cancer.* 2002;95:982–988.
10. Povoski SP, Olsen JO, Young DC, et al. Prospective randomized clinical trial comparing intradermal, intraparenchymal, and subareolar injection routes for sentinel lymph node mapping and biopsy in breast cancer. *Ann Surg Oncol.* 2006;13(11): 1412–1421.
11. Thompson M, Korourian S, Henry-Tillman R, et al. Intraoperative radioisotope injection for sentinel lymph node biopsy. *Ann Surg Oncol.* 2008;15(11):3216–3221.
12. Chagpar A, Martin RC, Chao C, et al. Validation of subareolar and periareolar injection techniques for breast sentinel lymph node biopsy. *Arch Surg.* 2004;139:614–620.
13. Thevarajah S, Huston TL, Simmons RM. A comparison of the adverse reactions associated with isosulfan blue versus methylene blue dye in sentinel lymph node biopsy for breast cancer. *Am J Surg.* 2005;189:236–239.
14. Kuerer HM, Wayne JD, Ross MI. Anaphylaxis during breast cancer lymphatic mapping. *Surgery.* 2001;129:119–120.
15. Simmons RM, Thevarajah S, Brennan MB, et al. Methylene blue dye as an alternative to isosulfan blue dye for sentinel lymph node localization. *Ann Surg Oncol.* 2003;10:242–247.
16. Purushotham AD, Upponi S, Klevesath MB, et al. Morbidity after sentinel lymph node biopsy in primary breast cancer: results from a randomized controlled trial. *J Clin Oncol.* 2005; 23:4312–4321.
17. Greene FL, Page DL, Fleming ID, et al. *AJCC Cancer Staging Manual.* 6th ed. New York, NY: Springer; 2002.
18. Lyman GH, Giuliano AE, Somerfield MR, et al. American Society of Clinical Oncology guideline recommendations for sentinel lymph node biopsy in early-stage breast cancer. *J Clin Oncol.* 2005;23:7703–7720.
19. VanZee KJ, Manasseh DME, Bevilacqua JLB, et al. A nomogram for predicting the likelihood of additional nodal metastases in breast cancer patients with a positive sentinel node biopsy. *Ann Surg Oncol.* 2003;10(10):1140–1151.
20. Mansel RE, Fallowfield L, Kissin M, et al. Randomized multicenter trial of sentinel node biopsy versus standard axillary treatment in operable breast cancer: the ALMANAC Trial. *J Natl Cancer Inst.* 2006;98:599–609.
21. Veronesi U, Paganelli G, Viale G, et al. A randomized comparison of sentinel-node biopsy with routine axillary dissection in breast cancer. *N Engl J Med.* 2003;349:546–553.
22. Giuliano AE, Haigh PI, Brennan MB, et al. Prospective observational study of sentinel lymphadenectomy without further axillary dissection in patients with sentinel node-negative breast cancer. *J Clin Oncol.* 2000;18:2553–2559.

Part III: Lymph Node Mapping and Dissection

11 Internal Mammary Sentinel Lymph Node Biopsy

Hiram S. Cody, III and Virgilio Sacchini

Introduction

- The predominant lymphatic drainage of the breast is to the axillary nodes but the internal mammary nodes (IMNs) have long been recognized as an alternate pathway (1,2).
- The historic rationale for "extended radical mastectomy" (ERM) (3), an operation that combined a full-thickness resection of the parasternal chest wall and IMN with a classic radical mastectomy (RM), was the observation by Urban (4) in 1951 of a very high rate of *parasternal chest wall recurrence* following RM in patients with inner quadrant breast cancers.
- The goal of ERM was to reduce the rate of local recurrence and, by improving local control, to improve survival. This goal was never met: Veronesi's randomized trial comparing ERM with RM demonstrates a 1.1% to 3.5% reduction in the 10-year rate of parasternal chest wall recurrence (5) but no difference in survival at 30 years' follow-up (6).
- The published experience with ERM (comprising 4,172 patients in 7 studies) (7) is instructive and relevant to the current era of sentinel lymph node (SLN) biopsy. IMN metastases
  - were present in 19% to 33% of all patients,
  - were more frequent in axillary node-positive (29%–52%) than node-negative (4%–18%) patients,
  - were equally frequent for central/medial versus lateral tumors if the axillary nodes were negative (8%–10% vs. 3%–13%), and
  - were more frequent for medial/central tumors if the axillary nodes were positive (36%–49% vs. 22%–26%).
- The principal reason for surgical staging of lymph nodes in breast cancer is prognostication. The prognosis of patients with metastases limited to the IMN or to the axillary nodes is comparable and is intermediate between that of patients with negative nodes and those with both IMN and axillary metastases (7–9). The identification of IMN metastases is, therefore, of particular importance for patients *who would not*

otherwise be candidates for systemic adjuvant therapy, that is, those with negative axillary nodes and tumors smaller than 1 cm. If one assumes that this subset (perhaps 5% of all patients) received systemic therapy, then less than 1% of all patients would experience a survival benefit.

■ A secondary goal of lymph node surgery is local control. Current treatment protocols for stage I to II breast cancer do not include any IMN treatment, and yet local recurrence in the IMN or parasternal area occurs in less than 1% of patients treated by either mastectomy (10) or breast conservation therapy (BCT) (11). The recent Oxford Overview (12), a landmark in the history of breast cancer treatment, clearly demonstrates a relationship between local control and survival, but only for those treatment strategies in which local recurrence was reduced by more than 10%. Local recurrence in untreated IMN is already rare, and for this reason, it is inconceivable that any further reductions in the rate of local recurrence could affect survival.

■ SLN biopsy, in which radioisotope and blue dye are used to map the first few lymph nodes draining the breast, has now replaced axillary dissection (ALND) as standard care for patients with operable breast cancer (13). SLN biopsy has also revived debate over the significance of nonaxillary lymphatic drainage, particularly to the IMN. In a remarkable series of 700 SLN biopsy procedures (done with meticulous lymphatic mapping by intratumoral injection), Estourgie et al.'s (14) reported results that largely recapitulate those from the era of ERM: by preoperative lymphoscintigraphy (LSG), 95% of patients drained to the axilla and 22% to the IMN. Among those with IMN drainage, nodes were seen most frequently in the third (36%), second (27%), and fourth (24%) interspaces.

 # INDICATIONS/CONTRAINDICATIONS

IM-SLN Biopsy

■ The above-mentioned data suggest that the benefit of IM-SLN biopsy will accrue to very few patients. Nevertheless, there are several clear indications for the procedure:

   ■ *Preoperative LSG showing drainage only to the IMN.* IMN drainage is almost always accompanied by axillary drainage, but for the few patients who map exclusively to the IMN, IM-SLN biopsy makes sense and allows the surgeon to avoid unnecessary exploration of the axilla.

   ■ *Preoperative LSG showing drainage to IMN and axillary nodes.* IM-SLN biopsy is reasonable in this setting if (a) the axillary SLN is benign on intraoperative examination and (b) the patient is not already a candidate for adjuvant chemotherapy on the basis of other criteria. While IM-SLN biopsy makes sense for any patient in whom a positive result would alter the plan for systemic therapy, this decision is increasingly based on factors other than lymph node status, among them ER/PR/her2 status, lymphovascular invasion, and (increasingly) gene expression profiling.

   ■ *Preoperative imaging (computed tomography [CT], magnetic resonance imaging, positron emission tomography) with evidence of IMN involvement.* Grossly enlarged IMN are usually amenable to CT-guided core biopsy and are thus a debatable indication for IM-SLN biopsy. As noted earlier, most patients with visible IMN metastases will be candidates for chemotherapy on the basis of other criteria. There are no data to suggest that surgical excision of grossly involved IMN (and specifically IM-SLN biopsy) will improve local control beyond that achieved by chemotherapy and radiotherapy (RT).

   ■ *"Reoperative" SLN biopsy with drainage to IMN.* SLN biopsy is feasible in patients who have had prior axillary surgery (either SLN biopsy or ALND) for breast cancer and present with local recurrence (15).

      ■ Lymphatic mapping in the reoperative setting is particularly useful since the prior surgery may have altered the lymphatic drainage of the breast unpredictably.

- We have observed nonaxillary drainage (most often to the IMN) in 30% of reoperative SLN biopsies vs. 6% of our "first-time" procedures (16).
- Ipsilateral recurrence in the conserved breast occurs in approximately 5% to 10% of all patients, and these are the patients for whom IM-SLN biopsy may ultimately prove to be most useful.

PREOPERATIVE PLANNING

- The success of SLN biopsy is maximized by a combination of radioisotope and blue dye mapping (17), and isotope is crucial for IM-SLN biopsy. ^{99m}Technetium is complexed to a variety of carrier particles (sulfur colloid in the U.S., colloidal albumin in Europe, and antimony in Australia) and injected into the breast either the day before or the morning of surgery; we have observed identical results with day-before or same-day isotope injection (18).
- The dermal lymphatics of the breast drain almost exclusively to the axilla and the deeper breast lymphatics drain to the IMN and axilla (19).
- The success of *axillary SLN* biopsy is maximized by *superficial* injections of isotope (intradermal, subdermal, or subareolar) and intraparenchymal/peritumoral injection is somewhat less successful. These results come from many observational studies and have been confirmed in a randomized trial (20).
- The success of *IM-SLN* biopsy is maximized by *deep* injections of isotope (intraparenchymal/peritumoral/intratumoral).
- Preoperative LSG is of arguable benefit if the goal at surgery is to identify axillary SLN (a handheld gamma probe is more sensitive that a full-field-of-view gamma camera) but is absolutely essential to identify nonaxillary patterns of lymphatic drainage, and particularly IM-SLN.
- In summary, for those clinical settings where IM-SLN biopsy is a priority, a combination of superficial and deep injections of isotope will maximize success overall, and preoperative LSG is mandatory.

SURGERY

Relevant Anatomy

- The IMN chain is confined just anterior to the extrapleural chest space approximately 2 to 3 cm lateral to the sternal border. Two IM veins parallel the IM artery, one medial and one lateral to it (Fig. 11.1).
- The IM artery runs through this same space along the lateral sternal border approximately 10 mm from the border at the first intercostal space increasing slightly to 20 mm at the sixth space.
- From the IM artery, derive the anterior intercostal arteries, two for each intercostal space, running between the two intercostal muscles, one inferior and the other superior, both anastomosed with the posterior intercostal artery (Fig. 11.1).
- Usually one IM lymph node is located per intercostals space in the same plane as the IM vessels (Fig. 11.2). In the first and second intercostal spaces, the lymph node is usually medial to the IM vessels, whereas in the third and fourth spaces, IM lymph nodes are lateral to the vessels (Fig. 11.2).

Injection of Blue Dye

- In the operating room, with the patient either sedated (for breast conserving surgeries) or under general anesthesia (for mastectomy), the chest is prepped and draped in the usual sterile manner.

Part III: Lymph Node Mapping and Dissection

Figure 11.1 Internal mammary anatomy.

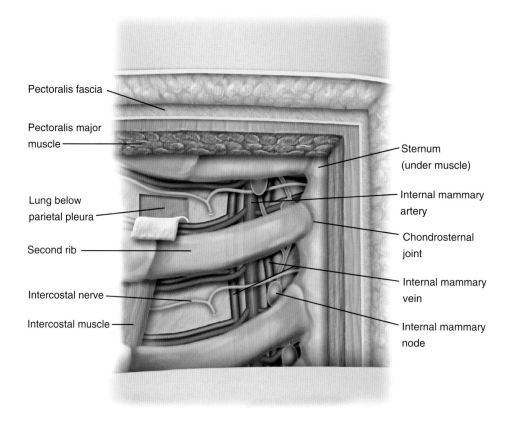

Pectoralis fascia

Pectoralis major muscle

Lung below parietal pleura

Second rib

Intercostal nerve

Intercostal muscle

Sternum (under muscle)

Internal mammary artery

Chondrosternal joint

Internal mammary vein

Internal mammary node

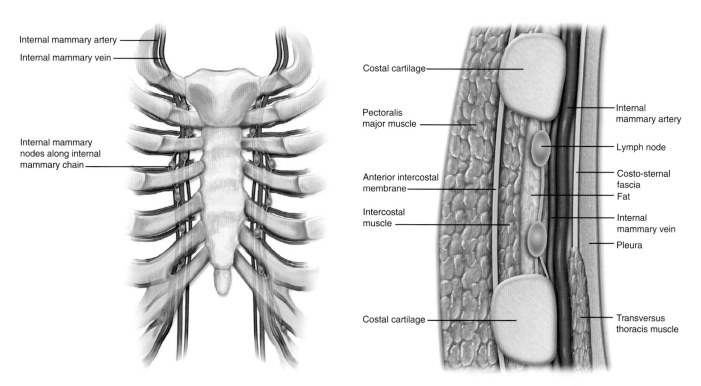

Internal mammary artery

Internal mammary vein

Internal mammary nodes along internal mammary chain

Costal cartilage

Pectoralis major muscle

Anterior intercostal membrane

Intercostal muscle

Costal cartilage

Internal mammary artery

Lymph node

Costo-sternal fascia

Fat

Internal mammary vein

Pleura

Transversus thoracis muscle

Figure 11.2 Internal mammary chain anatomy.

▓ Next, a subdermal injection of 1 to 5 cc of isosulfan blue dye is given in one of three ways:
  ▓ directly over the tumor
  ▓ just cephalad to the prior excision scar
  ▓ in the subareolar location.

As the dye fills the dermal lymphatics, particularly in cases of reoperative SLN biopsy, one can often see lymphatic flow as a blush extending laterally toward the axilla or medially toward the IMN.

Scanning the Breast

▓ By using a handheld gamma probe, we scan the breast, identifying and marking the following:
  ▓ the site of isotope injection
  ▓ any hot spots in the axillary or parasternal areas
  ▓ any hot spots in between (suggesting the presence of intramammary SLN).

Planning the Incision

▓ For patients having mastectomy, the skin incisions are marked out appropriately for conventional, skin-sparing, or skin-and-nipple-sparing mastectomy. If immediate reconstruction is planned, the incision is designed in collaboration with the plastic surgeon.

▓ For patients having BCT, a circumareolar or transverse skin-line incision is made relatively close to the tumor site but placed in such a way that if a completion mastectomy were required, the excision scar could be encompassed with minimal skin sacrifice. The breast incision should be of adequate length to allow good exposure for both the tumor excision and the IM-SLN biopsy.

▓ For mastectomy, the axillary SLN biopsy is usually done either through a small axillary counterincision or through the lateral portion of the mastectomy incision, prior to removal of the breast.

▓ For BCT, the axillary SLN biopsy is almost always done through a separate axillary incision (except perhaps for tumors very high in the axillary tail).

▓ For mastectomy, the IM-SLN biopsy is easily done through the mastectomy incision after removal of the breast.

▓ For BCT, the IM-SLN biopsy is done through the breast incision by dissecting in the retromammary fascial plane and retracting the breast medially as needed to expose the parasternal area. This is easily done even through lateral excision cavities. Some report using a separate parasternal breast incision for IM-SLN biopsy (21,22), but we have never found this to be necessary.

Exposing the IMN

▓ After identification of one or more hot spots parasternally (most commonly in the second, third, or fourth interspaces) (Figs. 11.3 and 11.4), the pectoralis major is split in the direction of its fibers (Fig. 11.5), exposing the intercostal muscles. These are carefully divided from the sternal border laterally for approximately 3 to 4 cm (Fig. 11.6). Lateral to this, the parietal pleura forms a single layer. Medially, the pleura splits into an anterior and posterior portion, with the IMN, IM artery, and IM veins lying between the anterior and posterior pleural leaflets (Fig. 11.7).

▓ After division of the intercostal muscles parasternally, the fatty tissue containing the IMN and IM vessels is seen directly beneath the thin anterior layer of the pleura. The lung may be seen moving beneath the pleura more laterally where the anterior and posterior pleural layers have fused. The anterior layer of pleura is carefully divided proceeding from the sternal border laterally.

▓ The goal is to expose the IMN and vessels but not to divide the pleura so far laterally that one enters the pleural cavity.

Part III: Lymph Node Mapping and Dissection

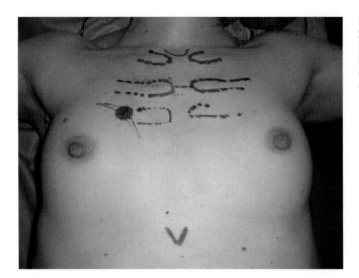

Figure 11.3 The tumor is at 2 o'clock position in the right breast, overlying the third rib. Lymphoscintigraphy has shown drainage to both axillary and internal mammary–sentinel lymph node.

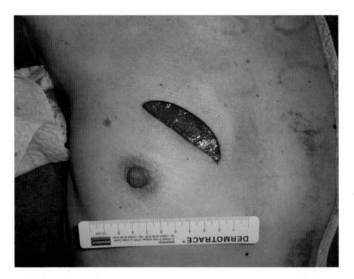

Figure 11.4 The tumor has been widely excised to the level of the pectoral fascia, overlying the second interspace, where the gamma probe has identified a hot spot.

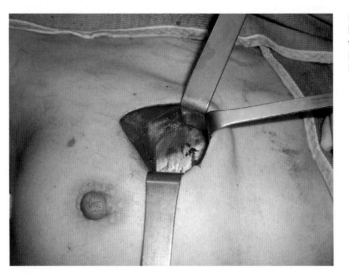

Figure 11.5 The pectoralis major has been separated in the direction of its fibers, exposing the intercostal muscles of the second interspace.

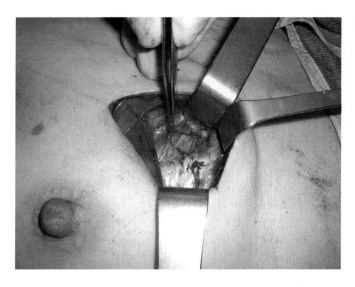

Figure 11.6 Dissection is performed through the intercostal muscles, proceeding from the sternal border laterally.

Excising the IMN

▤ The IMN area is carefully inspected and scanned to identify any blue and/or hot nodes, which, in general, are much smaller than axillary nodes and can be found either medial or lateral to the IM artery and (usually) paired IM veins (Fig. 11.8).

▤ The IMN are dissected free with gentle sharp and blunt dissection, taking care not to injure the vessels, removing if necessary the adjacent fatty tissue, and submitting each node as a separate specimen labeled by interspace of origin and position relative to the vessels (medial or lateral) (Figs. 11.9 and 11.10).

▤ The IMN are submitted for permanent pathology, not frozen section. Processing, as for axillary SLN, includes serial sections and staining with hematoxylin/eosin and anticytokeratins.

Problems with Identification and/or Excision

▤ IM-SLN biopsy is usually simple and straightforward, taking 5 to 10 minutes, but this is not always the case, and the surgeon must carefully weigh the small benefit of IM-SLN biopsy against the added morbidity of a more extended procedure.

▤ IM-SLNs that are inaccessible beneath the sternum or manubrium should be left in place.

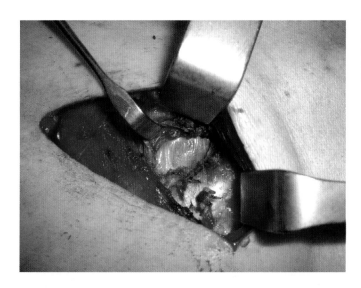

Figure 11.7 The anterior extension of the parietal pleura is seen overlying the internal mammary nodes and internal mammary vessels.

Part III: Lymph Node Mapping and Dissection

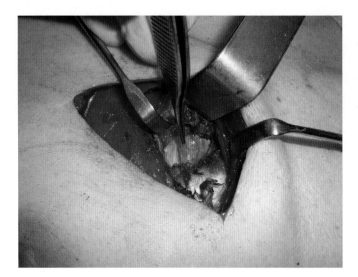

Figure 11.8 The pleura is carefully divided to expose the packet of fatty tissue that surrounds the internal mammary (IM) nodes, IM arteries, and IM veins, and staying within 2 and 3 cm of the sternal border to avoid entering the pleural cavity. No blue staining is apparent.

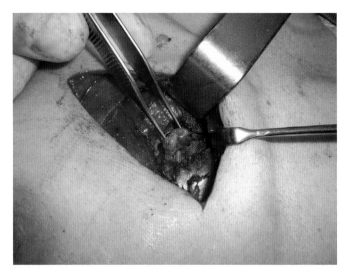

Figure 11.9 The internal mammary (IM) node with some adjacent fatty tissue is mobilized off the posterior extension of the parietal pleura, taking care not to enter the pleural cavity or to injure the IM vessels. The IM vein is visible medially at the sternal border, and the IM artery lateral to this, just posterior to packet of fatty tissue containing the IM-sentinel lymph node.

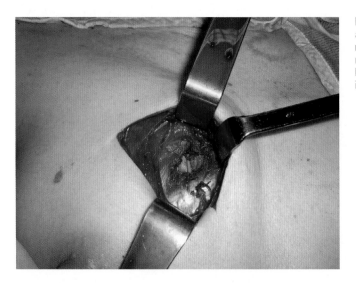

Figure 11.10 The operative field after removal of the internal mammary (IM)-sentinel lymph node and prior to closure. Just lateral to the IM artery, the pleura is bulging slightly but is intact.

- IM-SLNs that are inaccessible within a very tight interspace (usually the fourth or fifth) or behind the costal cartilages should, in general, also be left, although the removal of a small segment of costal cartilage for exposure is usually safe.
- IM-SLNs that are adherent to deeper structures or part of a large underlying tumor mass should be biopsied but not excised (more radical chest wall resections are reserved for patients who have failed chemotherapy and RT and should not in general be done de novo).
- Bleeding from small vessels is easily controlled with cautery, but significant bleeding from inadvertent injury to the IM arteries or veins may require ligation/clipping of the vessels (either through the adjacent interspaces or by resection of a costal cartilage for exposure).
- Inadvertent entry into the pleural cavity is easily recognized and treated. Some recommend suturing the pleural defect, but since the pleura is stretched tightly between the ribs, this is easier said than done. For patients under positive pressure ventilation, we prefer to hyperinflate the lungs and cover the pleural defect with a plug of moistened Surgicel, held in place by the overlying muscle layers. For patients under nonendotracheal anesthesia (i.e., breathing on their own), we simply evacuate the pneumothorax with a red rubber catheter, plug the pleural defect, and pull the catheter.

Wound Closure and Postoperative Care

- The intercostal muscles cannot be closed, but the pectoralis major is reapproximated over the IM-SLN biopsy site and the operative incisions are closed conventionally, with drains as needed.
- After IM-SLN biopsy, all patients have chest radiographs taken. Stable patients with pneumothorax are monitored with serial chest radiographs, and chest tubes are almost never required.

 COMPLICATIONS

- IM-SLN biopsy has little morbidity. In the six comparable series of IM-SLN biopsy (Table 11.1) (21,23–27), entry into the pleural cavity occurred in approximately 1% of patients, most of whom did not develop pneumothorax, and significant hemorrhage from the IM arteries or veins occurred in less than 1%.
- We have previously reported a similar rate of complications among 142 IM-SLN biopsy procedures done at our institution and the European Institute of Oncology (EIO) (28), and the EIO has recently updated its own experience in 663 patients, with similar results (29).

TABLE 11.1	Comparable Series of Internal Mammary–Sentinel Lymph Node Biopsy			
Author/year	**IMN imaged***	**IMN found***	**IMN positive***	**IMN-only positive***
Estourgie et al./2003[21] (*N* = 691)	**22%**	**19%** (86%)	**3%** (16%)	**1.3%** (43%)
Farrus et al./2004[23] (*N* = 120)	**17%**	**12%** (71%)	**1.6%** (13%)	0 (0)
Paredes et al./2005[24] (*N* = 391)	**14%**	**8%** (57%)	**2.8%** (35%)	**0.3%** (11%)
Leidenius et al./2006[25] (*N* = 984)	**14%**	**11%** (79%)	**1.8%** (16%)	**0.8%** (44%)
Madsen et al./2007[26] (*N* = 505)	**22%**	**17%** (77%)	**4%** (24%)	**1%** (25%)
Heuts et al./2007[27] *N* = 1008	**20%**	**14%** (70%)	**3%** (21%)	**0.9%** (30%)

*Bold percentages represent the proportion of the *total number of patients mapped,* percentages in parentheses represent the proportion *of the preceding column.*

Part III: Lymph Node Mapping and Dissection

RESULTS

- Selection bias affects most case series on IM-SLN biopsy, including our own (28), since the criteria for performing IM-SLN biopsy are not consistently clear. The most useful results come from the six series (comprising 3,699 patients), in which the authors systematically aimed to perform IM-SLN biopsy in *all patients who demonstrated IMN drainage* (Table 11.1) (21,23–27).
- IM-SLN were positive in 13% to 35% of patients in whom they were found at surgery; this proportion is similar to that identified by ERM (19%–33%) (7) and suggests that the staging accuracy of IM-SLN biopsy is reasonable; this of course could be proven with certainty only if all patients having an attempted IM-SLN biopsy also had a "backup chest wall resection" to examine the remaining IMN.
- Examined *as a proportion of the previous step* (Table 11.1), IM-SLNs
  - are imaged in 14% to 22% of patients,
  - are found at surgery in 57% to 86% of those imaged,
  - are positive in 13% to 35% of IM-SLNs found at surgery, and
  - are the sole site of nodal metastases in 11% to 44% of IM-SLN positives.
- Examined as *the proportion of all patients having SLN mapping*, IM-SLNs
  - were imaged in 14% to 22%,
  - were found at surgery in 12% to 19%,
  - were positive in 1.6% to 4%, and
  - were the only site of nodal metastasis in 0% to 1.3%.
- Of these few patients with nodal metastases limited to the IM-SLN, only a subset would be changed to systemic therapy—*those who were not already candidates for chemo- or hormonal therapy based on other criteria*—and only a minority of this subset would actually receive a survival benefit from the additional treatment (30).
- Some have argued that IM-SLN biopsy would allow greater selectivity in the use of RT, but if local recurrence develops in fewer than 1% of patients who received no IMN treatment at all (10,11), then we would argue that there is little reason to give RT in the first place.

CONCLUSIONS

- IMN metastases
  - are present in approximately 20% of all patients with invasive breast cancer,
  - are prognostically equivalent to axillary node metastases, and
  - even if untreated will rarely cause local recurrence.
- *As a proportion of all patients having SLN mapping*, IM-SLNs
  - were imaged in 14% to 22%,
  - were found at surgery in 12% to 19%,
  - were positive in 1.6% to 4%, and
  - were the only site of nodal metastasis in 0% to 1.3%.
- IM-SLN biopsy is reasonable for patients
  - with lymphatic drainage exclusively to the IMN and
  - with drainage to the IMN and axilla who would not otherwise receive systemic adjuvant therapy.
- IM-SLN biopsy for patients with suspiciously enlarged IMN is debatable.
- IM-SLN biopsy will play a growing role in the reoperative setting for the treatment of ipsilateral breast tumor recurrence, since prior axillary surgery may have altered the lymphatic drainage of the breast and nonaxillary drainage is much more frequent in this setting.
- Since both the benefit and the risk of IM-SLN biopsy are overall quite small, the challenge for the surgeon is to select for this operation only those patients who are most likely to benefit.

References

1. Stibbe EP. The internal mammary lymphatic glands. *J Anat.* 1918;52:258–264.

2. Handley RS, Thackray AC. Invasion of the internal mammary lymph glands in carcinoma of the breast (The Bradshaw Lecture). *Br J Surg.* 1947;1:15–20.

3. Urban JA. Radical mastectomy in continuity with en bloc resection of internal mammary lymph node chain: new procedure for primary operable cancer of breast. *Cancer.* 1952;5:992–1008.

4. Urban JA. Radical excision of the chest wall for mammary cancer. *Cancer.* 1951;4:1263–1285.

5. Veronesi U, Valagussa P. Inefficacy of internal mammary nodes dissection in breast cancer surgery. *Cancer.* 1981;47:170–175.

6. Veronesi U, Marubini E, Mariani L, et al. The dissection of internal mammary nodes does not improve the survival of breast cancer patients: 30-year results of a randomised trial. *Eur J Cancer.* 1999;35:1320–1325.

7. Klauber-DeMore N, Bevilacqua JB, VanZee KJ, et al. Comprehensive review of the management of internal mammary metastases in breast cancer. *J Am Coll Surg.* 2001;193:547–555.

8. Veronesi U, Cascinelli N, Bufalino R. Risk of internal mammary lymph node metastases and its relevance on prognosis of breast cancer patients. *Ann Surg.* 1983;198:681–684.

9. Cody HS, Urban JA. Internal mammary node status: a major prognosticator in axillary node-negative breast cancer. *Ann Surg Oncol.* 1995;2:32–37.

10. Fisher B, Redmond C, Fisher E. Ten-year results of a randomized clinical trial comparing radical mastectomy and total mastectomy with or without radiation. *N Engl J Med.* 1985;312:674–681.

11. Harris EE, Hwang WT, Seyednejad F, et al. Prognosis after regional lymph node recurrence in patients with stage I-II breast carcinoma treated with breast conservation therapy. *Cancer.* 2003;98:2144–2151.

12. Early Breast Cancer Trialists' Collaborative Group. Effects of radiotherapy and of differences in the extent of surgery for early breast cancer on local recurrence and 15-year survival: an overview of the randomised trials. *Lancet.* 2005;366:2087–2106.

13. Kim T, Giuliano AE, Lyman GH. Lymphatic mapping and sentinel lymph node biopsy in early-stage breast carcinoma. *Cancer.* 2006;106:4–16.

14. Estourgie SH, Nieweg OE, Olmos RA, et al. Lymphatic drainage patterns from the breast. *Ann Surg.* 2004;239:232–237.

15. Port ER, Fey J, Gemignani ML, et al. Reoperative sentinel lymph node biopsy: a new option for patients with primary or locally recurrent breast carcinoma. *J Am Coll Surg.* 2002;195:167–172.

16. Port ER, Garcia-Etienne CA, Park J, et al. Reoperative sentinel lymph node biopsy: a new frontier in the management of ipsilateral breast tumor recurrence. *Ann Surg Oncol.* 2007;14:2209–2214.

17. Cody HS, Fey J, Akhurst T, et al. Complementarity of blue dye and isotope in sentinel node localization for breast cancer: univariate and multivariate analysis of 966 procedures. *Ann Surg Oncol.* 2001;8:13–19.

18. McCarter MD, Yeung H, Yeh SDJ, et al. Localization of the sentinel node in breast cancer: identical results with same-day and day-before isotope injection. *Ann Surg Oncol.* 2001;8:682–686.

19. Tanis PJ, Nieweg OE, Valdes Olmos RA, et al. Anatomy and physiology of lymphatic drainage of the breast from the perspective of sentinel node biopsy. *J Am Coll Surg.* 2001;192:399–409.

20. Povoski SP, Olsen JO, Young DC, et al. Prospective randomized clinical trial comparing intradermal, intraparenchymal, and subareolar injection routes for sentinel lymph node mapping and biopsy in breast cancer. *Ann Surg Oncol.* 2006;13:1412–1421.

21. Estourgie SH, Tanis PJ, Nieweg OE, et al. Should the hunt for internal mammary chain sentinel nodes begin? An evaluation of 150 breast cancer patients. *Ann Surg Oncol.* 2003;10:935–941.

22. van der Ent FW, Kengen RA, van der Pol HA, et al. Halsted revisited: internal mammary sentinel lymph node biopsy in breast cancer. *Ann Surg.* 2001;234:79–84.

23. Farrus B, Vidal-Sicart S, Velasco M, et al. Incidence of internal mammary node metastases after a sentinel lymph node technique in breast cancer and its implication in the radiotherapy plan. *Int J Radiat Oncol Biol Phys.* 2004;60:715–721.

24. Paredes P, Vidal-Sicart S, Zanon G, et al. Clinical relevance of sentinel lymph nodes in the internal mammary chain in breast cancer patients. *Eur J Nucl Med Mol Imaging.* 2005;32:1283–1287.

25. Leidenius MH, Krogerus LA, Toivonen TS, et al. The clinical value of parasternal sentinel node biopsy in breast cancer. *Ann Surg Oncol.* 2006;13:321–326.

26. Madsen E, Gobardhan P, Bongers V, et al. The impact on post-surgical treatment of sentinel lymph node biopsy of internal mammary lymph nodes in patients with breast cancer. *Ann Surg Oncol.* 2007;14:1486–1492.

27. Heuts EM, Van der Ent FWC, von Meyenfeldt MF, et al. Internal mammary lymph node drainage and sentinel node biopsy in breast cancer—a study on 1008 patients. *Eur J Surg Oncol.* 2009;35:252–257.

28. Sacchini G, Borgen PI, Galimberti V, et al. Surgical approach to internal mammary lymph node biopsy. *J Am Coll Surg.* 2001;193:709–713.

29. Veronesi U, Arnone P, Veronesi P, et al. The value of radiotherapy on metastatic internal mammary nodes in breast cancer: results on a large series. *Ann Oncol.* 2008;19:1553–1560.

30. Early Breast Cancer Trialists' Collaborative Group. Effects of chemotherapy and hormonal therapy for early breast cancer on recurrence and 15-year survival: an overview of the randomised trials. *Lancet.* 2005;365:1687–1717.

Part III: Lymph Node Mapping and Dissection

12 Axillary Lymph Node Dissection

Elizabeth A. Shaughnessy

The axillary lymph node dissection emerged as a procedure separate from mastectomy when lumpectomy (or partial mastectomy or segmentectomy or tylectomy) became an established option for breast cancer patients with focal, resectable disease. The status of the axilla constitutes a stronger prognostic indicator than the tumor size (1); hence, knowledge of the extent of axillary involvement is critical in staging and, by inference, in treatment.

Historically, advocates for complete lymph node removal in the surgical management of disease date back to the 16th century. Our more modern surgical heritage extends back to Halsted, who advocated a complete axillary lymph node removal in his report of the radical mastectomy. He was strongly influenced by his colleague Charles Moore, whose concept of disease transmission in continuity via the lymphatics was adopted by Halsted in his development of the radical mastectomy (2,3). His publication of long-term survival following his results led to the foundation of the scientific method as applied to the field of surgery, which paved the way for clinical trials.

The advent of the sentinel node as a tool in the decision for further axillary management has led to fewer axillary lymph node dissections. This was the ultimate intent for the patient, since the full dissection is associated with potential lymphatic, neural, and vascular complications. The completion of an axillary lymph node dissection following a prior sentinel node biopsy lends further challenge to the surgical process, depending on the extent of the inflammatory reaction. Those currently in training and those who will train in the future will enter the workforce with less working familiarity with the process of an axillary lymph node dissection. It is incumbent upon those who possess a working familiarity to communicate it to the surgical generations of the future, learning from those more familiar with its nuances and challenges.

INDICATIONS/CONTRAINDICATIONS

An axillary lymph node dissection is performed within the context of a modified radical mastectomy for the treatment of inflammatory breast cancer and within the context of known positive ipsilateral lymph nodes for early breast cancer. In the context of a prior sentinel lymph node biopsy, this would be indicated by adenocarcinoma within the node. The NSABP B-32 trial randomized patients to completion axillary lymph node dissection versus completion axillary lymph node dissection only with the presence of a positive sentinel lymph node (4). Among those with any positive sentinel nodes, further nodal involvement was identified in 29% of the patients. With the growing incorporation of ultrasound as applied to breast, the identification of suspicious ipsilateral nodes has led to greater frequency in fine needle aspiration under ultrasound guidance of these nodes prior to any surgical procedure. This may lessen the overall cost of operative management, since a positive result would prompt an axillary lymph node dissection, whereas a negative result would prompt at least a sentinel lymph node biopsy.

On rare occasion, the injection of radioisotope or blue dye in the context of an axillary sentinel lymph node biopsy may fail to migrate to the axilla despite maneuvers to enhance such (warmth, massage, injection of parenchyma with sterile saline). The incidence of failure of these lymphatic markers to migrate has been documented as less than 3% in the context of community surgeons (4). Knowledge of axillary nodal involvement, as the prognostic factor of greatest impact, is needed for adequate staging; a completion axillary lymph node dissection would generally then be the default procedure.

The role of axillary lymph node dissection is under scrutiny relative to its role in early breast cancer. The question of whether to complete the axillary dissection becomes more complicated when dealing with a micrometastasis or single cells of those with restricted axillary access because of marked reduction in range of motion. In these cases, one may be unable to complete an axillary lymph node dissection, in the context of a positive sentinel lymph node, or one may pause to question the relative benefit. Certainly, adequate treatment of the axilla is indicated regardless, with radiotherapy often playing a larger role in regional control of the axilla (5).

The finding of negative sentinel node(s), if done appropriately, would not prompt a completion axillary lymph node dissection unless the operator was not confident of his or her ability to identify a sentinel lymph node, as when a surgeon may be in his or her learning curve or when circumstances bring the accuracy of the sentinel lymph node into question. Furthermore, surgeons today generally do not perform an axillary lymph node dissection in the context of ductal carcinoma in situ (DCIS), unless a sentinel lymph node biopsy was performed that demonstrated nodal metastases. Performance of a sentinel lymph node biopsy with the finding of comedo-type DCIS is supported (6), but performance of a sentinel lymph node before a mastectomy for extensive DCIS is also well founded.

PREOPERATIVE PLANNING

In the context of preoperative planning, assessment of the axilla, by either ultrasound and fine needle aspiration (FNA) or prior sentinel lymph node biopsy, may have taken place. There is a role for intraoperative sentinel node assessment, either by frozen section or by touch prep cytology, with completion axillary lymph node dissection to follow if positive. Known nodal involvement prompts studies to assess the extent of disease since nodal involvement is associated with a higher rate of distant disease (7); metastatic disease generally prompts systemic therapy, with surgical management only in select circumstances (8–9). These tests would include a bone scan and computed tomography scans of the chest and abdomen to assess the bone, lungs, and liver. Brain magnetic resonance imaging would be ordered selectively on the basis of patient symptoms.

Early education of the patient regarding drain management helps both to better prepare the patient and to support family or friends for the postoperative state. Finally, in scheduling a patient who has undergone neoadjuvant chemotherapy for surgery that will include a full axillary lymph node dissection, extra time needs to be budgeted beyond what is typical for that individual surgeon. A robust response to chemotherapy may generate an extensive scarring within the axilla, thickening fascial layers or obscuring anatomic landmarks that ultimately will slow surgical progress and dissection.

Finally, a discussion with the anesthesiologist prior to surgery may be warranted if you desire the patient not to be paralyzed during the course of surgery. If the patient is not paralyzed, testing large motor nerves can be done definitively.

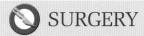 SURGERY

Relevant Anatomy

The axilla to be dissected is contained within an upside-down pyramid that runs from the axillary vein as the base and the walls of the pyramid from the serratus medially, the latissimus laterally, and the teres major posteriorly. The long thoracic nerve runs medially on the serratus at the level of the axillary vein and the teres major. The thoracodorsal nerve typically runs along the medial side of the thoracodorsal vessels and can be identified beginning at the takeoff of the thoracodorsal vessels from the axillary vein (Fig. 12.1).

Positioning

The positioning of the patient is key to one's success in both intraoperative exposure and postoperative patient recovery. Typically, the patient is placed in the supine position, with the ipsilateral arm on an armboard, at approximately a right angle to the body. Including the ipsilateral arm in the prepped field gives greater flexibility in future intraoperative exposure. Be attentive to the patient's preoperative upright posture. The patient with somewhat rounded, stooped shoulders may benefit from an additional blanket under the shoulders to bring the shoulders into their usual position, while the patient is supine (Fig. 12.2). If the shoulders are brought more forward with a blanket, then

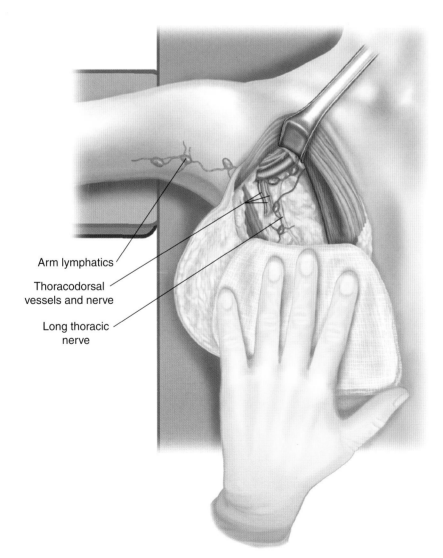

Arm lymphatics

Thoracodorsal
vessels and nerve

Long thoracic
nerve

Figure 12.1 Overview of axillary anatomy. The anatomy of the axilla includes a fat pad that is roughly an inverted pyramide containing lymphatics and lymph nodes inferior to the axillary vein. Critical neural structures include the thoracodorsal neurovascular bundle and the long thoracic nerve. The anterior border is defined by the pectoralis major muscle and the posterior border by the lattissimus dorsi muscle. Arm lymphatics can extend inferior to the axillary vein.

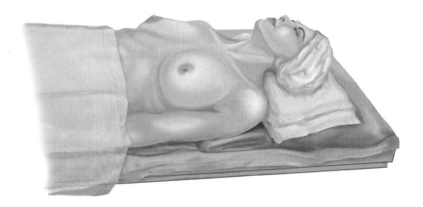

Figure 12.2 Positioning of the patient. Most patients are placed flat on the operating table. In the context of a patient with stooped shoulders because of large breasts, or in an older patient with stooped posture, the placement of padding under the upper torso and head can assist the anesthesiologist in the access of the airway for intubation, especially if the patient has an anterior airway. It may also help to reduce traction on the brachial plexus by maintaining the body posturing during the surgery.

additional supplemental padding should be placed on the arm boards to raise the upper extremities to the same level as the shoulder. This maneuver helps to prevent pulling along the nerves of the brachial plexus (Fig. 12.3).

I prefer the body to be positioned along the side of the table on the side to be approached operatively. Finally, for potential maneuverability medially under the pectoralis muscle, I position a rigid ether screen at the head of the operating table, with the crossing bar at approximately the level of the nose. This bar can be used later for suspending the arm brought up anterior to the face during the nodal dissection, if the pectoralis minor muscle is far more medial under the pectoralis major muscle (Fig. 12.4). The operating surgeon stands next to the operating table next to the thorax, whereas the assistant stands above the armboard, next to the head (Fig. 12.5).

Special Equipment

The special equipment may vary depending on the patient's anatomy or the needs of the case, especially if combined with other procedures. A headlamp should be considered if the patient is a larger individual and there will be an incision for the axillary lymph node dissection separate from an incision for the breast; it may be considered in the patient having a skin-sparing incision, where there will not be a separate incision for the axilla.

I prefer a right angle for blunt dissection, utilizing electrocautery for most dissections. If reduction of drainage is desired, the division of tissue can also be approached by using the harmonic scalpel to seal the lymphatics in the course of the dissection.

Figure 12.3 Positioning of the patient. If blankets or padding is maintained under the patient during the surgical procedure, then the upper extremity must be at the same height to avoid overextension of the brachial plexus.

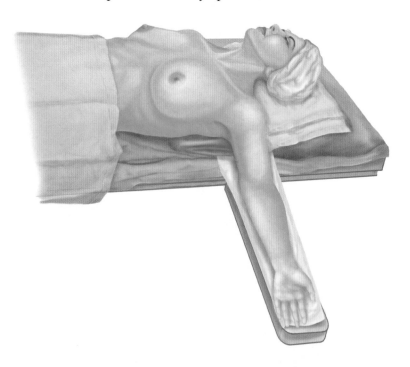

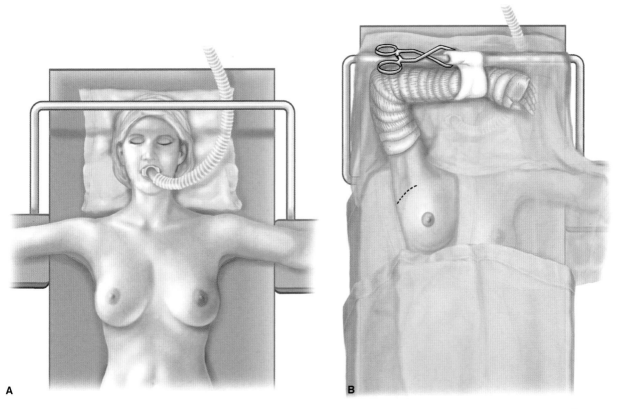

A

B

Figure 12.4 Positioning of the patient. The patient who is large may have a deep dissection within the axilla to complete at level II. To open up the axilla easily during the operation, a rigid ether screen is first attached to the table before the patient is prepped and draped. **A.** The crossbar is placed at approximately the level of the nose or slightly higher. Should higher axillary access be needed, the pectoralis muscles can be retracted more medially by suspending the hand and arm from the crossbar as shown. The upper extremity must be prepped into the field. **B.** The wrist is then wrapped with a towel and the towel folded over the drape and crossbar. A wide clamp, such as the mandibular clamp, is placed over the towel, drape, and crossbar, thereby suspending the arm over the upper chest and face. (Modified from Bland KI, Copeland EM II, eds. *The Breast: Comprehensive Management of Benign and Malignant Disorders.* 3rd ed. Philadelphia: WB Saunders, 2004.)

This usually takes more time; furthermore, there is a learning curve in terms of speed of use and coordination with one's assistant. The technique can be particularly valuable when approaching surgery in patients in whom you may be having difficulty with surgical oozing, who have a pacemaker or automated implantable cardioverter–defibrillator and one is concerned about electrical stimuli, or those who may be at risk of bleeding as they were on clopidogrel, warfarin, or aspirin.

Incision

The incision utilized may vary greatly, depending on the surgical management of the breast. As mentioned earlier, should a skin-sparing incision be used or should the patient's breast skin envelope remaining after mastectomy be of sufficient size, the opening from the mastectomy can be positioned over the axilla so as to allow the entire dissection through that opening; a separate incision may not be necessary. Similarly, within the incision utilized for a modified radical mastectomy done without skin-sparing, the full axillary lymph node dissection may be performed without additional incision (Fig. 12.6).

Alternately, a skin-sparing incision does not always allow for the dissection, and a separate counter incision is made in the axilla or as an extension of a prior sentinel lymph node biopsy incision. The incision made would be the same as one would use in conjunction with lumpectomy, extending from the anterior to the posterior axillary fold, preferably below the area bearing hair, in a preexisting skin fold (Fig. 12.7). When a separate incision is necessary, skin flaps need to be raised superiorly to the axillary fold and inferiorly to approximately the lateral extent of the inframammary fold.

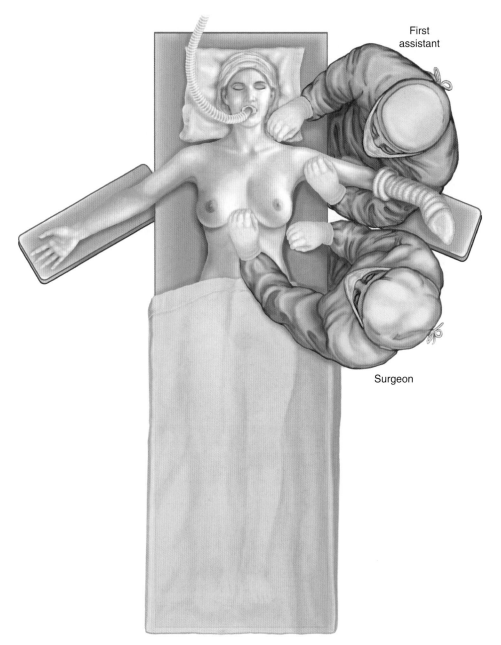

Figure 12.5 Positioning of the surgical team for the axillary lymph node dissection mirrors that of the simple mastectomy, with the assistant cephalad to the arm-board and surgeon caudad to it. (Modified from Bland KI, Copeland EM II, eds. *The Breast: Comprehensive Management of Benign and Malignant Disorders.* 3rd ed. Philadelphia: WB Saunders, 2004.)

First assistant

Surgeon

Defining Axillary Extent

The next steps within the axillary dissection focus on defining the borders of the axillary dissection. More easily, dissection along the lateral pectoral major border is performed, isolating this edge. The pectoralis major muscle is then retracted medially, exposing the pectoralis minor muscle.

At this point, an interpectoral dissection can be performed, especially if any Rotter nodes are suspected to be enlarged. At the medial surface of the pectoralis minor muscle, the advential tissues is carefully divided by using the electrocautery, taking care to preserve the muscle and the medial pectoral neurovascular bundle, which innervates both the pectoralis major and minor muscles, located near the superolateral aspect. The advential tissues are placed on traction laterally, utilizing a sponge, and the advential tissues carefully teased off the surface, maintaining these tissues in continuity with the axillary contents (Fig. 12.8).

The pectoralis minor muscle is then retracted medially as well, allowing for the division of the more posterior layers of the clavipectoral (or axillary) fascia. These

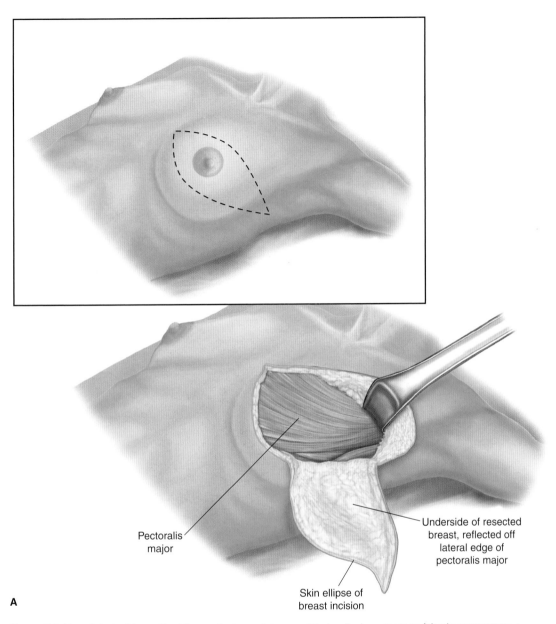

Pectoralis
major

Underside of resected
breast, reflected off
lateral edge of
pectoralis major

Skin ellipse of
breast incision

A

Figure 12.6 Use of the incision utilized for mastectomy. **A.** In a modified radical mastectomy (simple mastectomy + axillary lymph node dissection), an elliptical incision is utilized. The breast can be oriented with sutures or other device and excised separate from the axillary contents, or the breast can be classically maintained in continuity with the axillary contents. This will require transfer of the breast from resting on the lateral aspect of the operating table at times to resting on the chest wall. (*continued*)

fascial layers are then carefully divided, just deep to the pectoralis minor border. The attention is then turned to defining the lateral border of the latissimus dorsi muscle. With palpation, this border can be located and combined blunt dissection with electrocautery used to define this edge. Inferiorly, observe that the border pulls close to the chest wall. The dissection need not go farther in that direction. Superiorly, care is taken not to travel beyond the transition to the tendon of insertion as this brings the surgeon precariously close to the axillary vein. Within this dissection, one is likely to encounter branches of the intercostobrachial nerve, usually within 2 cm of the lower aspect of the axillary vein. It is typically difficult to spare branches that lie farther from the vein than a 0.5 cm. When encountering branches of this nerve that cannot be spared, ligation in continuity should be performed by utilizing clips or ties and dividing sharply to avoid

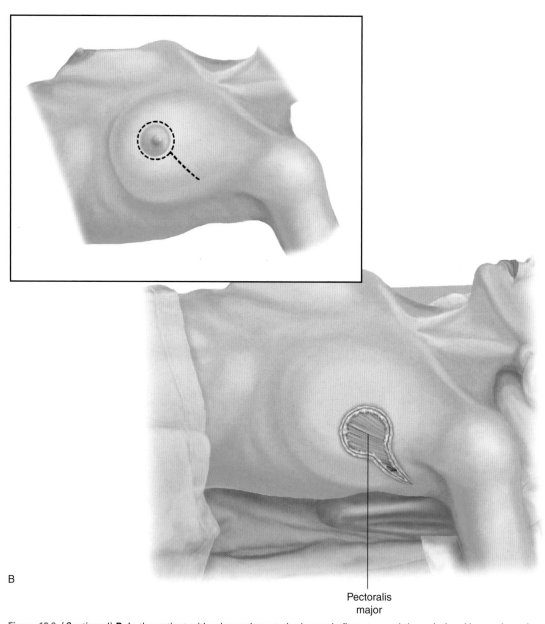

B

Pectoralis
major

Figure 12.6 (*Continued*) **B.** In the patient with a larger breast, the breast is first removed through the skin envelop prior to axillary lymph node dissection. The opening for the skin envelope may have sufficient loss of volume such that the opening can be placed over the axilla, allowing for a dissection without addition incision.

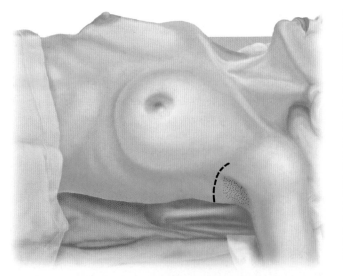

Figure 12.7 Use of a separate incision for axillary lymph node dissection. Should the patient having a skin-sparing incision have a small breast envelope, a counter incision within the axilla can be planned, generally without causing ischemia to the flap. The same incision can also be utilized if axillary lymph node dissection is performed in conjunction with a partial mastectomy or in another setting. The incision preferably is placed under the area bearing hair, following skin line folds or a preexisting skin fold, from the anterior axillary fold (pectoralis major muscle lateral edge) to the posterior axillary fold (latissimus dorsi muscle lateral edge).

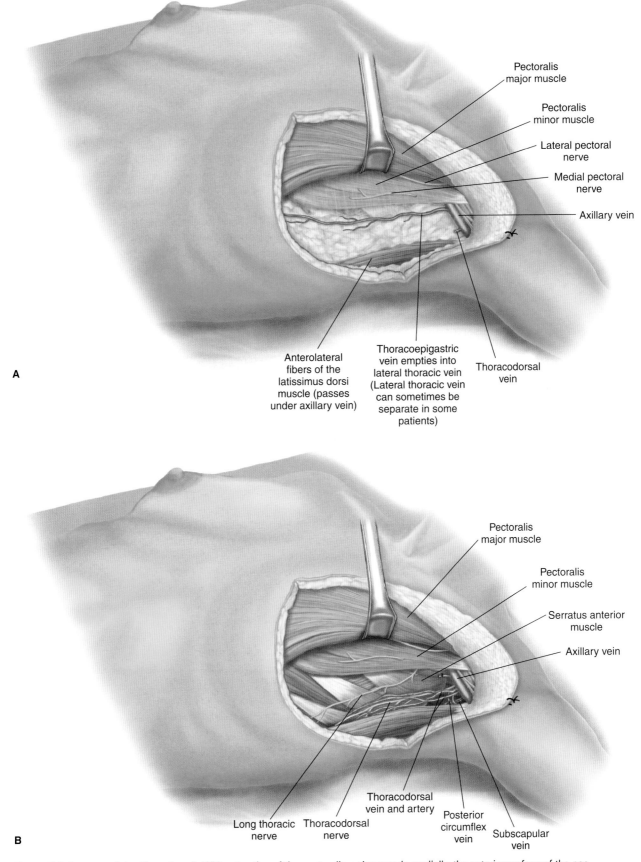

A

Pectoralis major muscle

Pectoralis minor muscle

Lateral pectoral nerve

Medial pectoral nerve

Axillary vein

Anterolateral fibers of the latissimus dorsi muscle (passes under axillary vein)

Thoracoepigastric vein empties into lateral thoracic vein (Lateral thoracic vein can sometimes be separate in some patients)

Thoracodorsal vein

B

Pectoralis major muscle

Pectoralis minor muscle

Serratus anterior muscle

Axillary vein

Long thoracic nerve

Thoracodorsal nerve

Thoracodorsal vein and artery

Posterior circumflex vein

Subscapular vein

Figure 12.8 Anatomy of the dissection. **A.** With retraction of the pectoralis major muscle medially, the anterior surface of the pectoralis minor muscle is visualized through adventitial tissue. The adventitia is incised along the medial anterior surface of the pectoralis minor muscle. With this adventitia placed on tension laterally, it can be slowly peeled off the anterior surface of the pectoralis minor muscle with the assistance of the electrocautery, keeping the adventitia and any Rotter nodes in continuity with the axillary contents. **B.** Once the lateral borders of the pectoralis major muscle and latissimus dorsi muscles have been exposed up to the level of the axillary vein, tension on the fat pad inferiorly helps to expose the inferior venous tributaries.

proximal and distal electrical conduction. Ligation of the nerve sheath may help to avoid neuroma formation postoperatively.

If one suspects that the axillary vein is near but cannot visualize its color or shape, certainly a pause in the dissection at that time would be prudent. One can reassess the approximate expected level of the axillary vein near the level of the medial arm, should the arm be out at a right angle to the body. Be aware that the axillary vein (10) can often be found to bifurcate, and rarely trifurcate, within the axillary space. Hence, transverse venous structures high in the axilla, even if they are not as large as expected for an axillary vein, should not be ligated as they may be part of a divided system.

With these two borders defined—anterior and posterior—the axillary contents are placed on gentle traction inferiorly, allowing one to catch a glimpse of the axillary vein between two fat lobules or planes that separate with the traction, if it has not yet already been identified. Once visualized, the clavipectoral fascia overlying the vein anteriorly is carefully divided by using blunt dissection and electrocautery, with the dissection carefully down to the anterior surface of the axillary vein. With the extent of the operative borders defined, the attention is then turned to the mobilization of the tissue in axillary level II.

Dissection of Axillary Level II

The pectoralis major and minor muscles are retracted medially for exposure. The acuity of the angle of the fibers of the pectoralis major muscle vary by individual; this leads to a greater or lesser amount of tissue within level II to dissect. For some, this distance may be so deep that maneuvers may be taken to obtain better exposure.

The table can be tilted away from the operating team so as to provide better exposure. It is here that the forearm, previously prepped in the field and wrapped in a stockinette, can be gently wrapped in a sterile towel about the wrist and suspended from the ether screen by using a large clamp. The clamp encompasses the towel folded over the drape and the screen (Fig. 12.9). This helps to relax the pectoralis muscles, allowing for their further retraction medially.

Again, traction is placed on the adventitial tissues below the axillary vein, and careful methodical dissection tissues is done, often with the assistance of the right angle clamp to blunt dissect away small amounts of tissue so as to identify lymphatics or small vessels that can be ligated. Care is taken to identify the location of the medial pectoral neurovascular bundle so as to better avoid it within the dissection. The mobilization includes the adventitia overlying the chest wall musculature but spares the fascia overlying it. The level II tissues are thus kept in continuity with the axillary contents as they are freed. Upon reaching the lateral extent of the chest wall, the surgeon then focuses on the completion of the axillary dissection.

Identification of Significant Neural and Vascular Structures and Dissection of Axillary Level I

Before the dissection begins, it is important to remember the courses of the long thoracic nerve (of Bell) and the thoracodorsal nerve lay posterior to the axillary vein. Whether the long thoracic nerve or the thoracodorsal nerve is dissected first is a matter of personal preference or, more likely, determined by the course of the operation and the ease with which one is able to identify these nerves.

Arbitrarily, this description begins at the chest wall, as this is where the previous discussion was left off. With the axillary vein's position known and seen, a small plane is dissected bluntly in the space below the medial aspect of the vein, approximately 1 to 1.5 cm away from the chest wall and parallel to it. This may be best begun with a clamp stretching the superficial tissues, but then this can be extended more deeply within the axillary fat pad, gradually, using two fingers, until reaching the midaxillary line. This is approximately the expected depth at which one expects to find the long thoracic nerve. A finger is inserted to the full depth of this dissection and turned so that the ventral (palmar) surface touches the chest wall. The finger is dragged along the chest wall in the posterior to anterior direction, feeling for the "violin string" rebound of the long thoracic nerve. It is not necessarily the case that you will be able to see the nerve

Figure 12.9 Positioning the patient.

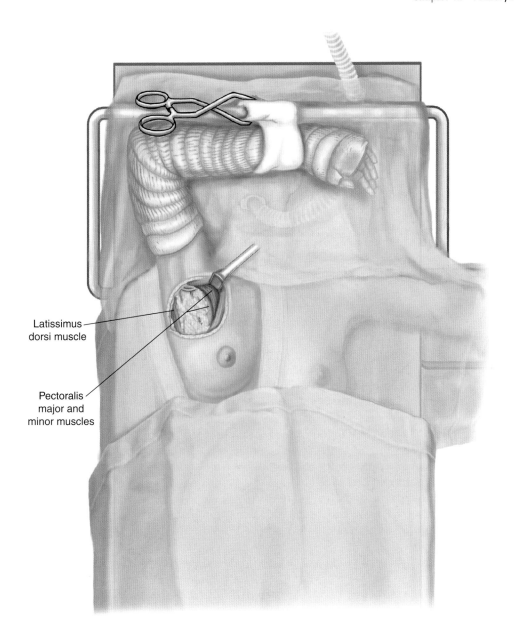

Latissimus dorsi muscle

Pectoralis major and minor muscles

Part III: Lymph Node Mapping and Dissection

in this first step of the dissection. If the nerve with its small vascular comitantes cannot be appreciated, either the dissection is not sufficiently posterior or the nerve is lateral to the plane developed, having been pushed there with the blunt dissection. First, extend the plane more posteriorly, and try again to feel for the nerve. If this is not successful, develop a new plane approximately 1 cm lateral to the first and repeat the maneuvers.

Once this nerve is identified, the plane is then extended for the length of the axillary field, keeping the long thoracic nerve intact and against the chest wall. Skeletonizing this nerve and its vascular bundle is discouraged; however, that stated, palpable lymph nodes should be mobilized laterally with the axillary contents. In doing so, the more transverse branches of the intercostobrachial nerve may be encountered; if they are not in immediate proximity of the axillary vein, it would be necessary to ligate them and divide sharply. In extending this plane inferiorly, the nerve is now better visualized. To confirm that the nerve's functional integrity is intact, it can be gently pinched with a tissue forceps such as a DeBakey forceps to activate the muscular contraction of the serratus anterior muscle. Interestingly, it has been my experience that this contraction is often difficult to initiate. I suspect that the nerve may take longer to repolarize and the dissection itself may cause some discoordinate depolarization. It may take several tries to pinch the nerve and confirm the integrity of the long thoracic nerve function in vivo.

In switching to the dissection of the thoracodorsal neurovascular, attention is directed to the venous tributaries to the axillary vein along the inferior surface. They are carefully identified and marginally dissected for a brief length (approximately 5 mm). Usually, midaxilla, there is a superficial larger tributary—the thoracoepigastric vein. Many times, this vein can be used as a marker for finding the deeper, more posterior, subscapular vein. The thoracodorsal vein is a tributary of this vein in most instances, with the circumflex and thoracodorsal vein branches combining to form the subscapular vein. On occasions, the thoracodorsal vein may actually merge with the thoracoepigastric vein at a distance of 1 to 2 cm from the axillary vein. Consequently, I do not divide the more superficial thoracoepigastric vein until such time as I have successfully identified the thoracodorsal neurovascular bundle.

In identifying a likely candidate for the thoracodorsal vein, the accompanying artery may have a variable relation to the vein; it could be medial, lateral, deep, or superficial to it. The nerve is nearly always medial to it. The nerve may course along and near the vein, beginning its path alongside the vein immediately inferior to the axillary vein, or it may take a more gradual angled course more medial, emerging from under the axillary vein more medially near the chest wall, near the long thoracic nerve at its more superior extent within the operative field. The nerve then may not be readily identifiable. Thus, it is generally safer then to begin the dissection from a lateral approach.

With a right angle or other clamp for blunt dissection, the tissue plane superficial and/or lateral to the candidate thoracodorsal neurovascular bundle is gently created, stretching the overlying tissues progressively toward the inferior aspect of the operative field. In doing so, the thoracodorsal nerve may more easily come into view. Confirmation of the presence of the nerve comes with a light pinch with the DeBakey forceps, confirming the contraction of the latissimus dorsi muscle. Once the path of the vascular bundle and that of the nerve are confirmed, the thoracoepigastric vein can be ligated and divided in proximity to the axillary vein, taking precautions to maintain a patent proximal branch if the thoracodorsal vein branches from it. Once the neurovascular bundle begins to "dive" more deeply, the dissection need not proceed more deeply. The tissue between this plane along the thoracodorsal neurovascular bundle and the edge of the latissimus dorsi muscle is then divided by using blunt dissection and electrocautery.

At this point, the remaining axillary contents are nearly ready to be excised from the axilla. In preparation for this, the tissues immediately inferior to the axillary vein are carefully dissected along its inferior aspect to the depth of the thoracodorsal neurovascular bundle. Be mindful that a branch of the intercostobrachial nerve may lie on the axillary vein's more inferior surface, and preserving it would be less morbid to the patient. Also, be aware that many of the lymphatics draining the ipsilateral upper extremity pass along the deep surface of the axilla, just inferior to the axillary vein. These may be apparent but small, tangled or draped (11), and possibly tented anteriorly if the patient is obese, pushed forward by a fat pad posterior to the depth of the thoracodorsal neurovascular bundle. Avoiding these, as long as it does not compromise removal of lymph nodes, may potentially help to reduce the incidence of postoperative ipsilateral upper extremity lymphedema.

The axillary contents are now ready for its excision. If a modified radical mastectomy was performed in this context, with the breast in continuity with the axillary contents, the breast or any axillary contents are gently lift anteriorly and medially, exposing the thoracodorsal neurovascular bundle. With the palmar surface of the dominant operating hand facing up, the index finger is placed over the neurovascular bundle and thus protecting it. The medial tissues, including the breast if applicable, are folded back over this positioned hand, exposing the now-visible long thoracic nerve. The tissues are then divided between the long thoracic nerve and the thoracodorsal neurovascular bundle by using electrocautery along the surface of the index finger, thereby avoiding both neural structures. Should there be any question as to their position as you proceed, do not hesitate to check and recheck. The axillary contents are then passed off the field to the pathologist for evaluation.

Anatomic Considerations

It is possible that a motor nerve may need to be sacrificed in the context of tumor involvement; however, neural invasion by tumor is usually accompanied by focal pain, giving the surgeon some indication that this may be the case and allowing for the potential discussion of nerve sacrifice preoperatively. Neural involvement by the tumor, however, may already affect the motor function preoperatively as though it had been sacrificed. The function will not be regained postoperatively, but the pain will resolve.

An anatomy atlas is certainly helpful in describing the most common anatomic structures, but there is considerable variability (10). Awareness of this variability allows for a safer, less morbid procedure for the patient and a smoother operation for the surgeon. As stated earlier, the axillary vein can often be bifurcated or rarely trifurcated. Consequently, the subscapular vein can be a tributary to the lower or upper branch; in my experience, it is more likely the upper branch. It is possible to locate these branches, but it likely will take extra time to do so. On occasion, there is no lateral thoracic vein against the chest wall, near the long thoracic vein; rather, there is a dominant thoracoepigastric vein that may then arch over to the chest wall to functionally drain the same region. In those cases, carefully preserve this venous branch, reflecting it medially or superiorly out of the way of the dissection once it is free of the axillary contents.

On very rare occasions, the long thoracic nerve may be very posterior. In that case, modify the dissection so that the axillary contents are removed only to the point of the midaxillary line, where the usual expected position of the long thoracic nerve would be, anticipating that a more posterior dissection could easily increase the risk of lymphedema.

In approximately 0.1% of cases, there is a lateral positioning of the thoracodorsal nerve relative to the thoracodorsal vein. In general, it does not complicate the dissection but may be confusing when one tries to test for intact function and discovers that the artery has been pinched. Rarely one may encounter a lack of a thoracodorsal neurovascular bundle proper; the thoracodorsal vein can course inferiorly to the latissimus dorsi, independent of a nerve or an artery. The artery can course separately along the lateral edge of the latissimus dorsi, a finding wholly uncharacteristic of this region, and the nerve can course medially, near (within 5 mm) and parallel to the long thoracic nerve. By preserving neural or vascular structures in unexpected positions, the anatomy can then be determined before anything critical is sacrificed.

Closure

Not surprisingly, the operative field needs to be inspected for hemostasis. Once this is ensured by whatever measures are necessary, consider placing a small clip at the uppermost of the dissection, on adventitial tissues at the apex of level II, to indicate to colleagues in radiation oncology as to the most medial aspect of the dissection. On the rare occasion that radiation is considered for the supraclavicular fossa in the adjuvant setting, the radiation oncologists may use the clips as an indicator of the extent of surgical removal in their planning of radiation fields. The field is then irrigated and inspected once again for adequacy of hemostasis before beginning the later steps of closure.

One may consider the placement of a catheter, such as that associated with the pain pump, for delivery of local anesthetic to the axilla for the first 2 to 3 days postoperatively. The insertion of the catheter system, based on the Seldinger technique, would be introduced from a medial approach, tunneling at least an inch through the subcutaneous adipose before entering the axilla superiorly over the lateral border of the pectoralis major muscle in the case of a separate axillary incision or over the superior aspect of the pectoralis muscle in the case of a modified radical mastectomy. The tip of the catheter should be gently coiled within the axilla; the external aspect of the catheter would be secured to the skin externally with Steri-Strips, tape and/or sterile plastic dressing.

Place a drain within the axilla, a flat 10 mm Jackson–Pratt drain or a round, channeled Blake drain, and bring this externally out through a stab wound in the low axilla above the bra line. In this manner, should a neuroma form at the drain exit site, it will not be frequently aggravated by the friction of a bra. The catheter is secured to the skin externally with a 3-0 nylon suture; the drain tubing is attached to a bulb. Trim the internal aspect of the drain bluntly approximately 2 to 3 cm inferior to the axillary vein. The axillary vein's position will drop with adduction of the arm, and one would prefer that the drain not be placed in direct contact if possible. If that contact does occur, a bluntly trimmed drain would be less likely to injure the vein than the one angled with a point.

Whether the axillary lymph node dissection was done in the context of skin-sparing and mastectomy or in conjunction with a mastectomy, the incision is closed per the closure techniques of the mastectomy (see Chapter 18: Simple Mastectomy). In the context of a separate axillary incision, proceed to close the skin in two layers. After placement of a skin hook at either extreme of the axillary incision to align the skin and facilitate closure, initially place an inverted simple suture within the deep dermis at the midpoint to help with maintenance of the alignment in the context of closure. As one may notice, the dermis of the axilla is very thin relative to the dermis of the breast and is thinner in the postmenopausal woman with decreased circulating estrogen level to maintain the skin and its appendages. Then close the deep dermis with a running simple suture of 3-0 Vicryl and follow with a subcuticular suture of 4-0 Monocryl. After cleansing and drying the incision and skin, place the dressing made either of Steri-Strips covered by gauze and a sterile plastic dressing or of Dermabond. Place antibiotic ointment around the drain exit site, and cover it with a sterile piece of gauze and sterile plastic dressing or tape.

 ## POSTOPERATIVE MANAGEMENT

Pain management is a greater issue with an axillary lymph node dissection than with a sentinel node biopsy. Administration of a combined narcotic/nonsteroidal anti-inflammatory drug such as acetaminophen and oxycodone (Percocet) or acetaminophen and hydrocodone (Vicodin) for 7 to 10 days is usually sufficient, although further pain management may be necessary should the drain remain in place longer than that duration.

It is wise to keep the patient at least overnight, for a 23-hour stay, to make sure that pain control is achieved. This also allows the patient the opportunity to learn aspects of drain management prior to discharge. The patient needs to be sent home with cups for measurement of the drainage volume and a drainage log to document the date and volume. While the drain is in place, the patient should not be allowed to drive; completion of a life-saving maneuver behind the wheel might be curtailed by a pause induced by the pain. Once the daily volume totals 30 mL or less, the drain is removed in the office setting. The site is then dressed with antibiotic ointment, gauze, and tape, switching to a bandage the next day. The patient is seen again a week later to make sure that a significant seroma has not formed in the interim.

Following removal of the drain, a brochure of exercises is offered to the patient, as prepared by our physical therapy department, to assist with the patient maintaining and improving her general strength and range of motion. As not every patient is sufficiently motivated or is hesitant to push herself, physical or occupational therapy should be arranged to assist the patient in returning to her prior strength and range of motion.

If the patient also had a breast procedure at the same time, or if the patient has a breast of sufficiently large size that it pulls on the axillary incision, the patient should wear a bra for the next 1 to 2 weeks to take the tension off the incision and to reduce the postoperative pain.

 ## COMPLICATIONS

Bleeding and infection remain the two most common complications following axillary lymph node dissection. Frequently, the statistics do not address the axillary lymph node dissection alone but in the context of a combined procedure with breast cancer management. The use of preoperative antibiotics in prospective, randomized studies and retrospective studies regarding management has been conflicting. Consequently, most individuals may limit the use of preoperative antibiotics to cases where wire localization of the breast is included or in high-risk individuals such as patients with diabetes mellitus. The inclusion of a drain increases the risk of perioperative infection to approximately 10% as the wound typically becomes colonized by bacteria within 4 days of its placement. The risk of leaving the drain in vivo must be balanced with the risk of pain and neurovascular compromise should the seroma fluid that accumulates compress the vasculature and neural structures of the underarm with adduction. With the placement of clips on apparent lymphatics during the dissection, the drain can usually be removed within a week, achieving less than 30 mL of drainage daily.

The reduction in lymph nodal tissue places the patient at increased risk of infection, primarily that of cellulitis. Since involvement of the draining lymphatics of the arm with infection may be a precipitating factor in the later onset of lymphedema, aggressive management of infection of that extremity is necessary to avoid this possibility.

The risk of a major blood vessel or motor neural injury is less than 1 in 1000. Certainly, laceration of the axillary vein requires immediate repair of the vein. A simple injury may be oversewn by using a 4-0 or 5-0 Prolene suture; more complex injuries may require intraoperative consultation with a vascular surgeon. Given the fragility of veins, the axillary vein is also at risk for compression or traction injury, especially given its proximity to the bulk of the axillary dissection. Injury to the long thoracic nerve can result in a winged scapula, with protrusion of the scapula. Injury to the thoracodorsal nerve weakens shoulder abduction and internal rotation, characteristic of latissimus dorsi function, but as vascular injury usually accompanies the neural injury, these vessels are then no longer available for use for potential free flap reductions and may lead to temporary vasocongestion, with later muscular atrophy. Injury to the medial pectoral neurovascular bundle is infrequent but can lead to eventual atrophy of the pectoral muscles, which can impact the overall cosmetic result. Finally, intercostobrachial nerve branches are routinely sacrificed in the context of the axillary lymph node dissection. Others report chronic neuropathic pain as a consequence of attempts to preserve these nerves. Traction on any sensory nerve can lead to temporary anesthesia, with returning function signaled by sharp stabbing pains and burning sensations. The time frame of neuropathy is on the order of weeks to months to resolve, whereas the growth of new nerves consequent to sacrificing branches of the intercostobrachial nerve is on the order of months to years. I suspect that division of nerves without occlusion of the nerve sheath may be associated with greater neuroma formation and persistent point tenderness; however, definitive studies would need to be done with long-term follow-up.

Lymphedema of the upper extremity is the dreaded risk that is less controllable in the context of this dissection. The incidence ranges from 10% to 27% depending on surgeon, extent of dissection, and the duration of follow-up. Obesity, age, and subsequent regional radiotherapy have been cited as risk factors for lymphedema. The development of lymphedema can be immediate, or it can be developed at any time later in the patient's lifetime. Participation in lymphedema therapy and aggressive physical therapy appears to offset this risk; however, later infection and scarring from lymphangitis or upper extremity trauma can prompt its onset. Lymphedema can occur in two different patterns—one of the medial proximal arm tissue only and one of the whole upper extremity. Adding the technique of axillary reverse mapping to the axillary lymph node dissection may be helpful in preventing lymphedema (See Chapter 13, Axillary Reverse Mapping).

The Stewart–Treves syndrome reflects the rare development of lymphangiosarcoma in the upper extremity affected by chronic lymphedema following axillary lymph node dissection. Generally, it is seen 10 to 20 years after treatment, and the patient has usually received regional radiotherapy as well. Limited studies suggest that there may be a genetic basis for this syndrome (12). Treatment options tend to be radical, often with poor results.

To the other extreme, the rare persistent lymphatic leak can occur, delaying drain removal, and the more rare chyle leak, supposedly from traction injury to the thoracic duct (13).

Axillary webs (14) are described as cords of tissue coursing from the surgical bed toward the arm, sometimes extending to the brachial fossa, forearm, or hand. These usually resolve with massage and physical therapy over time. This occurs in less than 10% of the patient and is generally self-limited.

RESULTS

The axillary lymph node dissection provides definitive nodal staging, a critical component of ultimate tumor stage. The combined breast cancer stage (tumor–nodal–distant metastases) ultimately guides the adjuvant therapies for treatment. Although not readily quantified, an underestimation of the nodal status would understage the patient, leading to less adequate therapy and a poorer outcome. In essence, this leads to a Will Rogers effect, shifting the stage and the outcome. This is what appears to be the case within a series of large Danish studies that examined the use of axillary radiation for local control. The authors noted that per stage, their patients' outcome did not compare with that found within the U.S. SEER data. These radiation oncologists also noted that the number of lymph nodes dissected within the axillary lymph node dissection did not contain as many nodes as that of the average dissection within SEER; they surmised that local control of the axilla was not adequate and introduced radiation to complete it. Not surprisingly, survival improved with local control (15–18).

Because the axillary lymph node dissection has been a defined method of management of axilla for nearly a century, very few studies have ever examined the outcomes of not completing the axillary lymph node dissection. Within the NSABP B-04 trial (19), the incidence of axillary recurrence within the group randomized to total mastectomy without axillary node dissection was 14% as compared with less than 2% within the group randomized to the modified radical mastectomy; the study failed to have sufficient power to address whether there was significant survival benefit from the axillary lymph node dissection.

CONCLUSIONS

The performance of an axillary lymph node dissection in the context of breast cancer metastatic to the regional lymph nodal basin is a challenging procedure. The procedure itself can provide adequate staging, regional local control, and possibly survival benefit for the individual with nodal disease.

References

1. Grube BJ, Giuliano AE. Observation of the breast cancer patient with a tumor-positive sentinel node: implications of the ACOSOG Z0011 trial. *Semin Surg Oncol.* 2001;20(3):230–237.
2. Halsted WS. I: the results of operations for the cure of cancer of the breast performed at the Johns Hopkins Hospital from June, 1889, to January, 1894. *Ann Surg.* 1894;20(5):497–555.
3. Halsted WS. I: a clinical and histological study of certain adenocarcinomata of the breast: and a brief consideration of the supraclavicular operation and of the results of operations for cancer of the breast from 1889 to 1898 at the Johns Hopkins Hospital. *Ann Surg.* 1898;28(5):557–576.
4. Krag DN, Anderson SJ, Julian TB, et al. For the National Surgical Adjuvant Brest and Bowel Project (NSABP): technical outcomes of sentinel-lymph-node resection and conventional axillary-lymph-node dissection in patients with clinically node-negative breast cancer: results from the NSABP B-32 randomised phase III trial. *Lancet.* 2007;8:881–888.
5. White JR. Axillary irradiation. In: Harris JR, Lippman ME, Morrow M, et al. eds. *Diseases of the Breast.* 4th ed. Philadelphia, PA: Wolters Kluwer/Lippincott Williams & Wilkins; 2010:570–577.
6. Yi M, Krishnamurthy S, Kuerer HM, et al. Role of primary tumor characteristics in predicting positive sentinel lymph nodes in patients lwith ductal carcinoma in situ or microinvasive breast cancer. *Am J Surg.* 2008;196(1):81–87.
7. Carlson RW, Allred DC, Anderson BO, et al. NCCN Breast Cancer Clinical Practice Guidelines Panel: breast cancer clinical practice guidelines in oncology. *J Natl Compr Cancer Network.* 2009;7(2):122–192.
8. Gnerlich J, Jeffe DB, Deshpande AD, et al. Surgical removal of the primary tumor increases overall survival in patients with metastatic breast cancer: analysis of the 1988–2003 SEER data. *Ann Surg Oncol.* 2007;14(8):2187–2194.
9. Babiera GV, Rao R, Feng L, et al. Surgical resection of the primary tumor, chest wall control, and survival in women with metastatic breast cancer. *Cancer.* 2008;113(8):2011–2019.
10. Anson BJ, McVay CB. Thoracic walls: breast or mammary region. In: Anson BJ, McVay CB, eds. *Surgical Anatomy.* 6th ed. Philadelphia, PA: Saunders; 1984:352–365.
11. Boneti C, Korourian S, Diaz Z, et al. Scientific Impact Award: axillary reverse mapping (ARM) to identify and protect lymphatics draining the arm during axillary lymphadenectomy. *Am J Surg.* 2009;198(4):482–487.
12. Roy P, Clark MA, Thomas JM. Stewart-Treves syndrome—treatment and outcome in six patients from a single centre. *Eur J Surg Oncol.* 2004;30(9):982–986.
13. Caluwe GL, Christiaens MR. Chylous leak: a rare complication after axillary lymph node dissection. *Acta Chir Belg.* 2003;103(2):217–218.
14. Moskovitz AH, Anderson BO, Yeung RS, et al. Axillary web syndrome after axillary dissection. *Am J Surg.* 2001;181(5):434–439.

15. Overgaard M, Jensen MB, Overgaard J, et al. Postoperative radiotherapy in high-risk postmenopausal breast-cancer patients given adjuvant tamoxifen: Danish Breast Cancer Cooperative Group DBCG 82c randomised trial. *Lancet*. 1999;353(9165): 1641–1648.

16. Rutqvist LE. Novel approaches using radiation therapies. *Recent Results Cancer Res*. 1998;152:255–264.

17. Overgaard M, Hansen PS, Overgaard J, et al. Postoperative radiotherapy in high-risk premenopausal women with breast cancer who receive adjuvant chemotherapy: Danish Breast Cancer Cooperative Group 82b Trial. *N Engl J Med*. 1997;337(14):949–955.

18. Van de Steene J, Soete G, Storme G. Adjuvant radiotherapy for breast cancer significantly improves overall survival: the missing link. *Radiother Oncol*. 2000;55(3):263–272.

19. Fisher B, Redmond C, Fisher ER, et al. Ten-year results of a randomized clinical trial comparing radical mastectomy and total mastectomy with or without radiation. *N Engl J Med*. 1985; 312(11):674–681.

Suggested Readings

Bland KI. Anatomy of the breast. In: Fischer JE, Bland KI, eds. *Mastery of Surgery*. 5th ed. Philadelphia, PA: Wolters Kluwer/ Lippincott Williams & Wilkins; 2007:482–491.

Grube BJ, Giuliano AE. Sentinel lymph node dissection. In: *Diseases of the Breast*. 4th ed. Philadelphia, PA: Wolters Kluwer/ Lippincott Williams & Wilkins; 2010:542–561.

Morrow M. Therapeutic value of axillary node dissection. In: Bland KI, Copeland EM, eds. *The Breast: Comprehensive Management of Benign and Malignant Disorders*. 3rd ed. St. Louis, MO: Saunders; 2004:1019–1030.

Vitug AF, Newman LA. Complications in breast surgery. *Surg Clin North Am*. 2007;87(2):431–451.

Part III: Lymph Node Mapping and Dissection

13 Axillary Reverse Mapping

V. Suzanne Klimberg

Introduction

The status of the regional lymph node(s) is a key prognostic variable, and therapeutic decisions are based on the presence or absence of breast cancer cells metastatic to the regional axillary lymph node(s). The basic technique of axillary lymph node dissection (ALND) has changed little over several decades; the principal features are that of an anatomical dissection. However, individual modifications of the ALND technique has resulted in the reported variations in the one of the most commonly reported complications of axillary surgery, lymphedema. Depending on the definition of lymphedema, the incidence has been reported as high as 50% dependent upon the radicality of the procedure and the necessity for adjuvant radiation. Sentinel lymph node biopsy (SLNB) was introduced a little over a decade ago as an initial procedure to determine the accurate presence of regional metastases and, thus, the need for the more extensive ALND. Therefore, allowing 70% to 80% of patients to forgo ALND. From its inception, SLNB has been assumed to be and appears to be less morbid in multiple small trials comparing the two procedures. The most recent studies of lymphedema after ALND report lymphedema in 7% to 77% of patients. Lymphedema after SLNB has been reported from 0% to 13%. National Surgical Adjuvant Breast and Bowel Project (NSABP) B-32 is a large randomized cooperative group trial that will be able to answer the question of whether there is a survival difference between the two procedures in patients with negative axillary lymph nodes and the extent of the difference in lymphedema between the two procedures. We have recently introduced axillary reverse mapping (ARM) as an added procedure to either SLNB or ALND to identify and protect lymphatics draining the arm in order to prevent the sequelae of lymphedema.

INDICATIONS/CONTRAINDICATIONS

We have recently described the variations in lymphatics draining the arm within the axilla. These variations in arm lymphatic drainage put the arm lymphatics at risk for disruption during SLNB and/or ALND. Therefore, mapping the drainage of the arm during SLNB or ALND would be indicated to decrease the likelihood of inadvertent disruption of the lymphatics. Axillary reverse mapping is a method of separating nodes draining the breast from those draining the arm in order to preserve arm lymphatics and prevent lymphedema.

Axillary reverse mapping may be used with any size lesion and when lymph node involvement is present and after neoadjuvant therapy. When previous axillary surgery has been performed such as SLNB without ARM, lymphatics may have already been disrupted and the value of ARM added to ALND in this scenario may be limited.

In patients with matted nodes, the drainage of the breast can back up into the lymphatics draining the arm, and the safety of ARM is unknown. In addition, matted breast nodes can entrap low-lying ARM lymphatics, making it impossible to preserve them.

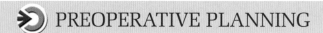

PREOPERATIVE PLANNING

Materials

Radioactive Materials

Any of the various materials previously established for the localization and SLNB may be used including but not exclusively technetium Tc 99m sulfur colloid (filtered or unfiltered) or technetium Tc 99m albumin. (See Chapter 10.)

Blue Dye

Five milliliters of 1% isosulfan blue dye (BD) is used for injection into the arm. When performing bilateral ARM procedures, this dose may be used for each side, or a single dose may be diluted with 5 ml of saline and divided for bilateral injection.

The Gamma Detector

The type of instrument used for detection of the sentinel lymph node (SLN) may be any of the marketed Food and Drug Administration (FDA)–approved devices with a collimated beam. The surgeon has the discretion of selecting a gamma detector that best serves his or her needs.

Radiation Safety

The handling, administration, and disposal of radioactive wastes should be performed in accordance with institutional policy. All radioactive specimens will be labeled with a sticker indicating the presence of radioactive materials. In all cases, strict precautions should be maintained according to radiation safety guidelines of handling open containers of radiopharmaceuticals. All materials used for injection (syringe, gloves, gauze) should be handled and disposed of in an appropriate container.

Relevant Anatomy

The anatomy of the lymphatic system draining the breast as it lies is the axilla is shown in Figure 13.1. In general the axillary triangle (level I axillary lymph nodes in which the lymphatics of the axilla sit is bordered by the serratus anterior and the pectoralis minor medially, the latissimus dorsi laterally, the axillary vein superiorly, and the teres major posteriorly (Fig. 13.2). Level II lymphatics are posterior to and in front of (Rotter's nodes) the pectoralis minor. Level III lymphatics are medial to the pectoralis minor. Recently, we described a method (ARM) that can demarcate the axillary lymph nodes draining the breast from those draining the arm within the axilla and the variations that have been identified (Fig. 13.3).

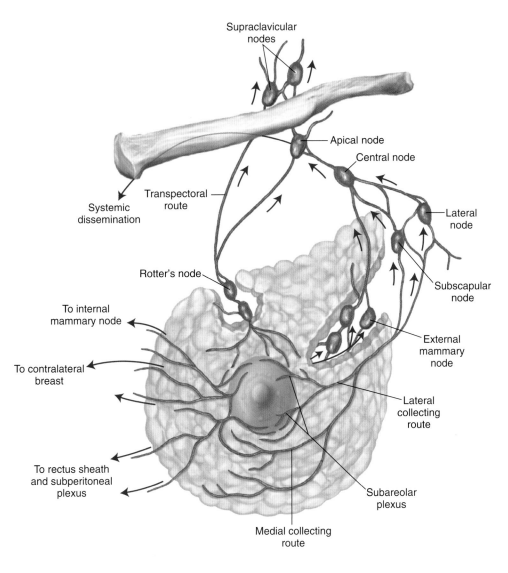

Figure 13.1 Lymphatic drainage of the breast.

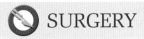 SURGERY

Surgical Technique

Positioning

The patient is placed supine with the arm extended at right angle as for any axillary procedure (Fig. 13.4).

Administration of the Radiopharmaceutical

Four milliliters or less of the radiopharmaceutical is injected into the breast. The injection will be given subareolarly/periareolarly or intratumorally in the dermis or peritumorally within 24 hours before surgery or intraoperatively after general anesthesia is obtained.

Injection of BD

Isosulfan blue is injected subcutaneously (5 cc) in the patient's ipsilateral upper volar surface of the arm at the time of the surgery, and an interval of at least 5 minutes is allowed for the dye to migrate to the lymph nodes prior to skin incision (Fig. 13.5). Massage and elevation of the arm may facilitate migration of the dye. It is always prudent to

Figure 13.2 Borders of axilla dissection.

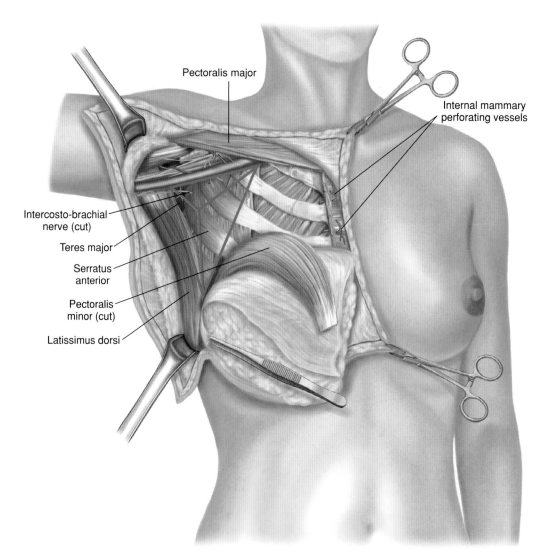

Pectoralis major

Internal mammary perforating vessels

Intercosto-brachial nerve (cut)

Teres major

Serratus anterior

Pectoralis minor (cut)

Latissimus dorsi

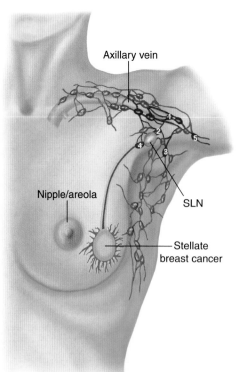

Axillary vein

Nipple/areola

SLN

Stellate breast cancer

Figure 13.3 Variations in ARM lymphatics. Axillary reverse mapping (ARM) technique combines radioactive localization of the SLN with blue dye mapping of the nodes draining the arm. Arm lymphatic variations: 1) Above or below the axillary vein; 2) Sling pattern; 3) Lateral apron; 4) Medial apron; 5) Twine or rope-like pattern.

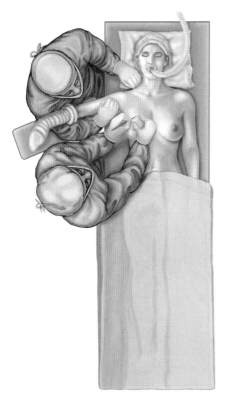

Figure 13.4 Position of patient for surgery with the arm at right angles to the table so that operator and assistant can stand opposite one another and juxtaposed to the patient during the procedure.

inform the anesthesiologist when the Lymphazurin is given, as it may cause the oxygen saturation to appear low.

Separation of SLN(S)/ALND and Blue ARM Nodes

Identification of the radioactive SLN should ideally be performed prior to incision of the skin and prior to BD injection. If the SLN cannot be located with radioactivity alone, then consideration should be given to using the BD in the breast to find the SLN. Once the axillary fascia is incised, care should be taken not to disturb any visible blue lymphatics usually emanating from the arm together with the axillary vessels and nerves. Using line-of-sight radioactive guidance, the SLN should be located within the axilla. Blue node/lymphatics should be identified and followed to their destination and

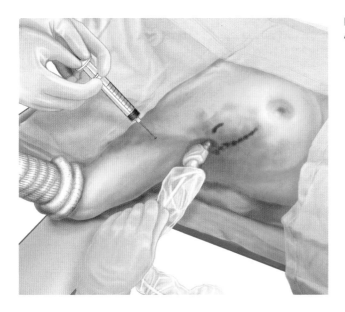

Figure 13.5 Injection of blue dye for ARM procedure.

Part III: Lymph Node Mapping and Dissection

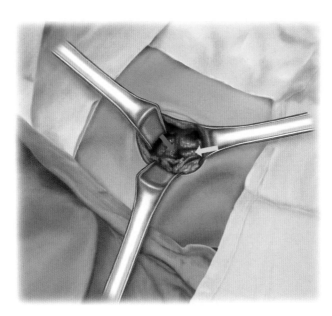

Figure 13.6 Blue ARM (*blue arrow*) node juxtaposed to hot SLN (*yellow arrow*).

separated from the hot SLN and the rest of the axillary lymph nodes if an ALND is to be performed. Multiple variations of blue ARM lymphatic have been identified and may be as much as 4 cm below the axillary vein and may consist of an apron of nodes and not just as a single node (Fig. 13.3). Blue lymphatics can be been seen from the SLN incision in more than one-third of the cases and may be juxtaposed to the SLN in approximately 5% to 6% of cases, in which case they can be dissected free of and protected during the SLN or ALND (Fig. 13.6).

Intraoperative Assessment of Blue Node

Assess the blue ARM node(s) for radioactivity. If the blue ARM node has greater than 10% of the counts of the hottest SLN, then it should be resected as an SLN. This occurs in 2% to 3% of cases. As is standard to SLNB to palpate and resect any suspicious lymph nodes in the axilla after removal of the hot node, also palpate the ARM node. If the ARM node gives any cause for suspicion, it should be resected for pathological analysis.

Hemostasis

During hemostasis, care should be taken to avoid injury (thermal or traumatic) to the blue nodes and associated lymphatics.

Closure

Close the fascia of the axilla followed by the dermis with 3–0 interrupted or running absorbable sutures. A skin suture is rarely necessary.

Dressing

Closure of the wound with skin glue is sufficient and allows the patient to shower immediately after surgery.

PEARLS AND PITFALLS

- Injection of BD in the volar surface of the arm allows quick migration of the dye (<5 minutes) while allowing the injection site to be hidden. Subcutaneous injection versus dermal gives the least risk of tattooing.
- Methylene blue should be efficacious for ARM, but it has only been used in a small number of cases. Methylene blue has been demonstrated to cause necrosis of the skin when injected intradermally or subcutaneously. For this reason, its use should be avoided. When use of methylene blue is necessary, make sure to dilute it five-fold.

■ Be sure to alert the anesthesiologist when the BD is given. Monitored oxygen desaturation appears to occur with BD injection. This requires no intervention.

■ If you suspect a BD reaction, give the patient 50 mg intravenous diphenhydramine (Benadryl). And 100 mg of methylprednisolone. Admit the patient for close observation for at least 24 hours. If a known allergy is present, premedicate with diphenhydramine and Solu-Medrol.

■ The blue ARM node may be attached to lymphatics that may or may not appear blue itself—be sure and take care to trace afferent and efferent lymphatics from blue nodes.

■ Most, but not all, lymphedema occurs within 4 years of axillary intervention. The patient should be monitored for lymphedema during regular visits and cautioned to avoid arm sticks and infection and to treat any arm infection early and aggressively. Bilateral volume displacement is the gold standard to monitor for lymphedema; however, many studies have used arm circumference 10 cm above and below the olecranon. An increase in 200 cc of volume or 2 cc arm circumference constitutes significant lymphedema.

POSTOPERATIVE MANAGEMENT

There are no special postoperative precautions or management of patients undergoing ARM above and beyond that of SLNB or ALND.

COMPLICATIONS

Radiation Exposure

The radiation exposure from this test is similar to the natural background radiation that is received in a year and is equivalent to that seen with SLNB.

Infection

Risk of infection has not been increased in the limited experience with this procedure nor would one expect it to be.

BD Allergic Reaction

The reported incidence of an allergic reaction to BD is 1.6%. Of note, only 0.4% develops a hypotensive reaction requiring pressor support. In such a case, the patient usually develops blue urticaria as an initial event and is appropriately treated with diphenhydramine and steroids given immediately intraoperatively. Patients with increased risk of BD reaction include those patients with known allergies to cosmetics. If an allergy to BD is suspected or known, the patient can be pretreated with diphenhydramine and steroids.

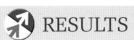# RESULTS

Lymphedema

There is limited but favorable reports of measurement of arm volumes after 6 months with and without preservation of ARM lymphatics (0% vs. 13%). Given that 2% to 3% of ARM lymphatics merge with SLN lymphatics in level I, the risk of lymphedema after any axillary sampling procedure can never be zero. The real long-term benefit of ARM added to SLN or ALND is yet to be determined.

✦ CONCLUSIONS

Axillary reverse mapping added to SLN and/or ALND appears to be safe and may prevent unnecessary lymphedema in a majority of patients.

Suggested Readings

Boneti C, Korourian S, Bland K, et al. Axillary reverse mapping: mapping and preserving arm lymphatics may be important in preventing lymphedema during sentinel lymph node biopsy. *J Am Coll Surg.* 2008;206:1038–1042.

Klimberg VS. A new concept toward the prevention of lymphedema: axillary reverse mapping. *J Surg Oncol.* 2007;14: 1890–1895.

Mansel R, Fallowfield L, Kissin M, et al. Randomized multicenter trial of sentinel node biopsy versus standard axillary treatment in operable breast cancer: the ALMANAC Trial. *J Natl Cancer Inst.* 2006;98(9):599–609.

Petrek JA, Senie RT, Peters M, et al. Lymphedema in a cohort of breast carcinoma survivors 20 years after diagnosis. *Cancer.* 2001;92:1368–1377.

Sakorafas G, Peros G, Cataliotti L. Sequelae following axillary lymph node dissection for breast cancer. *Expert Rev Anticancer Ther.* 2006;6(11):1629–1638.

Thompson M, Korourian S, Henry-Tillman R, et al. Axillary reverse mapping (ARM): a new concept to identify and enhance lymphatic preservation. *Ann Surg Oncol.* 2007;14(6);1890–1895.

Wilke LG, McCall LM, Posther KE, et al. Surgical complications associated with sentinel lymph node biopsy: results from a prospective international cooperative group trial. *Ann Surg Oncol.* 2006;13(4):491–500.

14 Partial Mastectomy

Sheryl G. A. Gabram

 INDICATIONS/CONTRAINDICATIONS

Definitions

Breast cancer surgery is trending in the direction of "less is more" as the number of patients newly diagnosed qualify for breast conservation surgery over mastectomy and sentinel lymph node biopsy instead of complete axillary lymph node dissection. Breast conservation treatment refers to removal of the breast cancer combined with radiation therapy to offer optimal local control, usually performed in association with axillary surgery. The surgical removal of the cancer from the breast may be referred to as lumpectomy, partial mastectomy, or quadrantectomy. Lumpectomy and partial mastectomy are essentially synonymous terms and indicate surgical removal of the tumor with the intent of obtaining a clear margin. In the United States, there is no ICD-9 code (Internal Classification of Diseases, 9th revision codes used for billing purposes) for lumpectomy, and therefore when reporting the operative details of performing breast sparing surgery, many surgeons will use the term "partial mastectomy" with ICD-9 code 19301. Quadrantectomy involves removal of a larger portion of breast tissue, a quadrant, often with overlying skin and removal of the breast tissue posteriorly from the pectoralis muscle. The latter technique has been popularized in Europe while in the United States, partial mastectomy/lumpectomy is performed more commonly.

Safety

The use of breast conservation treatment for early stage breast cancer has been tested in 6 worldwide prospective randomized clinical trials comparing lumpectomy/partial mastectomy (or quadrantectomy) to mastectomy. The long-term data indicate that when a negative margin is obtained, survival of breast sparing surgery compared to mastectomy is identical. In the United States National Surgical Adjuvant Breast and Bowel Project (NSABP) B-06 clinical trial, while the overall long-term survival was similar for those patients treated with lumpectomy, mastectomy, and lumpectomy with radiation, local control was markedly improved for those patients treated with radiation (in breast recurrence for lumpectomy with radiation of 14.3% vs. 39.2% for lumpectomy without radiation). Recurrence after mastectomy in this large trial was 10.2%, not significantly different for those patients treated with lumpectomy and radiation. The randomized trial from Milan on quadrantectomies also supports the safety of breast conservation for those patients meeting criteria for this procedure.

Indications

The indications for breast-sparing surgery include the following:

- Patients willing to receive radiation therapy with no contraindications
- Reasonable breast to tumor size ratio that would yield an acceptable cosmetic result after breast sparing surgery
- Localized disease assessed via breast imaging and clinical examination (disease limited to one quadrant)

Contraindications

The contraindications for breast sparing surgery include the following:

- Patient not a candidate for radiation therapy (such as those patients with scleroderma or other connective tissue diseases associated with skin involvement)
- Patient with history of prior therapeutic irradiation to the breast
- Patient unwilling to undergo radiation therapy
- Patient requiring radiation during pregnancy (pregnancy is an absolute contraindication to receiving radiation during pregnancy, thus creating a relative contraindication to Breast Conservation Therapy (BCT) during first and second trimesters)
- Two or more tumors in separate quadrants of the breast
- Evidence of diffuse breast involvement by imaging or clinical examination
- Persistently positive margins despite attempts at reasonable surgical re-excision
- Large tumor that would preclude a reasonable cosmetic outcome

 PREOPERATIVE PLANNING

Imaging

The clinical examination and imaging appearance of the tumor will determine whether breast conservation is feasible. It is important for surgeons to review all imaging to confirm localized disease that may or may not be associated with clinical findings. If the tumor is not palpable, a preoperative wire localization is necessary to identify the epicenter of the tumor for excision. Localization may also be necessary if the tumor is vaguely palpable, again to minimize the amount of breast tissue removed.

Increasingly, breast magnetic resonance imaging (MRI) is performed to determine the extent of the disease process especially in younger women as well as those women with extremely dense or heterogeneously dense breast tissue, where extent of the disease process may be underestimated by routine mammography. Some studies indicate that the use of this modality will change the operative plan in 16% of cases, with additional tumor identified in a multicentric fashion or the primary larger than suspected on routine mammography. The downsides of using breast MRI routinely is that no data have shown an improvement in survival for those patients who clinically are candidates for breast conservation. In the United States, insurance companies may not cover the charge of an MRI for all newly diagnosed breast cancer patients. Because the specificity is low, often a patient's surgery will be delayed if abnormalities on a breast MRI are uncovered that necessitate biopsy to either prove or disprove multicentricity. Currently, not all surgeons are advocates of routine MRI in planning for partial mastectomy.

Neoadjuvant Therapy (Systemic or Hormonal)

Another trend in breast cancer treatment is targeted individualized therapy depending on various tumor characteristics. This had led to an increase in delivering preoperative systemic chemotherapy or hormonal therapy to better document the treatment effect of a specific regimen prior to surgery. Performing surgery after neoadjuvant therapy will contribute significant information on tumor responsiveness of a particular regimen and help guide future systemic treatment. In addition, some patients will become candidates for breast conservation if treated with systemic therapy prior to surgery. Studies have shown that it is safe to offer upfront therapy (neoadjuvant chemo or hormonal treatment, also referred to as primary systemic chemotherapy or hormonal therapy) with only a minority of tumors progressing on therapy during such an approach. It is important for surgeons to clinically follow patients during neoadjuvant therapy to assess response to treatment and ensure that unresponsive tumors do not require a change in therapeutic intervention that may include a more immediate surgical procedure. Preoperative hormonal therapy is used for elderly patients and may take the place of surgery in a patient with multiple comorbid diseases who may be at high risk for surgery. For this elderly group, each case is decided upon on an individual basis and if the patient responds well to this approach, consideration for partial mastectomy in an outpatient setting under intravenous sedation in the operating room can take place at the point the tumor is no longer responding to the treatment regimen.

Role of Oncoplastic Surgical Techniques

Depending on the size of the partial mastectomy resection, some patients may benefit from oncoplastic surgical techniques in repairing the defect. This is an emerging field that offers patients an alternative to mastectomy, especially for very large defects in patients with generous breast tissue who may benefit from opposite breast reduction surgery (Fig. 14.1).

Factors involved in the surgical decision making for oncoplastic procedures after the performance of partial mastectomy include the following:

- *Timing of reconstruction in relation to radiation therapy:* It is ideal to consider oncoplastic surgery prior to partial mastectomy and radiation. Patients who present after completion of surgery and radiation are a challenge because if the defect is large, they may require transfer of significant amount of autologous tissue. In this setting, the remaining breast tissue has been exposed to radiation and wound healing may be

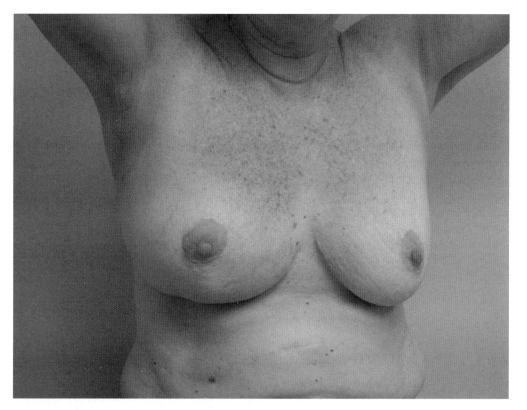

Figure 14.1 Right breast cancer with bilateral reduction surgery.

compromised. Often these patients have chosen breast conservation therapy because of a desire to have less versus more surgery. Sometimes, completion mastectomy and immediate reconstruction are the best options for significant defects.

■ *Status of tumor margins:* Oncoplastic techniques can be performed immediately after the partial mastectomy or delayed a week or two for final margin status determination (but before radiation is administered). If multicentric disease is suspected, the latter approach, with delay to confirm final margins, is advantageous. However, if disease appears localized, a unified procedure can be recommended, thus avoiding a second procedure in the operating room.

■ *Extent of breast skin and tissue resection:* This will be determined by the size of the tumor and proximity to the anterior skin margin. If reduction procedures are planned, the incisions for the partial mastectomy portion of the procedure can be in the same location of the reduction incisions. Careful planning between the surgical oncologist and the plastic surgery team is necessary for this approach. At the time of surgery, specimen mammography may be necessary to confirm that the entire lesion is resected with a visually acceptable margin.

■ *Breast size:* Patients with pendulous breasts may benefit from oncoplastic techniques even if the lesion for resection is small. Radiation to large breasts can be compromised and uneven dosages may occur in this group of patients. It is desirable to perform the partial mastectomy and bilateral reduction prior to radiation therapy as opposed to performing reduction surgery after the patient has completed all therapy.

■ *Ultimate cosmetic outcome:* An assessment needs to be made preoperatively if the patient would benefit from completion mastectomy versus wide partial mastectomy and reduction of the involved breast. If a patient does not meet criteria for postmastectomy radiation, the advantage to simple mastectomy and reconstruction may be to avoid radiation. Again, a co-ordinated informed discussion with the surgical oncologist, plastic surgeon, and patient taking into account the patient's expectations is necessary.

Patient Consideration

A detailed family history (three generations on both the maternal and paternal lineages) is necessary to determine if a patient may be at risk for the *BRCA1/BRCA2* genetic mutation. Characteristics of those at increased risk for *BRCA1/BRCA2* or other high penetrance mutations (p53 or PTEN) are displayed in Table 14.1. While breast conservation therapy is still an option for a patient diagnosed with the *BRCA1/BRCA2* genetic mutation, the role of bilateral mastectomies should be considered as well, because these patients are at higher risk for the development of new primaries on the involved side as well as contra lateral breast cancer. Genetic testing may delay surgery; however, if a patient is a candidate for neoadjuvant therapy, that treatment can proceed while the patient is referred for genetic counseling and possible testing.

Patients will often have predetermined desires regarding breast conservation surgery versus mastectomy. Data regarding the safety of breast conservation should be discussed with the patient. Even after these discussions, a group of patients will desire mastectomy and furthermore even request bilateral mastectomies (contralateral prophylactic mastectomy) with or without immediate reconstruction. While there is no survival advantage to this approach, an increasing trend of bilateral mastectomies in the setting of unilateral cancer has been identified.

Prevention of Acute Complications

There is ongoing debate about the role of prophylactic antibiotics for breast surgery. Several studies report the advantage of prophylactic antibiotics given as a one time dose 30 minutes prior to surgery, yet others have shown no benefit. High-risk patients, those who are obese, the elderly, and diabetic may be those who benefit from prophylactic antibiotics to a greater extent. Foreign body placement, wire localizations and clips for marking biopsy sites, may add to risk of infection and one may consider use of prophylactic antibiotics in these settings as well.

TABLE 14.1	**Indications for Referral to Genetics Counseling**

Family history, no personal history of cancer
   Non-Jewish family with any of the following:

- one case of breast cancer ≤50 in an FDR or SDR
- one FDR or SDR with both breast and ovarian cancer, at any age
- ≥ two cases of breast cancer in FDRs or SDRs if one is diagnosed at ≤50 or is bilateral
- one FDR or SDR with breast cancer diagnosed at ≤50 or bilateral and one FDR or SDR with ovarian cancer
- three cases of breast and ovarian cancer (at least one case of ovarian cancer) in FDRs and SDRs
- two cases of ovarian cancer in FDRs and SDRs
- one case of male breast cancer in an FDR or SDR if another FDR or SDR has breast or ovarian cancer

   Jewish family with any of the following:

- ≥ one ≥case of breast cancer ≤ 50 in an FDR or SDR
- ≥ one case of ovarian cancer at any age in an FDR or SDR
- ≥ one FDR or SDR with breast cancer at any age if another FDR or SDR has breast and/or ovarian cancer at any age
- ≥ one case of male breast cancer in an FDR or SDR

Family member with known gene mutation: *BRCA1/BRCA2*/p53/PTEN
Female with personal history of breast or ovarian cancer diagnosed ≤50 years of age, male with breast cancer at any age
Personal history of breast cancer, plus one or more of the following:

- Personal history of ovarian cancer
- Family history of ovarian cancer
- Family history of breast cancer diagnosed ≤50 years of age
- Family history of male breast cancer
- Family history of thyroid cancer, endometrial cancer, and/or Cowden syndrome
- Family history of sarcoma, adrenocortical cancer, brain tumors, leukemia/lymphoma
- Ashkenazi Jewish ancestry

FDR, first-degree relative; SDR, second-degree relative.

Prevention of bleeding and hematoma formation can take place by obtaining an accurate preoperative history of use of blood thinners such as daily aspirin or anti-inflammatory medications. If possible, these medications should be stopped 10 days to 2 weeks prior to surgery. Clopidogrel (Plavix) should be stopped a full week prior to surgery. Surgery should be delayed about 4 weeks after the last infusion of bevacizumab (Avastin) because of the potential of bleeding and dehiscence. Other agents that contribute to bleeding in breast patients are Vitamin E, ginseng, ginko biloba, and garlic. There is also a debate about closure of the partial mastectomy cavity. The conventional approach is double layer skin closure without deep sutures. Some surgeons prefer deep closure to decrease risk of hematoma formation, but this may compromise cosmetic appearance.

Unique Clinical Circumstances

The role of surgical resection for patients with stage IV breast cancer is an emerging area of surgical interest. In the past, resection of the primary tumor took place for bleeding, ulceration, ongoing infection, and necrosis or hygienic reasons. In retrospective studies, patients with stage IV breast cancer who have their tumor removed to a free margin may experience longer overall survival than those who are not resected. Ideally, a randomized prospective trial may determine which patients benefit from this approach; however, this type of study is limited by the number of patients presenting annually with stage IV breast cancer who could be enrolled in such a trial. If breast cancer is regarded as both a local and systemic disease, multimodal therapy including surgery for some stage IV patients may contribute to more optimal local control. Theoretically, resection of the primary tumor may inhibit further seeding of the blood with micrometastatic cells shed by the tumor, reduce overall tumor burden, and potentially prolong metastatic progression free survival. If the tumor is confined to a particular quadrant, partial mastectomy may be the surgical choice in these patients. Often stage IV patients have received some form of systemic therapy, chemotherapy or hormonal, prior to referral to the surgeon for resection of the primary, in an effort to determine how the tumor has responded to therapy. Close consultation with medical and, in some cases, radiation oncology is necessary in planning the multimodal treatment of stage IV patients.

Another unique clinical circumstance involves a patient who has had partial breast irradiation following lumpectomy and develops a new primary in another quadrant of the breast. This patient may be a candidate for a partial mastectomy for the second primary and then whole breast radiation. These are highly unusual situations, but with the increasing use of partial breast irradiation, these may occur in the future more commonly.

Pertinent Anatomy and Planning Technique of Incisions

The first step in planning for the location of a partial mastectomy incision is to remember that the patient may have to proceed with mastectomy if margins are not clear, and therefore placement of the partial mastectomy incision should be in close proximity to a potential future skin-sparing mastectomy incision. Curvilinear incisions following Langerhans lines are appropriate for upper hemisphere breast lesions while a vertically placed 6-o'clock incision can be used for those lesions between 5 to 7 o'clock (see Fig. 14.2). Some surgeons prefer circumareolar incisions to enhance cosmetic outcome. After incising the skin, it is optimal to dissect directly down to the lesion and avoid undermining thin skin flaps if possible. If a lesion is close to the skin and especially if retraction is present, a small portion of skin may need to be excised overlying the retraction. Skin removal creates a mastopexy effect and can contribute to slight asymmetry when compared to the contralateral breast Excision of extensive skin should be avoided unless coupled with oncoplastic surgical techniques for closure that address the contralateral breast as well. After removal of the specimen, correct orientation and marking for pathological assessment is a priority in the operating room. Some surgeons prefer, for simplicity, a short superior and long lateral silk suture for ease of processing in pathology. Note that radio-opaque markers exist for those specimens sent to imaging after removal (MarginMap uses caricatures for cranial, caudal, medial, lateral,

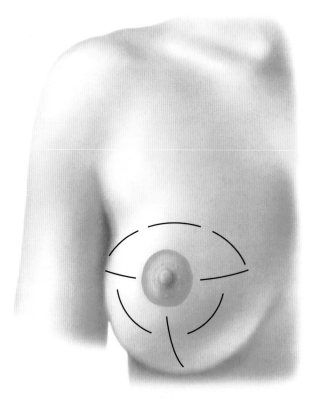

Figure 14.2 Orientation of incisions for lumpectomy/partial mastectomy excision procedure.

anterior/superficial, and deep that are easily viewed on specimen mammography), and these can be sutured in place, allowing the breast imager to report the proximity of a given margin to the surgeon in the operating room.

Margin Assessment

Intraoperatively margins can be assessed through specimen mammography providing valuable information to the surgeon when considering an immediate re-excision of a close margin. Some institutions perform frozen sections or touch preps on various margins; however, these techniques have their limitations based on expertise of the pathologist and final margin assessment by H&E staining remains the most accurate method. For purely invasive cancers, a microscopic 1-mm margin is sufficient. In those patients with ductal carcinoma in situ, a more diffuse process especially if an extensive intraductal component (ECI) is reported, ideally a 2-mm margin, should be obtained. In the United States, early randomized clinical trials used the definition of a negative margin as "tumor cells not touching the inked margin." This information can be taken into consideration when communicating with patients the role of re-excision for a close margin depending on the clinical setting. Emerging data in the era of multimodality therapy suggest that there is limited benefit in reduced local failure for margins greater than "no ink touching tumor."

Another technique practiced by some surgeons is to take additional shave margins at the time of the partial mastectomy, basing the depth of these additional margins on palpation of the tumor in the partial mastectomy specimen or on the imaging appearance of proximity to a given margin for nonpalpable disease. These shave margins can be taken in one location on the basis of the intraoperative assessment of the location of the tumor in the specimen or all "six" margins can be taken at the time of surgery (anterior, posterior, medial, lateral, superior, and inferior). Marking these elliptical shave margins is crucial in determining final margin status. One technique is to mark the elliptical margin with a stitch indicating the inside of the cavity. Data have shown that there is a reduced rate of returning to surgery for further re-excisions when shave margins are sent; however, this has to be balanced with the amount of tissue that is removed and the ultimate cosmetic outcome.

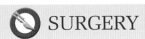

SURGERY

Overview of Sequence of Events for Partial Mastectomy

- Review imaging prior to procedure (Fig. 14.3): Determine location on the clock face of lesion in order to plan incision
- Place patient in supine position: Extend arms at 90 degrees or tuck at patient's side (Fig. 14.4)
- Induce anesthesia: Intravenous sedation or general
- Plan incision based on anatomy, location of lesion (Fig. 14.5)
- Inject local anesthetic (Fig. 14.6)
- Make incision with knife and avoid raising thin skin flaps: For wire localization cases, it is acceptable to make the incision closer to the lesion and then dissect out the wire and pull the wire through into the center of the incision (Figs. 14.7 and 14.8)
- Take tissue around specimen clinically approximating 0.5 to 1 cm
- Palpate cavity to ensure removal of any suspicious tissue (Fig. 14.9)
- Mark specimen for orientation (e.g., one short superior stitch, one long lateral, alternatively use sutured markers such as MarginMap —see Fig. 14.10)
- Send specimen for mammography to assess margins and need for re-excision (Fig. 14.11)
- Take additional cavity margins depending on results of specimen mammography and interest in shave margins (see Figs. 14.12 and 14.13)
- Close with single or double layer absorbable suture (Fig. 14.14)

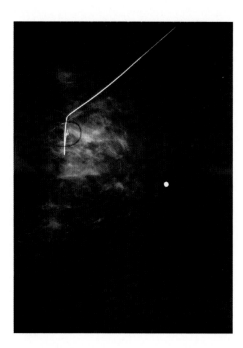

Figure 14.3 Review of imaging.

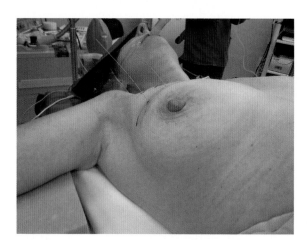

Figure 14.4 Placement of patient.

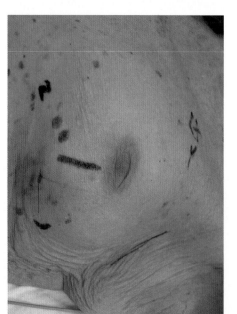

Figure 14.5 Planning incision.

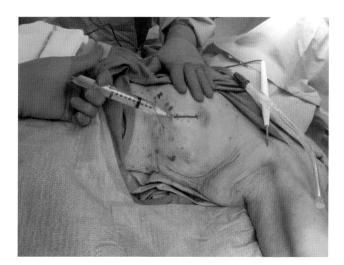

Figure 14.6 Injecting local anesthetic, pre-emptive analgesia.

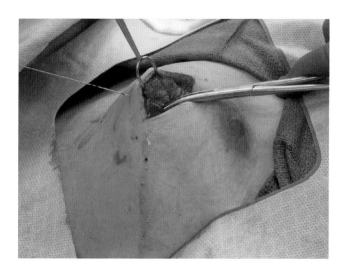

Figure 14.7 Pulling wire into center of cavity.

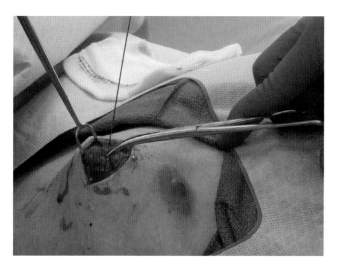

Figure 14.8 Wire in center of cavity preparing for dissection around wire.

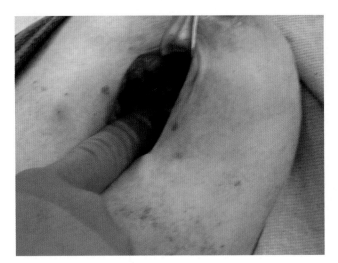

Figure 14.9 Palpating cavity after removal of specimen.

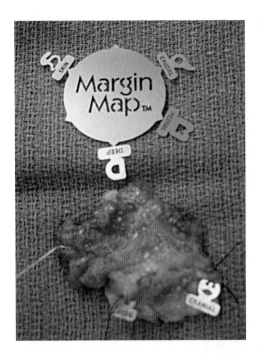

Figure 14.10 Orienting specimen for pathology.

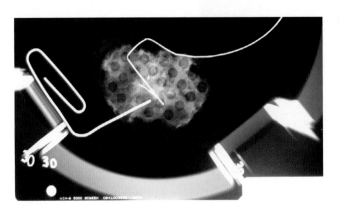

Figure 14.11 Specimen mammography.

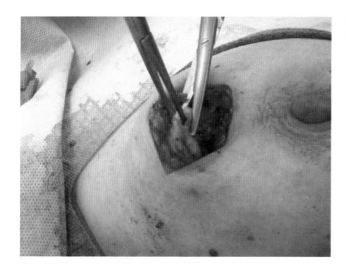

Figure 14.12 Excising shave margin, superior edge.

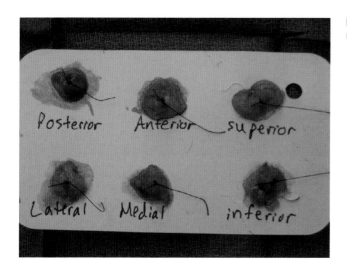

Figure 14.13 Orientation of shave margins (stitch on inside of cavity).

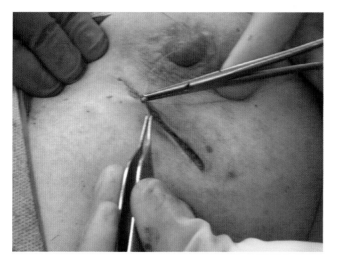

Figure 14.14 Double layer closure.

- Obtain postlumpectomy mammogram 1 to 3 weeks following surgery to ensure removal of all calcifications
- Order follow-up mammography on affected side every 6 months for 2 years and then annually

 POSTOPERATIVE MANAGEMENT

Postoperatively, a form-fitting bra or tank top is used to provide support during the healing phase. Most partial mastectomy cavities will fill with seroma fluid unless deep closure has taken place and these can be followed clinically. Aspiration should take place if the cavity if bulging or if the breast becomes diffusely erythematous, indicating poor lymphatic drainage that may improve with decompression of the seroma fluid. The diffuse erythema could represent cellulitis and if aspiration of the cavity takes place, cultures can be sent.

The pathology report should be reviewed carefully with attention directed to margin status. It is very appropriate to offer re-excision of a margin or margins if necessary on the basis of the amount of tissue excised at the first procedure and the amount of residual breast tissue. The breast to partial mastectomy cavity size needs to be taken into consideration if this is offered over mastectomy. Finally, the size of the invasive tumor is noted for staging purposes and if the tumor is estrogen or progesterone receptor positive and the lymph nodes are negative, consideration should be made to requesting further analysis of tumor characteristics with specific gene assays (Oncotype Dx or MammaPrint) to assist the medical oncologist in further decision making.

If the patient has multiple calcifications in the partial mastectomy specimen, while a specimen mammography was performed in the operating room, it still may be advantageous to obtain a postlumpectomy mammogram to document complete removal of suspicious residual calcifications prior to referral to radiation therapy. This will serve as a baseline mammogram for comparison 6 months later. It may be difficult to visualize calcifications if the partial mastectomy cavity has a large seroma and aspiration of the cavity may be indicated before performing mammography.

Referral to both medical and radiation oncology is recommended during the healing phase. It is important that the patient does not start radiation until medical oncology can determine the role of adjuvant therapy, especially chemotherapy as this is administered prior to radiation. Hormonal therapy is generally instituted after the completion of radiation therapy.

 COMPLICATIONS

Acute

Common early complications from partial mastectomy include wound infection ranging from cellulitis to abscess, and seroma or hematoma formation. The overall incidence can range from 1% to 20%. Localized cellulitis can be treated with oral antibiotics and the most common offending organism is Staphylococci. If the overlying erythema fails to resolve, aspiration of the partial mastectomy cavity should take place to rule out abscess formation (see Chapter 2). Frank abscesses ideally should be treated with multiple aspirations as long as improvement is documented as opposed to open treatment of the cavity, which will delay healing and potentially delay other treatments such as chemotherapy or radiation.

Uncommon early complications include pneumothorax from wire localization of the breast lesion, brachial plexopathy from malpositioning on the operating room table, and Mondor disease. Mondor disease is thrombosis of the thoracoepigastric vein and presents as a palpable cord coursing vertically from the lower breast to the upper abdomen. While symptoms will resolve with time, localized heat therapy and anti-inflammatory medication may facilitate quicker healing.

Late Complications

Late complications from partial mastectomy include chronic incisional pain and breast lymphedema. Risk factors identified for chronic pain include younger age, large tumor, radiation, chemotherapy, depression, and poor coping mechanisms. Successful management has been reported with serotonin uptake inhibitors such as amitriptyline and venlafaxine.

Breast lymphedema has the appearance of a diffuse cellulitis of the breast that disappears when the patient is placed in the supine position. The etiology is incompletely understood but most likely related to compromised lymphatic drainage as a result of extensive excision of breast tissue. If this condition presents in a delayed fashion, the surgeon needs to consider the possibility of local recurrence. For this delayed presentation, the next steps involve imaging and if negative, a punch biopsy to rule out breast cancer cells in cutaneous lymphatics. Treatment consists of aspiration of the seroma if large, local massage therapy after aspiration or if the cavity is already compresses, fitted compression garment and referral to occupational/physical therapy for assessment and care.

For those patients who undergo radiation therapy, a rare but notable long-term complication occurring approximately 3 to 12 years after treatment is angiosarcoma. The occurrence is rare, diagnosed in 1 of 2,000 primary breast cancers. The occurrence of reddish, purplish, or bluish nodules or discolorations of the skin that are multiple on the breast or chest wall is characteristic of this tumor. Imaging that includes mammography and a search for distant disease, is the next step noting that the most common site of metastasis is pulmonary. Surgically, the treatment is wide, simple mastectomy. If the mastectomy defect is large, wound coverage with flaps may need to be incorporated in the operative procedure to ensure complete resection of the disease with a wide margin (>1 cm). Chemotherapy is not well established and further work is warranted in this area, thus emphasizing the important role of wide surgical excision.

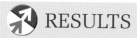 # RESULTS

Long-term Monitoring Plan

Treatable relapse of disease in a breast cancer patient occurs at an overall rate of 1% to 1.5% per year, but the rate for an individual is stage-specific and age-influenced. It is interesting to note that the majority of relapses are either self-detected or mammography screen-detected and not on clinical follow-up with the oncologist. For patients who have undergone breast conservation, the generally accepted recommendation for screening mammography of the ipsilateral breast is every 6 months for 2 years and then annually thereafter. While the data are limited on increasing survival with closer vigilance by screening mammography, the role of performing the first 6-month mammogram is to establish a baseline for following changes in the treated breast. The importance of self-vigilance should be emphasized with patients since changes on self-examination may be detected at intervals between clinical visits. Self-examinations should highlight the ipsilateral along with the contralateral breast and axillary surveillance. While more unusual, the appearance of diffuse skin nodules as a manifestation of recurrent disease needs to be monitored as well.

The role of MRI in screening for recurrent breast cancer for all patients is still under investigation. There is currently insufficient evidence for or against offering MRI screening for all patients with a personal history of invasive or noninvasive cancers. The potential for earlier detection exists; however, this may be at the expense of a higher number of benign biopsies. Ultimately, the decision to order MRI in patients treated with breast conservation as a method of more intense surveillance should be made on a case-by-case basis, and further data are expected to be forthcoming.

Treatment of Recurrence in the Conserved Breast

If recurrence is detected either by clinical examination or imaging, a biopsy is necessary to obtain tissue and characterize the tumor for further planning. The peak time for an ipsilateral breast tumor recurrence (IBTR) is 3 to 5 years after treatment and risk factors associated with this recurrence are as follows:

- Younger age
- Positive margins
- Tumor size
- High nuclear grade
- Lymphovascular invasion
- Extensive intraductal component (EIC)
- Omission of endocrine therapy or radiation therapy

When a patient is diagnosed with an IBTR, the risk for metastatic disease increases, and therefore the decision to obtain whole body imaging prior to any treatment is recommended. It is generally accepted that IBTR is a marker for, not a cause of distant disease; however, in patients who develop IBTR longer term and beyond the early peak, the concept that distant seeding from the IBTR may take place is a possibility. This is consistent with data that show survival benefit for radiation therapy in certain groups of patients.

For patients with breast conservation who have received whole breast radiation, the standard treatment for an IBTR is total mastectomy with or without immediate reconstruction. Depending on the characteristics of the tumor, if the patient is a candidate for chemotherapy, the option for neoadjuvant treatment prior to surgery to document the response of the tumor to treatment may be offered. Up to 50% of patients with an IBTR are at risk for systemic disease within 5 years of the IBTR. Those patients who are at higher risk for distant recurrence after an IBTR are those who had positive lymph nodes at the time of the initial surgery for the primary cancer, skin involvement in the recurrent cancer, and the presence of lymphovascular invasion in the recurrent cancer. These patients should definitely be considered for systemic therapy after their IBTR. Given the complexity of this decision making, multidisciplinary consultation for all patients with an IBTR is essential.

PEARLS AND PITFALLS

- Discuss safety of breast conservation and data on local recurrence
- Assess tumor to breast size ratio for adequate cosmesis
- Consider oncoplastic reduction techniques for large tumors
- Present option of neoadjuvant therapy if appropriate
- Review pathology report for determination of adequate margins
- Consider postlumpectomy mammography as an adjunct for margin clearance in cases with diffuse microcalcifications noted preoperatively
- Consider referral of patient to radiation oncology for pre-operative assessment
- Review pathology with patient and if margins clear, refer to radiation
- Inform patient of possibility of returning to the operating room for re-excision of lumpectomy bed or mastectomy if margins close or involved

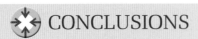

CONCLUSIONS

Partial mastectomy is a widely performed procedure for patients diagnosed with preinvasive and invasive breast cancer. Adherence to the important principles of selecting appropriate candidates, considering the role of neoadjuvant treatment, incorporating multimodal therapies to reduce recurrence rates, and careful follow-up are essential for the successful use of this approach in women diagnosed with breast cancer.

Suggested Readings

ACS Cancer Facts and Figures. http://www.cancer.org/downloads/STT/2008CAFFfinalsecured.pdf. Accessed January 2009.

Asad J, Jacobsen AF, Estabrook A, et al. Does oncotype DX recurrence score affect the management of patients with early-stage breast cancer? *Am J Surg.* 2008;196:527–529.

Cody HS. Current surgical management of breast cancer. *Curr Opin Obstet Gynecol.* 2002;14:45–52.

Dershaw DD. Mammogrpahy in patients with breast cancer treated by breast conservation (lumpectomy with or without radiation). *AJR Am J Roentgenol.* 1995;164:309–316.

Early Breast Trialists' Collaborative Group. Effects of radiotherapy and surgery in early breast cancer: an overview of the randomized trials. *N Engl J Med.* 1995;333:1444.

Fisher B, Anderson S, Bryant J, et al. Twenty–year follow-up of a randomized trial comparing total mastectomy, lumpectomy and lumpectomy plus irradiation for the treatment of invasive breast cancer. *N Engl J Med.* 2002;347(16):1233–1241.

Gralow JR, Burstein HJ, Wood W, et al. Preoperative therapy in invasive breast cancer: pathologic assessment and systemic therapy issues in operable disease. *J Clin Oncology.* 2008;26(5):814–819.

Grobmyer SR, Mortellaro VE, Marshall JH, et al. Is there a role for routine use of MRI in selection of patients for breast conserving cancer therapy? *J Am Coll Surg.* 2008;206:1045–1052.

Hampel H, Sweet K, Westman JA, et al. Referral for cancer genetics consultation: a review and compilation of risk assessment criteria. *J Med Genet.* 2004;41(2):81–91.

Hodgson NC, Bowen-Wells C, Moffat F, et al. Angiosarcomas of the breast: a review of 70 cases. *Am J Clin Oncol.* 2007;30:570–573.

ICD-9 Codes. http://icd9cm.chrisendres.com/icd9cm/. Accessed January 2009.

Jacobson F, Asad J, Boolbol SK, et al. Do additional shaved margins at the time of lumpectomy eliminate the need for re-excision? *Am J Surg.* 2008;196:556–558.

Komike Y, Akiyama F, Iino Y, et al. Ipsilateral breast tumor recurrence (IBTR) after breast conserving treatment in early breast cancer. *Cancer.* 2006;106:35–41.

Kronowitz SJ, Kuerer HM, Buchholz TA, et al. A management algorithm and practical oncoplastic surgical techniques for repairing partial mastectomy defects. *Plast Reconstr Surg.* 2008;122:1631–1647.

Lang JE, Babiera GV. Locoregional resection in stage IV breast cancer: tumor biology, molecular and clinical perspectives. *Surg Clin N Am.* 2007;87:527–538.

Montgomery DA, Krupa K, Cooke TG. Follow-up in breast cancer: does routine clinical examination improve outcome? A systematic review of the literature. *Br J Cancer.* 2007;97:1632–1641.

Morrow M, Harris JR. Primary Treatment of invasive breast cancer. In: Harris JR, Lippman ME, Morrow M, et al., eds. *Diseases of the Breast.* 2nd ed. 2000:526–527.

Newman LA, Mamounas EP. Reivew of breast cancer clinical trials conducted by the National Surgical Adjuvant Breast Project. *Surg Clin N Am.* 2007;87:279–305.

Saslow D, Boetes C, Burke W, et al. American Cancer Society guidelines for breast screening with MRI as an adjunct to mammography. *CA Cancer J Clin.* 2007;57:75–89.

Schwartz GF, Hughes KS, Lynch HT, et al. Proceedings of the international consensus conference on breast cancer risk, genetics, & risk management, April, 2007. *Cancer.* 2008;113:2627–2637.

Shen J, Hunt KK, Mirza NQ, et al. Predictors of systemic recurrence and disease specific survival after ipsilateral breast tumor recurrence. *Cancer.* 2005;104:479–490.

Tuttle TM, Habermann EB, Grund EH, et al. Increasing use of contralateral prophylactic mastectomy for breast cancer patients: a trend toward more aggressive surgical treatment. *J Clin Oncol.* 2007;25:1–7.

Veronesi U, Cascinelli N, Mariani L, et al. Twenty-year follow-up of a randomized study comparing breast-conserving surgery with radical mastectomy for early breast cancer. *N Engl J Med.* 2002;347(16):1227–1232.

Vitug AF, Newman LA. Complications in breast surgery. *Surg Clin N Am.* 2007;87:431–451.

15 Excision Followed by Radiofrequency Ablation (eRFA)

V. Suzanne Klimberg and Cristiano Boneti

Introduction

Lumpectomy followed by radiation is widely utilized for the treatment of breast cancer. At least 75% to 90% of recurrences occur at the previous lumpectomy site and positive margins are found in 20% to 55% of lumpectomy specimens. Radiation effectively lowers the risk at the site of the lumpectomy but is not as important in reducing ipsilateral elsewhere recurrences in the breast—giving rise to the concept and the effective treatment of brachytherapy that treats approximately a 1-cm area around the tumor bed with 100% radiation dose. Excision followed by radiofrequency ablation (eRFA), in a similar way, utilizes the radiofrequency ablation (RFA) to in effect extend the margins of the lumpectomy by 1 cm and ablate any undetectable residual disease. This procedure is designed to increase the margin in primary lumpectomy cavities without further excision, thereby avoiding additional tissue resection and maintaining optimum cosmesis in breast-conserving surgery (Fig. 15.1).

Significant preclinical and clinical data have demonstrated that RFA applied to a lumpectomy cavity can ablate a consistent centimeter around the cavity heating to 100°F for 15 minutes. This concept has been demonstrated using whole mount reconstruction of simulated lumpectomies in mastectomy specimens treated with eRFA. A multi-institutional trial in Italy showed that in vivo eRFA of invasive breast cancers followed by standard quadrantectomy showed at least a 1-cm circumferential ablation around the lumpectomy sites. It has also been shown effective in a pilot clinical trial in the United States to evaluate eRFA, 41 patients underwent lumpectomy followed by intraoperative RFA. Eleven of 41 patients had inadequate margins; however, only 1 required re-excision for a grossly positive margin. Biopsy of the cavity walls postablation demonstrated at least a 1-cm thick ablation. Seventeen of the 41 patients had postoperative radiation therapy. During the median follow-up of 24 months, there were no local recurrences. Two of the patients have had recurrence distant to the operative site. Recently, an update of this trial with 94 patients with nearly 2-year follow-up showed no in-site recurrences. A multi-institutional trial in the United States will further evaluate

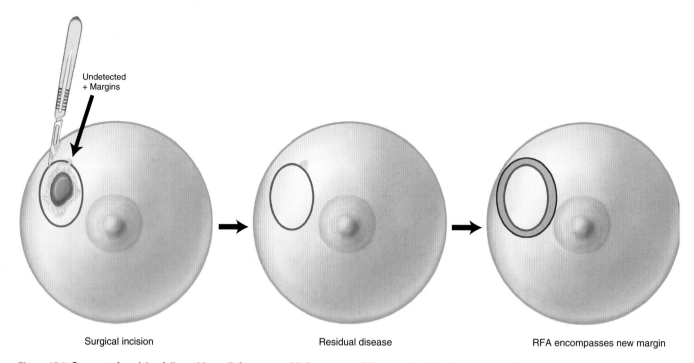

Undetected
+ Margins

Surgical incision   Residual disease   RFA encompasses new margin

Figure 15.1 Concept of excision followed by radiofrequency ablation to extend the margins of the lumpectomy site.

this procedure. In addition, Klimberg and colleagues have recently developed a method for following the in vivo ablation with Doppler. Because of the off-gassing of nitrogen, the zone of ablation as well as its proximity to the skin can be measured via the color Doppler. This allows not only assurance of a 1-cm thickness of ablation but a real-time way to avoid skin burns.

INDICATIONS/CONTRAINDICATIONS

The indications for eRFA—RFA after a lumpectomy for cancer (invasive or noninvasive cancer) include the following:

▨ Extend margin width without resecting additional tissue and by doing so decrease the possibility of re-excision for close margins.
▨ Ablate occult and otherwise undetectable disease in patients who cannot be treated with radiation therapy (XRT) (e.g., collagen vascular disease, comorbid diseases, prior XRT for conservative breast cancer treatment) or who refuse XRT or where XRT is of questionable value.

   Contraindications include the following:

▨ Patients with pacemakers (unknown risk)
▨ Patients with skin thickness after excision of less than 1.0 cm

PREOPERATIVE PLANNING

Order of Procedures

The radiopharmaceutical and/or blue dye is injected into the breast first or blue dye is injected into the arm for axillary reverse mapping (ARM). The sentinel lymph node biopsy is then performed (see Chapter 10) first. The excision or lumpectomy is then performed (see Chapter 14). Then, the excision bed can be prepared for eRFA (Fig. 15.2).

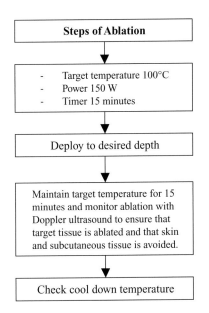

Figure 15.2 Steps of ablation procedure.

Radiofrequency Probe

The RITA StarBurst XL (AngioDynamics, Inc., Latham, NY) is the device used for all the procedures to date, but it should be possible to perform eRFA with any device that is able to monitor temperature. The tines of the array can be deployed up to 7 cm in diameter (Fig. 15.3). They are easily retracted for repositioning. The probe has four thermal tines spaced in between five tines for monitoring temperature. The sterile RFA probe is placed on the field separately. A sterile reusable connector cable is also placed on the field.

Generator Settings

The RFA generator is set to a power of 150 W, a temperature of 100°C—average of all and 15 minutes of ablation (three windows on left of generator) (Fig. 15.4). Five windows (to right within the circle) interactively indicate the five temperature tines.

Placement of Grounding Pads

Two grounding pads are placed for the eRFA and are placed away from the electrocautery grounding pads. They should also be placed away from any metal prosthesis—hip or otherwise.

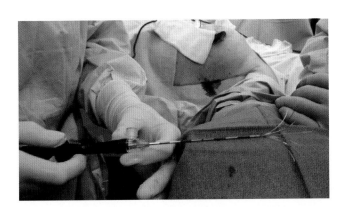

Figure 15.3 Adjustable RFA probe with five temperature tines and four heating tines.

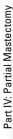

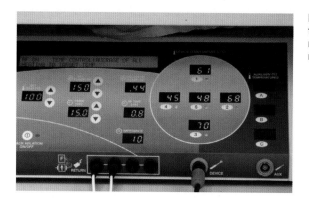

Figure 15.4 The RFA generator settings (to the left in picture) and the temperature monitoring windows (within the circle) on right.

Ultrasound/Doppler

Any standard ultrasound (US) with a Doppler mode can be used. A 7.5- to 10-MHz probe usually gives the appropriate depth to be monitored.

Relevant Anatomy

Figure 15.5 demonstrates the relevant anatomy of the overlying breast. The cosmetic result of any lumpectomy depends on the depth of the subcutaneous tissue underneath the incision. Thus, if only thin flaps will remain after the resection of a superficial tumor, it is best to resect an overlying ellipse of skin. If the tumor is deep and muscle is ablated, it is important to free that zone circumferentially in the plane of the retro-mammary fat pad so that the ablation is not fixed to the chest wall.

Figure 15.5 Relevant anatomy of the subcutaneous tissue breast and underlying pectoralis major.

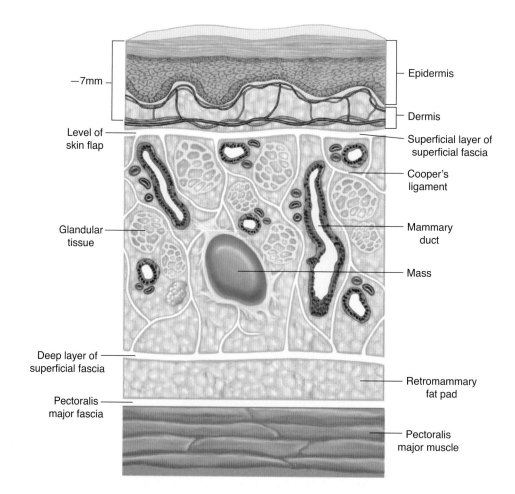

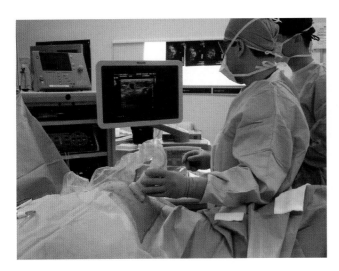

Figure 15.6 Positioning of the operator and assistant across from the mammograms, US/Doppler and RF generator.

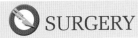

SURGERY

Surgical Technique

Anesthesia

Radiofrequency ablation can be performed under local with or without sedative, or general anesthesia. Local anesthesia is thought to actually facilitate the ablation, as impedance is lower in hydrated tissue.

Positioning

The patient is placed supine with the arm extended at right angle with the body positioned as with lumpectomy juxtaposed to the edge of the table such that the surgeon and assistant can stand on opposing sides of the arm and their view of the mammograms, RFA, and US/Doppler monitors is in line with view of patient (Fig. 15.6).

Preparation of the Excision Bed for Radiofrequency Ablation (eRFA)

- Use a 7.5- to 10-MHz probe to find the lesion and mark location of tumor (Fig. 15.7A and B).
- Make the incision directly over tumor. Take an ellipse of skin if tumor is less than 1 cm from the skin (Fig. 15.8A and B).

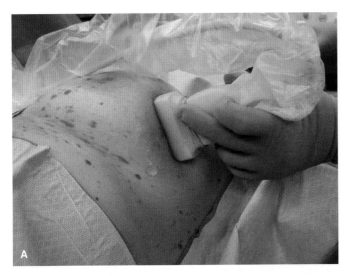
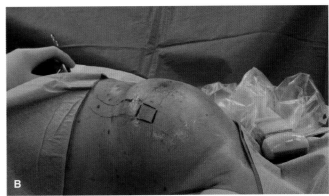

Figure 15.7 A. Demonstrates the use of a 7.5-MHz transducer in a transverse position to locate the underlying breast tumor. **B.** After using the probe in a longitudinal position as well, the exact location of the underlying tumor can be marked.

Part IV: Partial Mastectomy

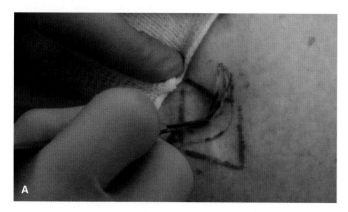 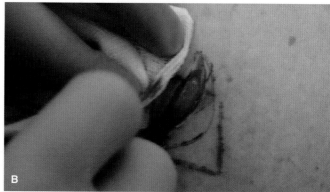

Figure 15.8 A. and **B.** Both demonstrate taking an ellipse of skin directly overlying a superficial tumor (≤1 cm).

■ Excise tumor with the aim of achieving a 1-cm tumor-free margin via US (Fig. 15.9).

■ After hemostasis is achieved, place a purse string in the cavity just above the level of the previous tumor and bring the cavity so that the opening is approximately 1 cm in diameter or about the width of the index finger (Fig. 15.10A and B).

Cavitary Positioning of the Radiofrequency Probe

■ Deploy the radiofrequency (RF) array in the tumor bed so that the tines enter the breast tissue of the lumpectomy bed to a depth of approximately 1 cm around what would have been the prior position of the tumor in regard to the skin and the chest wall (Fig. 15.11A and B).

■ Retract skin from ablation site to protect from the steam of the ablation (Fig. 15.11A).

Ablation Parameters

■ With the power at 150 W, the timer is set for 15 minutes and the RF probe is activated to 100°C average of all tines (circle on right) (Fig. 15.12).

■ If the depth of the tumor is greater than the depth of the deployed array, a "step" ablation may be necessary where the array is deployed and fired more than once to cover the margins around the tumor bed.

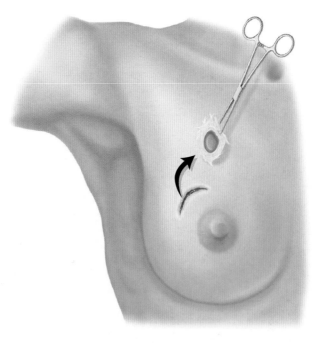

Figure 15.9 Concept of the removal of a tumor with a 1-cm margin around it.

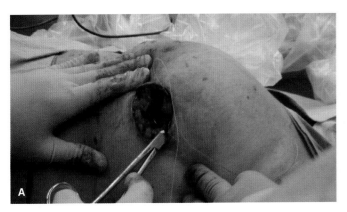

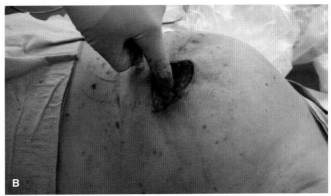

Figure 15.10 A. Demonstrates placement of a purse string just above the level of the tumor bed with a 3-0 absorbable suture. **B.** Demonstrates the 1-cm (approximately a finger's breadth) opening left after the purse string has been tied.

Intraoperative Real-time Imaging of Ablation Zone

The Doppler mode of any US can be used to determine width of ablation and to make sure ablation zone does not jeopardize the skin. The ablation zone lights up on Doppler secondary to off-gassing of nitrogen as the tissue is heated (Fig. 15.13A–C). Retract RFA probe if needed to protect the skin if the Doppler indicates the ablation is within 1 cm of the skin.

Cool Down

After the 15 minutes of ablation is complete, wait for 30 seconds. If temperature of the probes goes below 55°C, ablate at 100°C for 5 more minutes. When the timer runs out, the generator automatically goes into "Cool Down" mode for 30 seconds (0.5 minutes on the generator).

When the cool down is complete, check the temperatures to ensure that all are above 55°C. If not, continue ablation for 5 more minutes at target temperature of 100°C. (Alternatively, the device can be rotated 45 degrees to check temperatures and continue ablation, if necessary).

Postablation Irrigation

After cool down and confirmation of complete ablation, retract the RFA array and remove probe. Figure 15.14A and B reveal typical ablation in the cavity. This is more

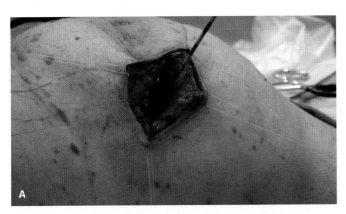

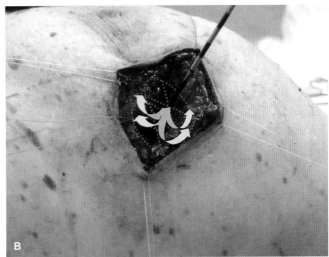

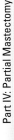

Part IV: Partial Mastectomy

Figure 15.11 A. Demonstrates a RFA array deployed into the wound with the skin carefully drawn back with sutures to avoid steam burns to the skin. **B.** Demonstrates the concept of the deployment of the tines 1 cm into the tumor bed and the effective ablation zone.

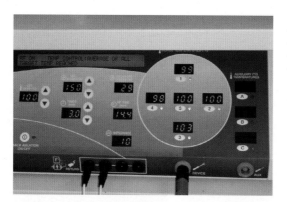

Figure 15.12 The RF generator demonstrates the temperatures in the ablation zone at the five temperature tines (within the circle to right) with the ablation in progress. The generator starts the timer when the average of all temperatures is at 100°C (some may be slightly less and others slightly more).

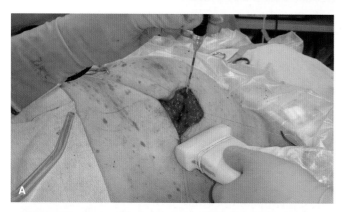

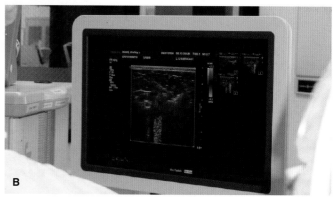

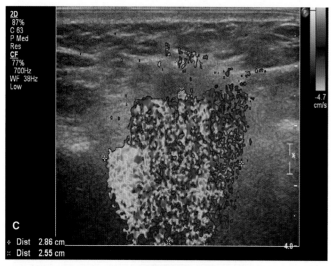

Figure 15.13 A. Demonstrates the positioning of the ultrasound (US) transducer for monitoring the ablation. **B.** Demonstrates the US/Doppler monitor as seen from the field at the beginning of ablation. **C.** The Doppler picture taken to measure the full extent of the ablation zone (2.86 × 2.55 cm with greater than 1 cm from skin).

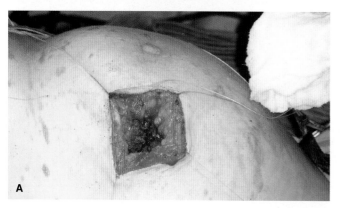

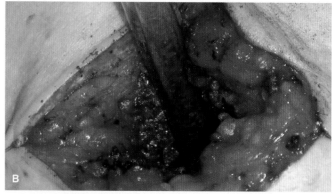

Figure 15.14 A. and **B.** Postablation, after removal of the RF probe, the area of ablation can often be easily recognized and may appear quite necrotic. In more fatty tissue, ablation may not be so apparent.

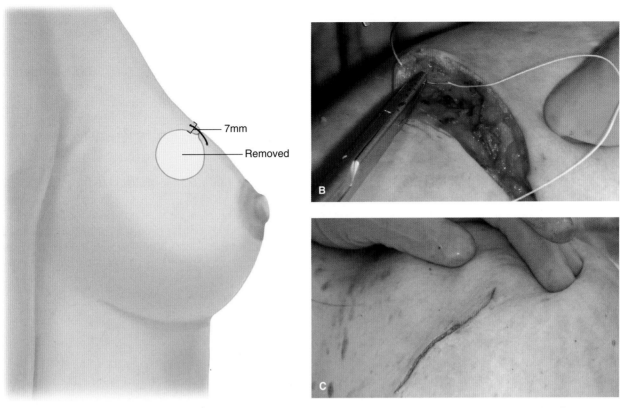

Figure 15.15 A. Concept of closure of lumpectomy cavity. **B.** Demonstrates closed subcutaneous layer closed and the first bite of the interrupted buried dermal stitch. **C.** Dermal layer closed.

readily apparent in more glandular tissue than in fatty tissue. Irrigate the wound with a mix of dilute hydrogen peroxide to remove debris.

Hemostasis
Electrocautery and stick are used as usual to achieve hemostasis.

Closure
The tumor bed is not usually closed because it would cause significant retraction. The subcutaneous tissue just below the skin (at least 7 mm) (Fig. 15.15A) is closed with 3-0 absorbable interrupted stitches, as is the dermal layer (Fig. 15.15B and C).

A 4-0 absorbable running subcuticular stitch is best to close the skin. A drain is unnecessary and may deter the cosmetic result.

Dressing
Closure of the wound with skin glue allows the patient to shower immediately after surgery and allows complete inspection of the wound for any signs of infection (Fig. 15.16).

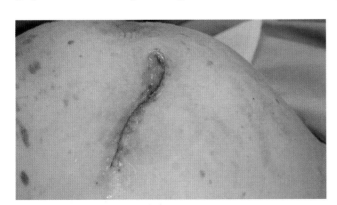

Figure 15.16 Demonstrates wound after closure with 4-0 running subcuticular stitch and dressing with skin glue.

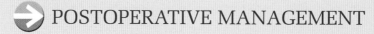 PEARLS AND PITFALLS

- The cosmetic result of any lumpectomy depends on the depth of the subcutaneous tissue underneath the incision. Excise an ellipse on skin over tumors 1 cm or less from the skin surface.
- Excise the tumor with a margin as you would normally do, creating the incision directly over the tumor.
- Steam from the ablation can cause a burn to the skin, so use sutures to retract the skin back.
- Be certain that all surfaces of the cavity are greater than 1 cm in thickness and use the Doppler to avoid skin burns. If the Doppler demonstrates you are getting to close to the skin, partially retract the RF array.
- Use a step ablation (overlap a deep with a more superficial ablation) for larger tumors. Although never necessary, the same RF probe can be used for up to five ablations.
- If the tumor is deep and muscle is ablated, it is important to free that zone circumferentially in the plane of the retromammary fat pad so that the ablation is not fixed to the chest wall.

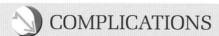 POSTOPERATIVE MANAGEMENT

Postoperative management is identical to that of any partial mastectomy. With the skin glue, patients may shower. There is no need for a pressure dressing although a sports bra is recommended to stabilize the breast for the first 48 hours.

COMPLICATIONS

Complications with eRFA appear to be at par with partial mastectomy except for the potential for the rare RF-related burn or for malfunction of the equipment. Use of Doppler should avoid this complication.

Postoperative pain does not appear to be different.

Skin Burns

Skin burns have been reported with nearly every ablation device or procedure. Burns are usually caused from the steam arising from the ablation zone and can be avoided by using sutures to retract the skin edges back from the site. A burn can also occur from a tine too close to the skin. These burns can be avoided by careful positioning and also continuous monitoring of the overlying skin with intraoperative Doppler US. If the ablation zone appears to close to the skin, the RF array may be repositioned.

Infection

Risk of infection has not been increased in the limited experience with this procedure.

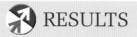 RESULTS

Avoid Re-excision

There is limited but favorable reports that the addition of eRFA can avoid re-excision for close (<3 mm) or focally positive margins in nearly 90 % of patients.

Treatment of Favorable Breast Cancers Without Radiation

Two-year follow-up on 94 patients with in situ or T1 and T2 grade I–III invasive ductal carcinoma treated with eRFA alone (no radiation) has demonstrated no recurrence at the site of the lumpectomy cavity. There were three ipsilateral occurrences elsewhere (>5 cm and different histology) and one contralateral occurrence. Similar to eRFA, radiation only decreases recurrence at the site of the original tumor, and in four randomized trials does not affect elsewhere recurrences in the ipsilateral breast.

✱✥ CONCLUSIONS

Excision followed by radiofrequency ablation added to standard excision or lumpectomy appears to be a safe method of extended margins to avoid re-excision and potentially treat favorable ductal carcinoma in situ and invasive breast cancer.

Suggested Readings

Aziz D, Rawlinson E, Narod SA, et al. The role of reexcision for positive margins in optimizing local disease control after breast-conserving surgery for cancer. *Breast J.* 2006;12(4):331–337.

Bland KL, Gass J, Klimberg VS. Radiofrequency, cryoablation, and other modalities for breast cancer ablation. *Surg Clin North Am.* 2007;87:539–550.

Buchholz TA. Radiation therapy for early-stage breast cancer after breast-conserving surgery [review]. *N Engl J Med.* 2009;360(1): 63–70.

Klimberg VS, Kepple J, Shafirstein G, et al. eRFA: excision followed by RFA—a new technique to improve local control in breast cancer. *Ann Surg Oncol.* 2006;13:1422–1433.

Klimberg VS, Korourian S, Henry-Tillman RS, et al. Obtaining negative margins after lumpectomy with eRFA prevents re-operation [abstract 6100]. *Breast Cancer Res Treat.* 2006;100(S1):S289.

Leong C, Boyages J, Jayasinghe UW, et al. Effects of margins on ipsilateral breast tumor recurrence after breast conservation therapy for lymph node-negative breast carcinoma. *Cancer.* 2004;100: 1823–1832.

Menes TS, Tartter PI, Bleiweiss I, et al. The consequence of multiple re-excisions to obtain clear lumpectomy margins in breast cancer patients. *Ann Surg Oncol.* 2005;12:881–885.

Singletary SE. Surgical margins in patients with early-stage breast cancer treated with breast conservation therapy. *Am J Surg.* 2002; 184:383–393.

Part IV: Partial Mastectomy

16 Breast Brachytherapy Device Placement

Peter D. Beitsch

 ## INDICATIONS/CONTRAINDICATIONS

Essentially all patients undergoing breast conservation therapy should have adjuvant radiation therapy. Traditionally, this has been whole breast irradiation, but over the last 15 years some patients have had only the perilumpectomy portion of their breast treated with radiation given over shortened periods of time—accelerated partial breast irradiation (APBI). Not all lumpectomy patients are candidates for APBI, but general recommendations have been put forth by both the American Society of Breast Surgeons and the American Brachytherapy Society (Table 16.1). Patients falling outside of these parameters can be treated on an individualized basis—always in consultation with the radiation oncologist.

Individual Brachytherapy Devices

Balloon Devices

MammoSite Balloon

The first generation of MammoSite balloon was approved by the U.S. Food and Drug Administration in May 2002. The balloon is made of silicone and has a single treatment lumen. It comes in two spherical sizes—4 to 5 cm and 5 to 6 cm—as well as a 5 cm elliptical size (Fig. 16.1). The main advantages of the MammoSite balloon are the comfort of the soft silicone and the familiarity of the device (it has been available the longest of any of the brachytherapy devices). The main disadvantages are the need for a minimum of 5 mm of skin-to-cavity distance (preferably >7 mm) and the soft balloon may not expand symmetrically, causing the central treatment lumen to be offset and therefore unusable. A second-generation device made of polyurethane is now available that overcomes the symmetry issue but not the skin spacing problem. A third-generation device with multiple catheters is available. The MammoSite ML has a central catheter and three catheters surrounding it. These multiple catheters allow the treatment plan to more precisely tailor the prescription dose to the cavity avoiding excess dose to the skin and chest wall. The balloon is filled with a combination of saline and a small amount of contrast such as Isovue.

TABLE 16.1	Patient Selection Criteria	
Criteria	American Brachytherapy Society	American Society of Breast Surgeons
Age	≥50	≥45
Histology	IDC	IDC, DCIS
Tumor size	≤3 cm	≥3 cm
Node status	neg	neg
Margins	neg	neg

Contura

SenoRx has developed a single-insertion device called the Contura with multicatheters within a balloon (Fig. 16.2). It comes in two sizes—a 4- to 5-cm diameter balloon and a 5- to 6-cm diameter balloon. It looks very similar to the MammoSite with similar insertion methods; however, the multiple catheters allow the treatment plan to more precisely tailor the dose to the cavity, avoiding normal structures such as heart, lung, rib, and skin (thus allowing a narrower skin-to-cavity distance). In addition, the device has suction parts at each end of the balloon to aspirate fluid and air from the cavity. The main disadvantage of Contura is the stiffness of the catheters, which can be uncomfortable to some patients. The balloon is filled with a combination of saline and a small amount of contrast such as Isovue.

By the end of 2009, approximately 6000 devices will have been placed and only short-term data are available for this device. The company has begun a registry trial with a targeted accrual of approximately 400 patients.

Multicatheter Bundled Devices

SAVI

Cianna has developed a single-insertion, multicatheter device called the SAVI (Fig. 16.3). It comes in 6-mini, 6, 8, or 10 catheters depending on the size of the lumpectomy cavity. The catheters are in direct contact with the lumpectomy walls. SAVI can be used in almost all cavities but is particularly suited for small (<30 cc) cavities (6-mini) and long, elliptical cavities. The multiple catheters allow the treatment plan to more precisely tailor the dose to the cavity, avoiding normal structures such as heart, lung, rib, and skin (thus allowing a narrower skin-to-cavity distance). Although there is a newer version of SAVI with more flexible catheters now available, the main disadvantage of the device

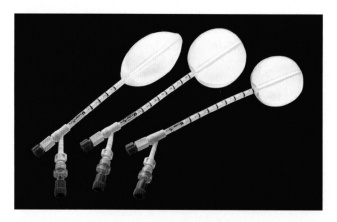

Figure 16.1 MammoSite balloon catheters.

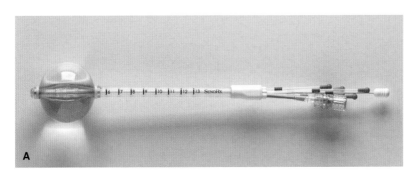

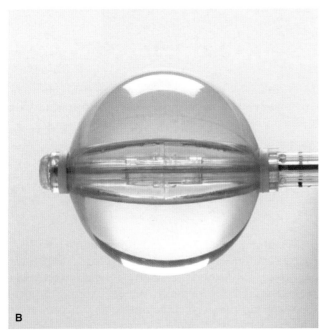

Figure 16.2 Contura balloon with multicatheters.

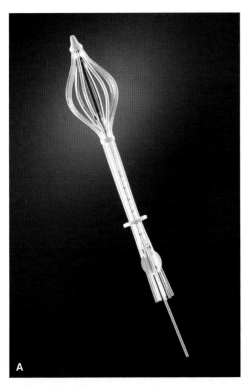

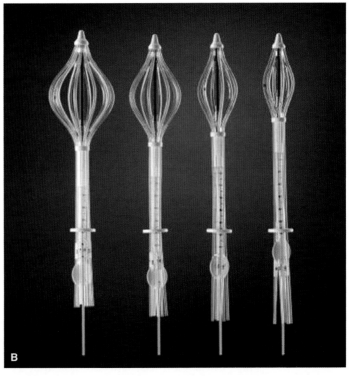

Figure 16.3 SAVI.

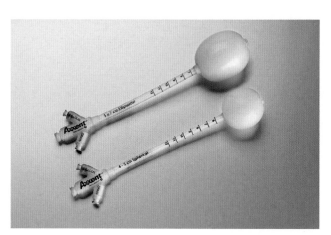

Figure 16.4 Axxent balloon devices.

is the stiffness of the catheters, which can be uncomfortable to some patients. By the end of 2009, approximately 3000 patients will have been treated with this device and only short-term treatment data are available.

New Brachytherapy Sources

Xoft

Xoft has developed a miniaturized X-ray radiation source, the Axxent system, that replaces the radioactive iridium seed and is delivered through their own single-catheter balloon devices (Fig. 16.4). The "source" is emitting radiation only when turned on and is of a much lower energy. This low-energy "source" allows the patient to be treated outside the radiation vault in places such as physician offices. The shielding required is similar to that needed for routine office X-rays. They have their own set of balloon applicators that have a barium-impregnated balloon and are inserted similarly to the MammoSite catheter. By the end of 2009, more than 500 devices had been used for treatment.

The EXIBT (Electronic Xoft Intersocietal Brachytherapy Trial) registry under the oversight of the American Brachytherapy Society, American Society of Breast Surgeons, and American College of Radiation Oncology has accrued 69 patients as of the end of 2009. Extensive treatment parameters (V150, V200, V300, etc.) have been collected along with short term/long term complication data and recurrence/survival data.

Zeiss

Zeiss has also developed a low-energy electronic radiation source that currently is used only intraoperatively; however, there are plans underway to develop balloon applicators for use in minimally shielded environments similar to the Xoft Axxent system. The TARGIT randomized study of intra-operative single dose radiation versus traditional whole breast irradiation has completed accrual. The results will be published in the near future.

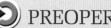 PREOPERATIVE PLANNING

Brachytherapy devices are usually placed postoperatively in the physician's procedure room. This allows the final pathology to be evaluated to ensure the patient is a good candidate for APBI. In addition, at least for the MammoSite balloon catheter, there may be a lower short-term infection rate and lower long-term seroma rate with postoperative placement.

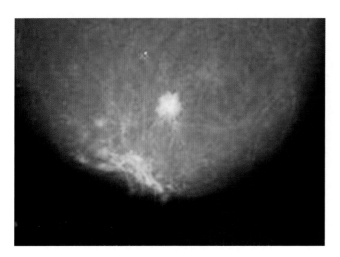

Figure 16.5 Fatty replaced mammogram with easily seen cancer.

Postoperative placement begins with the preoperative recognition that a patient is a potential APBI candidate. Once identified, APBI can be incorporated into the overall treatment discussion with the patient as a possibility for her postoperative adjuvant radiation. This is also a good time to have the patient consult with the radiation oncologist. This interdisciplinary interaction is crucial for successful APBI treatment.

Occasionally, preoperative workup includes breast magnetic resonance imaging to ensure there is no multicentric disease or the tumor is not larger than suspected. However, most APBI candidates are postmenopausal women with involuted breasts and fat density; mammograms show their cancers clearly (Fig. 16.5).

Pertinent Anatomy

The placement of a breast brachytherapy device requires a basic understanding of breast anatomy as well as a minimum level of ultrasound knowledge of the breast (Figs. 16.6 and 16.7). Ultrasound assessment includes skin-to-cavity distance, general gestalt of the shape, and actual dimensions of the cavity (height, width, and length) (Figs. 16.8 and 16.9). This evaluation of the cavity will aid in the choice of brachytherapy device as well as determining the size of the device needed.

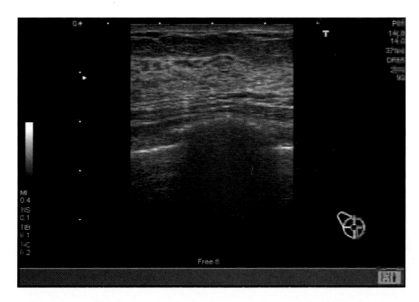

Figure 16.6 Normal sonographic anatomy.

Figure 16.7 Normal sonographic anatomy.

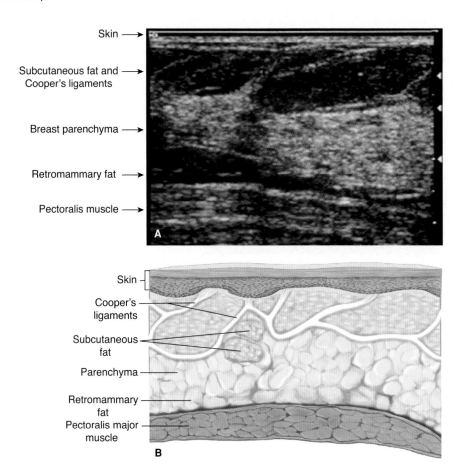

Skin ⟶

Subcutaneous fat and ⟶
Cooper's ligaments

Breast parenchyma ⟶

Retromammary fat ⟶

Pectoralis muscle ⟶

Skin

Cooper's ligaments

Subcutaneous fat

Parenchyma

Retromammary fat

Pectoralis major muscle

SURGERY

Successful office placement begins with proper surgical planning in the operating room. The surgeon needs to consider how he or she will place the brachytherapy device in the office at the time he or she is performing the lumpectomy. Considerations include the following:

1. Location of the incision—usually directly over the cancer although tunneling to the tumor is acceptable if this improves cosmesis (Fig. 16.10).

Figure 16.8 Sonographic appearance of lumpectomy cavity.

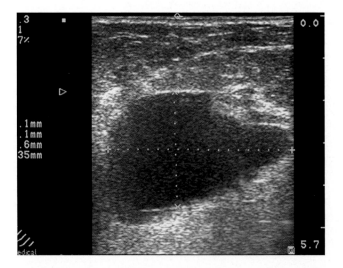

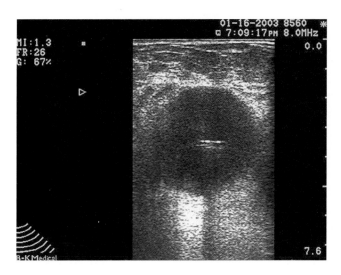

Figure 16.9 Sonographic image of bradytherapy balloon in lumpectomy cavity.

2. Taking a skin ellipse overlying the tumor—often done if the tumor is close to the skin surface (Fig. 16.11).
3. Subcutaneous closure—enough tissue is closed over the cavity to ensure adequate skin-to-cavity distance (although the newer multicatheter devices allow narrower skin-to-cavity distance, there is still a 2 to 3 mm minimum even for those devices) (Fig. 16.12).
4. Avoiding significant crevices or irregularly shaped cavities—this is to ensure that the brachytherapy device will be able to cover the lumpectomy cavity walls with the prescription dose of radiation (Fig. 16.13).

Newer oncoplastic techniques that obliterate all dead space including the lumpectomy cavity are usually not amenable to postoperative brachytherapy device placement. Mini-oncoplastic techniques that minimally rearrange the breast tissue and still maintain a cavity preserve post-operative APBI options. Use of a cavity evaluation device (CED) to maintain the lumpectomy cavity can also be used in conjunction with oncoplastic techniques to maintain a cavity post-operatively APBI. In addition, there are some intraoperative techniques that could be used to give the patient a single intraoperative radiation dose and then use oncoplastic techniques to close all dead space.

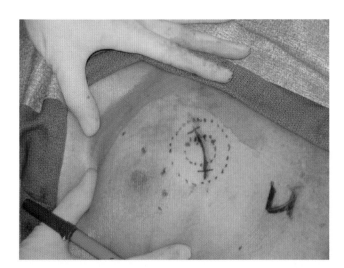

Figure 16.10 Lumpectomy incision directly over the cancer.

Part IV: Partial Mastectomy

Figure 16.11 Remove an ellipse of skin with superficial lesions to maximize skin spacing.

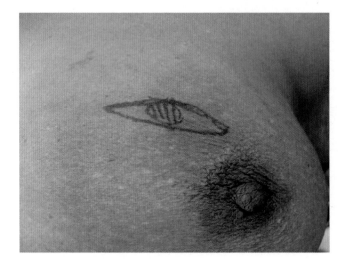

Figure 16.12 Adequate subcutaneous closure.

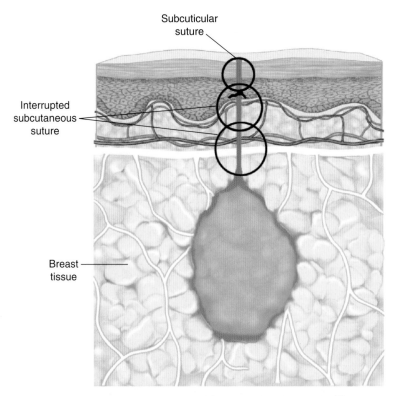

Figure 16.13 Sonographic image of irregular cavity with crevice on left side.

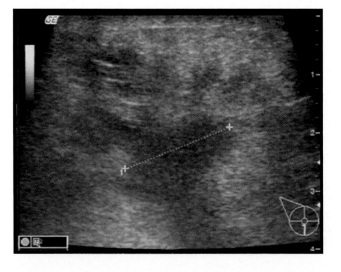

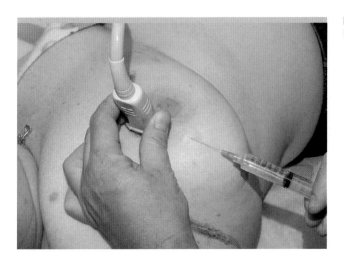

Figure 16.14 Cavity ultrasound and lidocaine injection.

 POSTOPERATIVE MANAGEMENT

Although all brachytherapy devices can be placed intraoperatively, postoperative placement is preferred since the final pathology report is available to ensure the patient has negative margins and is node negative. There are two main categories of devices— balloon based and bundled multicatheters. Indications for each device are similar as are the insertion techniques. However, each type has unique features and placement issues, which will be discussed now.

Balloon Insertion Technique

Lateral Insertion Technique

There are three techniques for postoperative balloon device placement. The most common technique is ultrasound-guided percutaneous implantation. This method involves sonographic visualization of the breast lumpectomy cavity. After skin and subcutaneous tissue infiltration with lidocaine (Fig. 16.14), an ~1 cm skin nick is made with a #11 blade several centimeters away from the lumpectomy incision (Figs. 16.15 and 16.16). Then, a sharp metal trocar (provided by the manufacturer) is inserted with ultrasound guidance into the lumpectomy cavity (Fig. 16.17). The cavity seroma decompresses through the trocar lumen (MammoSite) or with a syringe aspirated through the introducer sleeve (Contura) (Fig. 16.18) or through the trocar tract (Axxent). Then, the deflated balloon catheter is inserted into the cavity through the trocar track (Fig. 16.19). After the

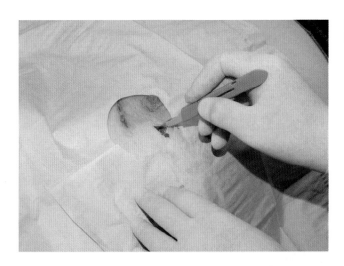

Figure 16.15 Sterile drape and lateral stab incision.

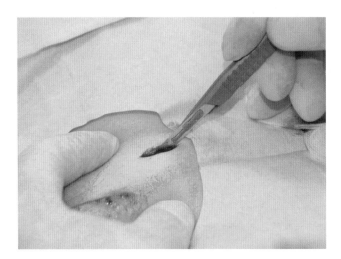

Figure 16.16 Sterile drape and lateral stab incision.

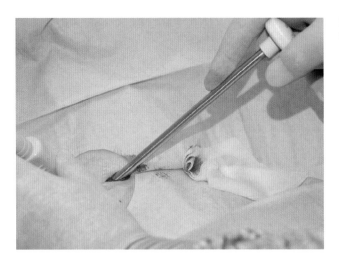

Figure 16.17 Trocar insertion under sono guidance.

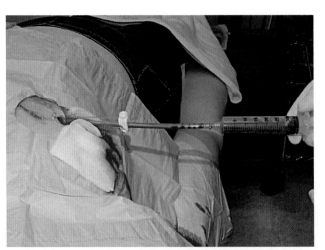

Figure 16.18 Aspirating the seroma through the introducer sleeve of the Contura.

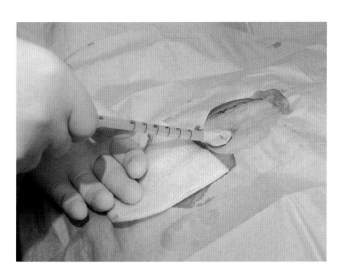

Figure 16.19 Balloon insertion.

balloon is inflated (Fig. 16.20), ultrasound is used to confirm balloon symmetry, balloon to cavity wall conformance, and balloon-to-skin distance (Fig. 16.21).

Scar Entry Technique

Another postoperative method is the scar entry technique. In this technique, the catheter is introduced through the healing lumpectomy incision. This involves slightly opening the lumpectomy incision and using a hemostat to develop a track into the lumpectomy cavity. The balloon is then placed directly into the lumpectomy cavity and inflated. Both sides of the wound are sutured to ensure the rest of the wound stays closed (Fig. 16.22).

CED Exchange

Proper postoperative placement for all the techniques begins in the operating room during the lumpectomy. The lumpectomy wound should be closed in multiple layers to provide as much subcutaneous tissue between the skin and the lumpectomy cavity (preferably at least 1 centimeter) (Fig. 16.12). One way to ensure optimal postoperative skin-to-cavity distance, as well as achieve cavity conformity, is to place a cavity evaluation device (CED)—a simple balloon without a central catheter that can be tunneled into the lumpectomy cavity through a separate lateral skin incision (Fig. 16.23). The CED acts as a placeholder until margin and nodal status are known and the patient is confirmed as a good candidate for brachytherapy device placement. The CED is considerably cheaper than the actual balloon devices and can be easily removed if the patient is not suitable for APBI. Most surgeons keep patients on antibiotics while the CED and subsequent brachytherapy devices are in place.

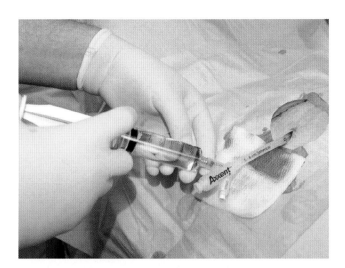

Figure 16.20 Inflating the balloon.

Part IV: Partial Mastectomy

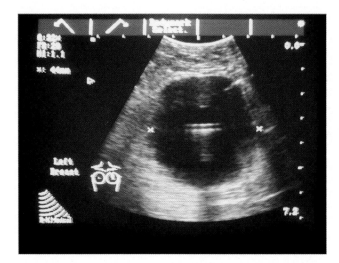

Figure 16.21 Ultrasound image of the balloon.

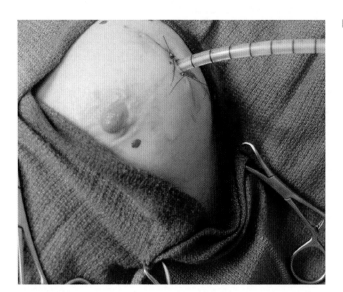

Figure 16.22 Scar entry technique.

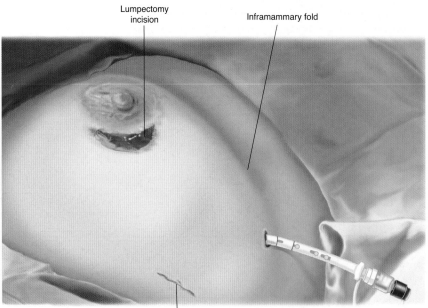

Figure 16.23 Cavity evaluation device placement.

Lumpectomy incision

Inframammary fold

Head of patient to left

Sentinal node incision in axilla

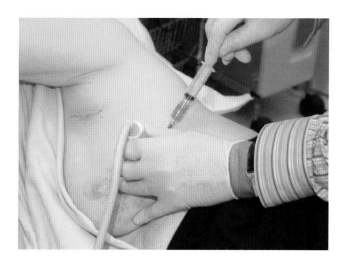

Figure 16.24 Lidocaine infiltration and seroma aspiration.

SAVI Technique

The bundled multicatheter devices are percutaneously placed with ultrasound guidance. The breast lumpectomy cavity is visualized and lidocaine is infiltrated in the skin and the track leading up to the cavity, usually entering the cavity as shown by the aspiration of a small amount of seroma fluid (Fig. 16.24). An ~1.2 cm skin nick is made with a #11 blade (usually a little larger than that used with the balloon devices) several centimeters away from the lumpectomy wound (Fig. 16.25). Then, a sharp trocar (provided by the manufacturer) is inserted with ultrasound guidance into the lumpectomy cavity (Fig. 16.17). The cavity seroma decompresses through the trocar tract. The undeployed SAVI device is inserted into the cavity through the trocar track (Fig. 16.26). The device is expanded to the edges of the cavity and locked in place. SAVI uses a deployment key that deploys and is removed, which locks the struts in place (SAVI, Figs. 16.27 and 16.28). The device is then sterilely dressed (Fig. 16.29).

After Device Placement

Once the device has been placed, the patient undergoes three-dimensional treatment planning utilizing computed tomography (CT) imaging. A typical scenario is device placement on Wednesday or Thursday and CT imaging on Friday. Treatment begins on Monday and continues twice a day until Friday. Either ultrasound or CT is used to verify device integrity/placement before every fraction of radiation. After the final treatment of 10 fractions totaling 34 Gy over 5 days, the radiation oncologist takes out the

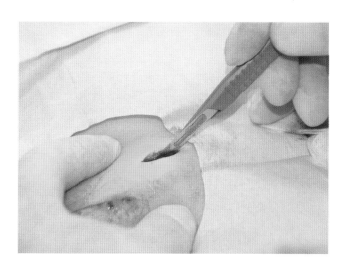

Figure 16.25 Lateral skin incision.

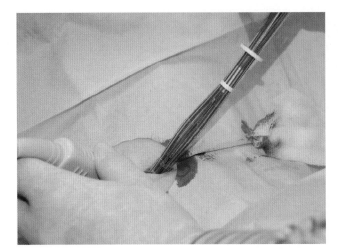

Figure 16.26 SAVI insertion.

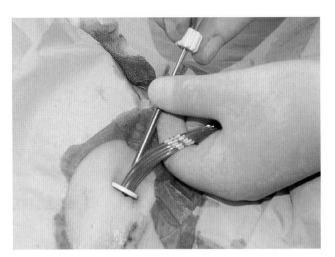

Figure 16.27 SAVI deployment.

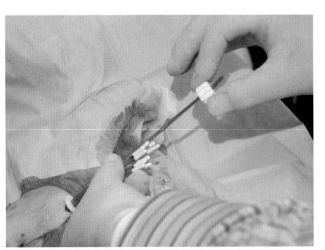

Figure 16.28 Removing the SAVI deployment key.

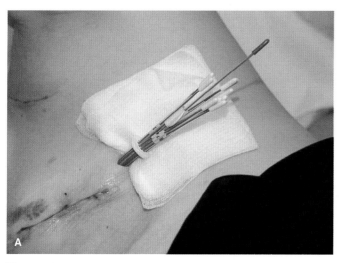
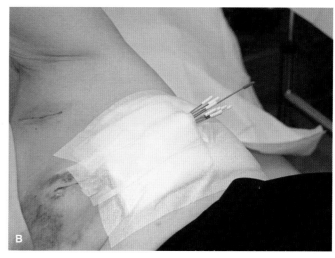

Figure 16.29 Sterile dressing.

device by deflating the balloon or retracting the catheters and gently removing the device from the breast.

 ## COMPLICATIONS

The majority of the data on brachytherapy devices is from the MammoSite device. Short-term toxicity with the MammoSite has been minimal, with mild erythema, pain, drainage, seroma, and ecchymosis seen occasionally and an infection rate of less than 10% with only the very rare infection necessitating balloon removal. Cosmetic results are good or excellent in ~90% of patients at 5 years.

 ## PEARLS AND PITFALLS

- When placing a CED in the operating room or a breast brachytherapy device in your office, there may be a significant amount of drainage from around the lateral insertion incision. Warning the patient will often save a midnight phone call.
- After placing a balloon device there may be fluid that is trapped between the balloon and the lumpectomy cavity wall. Gentle breast massage can be used to evacuate this fluid through the track and out of the lateral stab incision. This can be done at the time of insertion or when the patient gets her treatment planning CT scan.
- Both the Contura and Axxent balloon catheters have suction ports that can be used at anytime—in your office at the time of insertion, when the treatment CT scan is done, or anytime during the 5 days of treatment.
- If the MammoSite is being placed in the operating room, sometimes the skin-to-balloon distance is inadequate. This can be solved by reopening the wound, excising the thin skin flaps, and reapproximating additional subcutaneous tissue before closing the skin.
- As the lumpectomy cavity heals, it will become progressively more fibrotic and less distensible, eventually disappearing entirely. This healing fibrosis may make symmetrical deployment of the MammoSite balloon difficult (may be less of an issue with the Contura (polyurethane) stiffer balloon or the bundled multicatheter devices). This healing also means that there is a finite amount of time between the lumpectomy surgery and the placement of the MammoSite or other brachytherapy device (usually <4 weeks). Therefore, earlier placement of the MammoSite or other device is advisable.
- One of the advantages of brachytherapy is to get all the radiation therapy completed prior to the initiation of systemic therapy. However, to avoid radiation recall,

Part IV: Partial Mastectomy

chemotherapy should be delayed for a minimum of 3 weeks after the completion of the brachytherapy.

▦ Essentially, all cavities are irregular; however, the cavity walls can usually be pushed into a sphere by the balloon devices. The bundled devices can accommodate the irregular walls and the treatment plan will compensate for the irregularity.

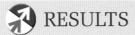 RESULTS

MammoSite Data

The company that developed the MammoSite balloon catheter began a registry just after U.S. Food and Drug Administration approval in May 2002. The MammoSite Registry was taken over by the American Society of Breast Surgeons in November 2003. The registry has 1400 patients (1449 treated breasts) with a median follow-up of more than 5 years as of the end of 2009. The 5-year actuarial ipsilateral breast tumor recurrence rate is 3.8% and axillary recurrence rate is 0.6%, which is comparable to the rates for whole breast irradiation.

 CONCLUSIONS

The use of APBI is increasing. This trend should continue since tumor size is continuing to decrease (thus allowing more women to meet selection criteria). APBI will become more widespread as surgeons and radiation oncologists offer it as a more convenient but safe alternative to the traditional 6 to 7 weeks of whole breast irradiation. The keys to successfully implementing a breast brachytherapy program include (i) interdisciplinary care with close coordination between the surgeon and the radiation oncologist, (ii) appropriate patient selection, (iii) intraoperative surgical planning which optimizes the postoperative device placement, and (iv) familiarity and knowledge of more than one device to choose the appropriate device for the individual patient.

Suggested Readings

1. Keisch M, Vicini F, Kuske R, et al. Initial clinical experience with the MammoSite breast brachytherapy applicator in women with early-stage breast cancer treated with breast-conserving therapy. *Int J Radiat Oncol Biol Phys.* 2003;55:289–293.
2. Zannis V, Walker L, Barclay-White B, et al. Postoperative ultrasound-guided percutaneous placement of a new breast brachytherapy balloon catheter. *Am J Surg.* 2003;186:383–385.
3. Dowlatshahi K, Snider H, Gittleman M, et al. Early experience with balloon brachytherapy for breast cancer. *Arch Surg.* 2004;139(6):603–607.
4. Keisch M, Vicini F, Kuske R, et al. Two-year outcome with the MammoSite breast brachytherapy applicator: factors associated with optimal cosmetic results when performing partial breast irradiation. *Int J Radiat Oncol Biol Phys* 2003;57(2)(suppl 1): S315.
5. Vicini F, Beitsch P, Quiet C, et al. First analysis of patient demographics, technical reproducibility, cosmesis and early toxicity by the American Society of Breast Surgeons MammoSite™ breast

brachytherapy registry trial in 1237 patients treated with accelerated partial breast irradiation. *Cancer.* 2004;104(6):1138–1148.
6. Zannis V, Beitsch P, Vicini F, et al. Descriptions and outcomes of insertion techniques of a breast brachytherapy balloon catheter in 1403 patients enrolled in the American Society of Breast Surgeons MammoSite breast brachytherapy registry trial. *Am J Surg.* 2005;190(4):530–538.
7. Jeruss JS, Vicini FA, Beitsch PD, et al. Initial outcomes for patients treated on the American Society of Breast Surgeons MammoSite clinical trial for ductal carcinoma-in-situ of the breast. *Ann Surg Oncol.* 2006;13(7):967–976.
8. Benitez PR, Keisch ME, Vicini F, et al. Five-year results: the initial clinical trial of MammoSite balloon brachytherapy for partial breast irradiation in early-stage breast cancer. *Am J Surg.* 2007;194(4):456–462.
9. Vicini F, Beitsch PD, Quiet CA, et al. Three-year analysis of treatment efficacy, cosmesis, and toxicity by the American Society of Breast Surgeons MammoSite® Breast Brachytherapy Registry Trial in patients treated with accelerated partial breast irradiation (APBI). *Cancer.* 2008;112(4):758–766.

17 Intraoperative Radiotherapy

Lydia Choi, Elisa Perego, and Virgilio Sacchini

Introduction

Rationale for Intraoperative Radiotherapy

The rationale for the use of segmental radiation therapy in place of whole-breast irradiation is based on the finding that approximately 85% of breast relapses are confined to the same quadrant of the breast as the primary tumor (1). Tumoral foci are usually near the primary tumor, and residual microscopic disease occurring in the same quadrant as the resection is often the cause of local disease recurrence. Phase I and II trials have demonstrated that single-dose intraoperative radiotherapy (IORT) for localized breast cancers can be applied without increasing the normal rate of complications after surgery. Other studies with brachytherapy with longer follow-up demonstrated that partial radiation therapy can be performed safely with good local control and good cosmesis in selected patients.

Advantages of IORT

The ability to deliver a single therapeutic dose of radiation to the tumor bed during surgery or within 5 days after surgery, thereby avoiding the standard 5- to 6-week external-beam treatment, may benefit patients through alleviating psychological distress, allowing earlier return to normal life, and reducing related expenses, including the cost of the procedure and other indirectly associated expenses.

Convenience and Cost

Shortening the course of radiotherapy from the standard 6-week regimen to a single-dose intraoperative technique lowers costs and allows more convenience for patients. It also increases compliance to 100% and eliminates the attrition rate during standard radiotherapy because of side effects or logistical difficulties in traveling to the radiation facility (1). It may allow more breast conservation in rural geographic areas where radiation facilities or transportation are not readily available and where many women must undergo mastectomy because of these secondary issues.

Accuracy

Precisely targeting therapy to the lumpectomy cavity with IORT also directs radiation to the site most likely to need therapy and spares the brachial plexus, heart, and lungs. It avoids an incorrectly directed boost of standard radiotherapy because of lack of clips or seroma to define the lumpectomy cavity accurately. Benda et al. (2) showed discrepancies between radiation oncologists in planning cavity boosts, with variation in targets of more than 1 cm. Radiation to the skin is also reduced by shielding and may be associated with improved cosmesis and possibly elimination of radiation-induced angiosarcoma.

Elimination of Delay in Receiving Radiotherapy

When radiation is delayed because of timing around chemotherapy, there is evidence to suggest increased local failure (3). Although data are conflicting, irradiating immediately renders arguments for or against giving chemotherapy first moot.

INDICATIONS/CONTRAINDICATIONS

Expanded Indications for Radiotherapy

Previously irradiated patients, either for Hodgkin disease or previous cancer, are generally considered to be ineligible for re-irradiation if they have recurrence. IORT has been found to be a promising option for these patients (4).

PREOPERATIVE PLANNING

Partial radiation therapy has been tested in several clinical phase I and II studies and is currently under investigation for phase III in a major nationwide National Surgical Adjuvant Breast and Bowel Project - Radiation Therapy Oncology Group (NSABP-RTOG) study randomizing breast cancer patients submitted to conservative surgery to receive conventional whole-breast external-beam radiation therapy or partial radiation therapy in the form of three-dimensional (3D) conformal external beam, brachytherapy with MammoSite or brachytherapy with iridium implants. Other trials in Europe such as the Electron Intraoperative radioTherapy (ELIOT) trial and TARGeted Intraoperative radioTherapy (TARGIT) trial are studying the delivery of partial radiation therapy during surgery, immediately after quadrantectomy, or lumpectomy.

As part of the TARGIT trial, criteria for IORT are defined as age greater than 40 years and unicentric invasive breast cancer less than 3 cm in size treatable by lumpectomy (5). The European Institute of Oncology trial limits participants to patients older than 48 years with unifocal small invasive cancer (maximum tumor diameter 2.5 cm).

Because IORT is still considered an experimental treatment for breast cancer, it has been limited outside of trials in use to older patients with early-stage cancer or patients who are not candidates for standard whole-breast irradiation, such as those previously irradiated or those with severe comorbidities (6). It has also been evaluated as a boost dose with standard radiotherapy to the whole breast, although when this is decided on as the course of treatment, a longer interval of 5 to 6 weeks between IORT and standard radiotherapy seems to be associated with reduced morbidity compared with intervals shorter than 4 weeks (7). Another use of IORT is as a dose to the nipple–areolar complex after nipple-sparing mastectomy. A total of 800 patients receiving IORT were compared with 200 receiving standard radiotherapy to the nipple–areolar complex with no significant difference in outcome, even when a group with close margins was evaluated (8).

Patients with bilateral breast cancer, multifocal or multicentric breast cancer, clinically positive lymph node metastasis, or extensive ductal carcinoma in situ (DCIS) are not candidates for IORT. Exclusion criteria for standard radiation also apply, such as collagen vascular disease and pregnancy, although a preliminary dose analysis of potential fetal radiation exposure in Milan showed negligible delivery to the fetus (9).

SURGERY

Relevant Surgical Anatomy

The boundaries of the breast include the clavicle superiorly, the sternum medially, and the latissimus dorsi posterolaterally. When brachytherapy is used, the lumpectomy is performed in a standard fashion, either with or without preoperative needle localization. In the United States this usually involves removal of less tissue than in Italy (the home of the ELIOT IORT trial) where quadrantectomy with removal of skin, parenchyma, and muscle fascia is often the norm. At least 1 cm of tissue from the tumor bed to either the skin or chest wall should remain after lumpectomy for the best cosmetic result from IORT.

There are two main methods of delivering IORT: electron beam through linear accelerators and brachytherapy. Several different machines are in use for delivering electron beams, and whereas previously these were stationary, currently most are portable. Mobile linear accelerators include Linac (Info&Tech, Rome, Italy), Novac7 (Hitesys Srl, Aprilia, Italy), Mobetron (IntraOp Medical Corp, Santa Clara, California), and Intrabeam (Zeiss, Inc, Oberkochen, Germany). These machines are portable electron delivery systems that can be moved into the operating room. Electron beams are delivered at variable energies (3, 5, 7, and 9 eV) with maximum energy of 10 to 12 MeV to limit possible exposure to other operating rooms (10).

The Intrabeam, which is the system used in the TARGIT trial, deserves mention for variation from this description. It is a photon radiosurgery system that has been approved by the Federal Drug Administration for use in any part of the body since 1999 (11). Photon radiosurgery also uses electron beams, but these are used to generate X-ray photons at the tip of a wand-like instrument that is inserted into the lumpectomy cavity. This results in delivery of radiation from the lumpectomy cavity outward, as with brachytherapy. The limit of this method is the superficial penetration of the radiation beam: only 2 mm of tissue surrounding the lumpectomy cavity receives the therapeutic dose of 20 Gy.

Procedure Steps

The method of IORT delivery determines the extent of breast dissection.

1. For all mobile linear accelerators, the lumpectomy or quadrantectomy is initially performed as usual. A skin incision is made, then dissection carried through subcutaneous fat and breast parenchyma to reach the tumor, which is removed with a 1 to 2 cm margin of normal surrounding tissue (Figs. 17.1 and 17.2).

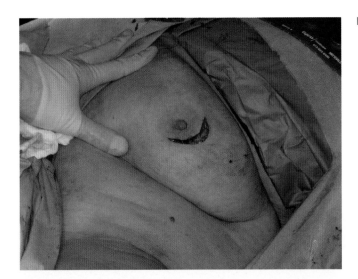

Figure 17.1 Lumpectomy incision.

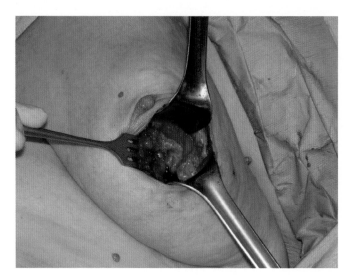

Figure 17.2 Lumpectomy cavity.

2. Skin and breast parenchyma must then be mobilized for protection during IORT delivery:
   a. Skin flaps are raised from the underlying breast tissue for a few centimeters circumferentially to allow retraction away from the radiation source.
   b. Breast parenchyma is then lifted free from the pectoralis muscle to allow insertion of a protective aluminum-lead disk over the pectoralis (Fig. 17.3).
   c. Once this is inserted, the breast parenchyma is temporarily closed over the disk with sutures and the skin is retracted (Fig. 17.4) before positioning of the radiation delivery tube (Fig. 17.5).
3. Radiation beams are collimated, or aligned, by a 5-mm-thick Perspex tube that has two parts: the sterile portion is placed in the operative field by the surgeon before connection to the distal portion, which is managed by the radiation oncologist. Electron beams are delivered perpendicular to the tissue for 2 minutes, with electron energies corresponding to the distance of penetration (Fig. 17.6).
4. After radiation delivery, the tube is removed and the lumpectomy incision closed as usual, with or without breast parenchymal closure (Fig. 17.7).

The other method of delivering IORT is brachytherapy. Radiation is delivered at high-dose rate through remote afterloading—in other words, a relatively high dose of

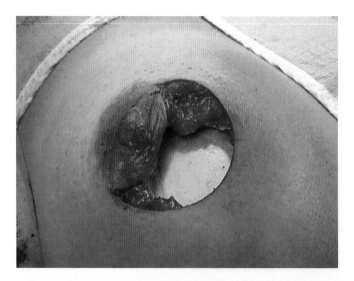

Figure 17.3 Lead disk insertion.

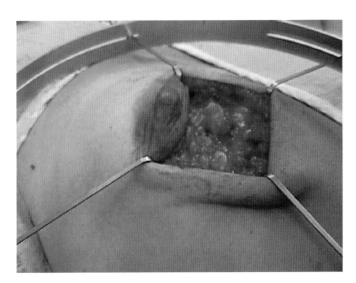

Figure 17.4 Closure of breast flaps and retraction of the skin.

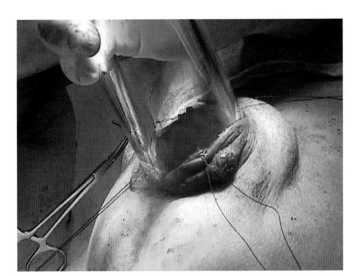

Figure 17.5 Cathodid tube insertion.

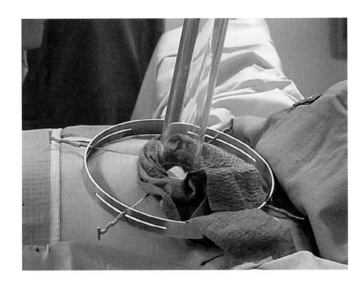

Figure 17.6 Skin retraction and radiation delivery.

Part IV: Partial Mastectomy

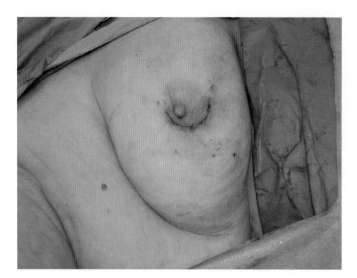

Figure 17.7 Skin closure.

radiation (20 Gy) is temporarily delivered through tubing connected to a Silastic template, which is inserted into the lumpectomy cavity. The main difference between this technique and the electron beam therapy is that the skin and chest wall do not have to be protected from the radiotherapy source because radiation is delivered internally to externally and diffuses sufficiently by the time it reaches the skin and muscle, thus avoiding significant toxicity (12).

1. With this method, the lumpectomy is again performed as usual. A 1 cm margin of normal breast tissue between the radiation source, skin, and chest wall is preferred. The skin is retracted using the Lone Star Retraction System (Fig. 17.8).
2. The sterile applicator is inserted into the lumpectomy cavity and the tubing connected to the radiation delivery source. The method used at our institution is to size the cavity with phantom Harrison–Anderson–Mick (HAM) applicators (Figs. 17.9 and 17.10). When the correct size is found, a corresponding real HAM applicator is inserted into the cavity (Fig. 17.11).
3. The skin edges are covered with sponges or towels to protect them from the radiation source (Fig. 17.12).
4. Computer-calculated dosimetry is used to determine the dwell time of the radiation source within the catheters and the total treatment time (Fig. 17.13).
5. The radiation source is delivered through the tubing into the applicators and left in place for the prescribed time (Figs. 17.14 and 17.15).

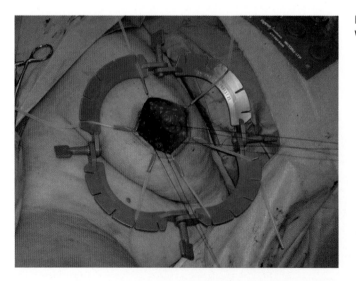

Figure 17.8 Retraction of the skin with Lone Star Retraction System.

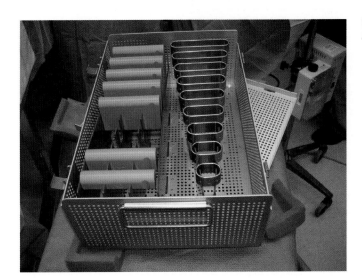

Figure 17.9 Phantom Harrison–Anderson–Mick applicator.

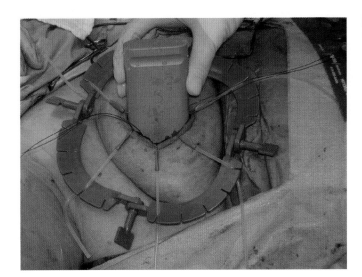

Figure 17.10 Find correct size Harrison–Anderson–Mick.

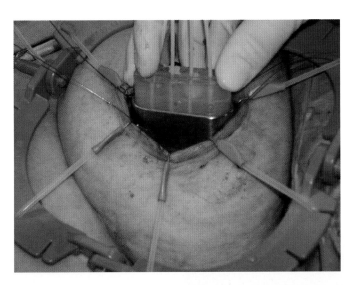

Figure 17.11 Real Harrison–Anderson–Mick applicator insertion.

Figure 17.12 Harrison–Anderson–Mick applicator complete insertion with skin protection.

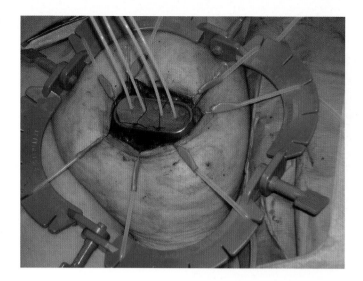

Figure 17.13 Intraoperative radiotherapy dosimetry.

(−15.00,1.53,7.86)

(−15.00,−1.47,7.86)

(0.00,1.53,7.86)

(0.00,−1.47,7.86)

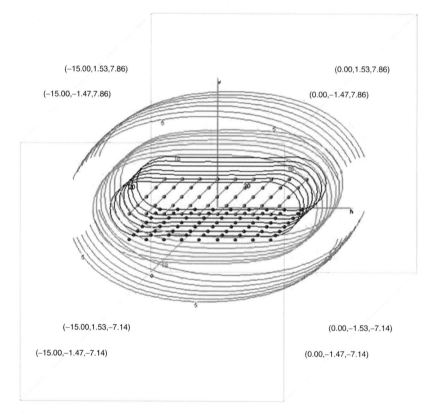

(−15.00,1.53,−7.14)

(−15.00,−1.47,−7.14)

(0.00,−1.53,−7.14)

(0.00,−1.47,−7.14)

Figure 17.14 After-loading machine.

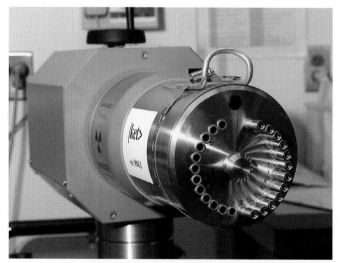

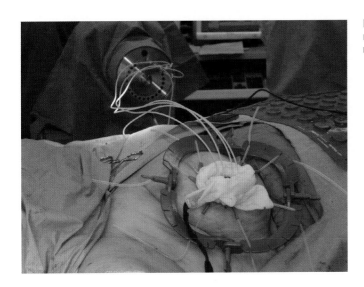

Figure 17.15 Wire connection to radiation source to after-loading machine.

6. When radiation delivery is completed, the source is removed and the lumpectomy incision closed as usual (Fig. 17.8).

 PEARLS AND PITFALLS

In summary, IORT can be used as a boost or as single-dose radiation therapy after breast-conservation surgery. The main advantages are convenience for the patient, lower cost, greater accuracy in delivery with less radiation to the skin and contralateral breast, elimination of delay in administering radiotherapy, and the possibility of expanding indications for radiation to previously irradiated patients.

In terms of eligibility for IORT, there are anatomic and patient considerations. Tumors too close to the skin or chest wall will not allow for IORT because a margin of 1 cm is needed between the skin or chest wall and the radiation source. Because of the experimental nature of IORT to date, older patients with small ductal tumors without an extensive intraductal component are ideal. Early trial results show comparable local recurrence rates, but follow-up is limited.

COMPLICATIONS

Positive margins on final pathology can be problematic when IORT is administered. Several methods are used to deal with this. The preference of the European Institute of Oncology, Milan has been to perform quadrantectomy to remove a generous portion of tissue and thus reduce positive margin rates. Other methods include frozen-section analysis of margins and waiting until final margins are assessed before administering IORT. In the brachytherapy trial at Memorial Sloan-Kettering Cancer Center, the specimen is examined grossly after sectioning for any close margins. The surgeon is informed if any margins appear to be close, and additional tissue is taken at the initial operation before beginning radiotherapy. All methods are associated with disadvantages, and reexcision of positive margins after radiotherapy has been given intraoperatively can result in poor wound healing.

Tumors too close to the skin or axillary tail, where there is insufficient breast parenchyma to shield skin or the chest wall, are not candidates for IORT. Lobular cancers have been excluded from some trials because of their higher likelihood of occult disease spreading beyond the immediate lumpectomy site.

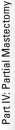

Part IV: Partial Mastectomy

TABLE 17.1		IORT Evaluated As a Replacement for the Boost Dose: Summary of Studies					
Trials	Patients, n	Median age, y (range)	Tumor size	N stage	Margin status	Median follow-up	5-y In-breast recurrence
Mannheim[6]	154	63 (30–83)	T1/T2	N0/N1	NA	34 mo	1.5%
Salzburg[14]	190	59	T1/T2	Up to N2	>3–5 mm	26 mo	0.0%
ISIORT[15]	1,031	NA	Up to T3	Up to N3	>2 mm	52 mo	0.6%
Montpellier[13]	50	59	≤3 cm	Up to N3	Clear	9 y	4.0% (10-y recurrence)

NA, not applicable; ISIORT, International Society of Intraoperative Radiation Therapy.

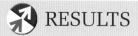 RESULTS

IORT As Boost

IORT has been evaluated as a replacement for the boost dose in several trials; selected trials are summarized in Table 17.1 (6,13–15).

The benefit of replacing the boost dose with IORT is to shorten radiotherapy by 1 week. Although follow-up is short term, recurrence rates have been extremely low. Longer follow-up is needed to determine true efficacy, but theoretically IORT as a replacement for the boost dose is reasonable and may even be more accurate since it is directed at the time of initial surgery. The study with the longest follow-up (Montpellier) has a low recurrence rate comparable with standard radiotherapy.

IORT As Sole Radiotherapy

Trials (Phase II)

Several trials have compared IORT with standard whole-breast irradiation. Although these are mostly single institutions and follow-up is limited, initial results are comparable with whole-breast irradiation.

European Institute of Oncology (Milan)   A 5-year follow-up using ELIOT has been reported at the European Institute of Oncology with good results. In this prospective analysis, all patients between July 1999 and December 2003 with tumors smaller than 2.5 cm undergoing breast-conserving surgery (or nipple-sparing mastectomy) were eligible for IORT with electrons, either as a single intraoperative dose (574 patients) or as a planned boost dose (16 patients) in addition to later standard radiotherapy. Patients with nipple-sparing mastectomy (111 patients) were given IORT as a retroareolar dose. Intraoperative dose with ELIOT was 21 Gy, the biologic equivalent of 58 to 60 Gy in standard radiotherapy. At 2-years follow-up, recurrence was very low (0.5%). Further follow-up is needed to confirm initial results. Other single-institution studies are summarized in Table 17.2 (16–18).

TABLE 17.2			Summary of Single-Institution Studies					
Trails	Patients, n	Age, y	Tumor size	N stage	EIC or lobular	Margin status	Median follow-up	5-y Local recurrence
Montpellier[13]	42	72	T1	N0	No	Micro neg	30 mos	5.0%
EIO[18]	574	59	<2.5 cm	N0, N+	Yes	NA	24 mos	0.5%
Baton Rouge[16]	67	60	T1, T2	N0, N+	No	Micro neg	28 mos	0.0%
MSKCC[17]	52	76	<2 cm	N0	No	Grossly clear 1.5 cm	31 mos	0.0%

EIC, extensive intraductal component; EIO, European Institute of Oncology, Milan; NA, not applicable; MSKCC, Memorial Sloan-Kettering Cancer Center; Micro neg, Microscopically negative margins.

Trials (Phase III)

Internationally, there are two ongoing international randomized trials to evaluate the effectiveness of IORT: the European Institute of Oncology trial based in Milan (ELIOT) and the TARGIT trial based in the United Kingdom.

European Institute of Oncology (Milan)   ELIOT is being evaluated in the ongoing European Institute of Oncology randomized trial. More than 400 patients were accrued from December 2000 to 2004. All patients were older than 48 years with biopsy-proven invasive breast cancer. Tumors had to be unicentric and smaller than 2.5 cm. Anyone with previous treatment for ipsilateral cancer or collagen vascular disease was excluded.

Preliminary results from phase II trial analysis in 2003 showed a very low incidence of adverse events. Morbidity related to ELIOT occurred in 2.5% of patients. The main adverse event was fibrosis or skin retraction. Locoregional recurrence was low, with one patient developing a new cancer in another quadrant. Two patients developed contralateral breast cancer and one developed distant metastases, at mean durations of 13 and 16 months after ELIOT, respectively. Follow-up of a larger group of 1,246 patients in 2008 showed similar results, with 2% local recurrence and 2% distant metastasis.

TARGIT (London)   The pilot study of 227 patients for TARGIT in 1998 showed that a single dose of 20 Gy of IORT delivered with electron beams (Intrabeam, Carl Zeiss MediTec, Jena, Germany) resulted in a low recurrence rate and incidence of adverse events. At a mean of 22-month follow-up, there were two local recurrences: one in another quadrant of the same breast and another with diffuse involvement of the breast 2 months after treatment. Cosmetic outcomes were determined to be excellent (19).

Recent results from the TARGIT phase III trial showed that in 854 women older than 45 years randomized to IORT, local recurrence was comparable with standard external-beam radiotherapy (1.2% vs. 0.95%) at 4 years with lower toxicity.

Brachytherapy Trials

Following the same principle, trials have also been started to evaluate the effectiveness of accelerated partial breast irradiation using brachytherapy: GEC-ESTRO in Germany, NSABP B-39 in the United States, and RAPID in Ontario, Canada.

NSABP B-39/RTOG 0413

Patients older than 40 years with stage 0, I, or II cancer with tumors up to 3 cm in size and three positive axillary lymph nodes are stratified by pre- or postmenopausal status, intention to receive chemotherapy, disease stage, and hormone-receptor status. Randomization is to either whole-breast irradiation or partial-breast irradiation by multicatheter brachytherapy (34 Gy), balloon catheter brachytherapy (Mammosite) (34 Gy), or 3D conformal external-beam radiation (38.5 Gy). All partial breast radiation will occur as twice-daily treatments of 3.4 to 3.85 Gy for 5 days.

GEC-ESTRO APBI (ERLANGEN)

Catheter-directed brachytherapy is being evaluated for equivalence to whole-breast radiation in this trial, with an accrual goal of 1,170 patients with early-stage breast cancer in 4 years. Patients older than 40 years with stage 0, I, or II cancer, including DCIS and lobular histology, are recruited. Cancer must be unicentric and unifocal, without lymphatic invasion, and excised to at least 2 mm clear margins. Because of this clear margin requirement, brachytherapy in this study is given during or after chemotherapy when adjuvant therapy is required.

The phase II trial for this randomized study included 274 patients accrued from 2000 to 2005 from several centers in Germany and Austria. At a mean follow-up of 3 years, there was a 0.7% local recurrence rate. Perioperative morbidity included implant infection

(3.3%) and hematoma (2.2%). Fibrosis and dermatitis occurred in 1.8% and 6.6% of patients respectively.

This study differs from others in that brachytherapy catheters are implanted in the lumpectomy cavity for 5 days while the therapy is delivered. A total of 32 Gy in eight fractions of 4 Gy twice daily are given. The mean time to therapy after lumpectomy is also 57 days, longer than in other studies.

RAPID (ONTARIO)

This study of accelerated partial-breast irradiation with 3D conformal external-beam radiation therapy is open to women older than 40 years with early-stage breast cancer. Tumors must be smaller than 3 cm in size and excised with negative margins. Axillary nodes should be negative except for immunohistochemistry (IHC) or cytokeratin-positive cells for inclusion in the trial.

Selected Groups (Elderly, Postradiation)

IORT is especially beneficial for the elderly. The Montpellier trial reports 2/94 recurrences, excellent cosmesis and quality of life, low toxicity, and 100% compliance with full therapy at a median follow-up of 30 months for patients older than 65 years (20).

The Mannheim group reports good results in a series of 17 patients previously irradiated for breast cancer or Hodgkin lymphoma (4). Recurrence would have mandated mastectomy in these patients, but with IORT they were able to have reconservation with no severe toxicity or recurrence. These results show that in a highly selected population, with a long disease-free interval (median 10 years), good outcomes can be achieved with re-irradiation.

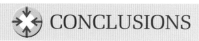 CONCLUSIONS

In selected patients with early-stage, unicentric breast cancer, IORT may be beneficial. Its advantages include lower cost, greater convenience, and possibly more accurate delivery of radiotherapy. Long-term efficacy is not yet known, and results of ongoing randomized trials are needed to determine equivalence with standard radiotherapy.

References

1. Athas WF, Adams-Cameron M, Hunt WC, et al. Travel distance to radiation therapy and receipt of radiotherapy following breast-conserving surgery. *J Natl Cancer Inst.* 2000;92(3):269–271.
2. Benda RK, Yasuda G, Sethi A, et al. Breast boost: are we missing the target? *Cancer.* 2003;97(4):905–909.
3. Fietkau R. [Effects of the time interval between surgery and radiotherapy on the treatment results]. *Strahlenther Onkol.* 2000;176(10):452–457.
4. Kraus-Tiefenbacher U, Bauer L, Scheda A, et al. Intraoperative radiotherapy (IORT) is an option for patients with localized breast recurrences after previous external-beam radiotherapy. *BMC Cancer.* 2007;7:178.
5. Holmes DR, Baum M, Joseph D. The TARGIT trial: targeted intraoperative radiation therapy versus conventional postoperative whole-breast radiotherapy after breast-conserving surgery for the management of early-stage invasive breast cancer (a trial update). *Am J Surg.* 2007;194(4):507–510.
6. Wenz F, Welzel G, Blank E, et al. Intraoperative radiotherapy as a boost during breast-conserving surgery using low-kilovoltage x-rays: the first 5 years of experience with a novel approach. *Int J Radiat Oncol Biol Phys.* 2010;77:1309–1314.
7. Wenz F, Welzel G, Keller A, et al. Early initiation of external beam radiotherapy (EBRT) may increase the risk of long-term toxicity in patients undergoing intraoperative radiotherapy (IORT) as a boost for breast cancer. *Breast.* 2008;17(6):617–622.
8. Petit JY, Veronesi U, Orecchia R, et al. Nipple sparing mastectomy with nipple areola intraoperative radiotherapy: one thousand and one cases of a five years experience at the European Institute of Oncology of Milan (EIO). *Breast Cancer Res Treat.* 2009;117(2):333–338.
9. Galimberti V, Ciocca M, Leonardi MC, et al. Is electron beam intraoperative radiotherapy (ELIOT) safe in pregnant women with early breast cancer? In vivo dosimetry to assess fetal dose. *Ann Surg Oncol.* 2009;16(1):100–105.
10. Beddar AS, Biggs PJ, Chang S, et al. Intraoperative radiation therapy using mobile electron linear accelerators: report of AAPM Radiation Therapy Committee Task Group No. 72. *Med Phys.* 2006;33(5):1476–1489.
11. Vaidya JS, Baum M, Tobias JS, et al. The novel technique of delivering targeted intraoperative radiotherapy (Targit) for early breast cancer. *Eur J Surg Oncol.* 2002;28(4):447–454.
12. Veronesi U, Gatti G, Luini A, et al. Intraoperative radiation therapy for breast cancer: technical notes. *Breast J.* 2003;9(2):106–112.
13. Lemanski C, Azria D, Thezenas S, et al. Intraoperative radiotherapy given as a boost for early breast cancer: long-term clinical and cosmetic results. *Int J Radiat Oncol Biol Phys.* 2006;64(5):1410–1415.
14. Reitsamer R, Peintinger F, Kopp M, et al. [Local recurrence rates in breast cancer patients treated with intraoperative electron-boost radiotherapy versus postoperative external-beam electron-boost irradiation: a sequential intervention study]. *Strahlenther Onkol.* 2004;180(1):38–44.

15. Sedlmayer F, Fastner G, Merz F, et al. [IORT with electrons as boost strategy during breast conserving therapy in limited stage breast cancer: results of an ISIORT pooled analysis]. *Strahlenther Onkol.* 2007;183(spec no 2):32–34.

16. Elliott RL, Deland M, Head JF, et al. Accelerated partial breast irradiation: Initial experience with the Intrabeam System. *Surg Oncol.* 2009 Nov 27 (Epub ahead of print). PMID: 19945859.

17. Sacchini V, Beal K, Goldberg J, et al. Study of quadrant high-dose intraoperative radiation therapy for early-stage breast cancer. *Br J Surg.* 2008;95(9):1105–1110.

18. Veronesi U, Orecchia R, Luini A, et al. Full-dose intraoperative radiotherapy with electrons during breast-conserving surgery: experience with 590 cases. *Ann Surg.* 2005;242(1):101–106.

19. Vaidya JS, Tobias JS, Baum M, et al. TARGeted Intraoperative radiotherapy (TARGIT): an innovative approach to partial-breast irradiation. *Semin Radiat Oncol.* 2005;15(2):84–91.

20. Lemanski C, Azria D, Gourgon-Bourgade S, et al. Intraoperative radiotherapy in early-stage breast cancer: results of the Montpellier phase II trial. *Int J Radiat Oncol Biol Phys.* 2010;76(3): 698–703.

Part IV: Partial Mastectomy

18 Simple Mastectomy

Elizabeth A. Shaughnessy

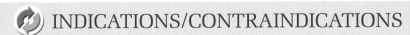

INDICATIONS/CONTRAINDICATIONS

Before the advent of sentinel node biopsy in the assessment of the axilla, the simple or total mastectomy was a procedure performed primarily in the context of extensive ductal carcinoma in situ. The procedure is now much more frequently utilized in a variety of contexts. Women with a family history or carriers of a deleterious mutation in BRCA1, BRCA2, or PTEN, armed with the knowledge that they may carry a genetic predisposition to develop breast cancer, are pursuing prophylactic mastectomy in increasing numbers, often paired with immediate reconstruction. Young women exposed to breast radiation before the age of 19, in the setting of mantle radiation for Hodgkin lymphoma, survived their malignancy only to find themselves at increased risk for medial breast cancers 10 to 20 years later (1). Rather than deal with yet another malignancy, many of these women are seeking bilateral prophlylactic mastectomy or bilateral mastectomy (one side prophylactic) with the diagnosis of a breast cancer. Contralateral prophylactic mastectomy following the initial diagnosis of a breast malignancy has significantly increased over the past 10 years (2,3), primarily due to patient preference, but also associated with the knowledge of increased risk with the above-mentioned genetic mutations.

Invasive carcinoma of the breast can be addressed by partial mastectomy or mastectomy if unifocal, usually with sentinel lymph node biopsy preceding it. In the presence of nodal involvement with breast cancer, surgical management of the breast may be paired with a full axillary lymph node dissection (see Chapter 12). Multicentricity would preclude partial mastectomy in the delivery of the standard of care. Multifocality may or may not allow for breast conservation, depending on the extent of disease. Although guidelines would suggest that resection of up to a quarter of the breast leaves an acceptable postoperative result, the perspective of the general public is one of increased expectations regarding the cosmetic end result. The use of breast magnetic resonance imaging (MRI) in assessing the extent of disease in a patient with dense tissues diagnosed with breast cancer is thought to be linked to a greater number of suspicious lesions identified within the breast, suggestive of multicentricity or multifocality. Consequently, more women opt for mastectomy rather than pursue additional biopsies that add to their anxiety or to the delay in access to systemic treatment. The incidence of a synchronous contralateral breast cancer in women with newly diagnosed breast cancer is reported as 3% to 4% (4) and is supported by MRI (5). Whether the second breast cancer would become clinically relevant in that woman's lifetime remains to be seen. Doing a routine MRI then, outside the context of a dense breast on mammography in a patient with a family history, would not be considered the standard of care.

In older patients with very large breasts, performance of a unilateral total mastectomy may be sufficient to throw off their sense of balance. Should a unifocal cancer need resection, strong consideration should be given to management with breast conservation to avoid the issue of imbalance. A multiplicity of medical problems may also serve to place the patient at high risk for complications from a general anesthetic; breast conservation would likely allow resection of a unifocal breast cancer under local anesthetic, with monitored anesthesia care. An absolute contraindication to total mastectomy as a method of managing the breast does not exist, except perhaps as an initial method of control with metastatic breast cancer or inflammatory breast cancer should the primary not require palliation. Generally speaking, mastectomy is done in the context of metastatic breast cancer for purposes of palliation. The data regarding whether to use it following an excellent response to chemotherapy for survival benefit is suggested by the data but not established firmly statistically (6–8).

Mastectomy is an option in the context of large breast sarcomas. In general, these can be managed using breast conservation, with attention to obtaining negative margins, unless recurrent or with the rare angiosarcoma, where margins of at least 3 cm are generally necessary and rarely obtained within the context of conservation (9).

Relative contraindications usually take the form of patients who present with inflammatory breast cancer, chest wall or skin involvement, and metastatic breast cancer. These patients generally would undergo chemotherapy initially as part of their therapy. A total mastectomy at a later date may or may not be indicated, depending on the response. Some patients cannot undergo a general anesthetic at the initial time of presentation, although there have been reports of use of the tumescent technique and performance of a total mastectomy undergoing local anesthesia. As patients live longer, we deal more frequently with patients who have had drug-eluting coronary artery stents placed, facing the contraindication to take the patient off clopidogrel out of concern that the stent could thrombose within the first 6 months. Patients have suffered myocardial infarction within a short time of receiving their diagnosis of breast cancer; a general anesthetic within the first few months will place that individual at increased risk of mortality under a general anesthetic. One can pursue treatment initially with systemic agents, in collaboration with a medical oncologist, with definitive resection to take place later.

Very rare issues of breast trauma under extenuating circumstances, with trauma incurred while taking aspirin, warfarin or clopidogrel, may require a mastectomy for full resection with negative margins.

Neoadjuvant therapy may enable the performance of a partial mastectomy when the patient presents with a large tumor relative to the size of the breast in approximately 25% to 30% of those who undergo chemotherapy first (10). Yet, the majority of these patients do not have a sufficiently complete response to allow breast conservation, which may not be evident before embarking on breast conservation. The clinician may be fooled into interpreting a greater response than is present, on the basis of physical findings. The mass present may be surrounded by small microscopic islands within the original tumor volume that will not yield negative margins upon full resection (nonconcentric response). The answer may not be known until the final pathology result returns. A completion total mastectomy may then be indicated.

PREOPERATIVE PLANNING

In the context of the patient who will undergo immediate reconstruction at the time of mastectomy, the surgeon needs to consider whether a sentinel lymph node should be included in the operative plan. The performance of a sentinel node, including blue dye, can be somewhat distracting in the dissection of the tissue planes but more so for the plastic surgeon; however, this issue is surmountable with time and frequency of experience. Intraoperative assessment of the sentinel node by touch preparation or by frozen section does not yield a positive result in all cases of metastatic disease to the sentinel nodes, sometimes the node may be too small to utilize for frozen section, and the final answer on permanent section takes several days. In anticipation of the reconstructive process, armed with the knowledge that a positive status for a sentinel node may not be known for several days, consider performance of the sentinel node in advance of the definitive extirpation. In that fashion, a completion axillary lymph node dissection can be performed at the time of mastectomy without concern for disruption of the reconstructed autologous tissue mound. Performance of an axillary lymph node dissection after tissue expander placement can be performed at a later date, especially if the approach was via muscle splitting as opposed to a lateral insertion approach. Yet the pectoralis muscles will be tighter, depending on the degree of expander fill, and may not allow as much abduction of the arm in positioning.

Further preoperative considerations would include the possibility of coordination with physicians or surgeons in other disciplines. If immediate reconstruction will be arranged at the time of the extirpation, then the patient must be seen by the plastic surgeon and a coordinated plan for surgery on a mutually available date should be established. If the patient is to have neoadjuvant chemotherapy, then coordination with the medical oncologist for initiation of the treatment and coordinated communication to streamline the patient's return for surgical planning. Should there be a question of postsurgical radiation, consultation with the radiation oncologist preoperatively should be considered before immediate reconstruction is pursued. Radiation can distort an autologous tissue flap; radiation of the chest wall in the presence of tissue expanders can often be done but is best planned with the radiation oncologist in light of any extenuating circumstances (11).

If a prophylactic mastectomy is planned, the breasts should be appropriately screened for an asymptomatic breast cancer, with a mammogram and possible breast MRI if appropriate. If done for breast cancer, a mammogram should be an integral part of the planning. A breast MRI may be considered if chest wall invasion or skin involvement is a concern, to delineate and potentially clinically stage the cancer.

In the immediate preoperative setting, prophylactic antibiotics, usually a cephalosporin administered approximately 30 minutes before incision, can reduce the rate of wound infection by 40% or more. In light of the fact that these surgeries are done under a general anesthetic, planning for deep venous thrombosis prophylaxis may include compression boots, an injection of subcutaneous heparin, or a single dose of low-molecular-weight heparin in the high-risk population.

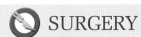 SURGERY

The intent of the total mastectomy is to remove the breast, sparing the lymph nodes. In the past, the anatomical extent of the breast was probably less well understood as evidenced by studies such as the NSABP B-04 study (12). This trial, in which women underwent mastectomy with or without axillary lymph node dissection, demonstrated an average of six lymph nodes with the breast specimen among those patients randomized to mastectomy alone. Clearly, how to remove the breast but spare the lymph nodes is not always a clear issue, but it is possible.

Studies that have examined local recurrences following total mastectomy indicate the areas where breast tissue is most likely retained are inferiorly and laterally in the tail of Spence. Certainly, this becomes a sticky issue when attempting to maintain the connective tissue of the inframammary fold in place for reconstructive purposes.

Positioning

The patient is placed in the supine position with the ipsilateral upper extremity on an armboard level with the table. I discourage the use of a roll along the lateral thorax as it places the arm in extension and abduction, placing the patient at risk for brachial plexopathy. Surgeon and assistant are at either side of the armboard; they can exchange

Figure 18.1 Positioning of the surgical team for the simple mastectomy, with the assistant cephalad to the armboard and surgeon caudad to it. (Modified from Bland KI, Copeland EM II, eds. *The Breast: Comprehensive Management of Benign and Malignant Disorders.* 3rd ed. Philadelphia, PA: WB Saunders, 2004.)

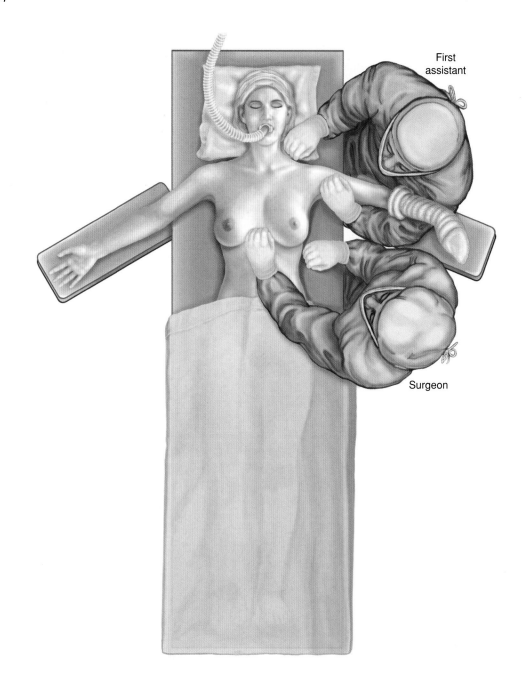

First
assistant

Surgeon

position, if so desired (Fig. 18.1). If desired, the foot of the table can be angled slightly to the site opposite the side for surgery to allow greater space between the armboard and anesthesia staff. This is utilized only for a unilateral approach.

PERIOPERATIVE MANAGEMENT

Incision

The upper anterior arm, breast, ipsilateral thorax, and lower neck are prepared and draped. The incision will vary, depending on whether skin-sparing is intended. If skin-sparing is not intended, an incision that allows for a flat closure against the chest wall will enable greater ease in wearing a breast prosthesis after healing. A variety of incisions have been described and are mentioned in Figure 18.2. Historically, the nipple and

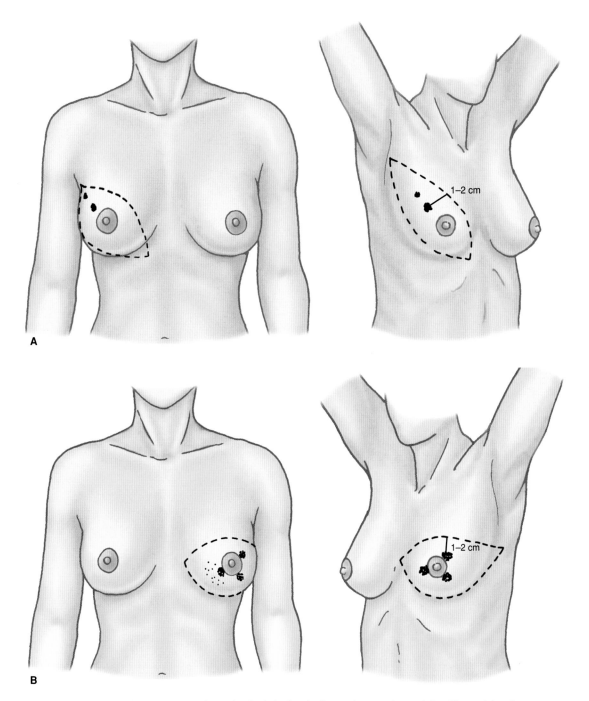

Figure 18.2 Historically, incisions were planned to include the nipple-areolar complex and the skin overlying the tumor, including the biopsy incision, within the planned ellipse. Multiple possibilities have been described, depending on where the tumor is located. **A.** The classic Orr oblique incision for the upper outer quadrant, directed cephalad along the anterior axillary fold. **B.** The classic Stewart incision extends to the anterior margin of the latissimus margin (posterior axillary fold). **C.** Modification of the incision described by Stewart, adapted to the upper inner quadrant. **D.** Further modification of the Orr incision, still oblique, but more vertically placed. **E.** Incision for lower outer quadrant. **F.** A more vertical modification to address more cephalad tumors. (Modified from Bland KI, Copeland EM II, eds. *The Breast: Comprehensive Management of Benign and Malignant Disorders.* 3rd ed. Philadelphia, PA: WB Saunders, 2004.) (*continued*)

areolar complex are included in the tissue excised, and the tumor generally lies deep to the skin excised. That stated, as long as the tumor is away from the skin, the surgeon typically utilizes an elliptical incision.

Inspect the breast and note its shape in the supine position. I note the extent to which the breast extends into the axilla laterally (Fig. 18.3). Choose a point under the hair-bearing area, along the posterior axillary fold, and mark it on the skin (Fig. 18.3A). If a

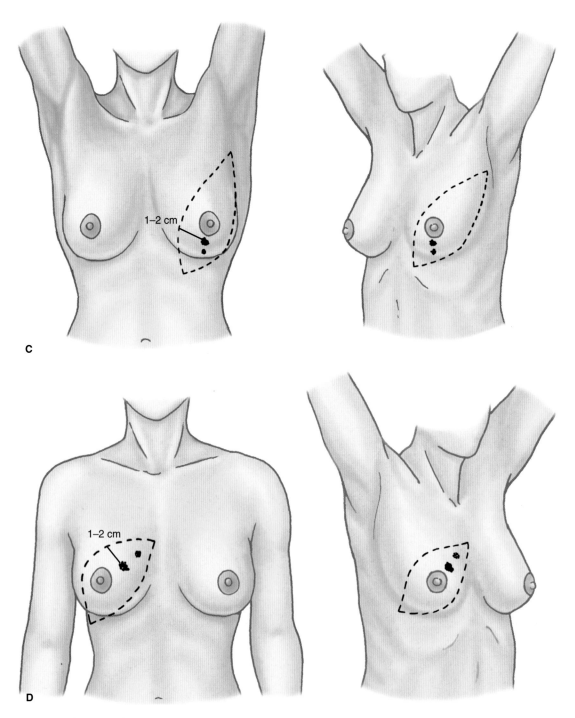

C

D

Figure 18.2 (*Continued*)

line was drawn through this point and the nipple, going to the opposite side of the breast (the lower inner quadrant), draw another point at the most medial aspect of the breast or slightly beyond. At a right angle relative to this imaginary line, first pull the breast gently down, and draw a line between these two points (Fig. 18.3B). When released, the skin displays an arc. Similarly, lift the breast up at a right angle to the imaginary line formed by the original two points and draw a straight line between these points. Once released, this results in a drawn ellipse. Before incising, check to make sure that sufficient skin is available for closure by approximating the skin with hands; rarely must I readjust what was planned. Care should be taken to prevent closing under tension.

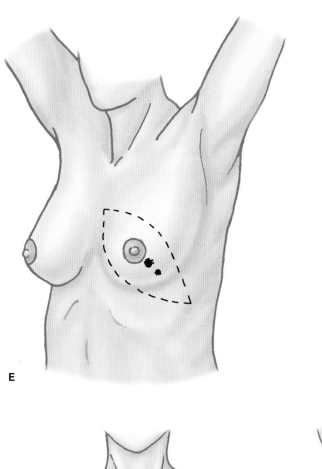

E

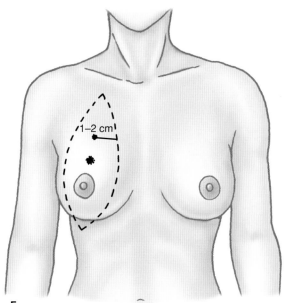

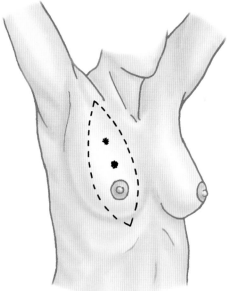

F

Figure 18.2 (*Continued*)

If skin-sparing is intended, several choices are possible (Fig. 18.4). Since skin-sparing is usually applied only when immediate reconstruction is coordinated, the incision I utilize is chosen in conjunction with the plastic surgeon with whom I am operating. The essence is that at least part of the incision, if not all, is close to the areolar border.

Raising the Skin Flaps

In utilizing an incision that traverses the skin of the hemithorax, the surgeon has a choice of several different retractors that can be utilized successfully—Adair tenaculae,

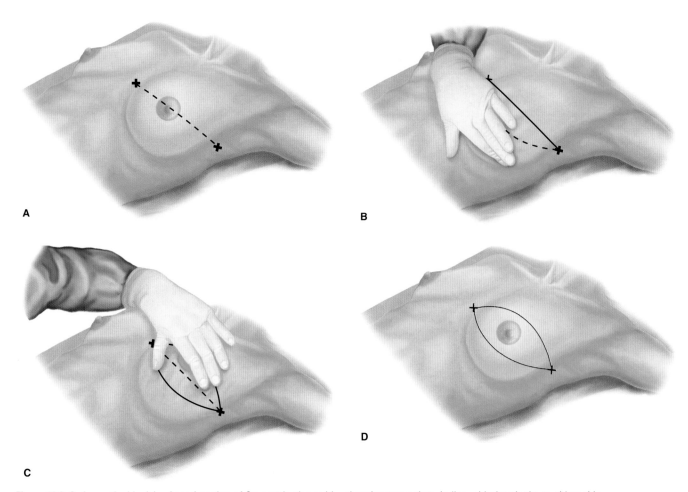

Figure 18.3 A. A practical incision based on that of Stewart is planned by choosing two points, in line with the nipple, to either side of the breast, with the lateral site along the posterior axillary fold, under the hairline. **B.** The breast skin is pulled down orthogonal to that imaginary line and a straight line drawn between the points. **C.** The breast is pushed up orthogonal to the imaginary line between the two points and a lower straight line drawn between the points below the nipple. **D.** With the breast relaxed, an ellipse has formed, which will close relatively flat against the chest.

skin rakes, or skin hooks. This usually reflects the surgeon's training and preference. Retraction focuses on lifting the skin at a right angle to the skin surface, with the surgeon placing gentle tension down toward the chest wall (Fig. 18.5). If the skin flap is bent back, there is a greater likelihood for the surgeon to injure the skin or create a "buttonhole." The tissue plane between the investing adipose of the skin and the investing adipose of the breast is by the slight white feathering of the connective tissue between these layers. In essence, this is followed down to the chest wall in the superior, medial, and inferior aspects. This may or may not be readily evident in the tissue dissection. Furthermore, the distance between the skin dermis and this connective tissue plane is relatively thinner at the areola and may be thicker as the distance from the areola increases. Laterally, the skin flap is dissected nearly to the lateral border of the latissimus dorsi muscle. In lifting the skin flap, I prefer to utilize electrocautery, widely sweeping to avoid any heat buildup along the tissues. The harmonic scissors can also be used to seal the vessels in the context of someone recently on clopidogrel, eptifibatide, or aspirin. Others utilize sharp dissection with the scalpel, or harmonic breast scalpel, which can be relatively easily applied as there is infrequent vascular communication between these two tissue planes, unless neoangiogenesis was induced by the tumor. Expect to find a large vein traversing these two planes in the upper inner quadrant and in the upper outer quadrant (13).

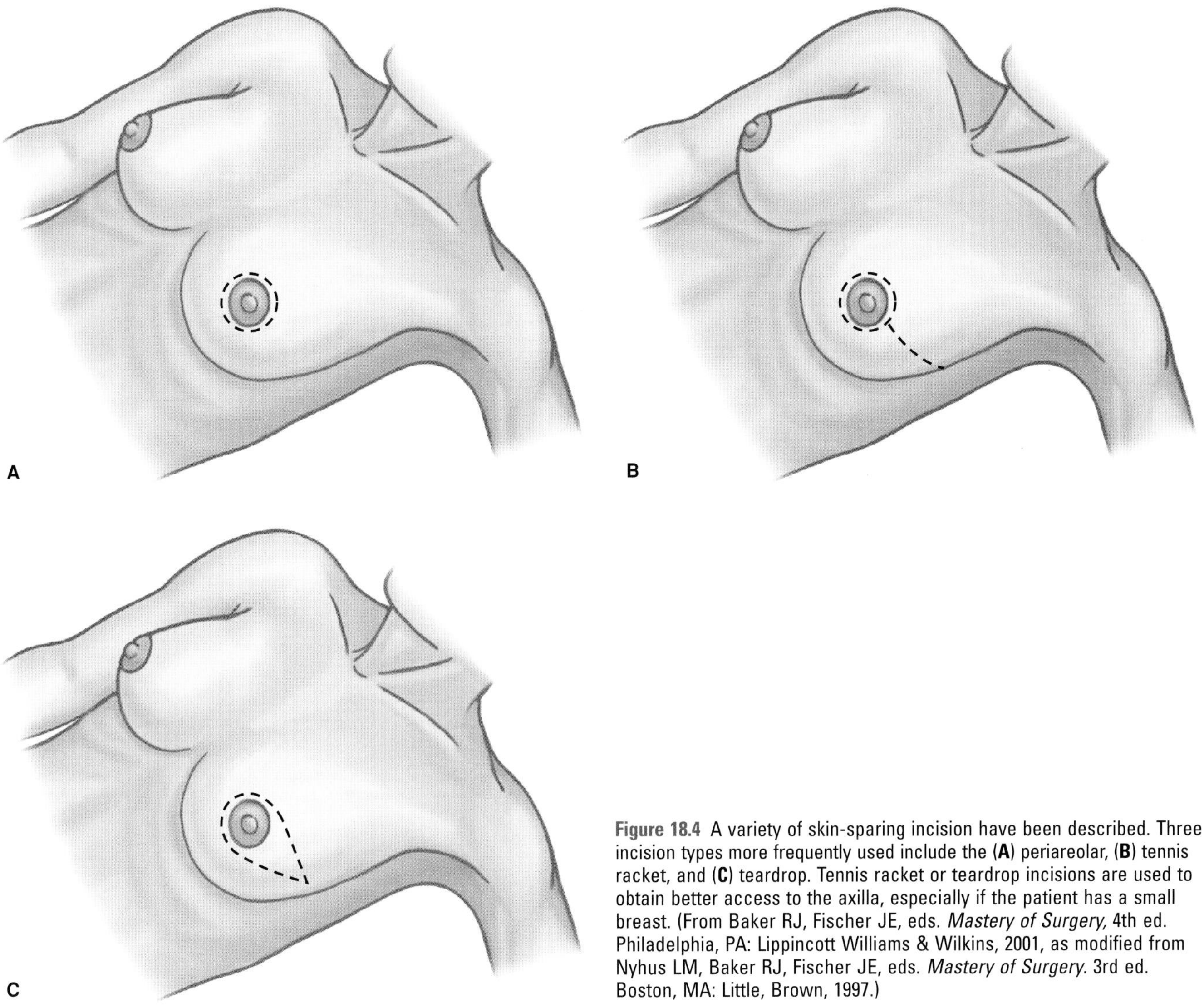

Figure 18.4 A variety of skin-sparing incision have been described. Three incision types more frequently used include the (**A**) periareolar, (**B**) tennis racket, and (**C**) teardrop. Tennis racket or teardrop incisions are used to obtain better access to the axilla, especially if the patient has a small breast. (From Baker RJ, Fischer JE, eds. *Mastery of Surgery,* 4th ed. Philadelphia, PA: Lippincott Williams & Wilkins, 2001, as modified from Nyhus LM, Baker RJ, Fischer JE, eds. *Mastery of Surgery.* 3rd ed. Boston, MA: Little, Brown, 1997.)

If a skin-sparing incision is utilized, the opening utilized will limit exposure. To prepare for this, both surgeon and assistant wear headlamps. Smaller retractors, such as the Joseph double skin hooks, are preferentially used because of the limited exposure. As with the typical elliptical incision, the skin flap is raised between the investing adipose of the skin and the investing adipose of the breast. The layer of investing adipose is thinner nearest the areolar border, with gradual thickening as the skin approaches the chest wall. In the patient with minimal subcutaneous adipose, this layer can be so thin as to place the skin at risk of injury; it is also difficult to see or locate. Many surgeons utilize the tumescent technique—the injection of saline within this plane circumferentially to expand it, possibly with epinephrine (14). If sentinel node biopsy has been performed in advance of the mastectomy by approximately a week, this often leads to a slight "autotumescence," with a small degree of edema acquired in the subcutaneous breast tissues, and further injection may not be necessary.

If surgeons have small fingers, then they likely can utilize them within the incision to place the breast tissue on traction. The dissection proceeds circumferentially. As it deepens toward the chest wall, assistants may switch to physically holding the skin, or should they have large fingers, a lighted retractor such as the C-Strang is invaluable (Fig. 18.6). Should surgeons have large fingers, tension on the breast tissue can be

Figure 18.5 Development of the skin flaps proceeds with retraction of the skin at a right angle to the table. With traction on the breast tissue, pressing down or pulling away from the skin flap, the tissue plane is more readily identifiable. The plane between the adipose of the skin and that of the breast is usually found 2 to 4 mm below the dermis. The adipose of the skin is the thinnest near the areola and slowly becomes thicker toward the chest wall. Adair breast tenaculae are depicted here in the retraction, but other methods are utilized as well.

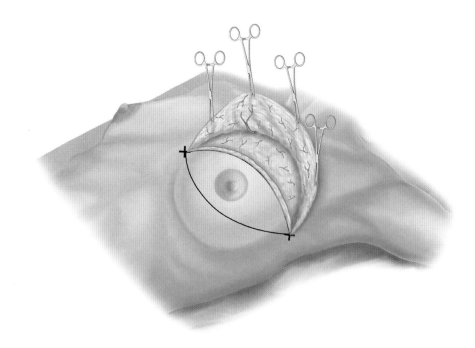

maintained by pulling on it with a skin rake or by pushing the tissue down with a tissue forceps. On rare occasion, when working medially, surgeons may note that the patient may have synmastia, with breast tissue from either side meeting over the sternum. In the context of unilateral mastectomy, then, I have chosen not to abruptly cut the tissue midline, which would lead to an abrupt shelfing effect, but taper it so that the tissue lies more smoothly against the chest wall.

As with the more open technique, more blood vessels will be encountered between the adipose investing the skin and the breast tissue along a vein in the upper inner quadrant (high internal mammary perforator) and another in the upper outer quadrant (variable branch of the axillary or lateral thoracic). Larger intercostal perforators will be encountered medially along the sternal border. These are usually between the second, third, and fourth intercostals spaces. If a dominant branch is going directly to the skin and can be avoided, do so for the sake of flap perfusion. If one of these vessels should bleed, it is preferable to isolate the vessel and tie a suture or place a suture ligature. As the vessels are emerging from under the muscle, a partially injured larger vessel may

Figure 18.6 Development of the skin flaps with a skin-sparing incision is similar to that of the larger incision, just in a smaller field. Tension is placed on the breast tissue by pulling down on the breast tissue toward the chest wall or by pulling the breast tissue away from the skin. The skin is initially retracted away from the chest wall, with skin rakes or hooks as the plane is developed. As the dissection progresses, one can switch to hand retraction, occasional rolling the flap forward or backward for access. One could also utilize a lighted retractor in the context of space restraint.

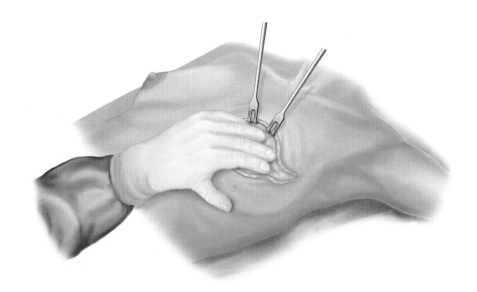

cease bleeding temporarily, but then start again later, only now retracted under the muscle. Chasing the vessel with the cautery could lead to rare instances of pneumothorax.

Through this entire dissection, the skin can be handled firmly but not with excessive traction. On occasion, the traction can also lead to reflex vascular contraction and relative ischemia. Remember, too, that cautery along the skin flap should be done sparingly so as to reduce the degree of heat injury to the skin flap. Heat injury can also be incurred with use of the harmonic breast scalpel.

Dissection of the Breast from the Chest Wall

The patient's acute pain from mastectomy seems proportional to pectoralis major muscle injury during dissection. This can be minimized by dissection the tissue off the muscle, utilizing electrocautery to travel in parallel to the muscle fibers. Traditionally, the muscle fascia is included with the specimen. I utilize two Allis clamps along the superior edge of the breast tissue for traction (Fig. 18.7). This lifts the tissue and exposes a white line of fascia along the muscle. In utilizing electrocautery, one can minimize muscle contraction during the dissection by traveling continuously along the muscle fibers in parallel. This sets up a tetanus, since the muscle does not get sufficient time to recover before stimulation is administered again.

In the context of the classical elliptical incision, the dissection is most easily performed by the surgeon by standing in the position above the armboard. Given the limited exposure of the skin-sparing incision, the breast is more easily taken off the muscle with the surgeon standing below the armboard (Fig. 18.8). Gradually, the breast tissue is reflected laterally, so that the breast remains attached along the lateral border of the pectoralis major muscle by the muscle fascia. At this point, if a skin-sparing incision was employed, most of the breast can usually be maneuvered out of the areolar incision, making access a little easier.

On very rare occasion, one may encounter the rare variant—sternalis muscle—seemingly an extension of the rectus abdominis muscle along the sternum described by Dobson in 1882 (15). Identified in less than 0.7% of radical mastectomy specimens (16), these fibers travel vertically along the lateral aspect of the sternum, inserting into ribs within the operative field. It can be spared relatively easily.

The remainder of the dissection takes place on the underside of the breast, as this tissue plane can be better visualized laterally. The muscle fascia is divided along the lateral edge of the pectoralis major muscle. With gentle tension on the breast tissue, the tissue plane of the axillary fascia can be identified. Electrocautery is utilized to slowly travel along this white plane, remaining superficial to the nodes but including

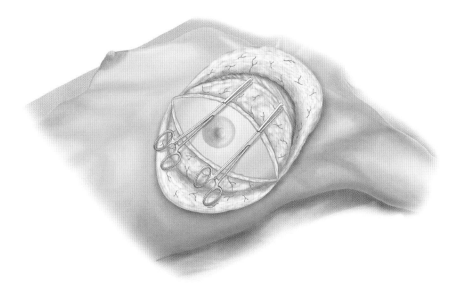

Figure 18.7 Mobilization of the breast off the chest wall can be aided by place of Allis clamps along the superior border of the breast, including the investing "fascia" of the muscle (perimysium). The tissue is pulled up or inferiorly with gentle traction. The dissection is performed utilizing electrocautery or sharp dissection, traveling in parallel to the chest wall muscle fibers. Since the pectoralis major muscle fibers splay, the angle of dissection shifts as one progresses within the dissection.

Figure 18.8 Positioning of the operating surgeon and assistant during the mobilization of the breast from the chest wall. **A.** The operating surgeon has greater access to the muscle fibers from a position cephalad to the armboard, in the context of an elliptical incision. **B.** When a skin-sparing incision has been utilized, the dissection is probably best initiated from a position caudal to the armboard, using a headlamp and possibly a light retractor since access is limited. (*continued*)

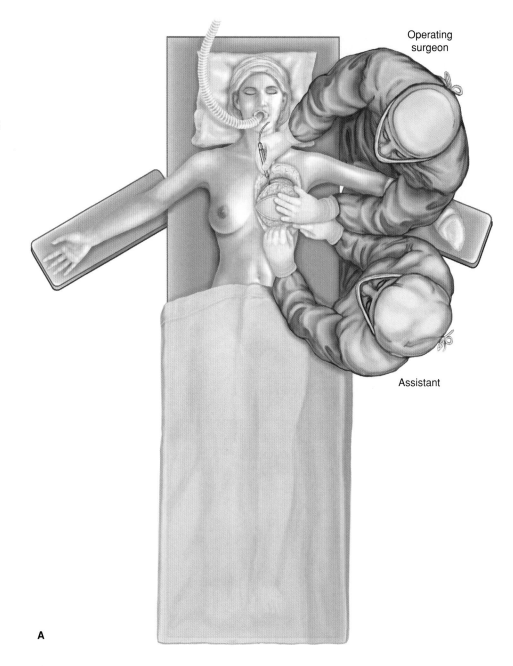

Operating surgeon

Assistant

A

the tail of Spence. Expect a number of lateral small blood vessels from the chest wall to be cauterized or divided with ties or clips. Before the tissue is completely removed, flip it back into its prior position to place sutures or clips to orient the specimen. Typically, once the tissue is passed off the field, it is weighed if immediate reconstruction is planned. The reconstructive surgeon utilizes the information to better provide symmetry.

Wound Closure

As per usual, hemostasis should be ensured before considering closure. The operative field is irrigated with sterile saline and checked once more. In the context of the patient who has a skin-sparing incision, I place a saline-soaked laparotomy sponge loosely within the skin envelope to prevent desiccation of the underlying tissues before turning the case over to my colleague in reconstructive surgery, or proceed with reconstruction if you are so trained.

Figure 18.8 (*Continued*)

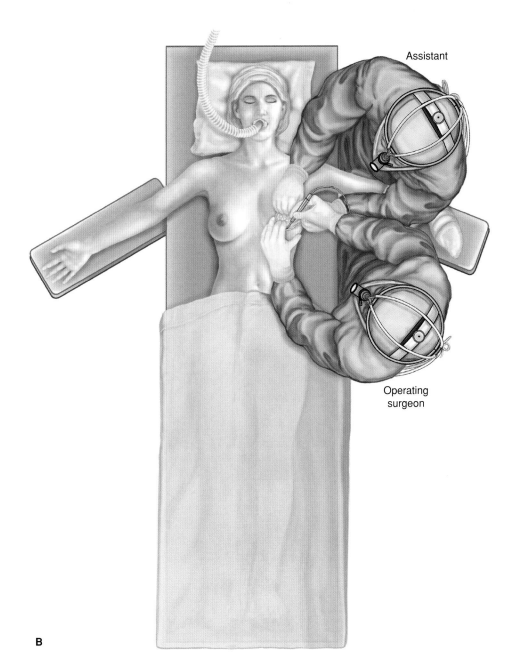

Assistant

Operating
surgeon

B

If the patient will not have immediate reconstruction, now is the time to assess the approximation of the skin flaps. Will they close easily, and without undue tension? If there is some redundant skin, this can be trimmed. Frequently, in the case of the older patient with a larger breast, the weight of the breast pulls on the lateral thorax skin, and eventually on the back. This forms a redundant fold of tissue that is not resected in the standard total mastectomy. If the incision itself is simply closed, this may lead to a winging of the skin fold laterally, which is a point of discomfort in wearing bras and in fitting a breast prosthesis (Fig. 18.9). A Y-plasty along the lateral aspect can be performed that will allow the lateral tissues to lie flatter against the chest wall (17). Additional difficulties such as insufficient skin to close may be approached by undermining the subcutaneous tissues inferiorly and sometimes superiorly to better mobilize them closer if tissues are nearly closed. Other options include the possibility of skin grafting (18).

A drain is usually placed under the chest wall skin flap and brought out through the inferior or superior axillary skin. I avoid the actual inframammary fold in case a neuroma would form at the site; after healing, the rubbing of a bra over a neuroma

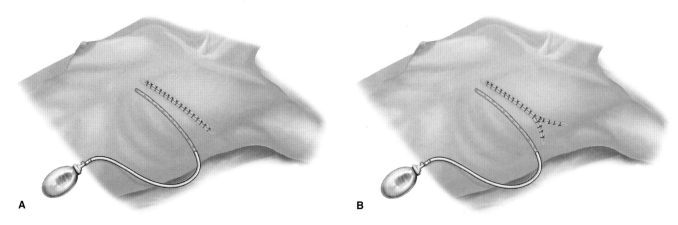

Figure 18.9 Closure of the incision, with a Jackson–Pratt drain exiting the skin of the low axilla and secured externally with a nylon suture. With the drain under the lower flap, it catches the fluid dependently. **A.** The incision with a simple closure of the ellipse. **B.** With a Y-plasty modification in the context of those larger individuals who have developed a ridge of tissue extending to the lateral thorax or back secondary to the weight of the breast over time. This closure results in reducing the excess tissue laterally, beyond the breast, which may stick out after closure. Closure of the skin-sparing incisions is not depicted, as it is generally used in the context of collaboration with a plastic surgeon who will reconstruct before closure.

would irritate the pain of a neuroma. My preference is a Jackson–Pratt drain or Blake channel drain. These are most likely to remain patent should there be large amounts of fluid. The drain is secured to the skin externally near the drainage site with a suture; I prefer to secure the drain by using a 3-0 nylon to reduce bacterial colonization that can come with use of braided sutures. I place the drain dependently under the inferior chest wall since most people are erect for the majority of the day. I trim the catheter to lay about 5 to 6 in. beyond the distant of the catheter to the patient's hip before the bulb is attached. This allows for a small amount of freedom of movement should the patient place the bulb in a pant pocket or pin the bulb to the waistband or shirt.

In closing the skin, I approximate the skin first with temporary interrupted staples. This allows for easing in of redundant skin and helps to prevent "dog ears." I prefer a running two-layer closure, removing the staples as I progress, as it helps to evenly distribute the tension along the incision and form a better seal for the drain. Dressings are then applied.

POSTOPERATIVE MANAGEMENT

The patient will generally stay overnight in light of the issue of drain management teaching, to ensure that the pain is well-controlled independent of intravenous pain medications and is not nauseated and can tolerate an usual diet. Compared with other surgeries outside of body cavities, there is a higher incidence of nausea with a general anesthetic in breast surgeries. With discharge, issues of postoperative management primarily revolve around the drain and when it is removed, as well as the skin flaps and their health in healing. Chronic incisional pain occurs infrequently, but decreased range of motion about the ipsilateral shoulder can also be associated. The management of the drain and its removal continues to be somewhat controversial. Early removal of the drain increases the chance that seroma formation will occur. Later removal increases bacterial colonization and infection rates.

In the United States, patients are frequently discharged with the drain in situ, whereas the drain is usually removed before discharge in Europe. The occasional study within the literature supports having the patient measuring and recording the volumes of output, so that total volumes per day could be assessed at the postoperative visit. The literature supports removing the drain once daily drainage reaches 30 to 40 mL/day, although volumes as high as 50 to 60 mL/day are acceptable. Using standard surgical techniques, this reduction in volume occurs in approximately 1 week with a total mastectomy only; should immediate reconstruction be involved, drainage may last somewhat longer. Although there is some experimental evidence to suggest that the possible use of fibrin glue during the operation may reduce the amount of time that drains are left in situ, the added cost of such techniques would be brought at minimal advantage.

Although there is some use of prophylactic oral antibiotics such as cephalexin among surgeons who place drains, this has not reduced the incidence of infection for total mastectomy. A cheap alternative that has not been studied prospectively is antibiotic ointment around the outside of the drain tubing at the exit site to reduce bacterial counts and to provide a greater seal against fluid capillary action along the tubing.

Massage of the incision line with a compound that contains vitamin E helps to reduce the formation of hypertrophic scars. The body continues to remodel the scar for over a year, so continued application is essential in the remodeling process. Massage of the chest wall is also of importance in the absence of immediate reconstruction. Scarring of the skin to the chest wall muscle, if associated with thick scar, may tether the muscle. Again, massage of the area is of importance.

It is important to stress to the patient that going about the usual daily activities is critical to help maintain shoulder flexibility. Exercises for ipsilateral shoulder range of motion could be provided; if restriction of motion is apparent, occupational therapy and physical therapy would be of benefit.

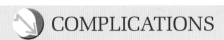 COMPLICATIONS

Infection

Given the placement of a drain and the larger extent of surgery, the rate of immediate postoperative wound complications for the patient undergoing total mastectomy is approximately 10% to 12%. Factors influencing this rate likely reflect compromise of the skin barrier, both by the incision and by the drain exit site, and are reflected in studies that document that the infection risk increases with the number of drains placed. Hence, the patient who undergoes skin-sparing and immediate reconstruction may have a higher risk of wound infection with increasing numbers of drains and increasing time under anesthesia (19), with infection rates of approximately 20%. Colonization of the wound with bacteria is approximately 30% at day 7, rising to 80% by day 14. The sooner the drain can be removed, the lower the incidence of infection. The management of the patient postoperatively involves monitoring the wound for signs of infection.

The organisms most frequently linked to wound infection include *Staphylococcus aureus*, and *S. epidermidis*. *Pseudomonas* species have been described, and rarely *Streptococcus*. Poor clean technique in drain management is suggested, with the identification of *Serratia* species as well. Multifactorial retrospective studies cite age as influencing the occurrence of infection, obesity, and skin necrosis of the flap. Smoking influences skin perfusion, and it is not surprising that there is almost a fourfold increase in wound infection in patients who smoke (20). Preoperative antibiotics and possible intraoperative redosing, depending on the case length, may be worthwhile in reducing the incidence of infection. Once the infection presents, mild cellulitis can be managed with oral antibiotics, yet may require intravenous therapy if the infection fails to respond. The rare infection progresses to an abscess and usually points at the sites of greatest weakness—the incision or former drain exit site. Abscess formation can be confirmed with aspiration of purulent fluid, as opposed to serous fluid. Abscess formation in this context is rare but seldom can be managed by aspiration alone; drainage by opening the original incision is most prudent (19).

Hemorrhage or Hematoma

The greater use of electrocautery in tissue dissection has greatly reduced the incidence of bleeding and hematoma formation in breast surgery, yet series report that this continues at a rate of 2% to 10% (19). In the case of a small wound such as a biopsy site, this may remain self-contained and be easily reabsorbed. However, in the context of a total mastectomy and immediate reconstruction, formation of a large hematoma may be painful and if tense, cause tissue necrosis.

Postoperative bleeding can be influenced by a number of medications that the patient may be taking, prescribed or over-the-counter. Nonsteroidal anti-inflammatory drugs that affect platelet function, such as aspirin, ibuprofen, or ketorolac, need be avoided for a week before surgery. Herbal preparations containing high concentrations of garlic, or with ginseng or gingko biloba, are associated with bleeding diatheses as well. Clopidogrel bisulfate (Plavix), an inhibitor of ADP-induced platelet aggregation, is used in the treatment of acute myocardial infarction, stroke and peripheral vascular disease. In those with recent drug-eluting coronary artery stent placement, continued use of clopidogrel bisulfate is recommended for the first 6 months to prevent stent thrombosis. It is preferable to stop the medication 1 to 2 weeks prior to surgery (the lifespan of platelets) or treat with neoadjuvant therapy until such time that the patient can safely be without the drug for surgery. Knowledge of what the patient ingests, prescribed or otherwise, will make for a smoother postoperative course if managed appropriately.

Seroma

The rich lymphatic supply to the breast is interrupted within the context of resection of the breast that, in conjunction with the large, raw surface under the skin can allow for a signification fluid accumulation. Drains are placed to evacuate these collections, allowing the surfaces to touch, adhere, and heal. Seromas after drain removal can occur, necessitating aspiration in 10% to 80% of the cases, depending on the series! This can be temporized by seroma aspiration in most cases, bypassing insertion of another drain. Yet, meticulous sterile technique should be applied as the incidence of infection with aspiration of seromas can be as high as 30%.

The persistent seroma is perplexing to both the patient and the surgeon. Approaches such as reduction in movement may temporize the issue but eventually lead to limited range of motion in the long term and potentially increase the risk of lymphedema, especially if full axillary lymph node dissection is included with mastectomy. Although some reports have described success with compression dressings, others have not found them to be helpful. It is certainly worth trying in the context of the persistent seroma. The use of sclerosants such as tetracycline have not been helpful and the data from sealants inconsistent (19). For the few patients with persistent seromas following mastectomy, my practice has not hesitated to refer them on for breast radiation when chest wall radiation is indicated, in light of the observation that seromas from partial mastectomies decrease with whole breast radiation. However, if the seroma is large, it may affect the ability to deliver the radiotherapy.

Flap Necrosis

Mastectomy flap necrosis is far more likely to occur among smokers as opposed to those who do not smoke (18.9% vs. 9.0%), and this rose to 21.7% if immediate reconstruction was performed (20) but was markedly less so if delayed reconstruction was pursued. In general, smokers have a higher risk of donor-site complications as well, as compared with nonsmokers or former smokers (25.6% vs. 14.2% vs. 10.0%).

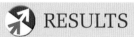 RESULTS

In general, the incidence of local recurrence is less for total mastectomy than for lumpectomy (partial mastectomy) with radiation. For those who undergo a total mastectomy for early breast cancer, stage 0, I, or II, locoregional recurrence risk is approximately 3% to 5.8% at 10 years. On the other hand, with more locally advanced disease such as stage IIIA disease, the risk of recurrence could be as high as 30% if radiation is not included (21).

This compares to a local recurrence risk of 7% to 14% among those undergoing breast conservation with radiation. The literature regarding the oncologic outcome of nipple-sparing mastectomy for breast cancer is sparse, but the more thorough analysis of occult nipple involvement demonstrated cancer in 21% of the specimens (22).

The last 5 to 10 years has brought a gentle surge in the performance of prophylactic mastectomy, in both the context of patients at increased risk for risk reduction and in the context of women who desire contralateral prophylactic mastectomy with their diagnosis of breast cancer (2,3). Hartman et al. (23) had previously demonstrated a minimal risk of local breast cancer with standard mastectomies but a slightly higher risk for subcutaneous mastectomies (nipple-sparing mastectomies), with greater than 90% risk reduction overall. This was echoed in the experience of documented by McDonnell et al. (24), whereas Van Geel (25) noted an even greater benefit to prophylactic mastectomy approaching 100% reduction in risk. Using SEER data, prophylactic mastectomy for BRCA1 or BRCA2 gene mutation carriers indicated a survival benefit and cost-effectiveness (26). For those whose lifetime risk of developing breast cancer is less than 25%, there was no calculated survival benefit, although one large series approached significance (27). Cost-effectiveness models have not been published in this context.

For those undergoing a total (or simple) mastectomy, the fitting of a breast prosthesis is most comfortable to the patient in the context of a flat chest, with a minimum of skin redundancy. For the surgeon to obtain this consistently is a challenge, but one that can be mastered.

CONCLUSIONS

The performance of a mastectomy, with or without skin-sparing requires patience and attention to tissue planes and vessel location to perform it well. The introduction of skin-sparing and the potential for coordination for immediate reconstruction makes this technique versatile. The technique has remained in the surgeon's armamentarium for over the past century, demonstrating its continued efficacy. At present, this technique shows no evidence of quickly retiring, just evolving. It is one that is well-tolerated by the patient.

References

1. Basu SKB, Schwartz C, Fisher SG, et al. Unilateral and bilateral breast cancer in women surviving pediatric Hodgkin's disease. *Int J Radiat Oncol Biol Phys.* 2008;72(1):34–40.
2. Tuttle TM, Haubermann EB, Grund EH, et al. Increasing use of contralateral prophylactic mastectomy for breast cancer patients: a trend toward more aggressive surgical treatment. *J Clin Oncol.* 2007;25(33):5203–5209.
3. Tuttle TM, Jarosek S, Habermann EB, et al. Increasing rates of contralateral prophylactic mastectomy among patients with ductal carcinoma in situ. *J Clin Oncol.* 2009;27(9):1362–1367.
4. Carmichael AR, Bendall S, Lockerbie L, et al. The long-term outcome of synchronous bilateral breast cancer is worse than metachronous or unilateral tumours. *Eur J Surg Oncol.* 2002;28: 388–391.
5. Lehman, CD, Gatsonic C, Kuhl C, et al. MRI evaluation of the contralateral breast in women with recently diagnosed breast cancer. *New Engl J Med.* 2007;256:1295–1303.
6. Rao R, Feng L, Kuerer HM, et al. Timing of surgical intervention for the intact primary in stage IV breast cancer patients. *Ann Surg Oncol.* 2008;15:1696–1702.
7. Babiera GV, Rao R, Feng L, et al. Effect of primary tumor extirpation in breast cancer patients who present with stage IV disease and an intact primary tumor. *Ann Surg Oncol.* 2006;13:776–782.
8. Khan SA, Stewart AK, Morrow M. Does aggressive local therapy improve survival in metastatic breast cancer? *Surgery.* 2002;132: 620–626.
9. Pencavel TD, Hayes A. Breast sarcoma—a review of diagnosis and management. *Int J Surg.* 2009;7(1):20–23.
10. Rastogi P, Anderson SJ, Bear HD, et al. Preoperative chemotherapy: updates of National Surgical Adjuvant Breast and Bowel Project protocols B-18 and B-27. *J Clin Oncol.* 2008;26(5): 778–785.
11. Kronowitz SJ, Robb GL. Breast reconstruction with postmastectomy radiation therapy: current issues. *Plast Reconstr Surg.* 2004;114:950–960.
12. Fisher B, Redmond C, Fisher ER, et al. Ten-year results of a randomized clinical trial comparing radical mastectomy and total mastectomy with or without axillary resection. *New Eng J Med.* 1985;312:674–681.
13. McVay CB. The thorax. In: *Anson & McVay Surgical Anatomy.* Vol 1. 6th ed. Philadelphia, PA: WB Saunders, 1984:356.
14. Paige KT, Bostwick J III, Bried JP. TRAM flap breast reconstruction: tumescent technique reduces blood loss and transfusion requirements. *Plast Reconstr Surg.* 2004;113(6): 1645–1649.
15. Dobson GE. Note on the rectus abdominis et sternalis muscle. *J Anat Physiol.* 1882;17:84–85.
16. Harish K, Gopinash KS. Sternalis muscle: importance in surgery of the breast. *Surg Radiol Anat.* 2003;25:311–314.
17. Hussien M, Daltrey IR, Dutta S, et al. Fish-tail plasty: a safe technique to improve cosmesis at the lateral end of mastectomy scars. *Breast.* 2004;13(3):206–209.
18. Arango A, Restrepo JE. A technique for skin grafting of postmastectomy defects. *Surg Gynecol Obstet.* 1978;147(2):245.
19. Vitug AF, Newman LA. Complications in breast surgery. *Surg Clin North Am.* 2007;87(2):431–451.
20. Chang DW, Reece GP, Wang B, et al. Effect of smoking on complications in patients undergoing free TRAM flap breast reconstruction. *Plast Reconstr Surg.* 2000;105(7):2374–2380.
21. Meretoja TJ, Rasia S, von Smitten KA, et al. Late results of skin-sparing mastectomy followed by immediate breast reconstruction. *Br J Surg.* 2007;94(10):1220–1225.

22. Brachtel EF, Rusby JE, Michaelson JS, et al. Occult nipple involvement in breast cancer: clinicopathologic findings in 316 consecutive mastectomy specimens. *J Clin Oncol.* 2009;27:4949–4955.

23. Hartman LC, Schnaid D, Woods JE, et al. Efficacy of bilateral prophylactic mastectomy in women with a family history of breast cancer. *N Engl J Med.* 1999;340(2):77–84.

24. McDonnell SK, Schaid DJ, Myers FJ, et al. Efficacy of contralateral prophylactic mastectomy in women with personal and family history of breast cancer. *J Clin Oncol.* 2001;19(19): 3938–3943.

25. Van Geel AN. Prophylactic mastectomy: the Rotterdam experience. *Breast.* 2003;12(6):357–361.

26. Grann VR, Panageas KS, Whang W, et al. Decision analysis of prophylactic mastectomy and oophorectomy in BRCA1-positive or BRCA2-positive patients. *J Clin Oncol.* 1998;16(3): 979–985.

27. Peralta EA, Ellenhorn JD, Wagman LD, et al. Contralateral prophylactic mastectomy improves the outcome of selected patients undergoing mastectomy for breast cancer. *Am J Surg.* 2000;180(6): 439–445.

Suggested Readings

Bland KI. Anatomy of the breast. In: Fischer JE, Bland KI, eds. *Mastery of Surgery.* Philadelphia, PA: Lippincott Williams & Wilkins, 2007: 482–491.

Chung AP, Sacchini V. Nipple-sparing mastectomy: where are we now? *Surg Oncol.* 2008;17:261–266.

Klimberg VS. Simple mastectomy. In: Klimberg VS, ed. *Atlas of Breast Surgical Techniques.* Philadelphia, PA: Saunders Elsevier, 2010: 184–201.

Margulies AG, Hochberg J, Kepple J, et al. Total skin-sparing mastectomy without preservation of the nipple-areola complex. *Am J Surg.* 2005;190(6):907–912.

Rotstein C, Ferguson R, Cummings KM, et al. Determinant of clean surgical wound infections for breast procedures at an oncology center. *Infect Control Hosp Epidemiol.* 1992;13(4):207–214.

Vitug AF, Newman LA. Complications in breast surgery. *Surg Clin North Am.* 2007;87(2):431–451.

19 Modified Radical Mastectomy and Total (Simple) Mastectomy

Kirby I. Bland

In 1867, Charles H. Moore (1) stated the following: "Sometimes the tumor only is removed; sometimes the segment of the breast (where the tumor lies) is taken away . . .; sometimes . . . the entire mamma. Mammary cancer requires the careful extirpation of the entire organ."

Introduction

Historical Aspects and Development of the Modified Radical Mastectomy

Modified radical mastectomy has evolved in American surgery as one of the most common surgical procedures completed by general surgeons and surgical oncologists. This procedure followed by some 60 years the development by William Stewart Halsted (2) and Willie Meyer (3) both of whom independently reported, in 1894, the successful therapy of advanced breast carcinoma with radical mastectomy. The synthesis of mastectomy techniques by Halsted and Meyer's predecessors in surgery and pathology, therefore, allowed them to achieve unprecedented success to obtain this objective without the availability of irradiation or chemotherapy. These techniques for the Halsted radical mastectomy provided evolution of modified radical techniques that allowed varying degrees of breast extirpation and lymphatic dissection (Table 19.1). The modified radical mastectomy has clearly defined complete breast removal, inclusion of the tumor and its overlying skin, and regional axillary lymphatics, with preservation of the pectoralis major muscle. Unequivocally, preservation of this muscle has provided better cosmesis of the chest wall and has variable outcomes to enhance motor function of the shoulder when pectoralis major preservation and neurovascular innervation is ensured (4).

TABLE 19.1	Historical Development of Modified Radical Mastectomy	
Author	Year	Surgery
Moore	1867	Segmental breast resection, selective axillary dissection
Volkmann	1875	Total breast extirpation, with removal of pectoralis major fascia, preservation of pectoralis major muscle
Gross	1880	Total mastectomy and complete axillary dissection
Banks	1882	Modified radical mastectomy, with pectoralis preservation
Sprengel	1882	Total mastectomy and selective axillary dissection
Kuster	1883	Total mastectomy and routine axillary dissection
Halsted	1894	Radical mastectomy
Meyer	1894	Radical mastectomy
Murphy	1912	Radical mastectomy, modified by pectoralis preservation
McWhirter	1948	Modified radical mastectomy with radiotherapy
Patey	1948, 1967	Modified radical mastectomy with resection of pectoralis minor
Madden	1972, 1965	Modified radical mastectomy with pectoralis preservation

In Bland et al. (4).

Of historical interest are the following:

▪ Glastein et al. (5) in the Consensus Development Conference on the Therapy of Breast Cancer stated that the modified technique was the standard of therapy for women with stages I and II breast cancer (5,6).
▪ This Conference group thereafter challenged others to suggest that the modified radical mastectomy was the "gold standard" on which other local original therapies would be compared (7–14).

PREOPERATIVE PLANNING

The modified radical mastectomy represents the most common operation done in general surgery as an ablative technique for cancer. This procedure entails

▪ *en bloc resection* of the breast, which is inclusive of the nipple–areolar complex, axillary lymphatics, and the overlying skin surrounding the tumor and
▪ primary closure, which may include reconstruction methods.

The variations of the technique were originally described by Auchincloss (15), Hanley (16), and Madden (17) and preserve the pectoralis major and minor muscles protecting their neurovascular innervation, with incomplete clearance of level III nodes that are medial and caudal to the axillary vein. The surgeon should ensure preservation of the medial pectoral neurovascular bundle, as this neurovascular complex commonly penetrates the pectoralis minor muscle with innervation of the pectoralis major.

The Patey technique involves removal of the pectoralis minor muscle to allow clearance of level III (medial–caudal) nodal group to ensure complete axillary node dissection (18,19). While the modified radical technique attempts to spare the medial and lateral pectoral nerves, the more extended nodal removal (to level III apical group) synchronous with resection of the pectoralis minor muscle makes pectoral nerve preservation more difficult to accomplish. Proportional loss of nerve innervation to the pectoralis major will induce atrophy of this muscle group.

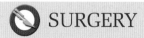 SURGERY

▪ **Anesthesia and positioning** (Fig. 19.1): The modified radical technique requires supine positioning prior to induction with general endotracheal anesthesia. Preferably,

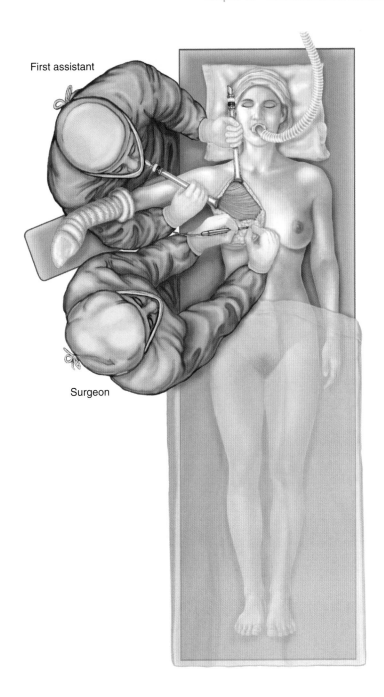

First assistant

Surgeon

Figure 19.1 Position of patient for left modified radical mastectomy at margin of operative table. The first assistant is cephalad to the arm-board and shoulder of the patient to allow access to the axillary contents without undue traction on major muscle groups. Depicted is the preferential isolation of the hand and forearm with an occlusive Stockinette cotton dressing secured distal to the elbow. This technique allows free mobility of the elbow, arm, and shoulder to avoid undue stretch of the brachial plexus with muscle retraction.

Part V: Mastectomy

the patient's hip and shoulder should be aligned with the edge of the operating table to allow simple access to the operating field without undue traction on muscle groups and to avoid stretch-injury to the brachial plexus. Further protection of the brachial plexus from shoulder retraction should be achieved by placing the ipsilateral arm onto a padded arm board with slight elevation of the ipsilateral hemithorax to allow complete rotation and movement of the relaxed shoulder in the operating field.

- **Preparation of the skin:** Prior to draping, the ipsilateral breast, neck, hemithorax, shoulder, axilla, and arm are prepped with standard povidone–iodine solution. In the case of iodine allergies, alternative sterile prep solutions are recommended. The prep should extend across the midline, inclusive of the complete circumferential prep of the ipsilateral shoulder, arm, and hand. We prefer isolation of the ipsilateral forearm and hand with Stockinette® dressing secured by Kling® or Kerlex® cotton rolls. Sterile drapes are placed to provide a wide operative field and are secured to the skin,

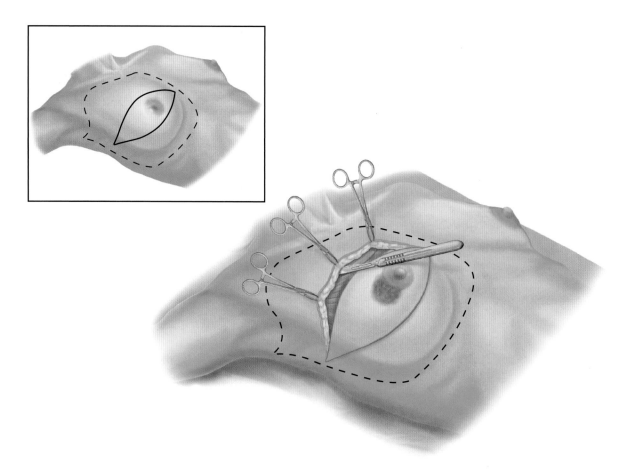

Figure 19.2 *Inset,* Limits of the modified radical mastectomy are delineated laterally by the anterior margin of the latissimus dorsi muscle, medially by the sternal border, superiorly by the subclavius muscle, and inferiorly by the caudal extension of the breast approximately 3 to 4 cm inferior to the inframammary fold. Skin flaps for the modified radical technique are planned with relation to the quadrant in which the primary neoplasm is located. Adequate margins are ensured by developing skin edges 3 to 5 cm from the tumor margin. Skin incisions are made perpendicular to the subcutaneous plane. Flap thickness should vary with patient body habitus but ideally should be 7 to 8 mm thick. Flap tension should be perpendicular to the chest wall with flap elevation deep to the cutaneous vasculature, which is accentuated by flap retraction.

preferably with staples. The first assistant is positioned craniad to the shoulder of the ipsilateral breast to provide retraction and arm mobilization without undue stretch traction on the brachial plexus. Following positioning and preparation, adequate mobility of the ipsilateral shoulder and arm should be confirmed prior to surgical incision (Fig. 19.2).

Skin Incision and Topographical Limits of Dissection

Figures 19.3 through 19.9 confirm the various locations of breast primaries in which adequate therapy with and without irradiation or chemotherapy necessitates total mastectomy. These incisions are planned when conventional techniques are to be utilized without planned immediate reconstruction. While previously recommended wide (radical) skin margins of greater than 5 cm were considered essential for local–regional control, current data would suggest that skin margins of 1 to 2 cm from the gross margin of the index tumor are necessary and adequate to ensure final pathology-free margins. Margins in excess of 2 cm are technically feasible for the majority of total mastectomies in which reconstruction (early or delayed) will not be completed. Clearly, preoperative planning and consideration of the types of incisions are essential for the general surgical oncologist. Preoperative consideration should be given to the skin-sparing technique when the patient desires reconstruction. The most commonly applied elliptical excision for central and subareolar breast primaries is the *classical Stewart incision*

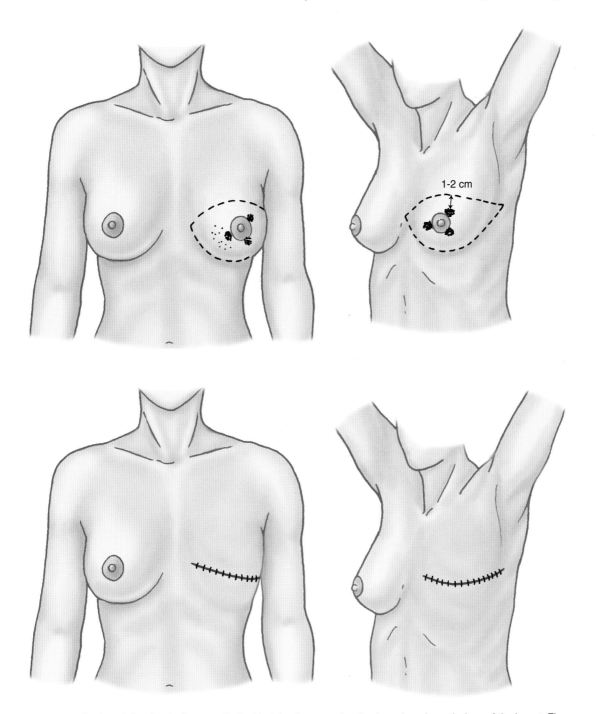

Figure 19.3 Design of the classic Stewart elliptical incision for central and subareolar primary lesions of the breast. The medial extent of the incision ends at the margin of the sternum. The lateral extent of the skin incision should overlie the anterior margin of the latissimus dorsi. The design of the skin incision should incorporate the primary neoplasm en bloc with margins that are 1 to 2 cm from the cranial and caudal edges of the tumor.

(Fig. 19.3) or the modification of the Stewart incision of the inner lower quadrant of the breast. For lesions in the upper outer quadrant, the *classical Orr incision* is preferred.

Limits of the modified radical procedure are as follows:

■ delineated *laterally* by the anterior margin of the latissimus dorsi muscle,
■ delineated *medially* by the sterno–caudal junction border,
■ delineated *superiorly* by the subclavius muscle, and
■ delineated *inferiorly* by the caudal extension of the breast to approximately 2 to 3 cm below the inframammary fold.

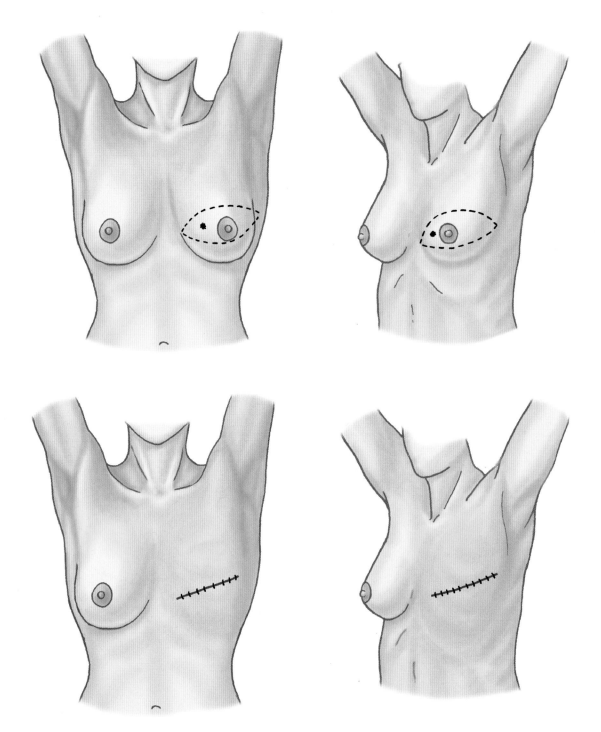

Figure 19.4 Design of the obliquely placed modified Stewart incision for cancer of the inner quadrant of the breast. The medial extent of the incision often must incorporate skin to the midsternum to allow a 1- to 2-cm margin in all directions from the edge of the tumor. Lateral extent of the incision ends at the anterior margin of the latissimus.

Skin incisions are planned perpendicularly to the subcutaneous plane; retraction hooks or towel clips are placed on skin margins to provide adequate perpendicular retraction to the plane of dissection. Retraction should be achieved with constant tension on the periphery of the elevated skin margin at right angles to the chest wall. An essential technique is that of "countertraction" of the operating surgeon against the assistant's retraction to maintain constant flap thickness and improve visualization within the operative field. Skin flap thickness will vary on the basis of patient body habitus, but it is ideally between

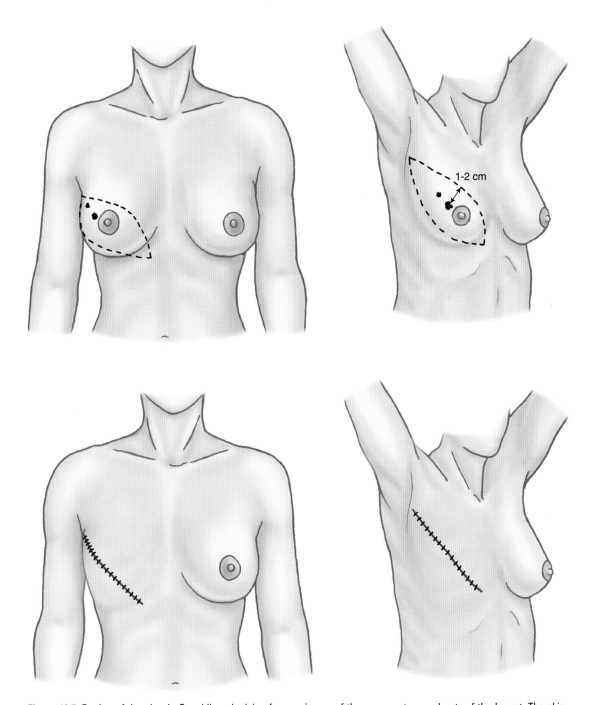

Figure 19.5 Design of the classic Orr oblique incision for carcinoma of the upper outer quadrants of the breast. The skin incision is placed 1 to 2 cm from the margin of the tumor in an oblique plane that is directed cephalad toward the ipsilateral axilla. This incision is a variant of the original Greenough, Kocher, and Rodman techniques for flap development.

6 and 8 mm. The interface for flap elevation is developed deep to the cutaneous vasculature with avoidance of the parenchymal vasculature and should be maintained evenly to achieve constant thickness, which will abrogate devascularization of tissue planes.

Topographical Anatomy

Figure 19.10 represents the topographical anatomy of levels I, II, and III of the axillary contents relative to the neurovascular bundle, pectoralis minor, latissimus dorsi, and

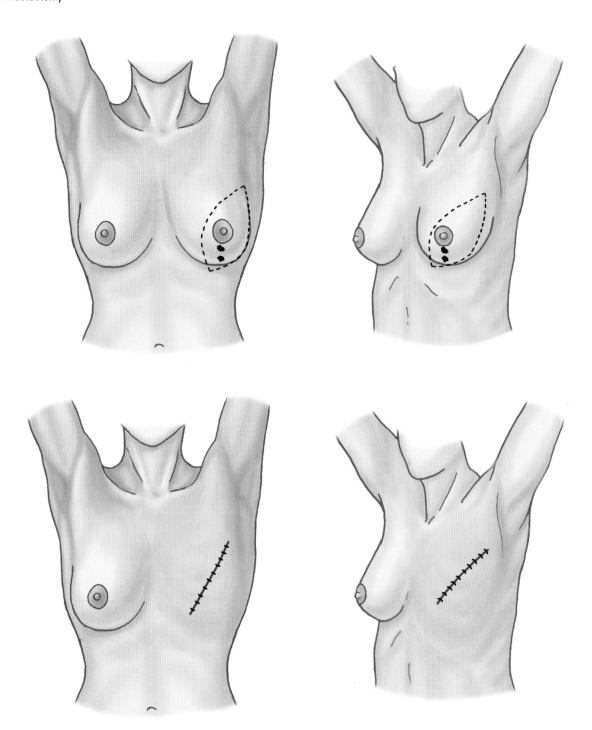

Figure 19.6 Variation of the Orr incision for lower inner and vertically placed (6 o'clock) lesions of the breast. The design of the skin incision is identical to that of Figure 20.4, with attention directed to margins of 1 to 2 cm.

posterior axillary space relative to the chest wall. Level I nodes comprise three principal groups of axillary nodes: the *external mammary group*, the *subscapular group*, and the *axillary vein* (*lateral group*). Level II, the *central nodal group*, is centrally placed upon and immediately beneath the pectoralis minor muscle and overlies the exposed axillary vein. The *subclavicular* (*apical*) *group* is designated level III nodes and represents that group of nodes cephalomedial to the pectoralis minor.

The conduct of the modified radical mastectomy, in contemporary terms, utilizes a dissection of level I and II nodes and spares the pectoralis major and minor muscles as

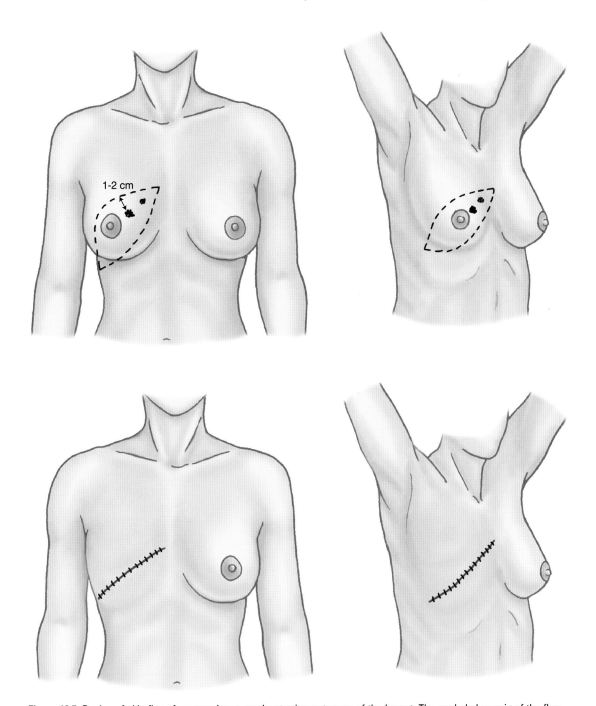

Figure 19.7 Design of skin flaps for upper inner quadrant primary tumors of the breast. The cephalad margin of the flap must be designed to allow access for dissection of the axilla. With flap margins 1 to 2 cm from the tumor, variation in the medial extent of the incision is expected and may extend beyond the edge of the sternum. On occasion, the modified Stewart incision can incorporate the tumor en bloc, provided that the cancer is not too high on the breast and craniad from the nipple–areola complex. All incision designs must be inclusive of the nipple–areola complex when total mastectomy is planned with primary therapy.

formerly described by Patey (Fig. 19.11). Removal of the breast is completed from cephalad to caudad with the inclusion of the pectoralis major fascia, as well as portional resection of the pectoralis major when tumor extension into the muscle is recognized clinically or radiographically. The pectoralis major fascia is dissected from the musculature in a plane parallel to the course of the muscle fibers. This technique avoids entry and exposure of muscle perforators and ensures minimal blood loss. The operator applies constant inferior traction on the breast and the fascia. Multiple perforated vessels will be encountered from

Figure 19.8 Incisions for cancer of the lower outer quadrants of the breast. The surgeon should design incisions that achieve margins of 1 to 2 cm from the tumor with cephalad margins that allow access for dissection of the axilla. The medial extent is the margin of the sternum. Laterally, the inferior extent of the incision is the latissimus.

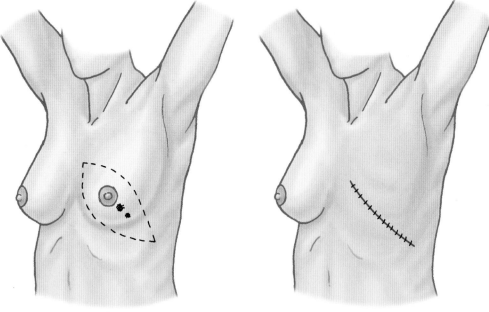

Figure 19.9 Depiction of skin flaps for lesions of the breast that are high lying, infraclavicular, or fixed to the pectoralis major muscle. Fixation to the muscle and/or chest wall necessitates Halsted radical mastectomy with skin margins at least 2 cm. Skin grafting is necessary when large margins of skin are resected for T_3 and T_4 cancers. Primary closure for T_1 and some T_2 tumors is often possible.

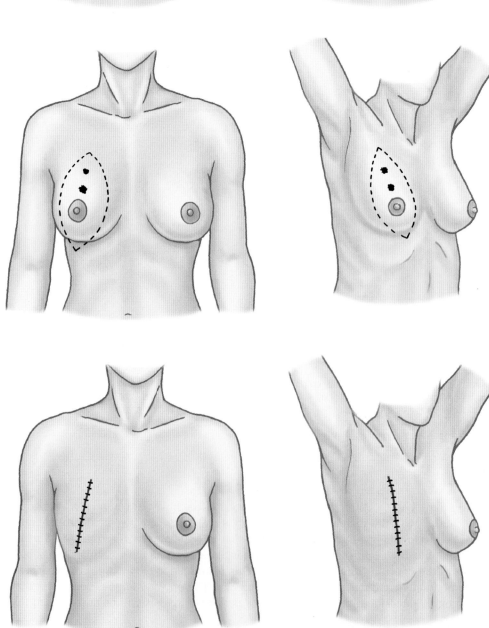

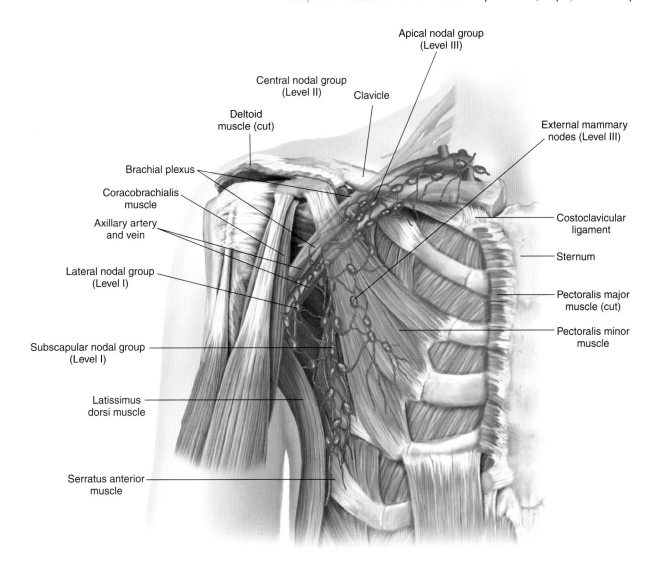

Figure 19.10 Topographic anatomic depiction of levels I, II, and III of the axillary contents with relation to the neurovascular bundle, pectoralis minor, latissimus dorsi, posterior axillary space, and chest wall. Level I comprises three principal axillary nodal groups: the external mammary group, the subscapular group, and the axillary vein (lateral) group. Level II, the central nodal group, is centrally placed immediately beneath the pectoralis minor muscle. The subclavicular (apical) group is designated level III nodes and is superomedial to the pectoralis minor muscle.

the lateral thoracic or anterior intercostals arteries that supply the pectoralis muscles. These perforators must be identified, clamped, divided, and ligated or clipped.

Resection of the pectoralis minor muscle is not necessary except for planned resection of clinically positive level III nodes. When such exposure is essential for planned resection of the pectoralis minor, the latter dissection begins with proper positioning such that the shoulder of the ipsilateral arm is abducted in the field. Figure 19.1 confirms the assistant holding the arm for relief of the brachial plexus. The borders of the pectoralis minor are digitally delineated and retracted to visualize the insertion of the pectoralis minor on the coracoid process where it can be divided with electrocautery (inset of Fig. 19.11). Care must be taken to identify and preserve the medial and lateral pectoral nerves as they penetrate the pectoralis minor in their course for neuronal innervation of the muscle groups. These nerves may be sacrificed if the pectoralis minor resection is planned. Following resection of the pectoralis minor muscle, superior visualization of level III nodes is ensured following resection of the insertion of this muscle on ribs 2 to 5. Protection of the full extent of the pectoralis vein as it courses beneath the pectoralis minor en route to entry between ribs 1 to 2 is essential to avoid venous

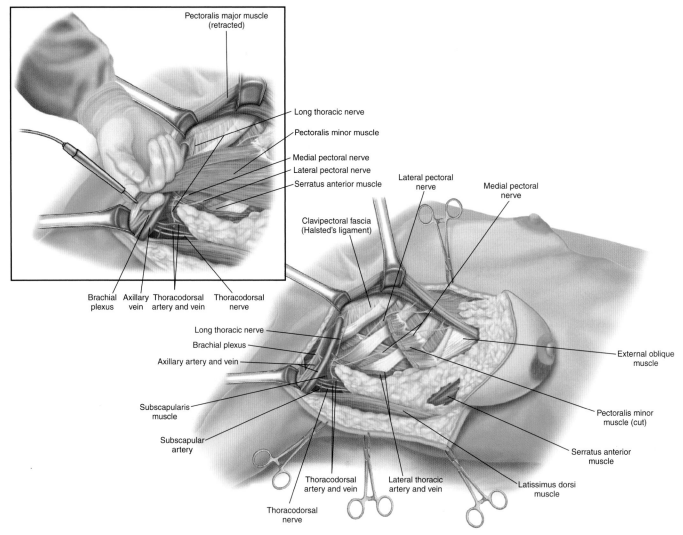

Figure 19.11 *Inset,* Digital protection of the brachial plexus for division of the insertion of the pectoralis minor muscle on the coracoid process. All loose areolar and lymphatic tissues are swept en bloc with the axillary contents. Dissection commences superior to inferior with complete visualization of the anterior and ventral aspects of the axillary vein. Dissection craniad to the axillary vein is inadvisable, for fear of damage to the brachial plexus and the infrequent observation of gross nodal tissue cephalic to the vein. Investing fascial dissection of the vein is best completed with the cold scalpel following exposure, ligation, and division of all venous tributaries on the anterior and ventral surfaces. Caudal to the vein, loose areolar tissue at the junction of the vein with the anterior margin of latissimus is swept inferomedially inclusive of the lateral (axillary) nodal group (level 1). Care is taken to preserve the neurovascular thoracodorsal artery, vein, and nerve in the deep axillary space. The thoracodorsal nerve is traced to its innervation of the latissimus dorsi muscle laterally. Lateral axillary nodal groups are retracted inferomedially and anterior to this bundle for dissection en bloc with the subscapular (level 1) nodal group. Preferentially, dissection commences superomedially before completion of dissection of the external mammary (level 1) nodal group. Superomedial dissection over the axillary vein allows extirpation of the central nodal group (level 2) and apical (subclavicular; level 3) group. The superomedial-most extent of the dissection is the clavipectoral fascia (Halsted's ligament). This level of dissection with the Patey technique allows the surgeon to mark, with metallic clip or suture, the superior-most extent of dissection. All loose areolar tissue just inferior to the apical nodal group is swept off the chest wall, leaving the fascia of the serratus anterior intact. With dissection parallel to the long thoracic nerve (respiratory nerve of Bell), the deep investing serratus fascia is incised. This nerve is closely applied to the investing fascial compartment of the chest wall and must be dissected in its entirety, cephalic to caudal to ensure innervation of the serratus anterior and avoidance of the "winged scapula" disability.

injury. Retraction of all nodal groups from the inferior and ventral surface of the axillary vein at the apical-most extent of the nodes ensures complete resection of level III. When level III dissection is necessary, this level should be tagged or clipped to indicate the highest resection level.

Contemporary therapeutic principles require planned resection of only levels I and II; thus resection of the pectoralis major and minor in most circumstances can be avoided, except with clinically positive or radiographically evident nodal disease at level III.

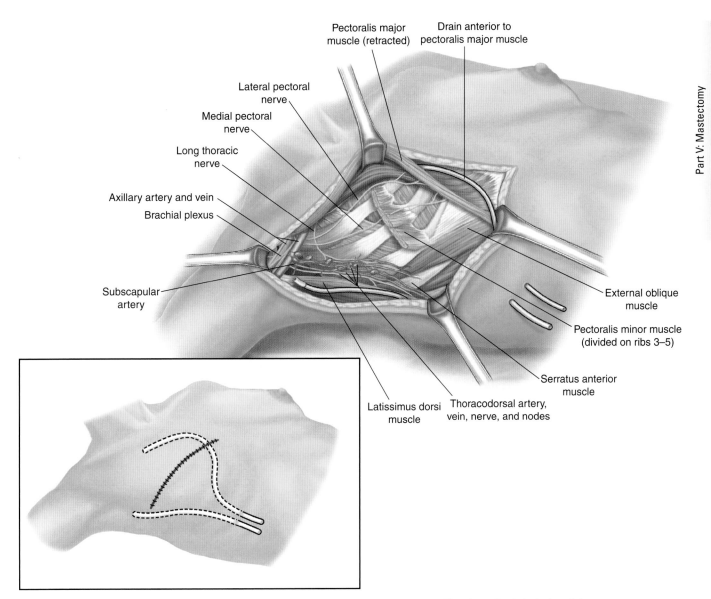

Figure 19.12 The completed Patey axillary dissection variant of the modified radical technique. The dissection is inclusive of the pectoralis minor muscle from origin to insertion on ribs 2 to 5. Both medial and lateral pectoral nerves are preserved to ensure innervation of pectoralis major. With completion of the procedure, remaining portions of this muscle are swept en bloc with the axillary contents to be inclusive of Rotter's interpectoral and the retropectoral groups. *Inset,* Following copious irrigation with saline, closed-suction silastic catheters (10 French) are positioned via stab incisions placed in the inferior flap at the anterior axillary line. The lateral catheter is placed approximately 2 cm inferior to the axillary vein. The superior, longer catheter placed via the medial stab wound is positioned in the inferomedial aspect of the wound bed anterior to the pectoralis major muscle beneath the skin flap. The wound is closed in two layers with 3-0 absorbable synthetic sutures placed in subcutaneous planes. Undue tension on margins of the flap must be avoided; it may necessitate undermining of tissues to reduce mechanical forces. The skin is closed with subcuticular 4-0 synthetic absorbable or nonabsorbable sutures. After completion of wound closure, both catheters are connected to bulb suction. Light, bulky dressings of gauze are placed over the dissection site and taped securely in place with occlusive dressings. The surgeon may elect to place the ipsilateral arm in a sling to provide immobilization.

Dissection of Axillary Lymph Nodes

Dissection of axillary nodes (Fig. 19.12) is performed en bloc to prevent disruption of lymphatics in the axillary space. The surgeon should begin the dissection medially with extirpation of the central (level II) groups and sometimes with apical node (level III) groups when clinically indicated. The cephalomedial-most extent of the dissection is marked at the costoclavicular ligament for the pathologist to examine for extension of nodal disease, which may have subsequent therapeutic and prognostic implications.

With proper elevation of superficial fascia on the anterior surface of the vein near the brachial plexus, the superficial content of fascia of the vein can be cleared on its ventral and anterior surfaces inclusive of level II nodes and with exposure of craniomedial nodes of level III in circumstances in which the pectoralis minor is resected. Inferior retraction of level II and III nodes en bloc with level I node removal is conducted in a craniad to caudal manner and parallel with the thoracodorsal neurovascular bundle. The loose areolar tissue of the juncture of the axillary vein and the anterior margin of the latissimus is swept inferomedially to include the lateral (axillary) nodal group, a portion of the level I group.

■ Care must be taken to identify and preserve the *thoracodorsal neurovascular bundle* in its entire length with muscular innervation at the central level of the latissimus dorsi. This neurovascular bundle lies deep in the axillary space and is fully invested with loose areolar tissue and nodes of the lateral nodal group. The subscapular nodal group (also level I) is identified between the thoracodorsal neurovascular bundle and the chest wall. This group is swept caudad en bloc with the attached lateral nodal group in a caudad fashion. Preservation of the thoracodorsal neurovascular bundle is necessary for subsequent breast reconstruction that employs the myocutaneous flap of the latissimus dorsi.

■ Once the chest wall has been cleared of the cephalad and craniad attachments of the breast and has been disarticulated leaving only the tissues of the axilla, the *long thoracic nerve* (respiratory nerve of Bell) must be identified and preserved to avoid permanent disability with the "winged scapula" and muscle apraxia from denervation of the serratus anterior muscle. The location of this nerve is consistently found applied to the investing fascia of the serratus anterior and courses along the chest wall anterior to the teres major and subscapularis muscle.

■ Contents that are anterior and lateral to the nerve are divided and lifted en bloc with the breast and axillary contents. Before dividing the inferior-most extent of the axillary contents, the long thoracic nerve, as well as the thoracodorsal neurovascular bundles, must be visualized and preserved.

■ Before removal of the dissected contents from the operating table, the surgeon should ensure orientation of the breast specimen with identification of the axillary contents. This can be done with suture in the axilla or in the clock face of the areolar to ensure a cephalad and caudad margin with relativity of the lateral and medial surfaces of the breast.

Wound Closure

■ Closed-suction silastic catheters (10 French) are placed via separate stab wounds entering the inferior flap near the anterior axillary line. Placement of the lateral catheter in the axillary space approximately 2 cm inferior to the axillary vein on the ventral surface of the latissimus dorsi muscle ensures drainage of the axilla space. The longer second catheter is placed medially and inferiorly to the wound bed to provide continuous drainage of blood and serum from the space between the skin flaps and the chest wall. Both catheters should be secured in place with separate 2-0 or 3-0 nonabsorbable nylon sutures.

■ The wound is closed in two layers, first with absorbable 2-0 synthetic suture to approximate the subcutaneous tissues ensuring bites in the cutis reticularis of the skin flap and absorbable 4-0 synthetic subcuticular sutures for skin closure. Alternatively, the skin may be stapled. Steri-strips® are applied perpendicular to the wound when nonabsorbable 4-0 synthetic closure of the subcuticular skin is accomplished. Suction catheters are connected to bulb reservoirs for negative pressure.

➡ POSTOPERATIVE MANAGEMENT

■ Operating dressings may remain intact for 72 hours unless there is concern for tissue viability or bleeding saturation of dressings. Suction catheters should remain in place for approximately 5 to 7 days or until drainage becomes serous and less than 20 to 25 cc per catheter over a 24-hour interval. Vigorous shoulder activity together with arm range of motion exercises should be delayed until drainage catheters are removed and should not be initiated aggressively. Range of motion exercises may be initiated the day following drainage removal but should be done progressively to avoid elevation of the adherent flaps on the chest wall.

With protracted serous or serosanguinous drainage, continued suction may be utilized via the lateral-most (dependent) catheter. Long-term catheter use requires the patient to be instructed in hygienic care of the catheter and skin wound, as well as frequent dressing changes.

COMPLICATIONS

Çinar et al. (20) have investigated the effects of early-onset rehabilitation on shoulder mobility, functional status, and lymphedema in patients who have had modified radical mastectomy. These investigators suggest that improvement in measurements of flexion, abduction, and adduction motion of the shoulder joint and the functional scores were better following home exercise program management after removal of drains. Thus, early-onset rehabilitation following modified radical mastectomy will provide improvement in shoulder mobility and functional capacity without initiating adverse effects in the postoperative period.

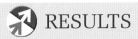 RESULTS

Prospective Trials of Modified Radical Mastectomy

Two independent, prospective, randomized trials conducted in the 1970s by Turner (21) in England and Maddox in Alabama (22,23) compared the Halsted radical with the modified radical technique. Turner et al. (21) evaluated 534 patients with T_1 or T_2 (N_0 or N_1) carcinoma of the breast to demonstrate that at a median follow-up of 5 years, no significant differences were evident for disease-free survival, overall survival, or local–regional control rates (Table 19.2).

Moreover, the analysis by Maddox et al. (22,23) comparing modified radical technique with radical technique for 311 patients with stages I to III disease demonstrated no significant differences at 5-year survival rates but did confirm significant decrease in local–regional recurrence rates when radical mastectomy was utilized (Table 19.3). All patients with positive nodes in the analysis by Maddox et al. (22,23) were randomized to receive chemotherapy. This study confirmed a trend toward enhancement of overall survival following the radical mastectomy, which was superior to the modified technique after 5 years (84% vs. 76%, respectively) and became even more evident at 10 years (74% vs. 65%, respectively; Fig. 19.13). While no significant differences in overall survival

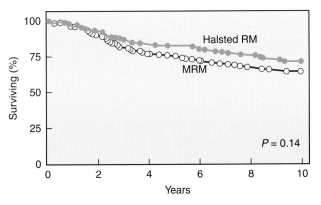

Figure 19.13 Overall survival of patients who underwent radical (red circles, $n = 136$) and modified radical (blue circles, $n = 175$) mastectomy ($P = 0.14$). (Re-created with permission from Maddox WA, Carpenter JT Jr, Laws HT, et al. *Arch Surg.* 1987;122(11):1317–1320. Copyright © 1987, American Medical Association. All rights reserved.)

TABLE 19.2	Manchester Trial Results: Overall Survival, Disease-Free Survival, and Local and Distant Disease-Free Survival Rates (%) for Radical and Modified Radical Mastectomy According to Clinical and Pathological Stage at Entry

	No. of patients followed up	Overall survival (5 y)	Disease-free local recurrence (5 y)[a]	Disease-free distant metastases (5 y)[a]	Overall disease-free survival (5 y)[a]
All cases					
Radical	278	70	75	63	58
Modified	256	70	79	63	58
Clinical stage I					
Pathologic stage I					
Radical	119	80	85	79	69
Modified	108	79	90	79	71
Pathologic stage II					
Radical	52	57	57	52	39
Modified	49	62	74	62	57
Clinical stage II					
Pathologic stage I					
Radical	41	85	91	79	79
Modified	38	78	88	71	70
Pathologic stage II					
Radical	64	55	59	47	38
Modified	59	55	56	45	30

[a]Figures indicate the percentages of patients not experiencing each event regardless of any other outcome.
Reproduced with permission from Turner et al. (21) Copyright The Royal College of Surgeons of England.
In Bland et al. (4).

between the procedures was evident with small cancers, ultimate survival rate benefit for patients with T_2 or T_3 was superior following radical technique (Fig. 19.14).

In the evaluation by Morimoto et al. (24) of Japan, similar comparisons of the two techniques with stage II disease receiving postoperative chemotherapy confirmed no significant differences in 5-year survival, overall survival, or local recurrence in the two groups (Table 19.4). Of note, nodal metastasis did adversely affect 5-year survival in both groups.

Additional prospective studies confirming the similarity of outcomes with the modified technique were reported by Staunton et al. (25) of St. Bartholomew's Hospital in London and converted to a 20-year follow-up for 193 patients. Approximately, 40% of patients received hormonal treatment and 9% received chemotherapy with a small

TABLE 19.3	University of Alabama Prospective Randomized Trial to Compare the Halsted Radical Mastectomy with the Modified Radical Mastectomy: Local Recurrence Rates of the Two Techniques

	Modified radical mastectomy						Halsted radical mastectomy					
			Local recurrence						Local recurrence			
			5 y		10 y				5 y		10 y	
Disease stage	No. of patients	%	No.	%	No.	%	No. of patients	%	No.	%	No.	%
I	43	13.8	4	9.3	NA	NA	37	11.9	2	5.4	NA	NA
II	112	36	8	7.1	NA	NA	83	26.7	3	3.6	NA	NA
III	20	6.4	4	20[a]	NA	NA	16	5.1	1	6.3[a]	NA	NA
Total	175	56.2	16	9.1[b]	20	11.4[c]	136	43.7	6	4.4[b]	8	5.8[c]

NA, Not available.
[a]$P = 0.09$; [b]$P = 0.04$; [c]$P = $ NS.
Modified with permission from Maddox et al. (22) and Maddox et al. (23).
In Bland et al. (4).

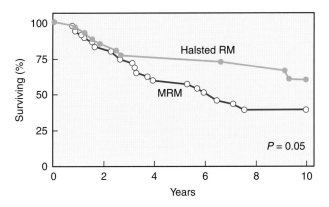

Part V: Mastectomy

percentage (6%) undergoing radiation as part of the initial treatment. The 5-, 10-, and 15-year survival rates of T_1/T_2 N_0 clinical stage I breast cancers were 90%, 79%, and 74%, respectively; for stage II (T_1/T_2 N_1) patients, these rates were 81%, 64%, and 60%, respectively. For stage III (T_3 N_0/N_1) cancers, these rates were 78%, 70%, and 0%, respectively. Given the excellent outcomes for control of disease, these authors concluded that the therapeutic outcomes with minimal morbidity allow the modified radical mastectomy to be considered the superior choice in treating the patient with primary operable cancer of the breast.

Total (Simple) Mastectomy

The clinical and surgical application of the term "total mastectomy" is synonymous with simple mastectomy. This procedure represents a modification of the modified radical mastectomy, in that preservation of the pectoralis muscles is ensured, but the axillary lymph nodes are dissected only at the level of the axillary tail of Spence nodes (level I). The rationale for this modification of technique is based upon the hypothesis that breast cancer is a systemic disease and outcomes are affected by complex host–tumor interactions. Thus, variations in local–regional therapies are unlikely to affect survival outcomes substantially, but rather biological host–tumor relationships are the principal drivers of metastatic dissemination (10,26–33). Thus, total mastectomy advocated the use of regional node dissection to treat local disease that appears clinically and anatomically confined to the breast by imaging techniques.

Prospective Trials of Total Mastectomy With or Without Irradiation

One of the largest clinical trials that evaluated total mastectomy with or without irradiation was the Cancer Research Campaign Clinical Trial (34–36). In the evaluation of 2,243 patients with a mean follow-up of 11 years, results confirm no statistical differences in overall survival benefits between the two techniques (Fig. 19.15). However,

TABLE 19.4	University of Tokushima Prospective Trial to Compare Modified Radical Mastectomy with Extended Radical Mastectomy in Patients with Stage II Disease Treated with Chemotherapy				
Operation	No. of patients	5-y DFS	5-y DFS for positive nodes	5-y OS	5-y OS for positive nodes
MRM	96	87.2	75.6	93.2	84.4
ERM	96	82.7	73.3	92.4	87.8

DFS, disease-free survival; OS, overall survival; MRM, modified radical mastectomy; ERM, extended radical mastectomy
Modified from Morimoto et al. (24).
In Bland et al. (4).

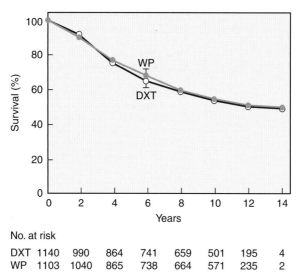

Figure 19.15 All evaluable patients: survival in watch policy (WP) and radiotherapy groups (DXT) ($\chi^2 = 0.02$, $P = 0.88$, hazard ratio [HR] = 1.0). "No. at risk" represents the number of patients alive at entry and biennially thereafter. This number decreases in the later years, because there are fewer patients with relevant trial times. Vertical bars indicate the 95% confidence intervals. (Re-created with permission from Berstock DA, Houghton J, Haybittle J, et al. *World J Surg.* 1985;9(5):667–670.)

No. at risk

DXT	1140	990	864	741	659	501	195	4
WP	1103	1040	865	738	664	571	235	2

these investigators confirmed a higher recurrence rate in the total mastectomy-only group versus the total mastectomy and irradiation group (Fig. 19.16). Recurrence rates appear to be proportional to tumor grade, and prophylactic irradiation was proposed to treat patients at high risk for recurrence. With subsequent follow-up of this trial at 19 years by Houghton et al. (37), local recurrence was significantly reduced by the addition of irradiation to total mastectomy. Nonetheless, survival rates remain similar between the two therapy groups, and there were more non–breast cancer deaths observed within the irradiated cohort.

By all standards, the trials of the National Surgical Adjuvant Breast and Bowel Project (NSABP) have played major roles to determine the appropriate surgical course for patients with breast cancer. In the B-04 trial of the late 1970s, 1,655 patients with an average follow-up of 11 years were reported by Fisher et al. (28). This study compared total mastectomy with and without axillary radiation with radical mastectomy. Final analysis confirmed no differences in disease-free survival rates between the groups with *clinically negative nodes*; there were no differences in disease-free overall survival rates between total mastectomy with *irradiation* and radical mastectomy for patients with *positive lymph nodes* (Fig. 19.17).

NSABP B-04 confirmed that for patients with node-negative disease who had local recurrence, rates of recurrence were lowest following total mastectomy with irradiation (Fig. 19.18). For patients with positive lymphatics, the local, regional, and distant recur-

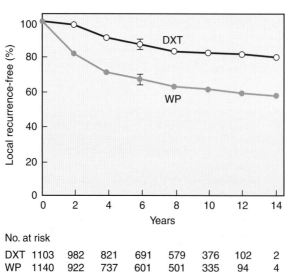

Figure 19.16 All evaluable patients: local recurrence-free in watch policy (WP) and radiotherapy groups (DXT) ($\chi^2 = 120.93$, $P < 0.001$, hazard ratio [HR] = 2.69). "No. at risk" represents the number of patients alive at entry and biennially thereafter. This number decreases in the later years, because there are fewer patients with relevant trial times. Vertical bars indicate the 95% confidence intervals. (Re-created with permission from Berstock DA, Houghton J, Haybittle J, et al. *World J Surg.* 1985;9(5):667–670.)

No. at risk

DXT	1103	982	821	691	579	376	102	2
WP	1140	922	737	601	501	335	94	4

Part V: Mastectomy

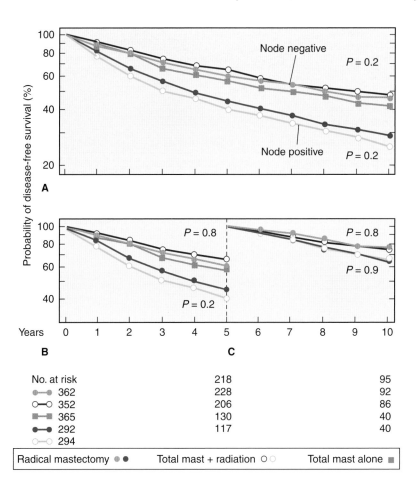

No. at risk

●—● 362	218	95
○—○ 352	228	92
■—■ 365	206	86
●—● 292	130	40
○—○ 294	117	40

Radical mastectomy ● ●   Total mast + radiation ○ ○   Total mast alone ■

Figure 19.17 Disease-free survival for patients treated with radical mastectomy (solid circles), total mastectomy plus radiation (open circles), or total mastectomy alone (solid square). Disease-free survival through 10 years (**A**), during the first 5 years (**B**), and during the second 5 years for patients free of disease at the end of the fifth year (**C**). There were no significant differences among the three groups of patients with clinically negative nodes or between the two groups with clinically positive nodes. (Re-created with permission from Fisher B, Redmond C, Fisher ER, et al. *N Engl J Med.* 1985;312(11):674–681. Copyright © 1985, Massachusetts Medical Society. All rights reserved.)

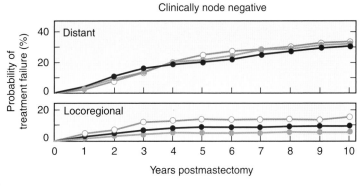

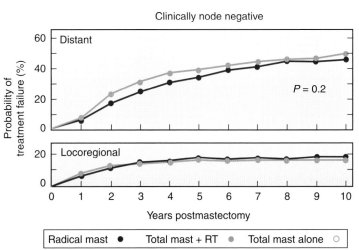

Radical mast ●   Total mast + RT ●   Total mast alone ○

Figure 19.18 Local or regional and distant treatment failures as the first evidence of disease in patients with clinically negative and positive nodes who were treated with radical mastectomy (red circles), total mastectomy and radiation (blue circles), or total mastectomy alone (open green circles). For node-negative patients, there were no significant differences in distant disease occurring as a first treatment failure among the three groups, whereas local and regional disease was best controlled in the group receiving radiation. For node-positive patients, there was no significant difference in distant or local and regional disease between the two groups. (Re-created with permission from Fisher B, Redmond C, Fisher ER, et al. *N Engl J Med.* 1985;312(11):674–681. Copyright © 1985, Massachusetts Medical Society. All rights reserved.)

Figure 19.19 Distant disease-free survival and overall survival for patients treated with radical mastectomy (solid circles), total mastectomy and radiation (open circles), or total mastectomy alone (solid square). **Top panel.** Disease-free survival through 10 years **(A)**, during the first 5 years **(B)**, and during the second 5 years for patients free of distant disease at the end of the fifth year **(C)**. **Bottom panel.** Disease-free survival through 10 years **(A)**, during the first 5 years **(B)**, and during the second 5 years for patients alive at the end of the fifth year **(C)**. There were no significant differences among the three groups of patients with clinically negative nodes or between the two groups with positive nodes. (Re-created with permission from Fisher B, Redmond C, Fisher ER, et al. *N Engl J Med*. 1985;312(11):674–681. Copyright © 1985, Massachusetts Medical Society. All rights reserved.)

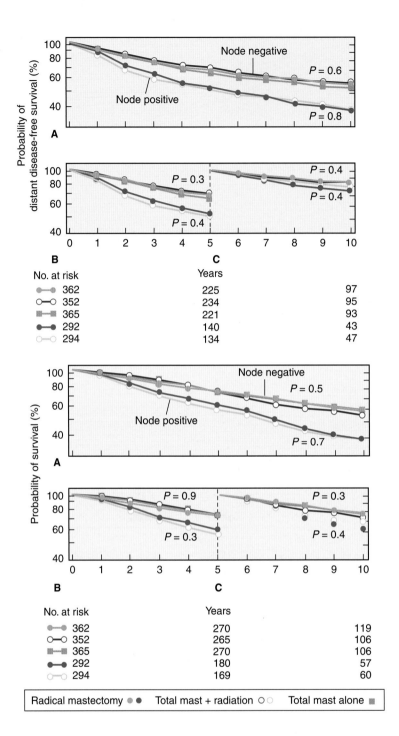

rence rates were comparable for patients treated by either simple mastectomy plus irradiation or by radical technique. Moreover, the trial confirmed results following 5 years accurately predict the outcomes at 10 years (Fig. 19.19).

Prophylactic Total Mastectomy in the High-Risk Patient

The sequencing of the human genome with advances in molecular biology and nanotechnology has enhanced the ability of the physician-scientist to predict risk for breast cancer. Furthermore, identification and confirmation of the role of the BRCA-1 and BRCA-2 genes associated with breast cancer confirms an objective methodology to identify patients at the highest risk for development of the disease (38–42). Once the mutation of BRCA-1/-2 gene is evident, the significant probability of risk for developing breast cancer at an earlier age and perhaps bilaterally is evident (40,43–46). Despite

TABLE 19.5	Indications for Prophylactic Total Mastectomy: Society of Surgical Oncology Position Statement (1995)	
Patients with no history of breast cancer	**Patients with unilateral breast cancer**	
Atypical hyperplasia	Presence of lobular carcinoma in situ	
Any history of lobular carcinoma in situ	Large breast that is difficult to evaluate	
History of relative with premenopausal breast cancer	Diffuse microcalcifications	
Dense, nodular breasts in association with:	Risk factors: Atypical hyperplasia	
Atypical hyperplasia	Family history in first-degree relative	
Family history of premenopausal breast cancer	Age <40 years at diagnosis	

From Bilimoria M, Morrow, M. *CA Cancer J Clin.* 1995;45(5):263–278 with permission. Copyright 1995 American Cancer Society: Reproduced with permission of Wiley–Liss, Inc., a subsidiary of John Wiley & Sons, Inc. In Bland et al. (4).

these confirmations, the most effective prevention for breast cancer is prophylactic mastectomy, but prospective data are limited. Guidelines proposed by the position statement of the Society of Surgical Oncology published in 1995 are included in Table 19.5.

The first prospective trial that examines BRCA-1/-2 mutations was completed by Meijers-Heijboer et al. (39) who compared prophylactic mastectomy with regular surveillance. Patients undergoing prophylactic mastectomy had no incidence of breast cancer, whereas the surveillance group developed cancer at a rate that was comparable to that of other patients with the same genetic mutation. Despite its short-term mean follow-up, the results are positive for the prophylactic technique but should be interpreted in light of the short duration of this follow-up. Previous retrospective analyses of the high-risk patient were conducted by Mayo Clinic surgeons, Hartmann et al. (47) and McDonnell et al. (48). At a mean follow-up of 14 years, the study by Hartmann et al. (47) confirmed that only 7 of 639 patients developed breast cancer following *prophylactic mastectomy.* Of significant importance are the technique utilized and the differentiation of the *subcutaneous (incomplete central) mastectomy* with that of the *total mastectomy* technique in which all tissues at risk are removed. Subcutaneous mastectomy has afforded excellent cosmetic results, but it should not be considered an oncologic procedure. The most quoted of these two papers by McDonnell et al. (48) examines the efficacy of the contralateral prophylactic mastectomy in women with a personal and familial history of breast cancer. This paper is important in that there was a reduction in risk of contralateral breast cancer in these patients by approximately 90% following the preventative procedure.

CONCLUSIONS

- Modified radical mastectomy implies removal of the breast, regional lymphatics, and pectoralis minor muscle.
- Preservation of the pectoralis major muscle enhances volume and contour of the chest-wall deformity.
- Limits of the lymphatic dissection include levels I and II, with preservation of level III (unless palpable nodes evident).
- Preservation of the thoracodorsal neurovascular bundle and long thoracic nerve enhances shoulder and arm functionality.
- Results of modified radical mastectomy are equivalent to those of the Halsted radical procedure.

References

1. Moore CH. On the influence of inadequate operations on the theory of cancer. *R Med Chir Soc Lond.* 1867;1:244.
2. Halsted WS. The results of operations for the cure of cancer of the breast performed at the Johns Hopkins Hospital from June 1889 to January 1894. *Arch Surg.* 1894;20:497.
3. Meyer W. An improved method for the radical operation for carcinoma of the breast. *Med Rec NY.* 1894;46:746.
4. Bland KI, Chang HR, Prati R, et al. Modified radical mastectomy and total (simple) mastectomy. In: Bland KI, Copeland EM, eds. *The Breast: Comprehensive Management of Benign and Malignant Diseases.* 4th ed. Philadelphia, PA: Saunders Elsevier, 2010:803–822.

5. Glastein E, Straus K, Lichner A. Results of the NCI early breast cancer trial. In: Proceedings of the National Institutes of Health Consensus Development Conference, June 18–21, 1990:32.

6. Moxley JH III, Allegra JC, Henney J, et al. Treatment of primary breast cancer: summary of the NIH Consensus Development Conference. *JAMA*. 1980;244(8):797–800.

7. Bader J, Lippmann ME, Swain SM. Preliminary report of the NCI early breast cancer (BC) study: a prospective randomized trial comparison of lumpectomy and radiation to mastectomy for stage I and II BC. *Int J Radiat Oncol Biol Phys*. 1987;12 (suppl):160.

8. Blichert-Toft M. A Danish randomized trial comparing breast conservation with mastectomy in mammary carcinoma. *Br J Cancer*. 1995;62(suppl 12):15.

9. Sarrazin D, Le MG, Arriagada R, et al. Ten-year results of a randomized trial comparing a conservative treatment to mastectomy in early breast cancer. *Radiother Oncol*. 1989;14(3): 177–184.

10. Fisher B, Anderson S, Redmond CK, et al. Reanalysis and results after 12 years of follow-up in a randomized clinical trial comparing total mastectomy with lumpectomy with or without irradiation in the treatment of breast cancer. *N Engl J Med*. 1995;333(22):1456–1461.

11. Robinson GN, van Heerden JA, Payne WS, et al. The primary surgical treatment of carcinoma of the breast: a changing trend toward modified radical mastectomy. *Mayo Clin Proc*. 1976; 51(7):433–442.

12. Sarrazin D, Le MG, Fontaine MF, Arriagada R. Conservative treatment versus mastectomy in T_1 or small T_2 breast cancer: a randomized clinical trial. In: Harris JR, Hellman S, Silen W, eds. *Conservative Management of Breast Cancer*. Philadelphia, PA: JB Lippincott, 1983.

13. Veronesi U, Valagussa P. Inefficacy of internal mammary nodes dissection in breast cancer surgery. *Cancer*. 1981;47(1):170–175.

14. Veronesi U, Banfi A, Del Vecchio M, et al. Comparison of Halsted mastectomy with quadrantectomy, axillary dissection, and radiotherapy in early breast cancer: long-term results. *Eur J Cancer Clin Oncol*. 1986;22(9):1085–1089.

15. Auchincloss H. Significance of location and number of axillary metastases in carcinoma of the breast. *Ann Surg*. 1963;158: 37–46.

16. Handley RS. The conservative radical mastectomy of Patey: 10-year results in 425 patients' breasts. *Dis Breast*. 1976;2:16.

17. Madden JL. Modified radical mastectomy. *Surg Gynecol Obstet*. 1965;121(6):1221–1230.

18. Patey DH, Dyson WH. The prognosis of carcinoma of the breast in relation to the type of operation performed. *Br J Cancer*. 1948;2(1):7–13.

19. Patey DH. A review of 146 cases of carcinoma of the breast operated on between 1930 and 1943. *Br J Cancer*. 1967;21(2): 260–269.

20. Çinar N, Seçkin Ü, Keskin D, et al. The effectiveness of early rehabilitation in patients with modified radical mastectomy. *Cancer Nurs*. 2008;31(2):160–165.

21. Turner L, Swindell R, Bell WGT, et al. Radical vs. modified radical mastectomy for breast cancer. *Ann R Coll Surg Engl*. 1981;63(4):239–243.

22. Maddox WA, Carpenter JT Jr, Laws HL, et al. A randomized prospective trial of radical (Halsted) mastectomy versus modified radical mastectomy in 311 breast cancer patients. *Ann Surg*. 1983;198(2):207–212.

23. Maddox WA, Carpenter JT Jr, Laws HT, et al. Does radical mastectomy still have a place in the treatment of primary operable breast cancer? *Arch Surg*. 1987;122(11):1317–1320.

24. Morimoto T, Monden Y, Takashima S, et al. Five-year results of a randomized trial comparing modified radical mastectomy and extended radical mastectomy for stage II breast cancer. *Surg Today*. 1994;24(3):210–214.

25. Staunton MD, Melville DM, Monterrosa A, et al. A 25-year prospective study of modified radical mastectomy (Patey) in 192 patients. *J R Soc Med*. 1993;86(7):381–384.

26. Fisher B, Fisher ER. Experimental evidence in support of the dormant tumor cell. *Science*. 1959;130:918–919.

27. Fisher B, Fisher ER. Transmigration of lymph nodes by tumor cells. *Science*. 1966;152(727):1397–1398.

28. Fisher B, Redmond C, Fisher ER, et al. Ten-year results of a randomized clinical trial comparing radical mastectomy and total mastectomy with or without radiation. *N Engl J Med*. 1985; 312(11):674–681.

29. Fisher ER, Fisher B. Host influence on tumor growth and dissemination. In: Schwartz E, ed. *The Biological Basis of Radiation Therapy*. Philadelphia, PA: JB Lippincott, 1966.

30. Fisher B, Fisher ER. The interrelationship of hematogenous and lymphatic tumor cell dissemination. *Surg Gynecol Obstet*. 1966; 122(4):791–798.

31. Fisher B, Redmond C, Fisher ER. The contribution of recent NSABP clinical trials of primary breast cancer therapy to an understanding of tumor biology: an overview of findings. *Cancer* 1980; 46(4 suppl): 1009–1025.

32. Fisher B, Redmond C, Poisson R, et al. Eight-year results of a randomized clinical trial comparing total mastectomy and lumpectomy with or without irradiation in the treatment of breast cancer. *N Engl J Med*. 1989;320(13):822–828.

33. Fisher B, Saffer EA, Fisher ER. Studies concerning the regional lymph node in cancer VII: thymidine uptake by cells from nodes of breast cancer patients relative to axillary location and histopathologic discriminants. *Cancer*. 1974;33(1):271–279.

34. Management of early cancer of the breast: report on an international multicentre trial supported by the Cancer Research Campaign. *Br Med J*. 1976;1(6017):1035–1038.

35. Berstock DA, Houghton J, Haybittle J, et al. The role of radiotherapy following total mastectomy for patients with early breast cancer. *World J Surg*. 1985;9(5):667–670.

36. Elston CW, Gresham GA, Rao GS, et al. The Cancer Research Campaign (King's/Cambridge) Trial for early breast cancer: clinico-pathological aspects. *Br J Cancer*. 1982;45(5):655–669.

37. Houghton J, Baum M, Haybittle JL. Role of radiotherapy following total mastectomy in patients with early breast cancer. The Closed Trials Working Party of the CRC Breast Cancer Trials Group. *World J Surg*. 1994;18(1):117–122.

38. Lerman C, Narod S, Schulman K, et al. BRCA1 testing in families with hereditary breast-ovarian cancer: a prospective study of patient decision making and outcomes. *JAMA*. 1996;275(24): 1885–1892.

39. Meijers-Heijboer EJ, Verhoog LC, Brekelmans CT, et al. Presymptomatic DNA testing and prophylactic surgery in families with a BRCA1 or BRCA2 mutation. *Lancet*. 2000;355 (9220):2015–2020.

40. Meijers-Heijboer H, van Geel B, van Putten WL, et al. Breast cancer after prophylactic bilateral mastectomy in women with a BRCA1 or BRCA2 mutation. *N Engl J Med*. 2001;345(3): 159–164.

41. Miki Y, Swensen J, Shattuck-Eidens D, et al. A strong candidate for the breast and ovarian cancer susceptibility gene BRCA1. *Science*. 1994;266(5182):66–71.

42. Wooster R, Bignell G, Lancaster J, et al. Identification of the breast cancer susceptibility gene, BRCA2. *Nature*. 1995;378(6559): 789–792.

43. Ford D, Easton DF, Stratton M, et al. Genetic heterogeneity and penetrance analysis of the BRCA1 and BRCA2 genes in breast cancer families. The Breast Cancer Linkage Consortium. *Am J Hum Genet*. 1998;62(3):676–689.

44. Struewing JP, Hartge P, Wacholder S, et al. The risk of cancer associated with specific mutation of BRCA1 and BRCA2 among Ashkenazi Jews. *N Engl J Med*. 1997;336(20):1401–1408.

45. Verhoog LC, Brekelmans CT, Seynaeve C, et al. Survival and tumour characteristics of breast cancer patients with germline mutations of BRCA1. *Lancet*. 1998;351(9099):316–321.

46. Verhoog LC, Brekelmans CT, Seynaeve C, et al. Survival in hereditary breast cancer associated with germline mutations of BRCA2. *J Clin Oncol*. 1999;17(11):3396–3402.

47. Hartmann LC, Schaid DJ, Woods JE, et al. Efficacy of bilateral prophylactic mastectomy in women with a family history of breast cancer. *N Engl J Med*. 1999;340(2):77–84.

48. McDonnell SK, Schaid DJ, Myers JL, et al. Efficacy of contralateral prophylactic mastectomy in women with a personal and family history of breast cancer. *J Clin Oncol*. 2001;19(19): 3938–3943.

49. Bland KI, McCraw JB, Copeland EM III, et al. General principles of mastectomy: evaluation and therapeutic options In:

Bland KI, Copeland EM III, eds. *The Breast: Comprehensive Management of Benign and Malignant Diseases.* 4th ed. Philadelphia, PA: Saunders Elsevier, 2010:747–778.

50. Murphy JB. Carcinoma of breast. *Surg Clin.* 1912;1:779.

51. McWhirter R. The value of simple mastectomy and radiotherapy in the treatment of cancer of the breast. *Br J Radiol.* 1948; 21(252):599–610.

52. Madden JL, Kandalaft S, Bourque RA. Modified radical mastectomy. *Ann Surg.* 1972;175(5):624–634.

53. Volkmann R. Geschwülste der mamma (36 Fälle) Beitrage zur Chirurgie. *Leipsig.* 1895:310.

54. Gross SW. *A Practical Treatment of Tumors of the Mammary Gland Embracing Their Histology, Pathology, Diagnosis, and Treatment.* New York, NY: D Appleton, 1880.

55. Banks WM. On free removal of mammary cancer with extirpation of the axillary glands as a necessary accompaniment. *BMJ.* 1882;2:1138.

56. Sprengel O. Mittheilungen über die in den Jahren 1874 bis 1878 aur der Volkmann'schen Klinik operativ behandelten 131 Falle von Brust-carcinom. *Archir F Klin Chir* 1882;27:805.

57. Kuster E. Zur behandlung des brustkrebses verhandlungen der deutschen gesellschaft für Chirurgie. *Leipsig.* 1883:288.

20 Radical Mastectomy

Kirby I. Bland

Introduction

The origin of the Halstedian procedure was one of an oncologically designed procedure that embraces local–regional control of disease. Thereafter, Halsted's utilization of the techniques, which was a consolidated synthesis of the development and writings of multiple surgeons who preceded him, allowed him to achieve local and regional recurrence rates of 6% and 22%, respectively, with this en bloc approach (1–3). Meyer (4), in a simultaneous publication, suggested that reduction in local recurrence rates to 6% from rates of 54% to 82% acknowledged by European surgeons was a masterful contribution to the treatment of this organ. Table 20.1 compares these operations available to European surgeons during the Halstedian era, with an accompanying 3-year estimated "cure" rate for breast cancer.

In its final anatomical design, the technique of the Halsted radical procedure espoused by both Halsted and Meyer embodied the following concepts and principles:

- wide excision of the skin, covering the defect with Thiersch grafts;
- routine resection of *both* pectoral muscles;
- routine axillary dissection (Levels I, II, III); and
- resection of all tissues en bloc, providing wide skin and surgical margins for all margins of tumor growth.

INDICATIONS/CONTRAINDICATIONS

The design and application of cytoreduction of the advanced primary mammary neoplasm has provided the medical oncologists and surgeons a vast increase in the latitude of application of less radical procedures in the therapy of carcinoma of the breast. Although modern pharmacology and breast irradiation enhance the probability of these cytoreductive events, especially with the combinations of targeted chemotherapeutic agents, the Halsted radical mastectomy is occasionally essential to achieve local–regional control of the breast, axilla, and chest wall. Quite simply put, these adjuvant therapies were the major advances that allowed less radical procedures to achieve enhanced local–regional control and survival without application of the Halsted or modified radical techniques.

TABLE 20.1	Chronology of the Mastectomy for Treatment of Breast Cancer with Expectant (Average) 3-Year "Cure Rates"			
Type of operation	**Study**	**Year**	**No. of cases**	**3-yr cures (%)**
Simple mastectomy	Winiwarter (Billroth)[a]	1867–1875		4.7
Average				**4.7**
Complete mastectomy	Oldekop[b]	1850–1878	229	11.7
and axillary	Dietrich (Lucke)[c]	1872–1890	148	16.2
dissection in	Horner[d]	1881–1893	144	19.4
most cases	Poulsen[e]	1870–1888	110	20
	Banks[f]	1877	46	20
	Schmid (Kuster)[g]	1871–1885		21.5
Average				**18.1**
Complete (total)	Sprengel (Volkmann)[h]	1874–1878	200	11
mastectomy, axillary	Schmidt[i]	1877–1886	112	18.8
dissection, removal	Rotter[j]		30	20
of pectoral fascia	Mahler[k]	1887–1897	150	21
and greater or	Joerss[l]	1885–1893	98	28.5
lesser amounts of				
pectoral muscle				
Average				**19.9**
Modern radical	Halsted[m]	1889–1894	76	45
mastectomy	Halsted[n]	1907	232	38.3
	Hutchison[o]	1910–1933		39.4
Average				**40.9**

[a]Data from Billroth (5); [b]Data from Oldekop (6); [c]Data from Lucke (7); [d]Data from Horner (8); [e]Data from Poulsen (9); [f]Data from Banks (10); [g]Data from Kuster (11); [h]Data from Volkmann (12); [i]Data from Schmidt (13); [j]Data from Rotter (14); [k]Data from Mahler (15); [l]Data from Joerss (16); [m]Data from Halsted (1); [n]Data from Halsted (2); [o]Data from Hutchison (17). From Bland and Copeland (18) with permission.

PREOPERATIVE PLANNING

Table 20.2 acknowledges current indications for the use of the Halsted radical mastectomy for patients presenting with advanced local–regional disease.

■ Major transitions from the Halstedian approach for breast cancer therapy have occurred as a result of the equivalent local–regional control that is evident with alternative breast conservation principles (19).

■ Unequivocally, with the increasing application of appropriate breast conservation surgery in eligible patients has been a redefinition for indications of the Halsted procedure.

■ Included in Table 20.2 is treatment of local recurrence following the conservation approach in the presence and/or absence of regional disease. In this circumstance, the radical mastectomy may be indicated when disease *invades the pectoralis major* muscle. Surgical dogma would suggest that this represents a "salvage mastectomy" necessary for large, bulky recurrences, especially for posterior lesions that recur with fascial or muscle fixation. In contemporary practice of surgical oncology, the medical or surgical oncologist should expect this event to occur in less than 2% to 5% of presenting patients following conservation approaches.

■ Furthermore, the radical surgical procedure may be the only available technique for local–regional control of locally advanced (fixed, ulcerated) disease, especially in patients who have received prior therapy with total breast irradiation and/or multimodal cytotoxic therapy (20–22).

■ There is no current indication for an *extended radical mastectomy* held in the contemporary practice of breast surgery. However, for long durations, there were proponents of the extended procedure as an advantage over the Halsted radical procedure with its principal advantage for lesions of the medial upper or lower quadrants in which the radical procedure, together with internal mammary nodal dissection,

TABLE 20.2	Relative Indications for the Halsted Radical Mastectomy[a]

Advanced locoregional disease with fixation to pectoralis major muscle (T_2, T_3, T_{4a-c}; stages IIIA, IIIB, IIIC), when refractory to induction chemotherapy and irradiation

Advanced locoregional disease with skin ulceration (T_{4b}; stage IIIb) unresponsive to radiochemotherapy

Recurrent advanced, locoregional disease (T_2, T_3, T_4) after partial (segmental) mastectomy with tumor fixation to pectoralis major muscle ("salvage" mastectomy)

For completion of the radical procedure with locoregional recurrence after modified/segmental mastectomy when tumor invades chest wall and is refractory to cytoinduction chemotherapy

High-lying advanced peripheral lesions near clavicle/sternum with tumor fixation to muscle (stages IIA, IIB; stages IIIA, IIIB)

[a]All presentations of advanced locoregional disease should receive induction cytotoxic drug therapy, radiotherapy, or both before radical mastectomy. Staging to rule out systemic disease should precede induction therapy.
From Bland and Copeland (18) with permission.

enhanced survival (23–26). In most North American, South American, and European clinics, the extended procedure has been fully abandoned.

SURGERY

Following induction of general endotracheal anesthesia, the patient is carefully positioned with a cooperative anesthesiologist and surgeon to ensure that the patient is positioned supine on the operating table near its margin.

■ The ipsilateral and involved arm should have careful inspection such that the shoulder contour overlies the placement of a padded arm board and allows the ipsilateral hemithorax and shoulder to be slightly elevated on a sheet roll. This latter maneuver ensures avoidance of subluxation and abduction of the shoulder with potential stretch of the brachial plexus. Such stretch injury to the brachial plexus may initiate motor denervation (transient or prolonged) of the shoulder and arm. This complication is best avoided by padding the arm board to allow elevation of the forearm and hand, as well as providing a relaxed anatomical position (Fig. 20.1).

■ The operator should confirm that the ipsilateral arm and shoulder have free mobility for adduction across the chest wall; moreover, the elbow should be easily flexed and extended without undue tension (Fig. 20.2).

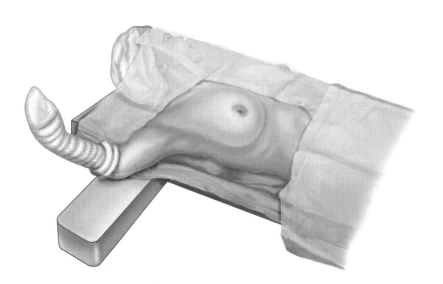

Figure 20.1 Typical position for draping patient for operations of cancer of the right breast. The ipsilateral hemithorax is positioned at the margin of the operative table with a sheet roll that provides slight elevation to the ipsilateral shoulder and hemithorax. This position potentially prevents subluxation and abduction of the shoulder with stretch of the brachial plexus. Draping of the periphery of the breast is inclusive of the supraclavicular fossa and the entire shoulder to allow adequate mobility for adduction of the shoulder and arm across the chest wall. The elbow should be easily flexed and extended without undue tension.

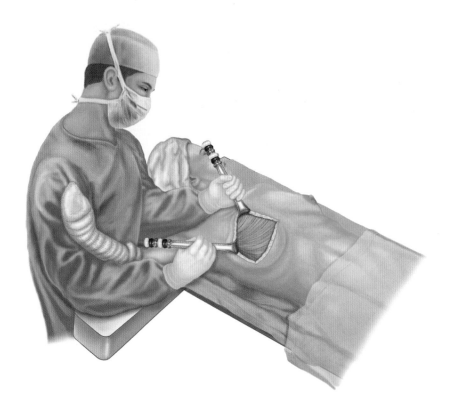

Figure 20.2 Position of the first assistant for right radical mastectomy. The surgical assistant, positioned cephalad to the armboard and shoulder, is able to provide traction, control, and protection of the arm and shoulder. Undue traction of chest wall musculature with potential damage to the brachial plexus can be avoided by ensuring free mobility of the shoulder and elbow that is being controlled by the first assistant.

Prior to commencement of the surgical incision, the ipsilateral arm is placed in a relaxed, extended position on the armboard to allow proper planning of the incision. Incisions are made on the basis of guidelines discussed in this chapter. The two most common incisions employed for the Halsted radical mastectomy are the *classical Orr* and *Stewart incisions* and are illustrated in Figures 19.10 through 19.16 in chapter 19 (Modified Radical Mastectomy). Planned tissue dissections and flap elevations may be completed with electrocautery, cold scalpel, or aluminum garnet (Nd:YAG) laser scalpel (27).

As reflected in Table 20.2, relative indications for the Halsted radical mastectomy must be applied and have decreasing usage in American surgery due to the increasing application of neoadjuvant chemotherapy with tumor cytoreduction. However, tumors that were T2, T3, or T4 with gross fixation (involvement) of the skin overlying the pectoralis major muscle (Fig. 20.3, inset) and for peripheral high-lying lesions that are fixed near the clavicle to the pectoralis major and are not otherwise candidates for radiation therapy would be considered for the procedure. Furthermore, stages IIIa, IIIb, and IIIc would be candidates for the Halsted radical mastectomy when these individuals were refractory to induction chemotherapy and/or irradiation. It is rare in conventional medical oncology to present with advanced local–regional disease and skin ulceration (T4b; stage IIIb) with tumors that are unresponsive to chemotherapy as formally noted in the medical literature. More commonly seen today is advanced local–regional disease in which there has been evident tumor fixation to the pectoralis major following segmental mastectomy and whole breast irradiation. Fixation to the pectoralis major muscle in this circumstance should have planned partial or total resection of the pectoralis major, even when radiographic evidence (mammogram, MRI [magnetic resonance imaging]) confirms evidence of cytoreduction.

It is the typical exposure of the craniolateral-most aspect of the wound that allows the identification and exposure of the humeral insertion of the pectoralis major muscle with continuation of the dissection in a central superiomedial direction with muscular elevation to allow exposure of the pectoralis minor. The insertion of the pectoralis major on the humerus is transected and rotated medially. This muscle has its origin on ribs 1 to 6 near the sternocostal junction. The surgeon must thereafter be aware of the anatomical

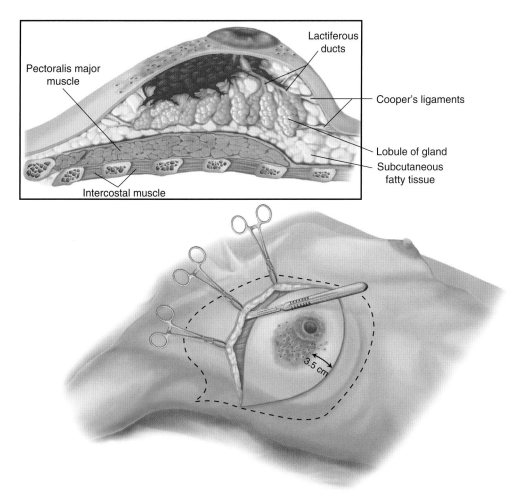

Pectoralis major
muscle

Lactiferous
ducts

Cooper's ligaments

Lobule of gland

Subcutaneous
fatty tissue

Intercostal muscle

3.5 cm

Part V: Mastectomy

Figure 20.3 Inset, Large breast lesions (T2, T3, T4) may present with gross fixation to the skin and/or pectoralis major musculature. The radical mastectomy is designed to encompass wider skin flaps than the modified technique. The margins designed and developed should encompass normal skin and breast parenchyma 3 to 5 cm from the periphery of the tumor. This wider margin ensures tumor clearance and facilitates skin closure without redundancy of tissue flaps. The design of elevated flaps is inclusive of skin margins at the periphery of the breast on the chest wall. The broken line indicates the limits of the dissection and includes the following: superior, the inferior border of the clavicle at the subclavius muscle; lateral, the anterior margin of the latissimus dorsi muscle; medial, midline of the sternum; and inferior, the inframammary fold with extension of dissection to the cephalic extension of the aponeurosis of the rectus abdominis tendon.

position of the cephalic vein and its relationship to the deltopectoral triangle. Thereafter the dissection commences medially with resection of the pectoralis major at its craniad clavicular attachments. This maneuver allows the surgeon direct exposure to the axilla. Thereafter, the tendonious portion of the pectoralis minor may be identified, encircled digitally, and stripped back to its insertion on the coracoid process of the scapula (Fig. 20.4). The pectoralis minor is likewise digitally elevated from the axilla with careful elevation from the axilla taking care to avoid injury to the axillary vein. Division and ligature of perforating muscular branches from the thoracoacromial artery and vein must be ensured. The *medial* (anterior thoracic) *pectoral nerve* commonly penetrates the pectoralis minor prior to innervation of the pectoralis major, and it should be ligated and divided on its posterior surface of origin from the medial cord of the brachial plexus.

The surgeon thereafter commences medial rotation and resection of the pectoralis major and minor from the chest wall en bloc. As the medial resection of the pectoralis major continues, the *lateral* (anterior thoracic) *pectoral nerve* with origin from the lateral cord (and is located medially in the neurovascular bundle) should be identified and ligated. We prefer to continue the dissection in the superiomedial-most aspect of the elevated flap such that the pectoralis major is divided from its medial origin at the costosternal junction of ribs 2 to 6 (Fig. 20.5). Resection of both pectoralis musculature will invariably allow the surgeon to encounter multiple perforator vessels (lateral thoracic, anterior, intercostals arteries) at its periphery and that are end arteries into the pectoralis major and minor muscles. Perforator branches from the intercostal muscles that take origin from the intercostal arteries and vein are also encountered. It is essential that the operator individually clamp and ligate with nonabsorbable 2-0 or 3-0 suture

Figure 20.4 Exposure of the super-olateral aspect of the mastectomy wound following division of the humeral insertion of the pectoralis major muscle. The insertion of the pectoralis minor on the coracoid process of the scapula is transected and rotated medially with en bloc dissection of Rotter's interpectoral nodes. Technically, the dissection commences on the anterior and ventral aspects of the axillary vein to incorporate levels I to III nodes. Division of the pectoralis major and minor tendons allows the surgeon direct access to the floor of the axilla.

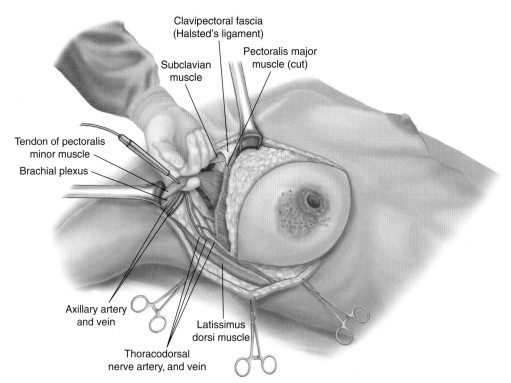

all divided tributaries with division of the pectoral muscles. With inferiomedial traction of the specimen and the operator's hand posterior to the specimen lying on the chest wall, the axillary contents may be fully exposed. The origin of the pectoralis minor on ribs 2 to 5 is thereafter visualized and is divided, ideally with electrocautery, at its insertion into the sternocostal junction. With this maneuver, *Rotter's interpectoral nodes* are swept en bloc into the specimen and allow full visualization of the course of the axillary vein to the level of *Halsted's ligament (costoclavicular),* which is recognized as a condensation of the *clavipectoral fascia.* Thereafter, *Level III (apical, subclavicular) nodes* are

Figure 20.5 Superomedial dissection of the elevated pectoralis minor and pectoralis major muscles en bloc with the breast. The breast parenchyma remains intact with the pectoralis major fascia. Illustrated is the medial extent of the dissection along the costoclavicular margin with division of insertion of the pectoralis major on ribs 2 through 6 and the pectoralis minor on ribs 2 through 5. Multiple perforator branches from the intercostal muscles are encountered at the origin of the intercostal arteries and veins. Following superomedial and inferomedial dissection, the axillary contents are fully exposed to allow completion of the Patey axillary dissection of levels I to III nodes.

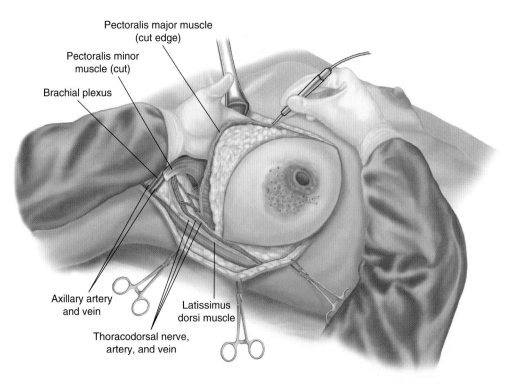

dissected at this level and should be individually clipped or tagged to indicate the highest level of dissection.

As the tendonious portion of the latissimus dorsi muscle is the point of juncture prior to beginning the dissection of the axillary vein, all tissues in this plane must be cleared of the *lateral (axillary) nodal group* (Level I). Care is taken to preserve the thoracodorsal artery, nerve, and vein. The surgeon must be aware of the origin of the *thoracodorsal nerve*, which is uniformly medial to the thoracodorsal artery and vein. This nerve originates from the posterior cord and may run a variable course in the central axillary space and may even cross anterior or posterior to the thoracodorsal artery and vein as it courses inferiolaterally to innervate the latissimus dorsi muscle in its central muscular portion. As the axillary dissection commences, the operator will often encounter, at a minimal, two branches of the intercostobrachial nerves, which traverse the axillary space at right angles to the latissimus and chest wall. These nerves, which are sensory to the medial arm and axilla with fibers from the lateral cutaneous branches of the second and third intercostal nerves, may be sacrificed without prolonged morbidity aside from paresthesia and hypesthesia of the axilla and medial arm skin. We prefer to sweep the *lateral (axillary) nodal group* caudad and parallel to the thoracodorsal neurovascular bundle and to be incorporated en bloc with the *subscapular nodal group (Level I)* that is medially placed between the thoracodorsal nerve and the lateral chest wall. With dissection of these two nodal basins and their investing areolar tissues, the posterior boundary of the axillary space is delineated following exposure of the teres major muscle. Medial dissection with clearing of the ventral surface of the axillary vein further allows direct visualization of the subscapularis muscle, which is medially placed near the chest wall and medial to the teres. Inferior dissection of the *external mammary nodal group* of *Level I* is deferred until completion of dissection of the *central nodal group (Level II)* and the *apical* or *subclavicular Level III nodes.* Following clearing of the superiomedial nodal contents, the costoclavicular (Halsted ligament) area allows these nodal groups to be retracted inferiorly with the dissected muscles. Thereafter, nodal dissection begins on the chest wall with en bloc dissection of the *external mammary nodal group (Level I)* that is medial and contiguous with the tail of Spence of the breast. The operator is reminded to dissect in the cephalad to caudad direction, parallel with the thoracodorsal neurovascular bundle, sweeping all contents en bloc. This maneuver is important in dissection to prevent neural injury and allows direct access to the venous tributaries posterior to the axillary vein. Thereafter the surgeon will encounter the chest wall and exposure of the fascia of the serratus anterior. This maneuver is essential to allow high-level identification below the axillary vein of the *long thoracic nerve (respiratory nerve of Bell),* which provides motor innervation to the serratus anterior. This nerve courses consistently along the lower lateral chest wall, just superficial to the teres major over the subscapularis musculature. Following incision of the serratus anterior fascia, this nerve is dissected throughout its course in the medial axillary space from its superiormost origin near the chest wall to its innervation of the serratus anterior following proper exposure.

Thereafter, the axillary contents anterior and medial to the long thoracic nerve are swept inferiomedially en bloc with the specimen. The surgeon should defer division of the inferior boundary of the axillary content dissection until the preserved innervation of the long thoracic and the thoracodorsal nerves are visualized.

Any points of origin of the pectoralis major from the first through the sixth ribs are left intact with the medial dissection completely divided such that an en bloc resection of the pectoralis major is accomplished over the retromammary bursa. The surgeon continues the dissection in an avascular plane to sweep the breast and axillary contents toward the aponeurosis of the rectus abdominis muscle to complete extirpation of the specimen as an en bloc procedure (Fig. 20.6).

Two closed-suction catheters (flat 10 mm Jackson-Pratt) are placed via separate incisions that enter the inferior margin of the flap at approximately the anterior axillary line with the second lateral catheter placed approximately 2 cm below the axillary vein. Drains are secured at skin level with 3-0 nonabsorbable nylon sutures. Suction catheters should not be secured to the chest wall to abrogate the potential for muscle injury and hemorrhage with removal.

Figure 20.6 The complete Halsted radical mastectomy with residual margins of the pectoralis major and minor muscles. Ideally, preservation of the long thoracic nerve ensures innervation of the serratus anterior. Innervation of the latissimus dorsi muscle is ensured with preservation of the thoracodorsal nerve that accompanies the neurovascular bundle of the posterior axillary space. Inset depicts position of closed-suction catheters (18 to 20 French) placed through separate stab wounds that enter the inferior margin of the flap at approximately the anterior axillary lines.

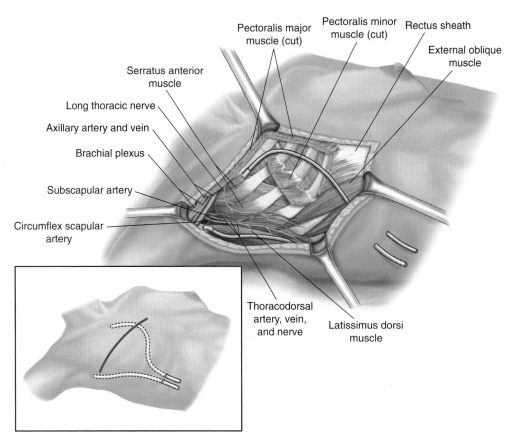

Prior to flap closure, skin margins are carefully inspected to evaluate for devascularization that results from trauma of dissection or tangential incisions that contribute to skin necrosis and wound dehiscence. We prefer closure with interrupted 2-0 absorbable synthetic sutures placed in subcutaneous tissues with purchase of the cutis reticularis of the skin without tension. Optionally, the skin may be closed with subcuticular 4-0 synthetic absorbable sutures or stainless steel staples. Steri-strips® are applied across (perpendicular to) the incision when subcuticular sutures are used in closure. After irrigation, the closed-suction catheters are thereafter connected and maintained on continuous low to moderate suction with large, plastic, vacuum reservoirs. Closure of dead space by suturing of skin flaps to underlying muscle combined with early removal of closed-suction drainage has been reported by O'Dwyer et al. (28) to diminish the incidence of seroma formation. We prefer to use light, bulky dressings applied with adherent sealed closure of the surgical incision. Some surgeons prefer compression dressings over flaps, and thus, wrapping of the chest wall with compression dressings. This practice may initiate central damage to the flaps with the potential of necrosis if undue pressure is applied with taping. Typically, wound catheters may be removed when drainage becomes predominantly serous and has decreased to a maximum of 20 to 25 cc during a 24-hour interval. Shoulder exercises are initiated on the day following removal of the drainage catheters.

Alternative Closure of Flap Defects

With use of the classical Halstedian operation and sacrifice of large volumes of skin centrally, alternative measures are essential to close the central defect. However, with the conventional cytoreductive chemotherapeutic neoadjuvant principles used today, such maneuvers are rarely necessary and flap closure can usually be accomplished as a primary procedure. However, should defects be sizable and alternative closure is essential, one could consider using either myocutaneous flaps (latissimus dorsi or rotational

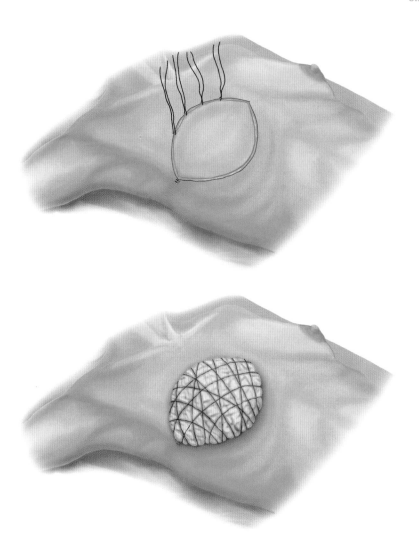

Part V: Mastectomy

Figure 20.7 **Top.** Large defect that is expectant with creation of large skin flaps inclusive of the periphery of the breast for T3 and T4 lesions with fixation to the pectoralis major. Such large defects must be grafted with split-thickness skin (0.018 to 0.020 in) that is preferably obtained through a dermatome from skin of the anterior/lateral thigh or buttock. An additional option for closure is the myocutaneous latissimus dorsi flap. **Bottom.** The partial-thickness skin graft held in position with a compression stent created with cotton gauze mesh. These large skin defects do not require catheter drainage. Alternatively, compression foam mesh as the stent may be applied over the split-thickness skin graft. Foam mesh may be stapled in place at the margin of the skin defect.

flaps) and/or the placement of skin grafts. In the latter circumstance, the defect may be grafted with split-thickness skin grafts (0.018–0.02 in) procured with a dermatome from the anteriolateral thigh or buttock (Fig. 20.7).

To immobilize the skin graft and enhance the probability of adherence (with "graft take" to the chest wall), the partial-thickness graft is stented with bolsters (Fig. 20.7) or compression-foamed mesh, which may be stapled to the peripheral wound edges. In such closures, catheters are not necessary when skin grafts are applied to the defect. The stents placed over the split-thickness skin graft are not removed until day 5 or 6 postoperatively, unless undue drainage (serum, blood, suppuration) from beneath the grafts is evident. This practice increases the probability of graft adherence, which is further enhanced when postoperative shoulder immobilization for large defects is ensured.

When patients do not require postoperative irradiation following Halsted radical mastectomy, these patients may be offered immediate breast reconstruction following the radical procedure. Breast reconstruction allows for cosmetic enhancement of the patient with maintenance of form and functional restoration. This alternative is being applied more commonly internationally (29,30). However, with the presence of adverse biological features and the inexact probability of positive margins, the surgeon must defer the reconstruction. Nonetheless, the Wells prospective trial conducted by Patel et al. (31) with follow-up over 10 years suggests that an immediate reconstruction is widely applicable and technically feasible and can be conducted with long-term outcomes that are not detrimental to local recurrence of metastatic disease. Morrow et al. (32) detailed the factors that influenced the use of breast reconstruction postmastectomy in a National Cancer Data Base (NCDB) study by the American College of Surgeons. Reconstruction

TABLE 20.3	Percentage of Breast Cancer Cases with Partial (Segmental) Mastectomy by U.S. Census Region, 1990, Stage 0 and I Cases		
Region	1985	1988	1990
New England	39.9	44	52.6
Mid-Atlantic	16.4	33.6	48.9
South Atlantic	27.8	27.2	32
East North Central	19.6	25.9	40.7
East South Central	28.3	16.3	17.5
West North Central	14.1	20.1	24.2
West South Central	25.8	20.6	28.8
Mountain	14.5	25	40.1
Pacific	34.1	36	41.3
All regions	25.8	29.8	38.1
No. of cases	5,592	12,420	18,641

From Winchester et al. (33).
From Bland and Copeland (18) with permission.

was an *underutilized* option for the management of 155,463 patients who were studied by the NCDB between 1985 and 1990. In addition, 68,348 patients evaluated between 1994 and 1995 had similar experience, in that this was an underutilized consideration. With the advancement and utility of myocutaneous reconstruction, with or without implants, the use of immediate reconstruction has increased between 1985 and 1995 from 3.4% to 8.3%. Unequivocally, considerations of the patient's decisions for reconstructive surgery include income, age, geographic location, hospital size and type, and tumor stage. These reports emphasize the importance of patient education as an essential component to address and provide proper patient consultation and information for options that include reconstruction risk, recurrence, and long-term morbidity.

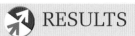 RESULTS

Trends and Patterns of Care (1985–2002)

National Cancer Data Base of the American College of Surgeons Commission on Cancer

Since 1985, the NCDB of the Commission on Cancer of the American College of Surgeons has tracked therapy trends for breast cancer. Such data are included in Tables 20.3 and 20.4, which identify the increasing usage of breast conservation for early disease (T_1, T_2, stage 0) by U.S. Census Region conducted in 1990 (33). Thus, the trends and patterns of care by board-certified fellows of the college reflect decreasing application of

TABLE 20.4	Percentage of Breast Cancer Cases by Type of Surgery by Year of Diagnosis		
Operation	1985	1988	1990
Radical mastectomy	1.9	1.5	0.6
Modified radical mastectomy	63.2	64.8	59.7
Total mastectomy	3.4	3.8	2.8
Partial (segmental) mastectomy	18.4	22.2	28.4
Subcutaneous mastectomy	0.5	0.5	0.5
Surgery type unknown	3.5	1	1.1
No surgery	7	5.4	4.5
Unknown if surgery done	2.1	0.8	2.4
Total	100	100	100
No. of cases	14,509	26,465	39,869

From Winchester et al. (33).
From Bland and Copeland (18) with permission.

TABLE 20.5	**Stage Distribution of Patients by Surgical Procedures**

Operation	Median age (yr)	Stage unknown (%)	PAJCC stage (%)							No. of patients
			0	I	IIA	IIB	IIIA	IIIB	IV	
<Total, no nodes	69.2	34.6	22.2	4.7	2.5	1.1	0.7	4.8	19.4	3,319
<Total, nodes	59.4	6.2	7.9	19.8	11.9	8.2	3.7	3.6	5.7	5,095
Subcutaneous	56.5	0.6	2	0.2	0.2	0.3	0.2	0.4	0.6	157
Total, no nodes	71.8	9.6	11	2	2.2	1.3	0.9	7.5	8.5	1,519
Total, nodes	63	21.2	52.4	71	81.1	87.6	90.3	75.5	39.5	28,960
Radical	60.8	0.8	0.4	0.5	0.9	1	2.2	3.1	1.8	392
Extended	55	0	0.1	0	0	0	0.2	0.3	0.2	17
Surgery type unknown	62.4	26.1	3.8	1.3	0.9	0.5	1.5	4.4	22.5	1,863
No. of patients	—	3,980	2,484	13,600	10,614	5,871	1,786	1,527	1,773	—

PAJCC, Pathologic American Joint Committee on Cancer; <Total, less than total mastectomy.
Each column represents the percentage of patients with that stage disease who had the operation listed in that row; that is, 22.2% of patients with stage 0 disease were treated by less than total mastectomy without a node dissection.
Permission requested from Osteen et al. (34).
From Bland and Copeland (18) with permission.

radical mastectomy in 1985, 1988, and 1990 to 1.9%, 1.5%, and 0.6%, respectively. Simultaneously was a pattern for decreasing use of the modified radical mastectomy also in favor of application of more conservative procedures with decrease from 63.2%, 64.8%, and 59.7% for surgeons using the procedure in 1985, 1988, and 1990, respectively (Table 20.4). Thus, as one can see, the explanation for decreasing use of the radical procedure was found in the shift to segmental (partial) mastectomy, which represented 28.4% of mastectomies in 1990 (33).

In the 1990 surveys of the college, the criteria upon which the surgeon based selection of the operative procedures are depicted in Tables 20.5 and 20.6. These illustrate stage, age distribution, and geographic variation for use of the various techniques (Table 20.6). Radical and extended radical techniques were rarely used except in advanced local–regional disease (stages IIIa and IIIb). Thus, the majority of U.S. surgeons by 1990 replaced the radical procedure with the modified radical approach (Patey, Auchincloss-Madden) (34,35). We (36) have previously reported that the percentage and number of cases being treated at an earlier stage, as reported by the NCDB from 1985 to 1995, indicate that stage migration to an earlier, more curable stage is evident (Table 20.7).

TABLE 20.6	**Frequency of Surgical Procedures by Region**

Operation	Region (% treated by operation type)									
	Canada + U.S. Pass	New England	Middle Atlantic	South Atlantic	East North Central	East South Central	West North Central	West South Central	Mountain	Pacific
<Total, no nodes	4.7	13	10.2	6.8	7.4	4.1	5.6	6.1	6	8.2
<Total, nodes	11.8	17.5	13.8	11.6	10.8	6.1	9.9	8.2	11.3	4.9
Subcutaneous	0.9	0.3	0.2	0.3	0.4	0.5	0.4	0.5	0.5	0.5
Total, no nodes	3.3	44	4.3	3.7	3.4	3.3	3.6	3.5	3.9	3
Total, nodes	66	58	64.6	72.4	72.2	79	74.5	75.5	72.9	68.3
Radical	5.2	0.7	1	0.9	0.7	2.5	1.2	1.4	1.3	0.4
Extended	—	—	—	0.1	0.1	—	—	—	—	—
Surgery type unknown	8	6	5.8	4.2	5.2	4.5	4.8	4.8	4.2	4.5
No. of patients	212	4,137	6,782	5,287	7,836	2,213	3,288	2,886	1,946	6,958

<Total, less than total mastectomy.
Permission requested from Osteen et al. (34).
From Bland and Copeland (18) with permission.

TABLE 20.7	Percentage and Number of Cases by Combined AJCC Stage Group and Year of Diagnosis					
	1985		**1990**		**1995**	
PAJCC/CAJCC stage	*n*	%	*n*	%	*n*	%
Stage 0	2,249	7.4	8,968	11.2	14,790	14.3
Stage I	10,705	35.1	31,797	39.8	43,363	41.9
Stage II	11,959	39.2	27,922	35	33,315	32.2
Stage III	3,554	11.6	6,832	8.6	7,616	7.4
Stage IV	2,050	6.7	4,299	5.4	4,377	4.2
Total	30,517	100	79,818	100	103,461	100
Unknown	12,519		9,154		4,562	
Cases	43,036		88,972		108,023	

AJCC, American Joint Committee on Cancer; PAJCC, Pathologic American Joint Committee on Cancer; CAJCC, Clinical American Joint Committee on Cancer
From Bland et al. (36).
From Bland and Copeland (18) with permission.

Convincing are the evolving trends to earlier disease stage (stages 0–I). In contrast, a decrease from 39.2% for stage II (1985) to 32.2% (1995) was evident during this decade. Furthermore, there is a decrease in stage III disease from 11.6% (1985) to 7.4% in 1995 within the same interval. These trends are likely the result of an increasing application of high-quality mammography screening, as well as patient education as promulgated by the synchronous effort of the American Cancer Society and the American College of Surgeons. Table 20.8 reflects the relative survival by combined AJCC (American Joint Committee on Cancer) stage and treatment from 1985 to 1990. Evident again is the decreasing use of the modified radical technique with or without radiation therapy in early stage disease (stages 0–I), with essentially no application of the Halsted procedure by U.S. surgeons. Convincingly, the most commonly used procedure for stage II, III, and IV disease is the modified radical mastectomy with or without irradiation (36). Moreover, surgeons are increasingly unlikely to use the subcutaneous mastectomy for other than stage 0 disease, as this is not an oncological procedure (36).

Figures 20.8 and 20.9 depict trends of U.S. surgeons as reported by the NCDB for choice of operation relative to AJCC stage of disease. Decreasing applications of the modified radical or the Halsted procedure is evident in stages 0–II (Fig. 20.8), with concurrent increase in breast conservation for those stages (Fig. 20.9).

Figure 20.8 Percentage of breast cancers receiving modified or radical mastectomy during initial course of therapy by American Joint Committee on Cancer stage of disease in cases diagnosed between 1985 and 1998, according to National Cancer Data Base.

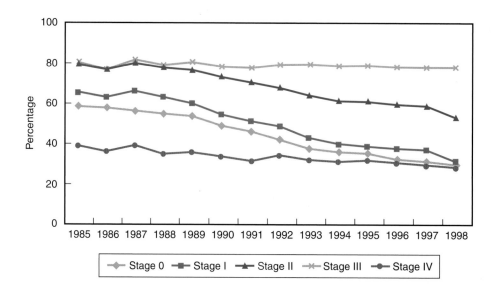

TABLE 20.8   Relative Survival of Breast Carcinoma Patients by Combined AJCC Stage and Treatment, 1985–1990

Stage	Treatment mastectomy	Radiation therapy	Systemic therapy	Entering patients	Years survived											SE
					0	1	2	3	4	5	6	7	8	9	10	
0	Partial, no axillary dissection	No	No	2,027	100	100	99	99	99	99	98	98	98	98	98	3
0	Partial, no axillary dissection	Yes	No	638	100	100	100	100	100	100	100	99	99	99	99	6
0	Partial with axillary dissection	Yes/No	Yes/No	876	100	100	99	99	98	99	99	96	93	93	92	4
0	Subcutaneous/total	Yes/No	Yes/No	1,086	100	100	100	100	99	99	99	96	94	90	90	4
0	Modified radical	No	No	3,451	100	100	100	100	100	100	100	97	97	97	97	2
0	None	Yes/No	Yes/No	479	100	96	93	91	91	91	91	90	92	91	86	6
0	Other treatment			824	100	97	95	93	93	91	90	88	87	87	87	4
0	All treatment			9,381	100	100	99	99	99	99	99	96	95	95	95	1
I	Partial, no axillary dissection	No	No	1,684	100	97	95	93	90	87	81	75	73	71	66	5
I	Partial, no axillary dissection	Yes	No	1,284	100	100	100	99	97	96	94	90	87	86	85	4
I	Partial, no axillary dissection	Yes	Yes	512	100	95	91	88	84	78	76	61	58	58	58	12
I	Partial with axillary dissection	No	No	1,242	100	100	98	96	94	94	91	88	86	86	85	4
I	Partial with axillary dissection	Yes	No	5,469	100	100	100	100	100	100	99	97	96	96	94	1
I	Partial with axillary dissection	Yes	Yes	2,800	100	100	100	100	100	100	95	89	86	86	86	6
I	Modified radical	No	No	14,200	100	100	100	100	100	99	97	93	93	92	92	1
I	Modified radical	No	Yes	5,062	100	100	100	99	98	97	95	91	89	87	84	3
I	Other treatment			4,899	100	98	96	94	92	90	89	86	84	83	81	2
I	All treatment			37,152	100	100	99	99	98	97	95	92	90	89	88	1
II	Partial with axillary dissection	Yes	Yes	2,911	100	100	97	95	92	88	85	81	78	75	72	3
II	Modified radical	No	No	9,861	100	99	96	93	89	86	82	78	75	72	71	1
II	Modified radical	No	Yes	11,835	100	100	95	91	87	83	79	72	70	67	65	1
II	Modified radical	Yes	Yes	1,780	100	98	91	84	77	71	68	62	58	54	51	3
II	Other treatment			7,962	100	96	91	87	82	78	75	69	67	64	62	1
II	All treatment			34,349	100	99	94	91	86	83	79	73	70	68	66	1
III	Modified radical	No	No	1,372	100	91	82	74	68	63	60	55	51	50	47	3
III	Modified radical	No	Yes	2,702	100	96	83	72	64	58	52	46	45	41	38	2
III	Modified radical	Yes	Yes	1,594	100	95	82	70	60	53	48	41	36	35	31	3
III	Other treatment			2,844	100	85	70	60	50	44	40	35	32	29	28	2
III	All treatment			8,512	100	92	79	68	60	54	50	44	41	38	36	1
IV	Partial, no axillary dissection	Yes/No	Yes/No	882	100	61	40	26	21	14	10	8	5	4	4	2
IV	Partial with axillary dissection	Yes/No	Yes/No	305	100	74	43	33	25	18	17	14	12	12	12	3
IV	Subcutaneous/total	Yes/No	Yes/No	382	100	63	43	31	21	15	12	12	9	8	6	3
IV	Modified radical	No	No	289	100	71	47	40	31	27	26	22	19	16	15	4
IV	Modified radical	No	Yes	681	100	79	54	41	29	22	17	13	12	11	11	2
IV	Modified radical	Yes	Yes	458	100	78	54	41	33	24	19	14	14	12	12	3
IV	None	No	No	352	100	32	21	14	10	9	9	7	7	7	7	2
IV	None	Yes	No	142	100	46	29	21	10	9	6	4	4	4	4	3
IV	None	No	Yes	800	100	56	37	22	14	9	7	4	4	4	4	1
IV	None	Yes	Yes	508	100	54	35	23	14	8	5	2	1	1	1	1
IV	Other treatment			629	100	76	38	29	20	16	12	10	9	7	3	2
IV	All treatment			5,428	100	63	42	30	21	16	12	10	8	7	7	1

AJCC, American Joint Committee on Cancer; SE, standard error.
Modified from Bland et al. (36).
From Bland and Copeland (18) with permission.

Figure 20.9 Percentage of breast cancers receiving partial mastectomy during initial course of therapy by American Joint Committee on Cancer stage of disease in cases diagnosed between 1985 and 1998, according to National Cancer Data Base.

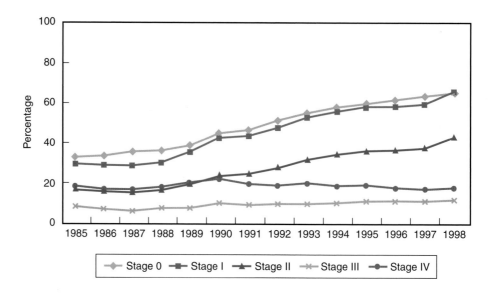

References

1. Halsted WS. The results of operations for the cure of cancer of the breast performed at the Johns Hopkins Hospital from June, 1889, to January, 1894. *Ann Surg.* 1894;20:497.
2. Halsted WS. The results of radical operations for the cure of cancer of the breast. *Ann Surg.* 1907;25:61.
3. Cooper WA. The history of the radical mastectomy. In: Hoeber PB, ed. *Annals of Medical History.* Vol 3. New York, NY: Paul B. Hoeber, 1941.
4. Meyer W. An improved method of the radical operation for carcinoma of the breast. *Med Rec.* 1894:746–746.
5. Winiwarter V. *Beiträge Zur Statistik D. Carcinome.* Stuttgart, Germany: Gedruckt bei L. Schumacher, 1878.
6. Oldekop J. Statistiche zusammenstellung von 250 fällen von mamma-carcinom. *Arch F Klin Chir.* 1879;24:536.
7. Dietrich G. Beitrag zur statistik des mammacarcinom. *Duch Z F Chir.* 1892;33:471.
8. Horner F. Ueber die Endresultate von 172 operierten Fällen maligner Tumoren der weiblichen Brust. *Beitr Z Klin Chir.* 1894;12:619.
9. Poulsen K. Die geschwülste der mamma. *Arch F Klin Chir.* 1891;42:593.
10. Banks M. A plea for the more free removal of cancerous growths. In: Liverpool and Manchester Surgical Reports, 1878:192–206.
11. Schmid H. Zur statistik der mammacarcinome und deren heilung. *Dtsch Z F Chir.* 1887;26:139.
12. Sprengel O. 131 Fälle von brust-carcinom. *Arch F Klin Chir.* 1882;27:805.
13. Schmidt GB. Die geschwülste der brustdrüse. *Beitr Z Klin Chir.* 1889;4:40.
14. Rotter J. Günstigere dauererfolge durch eine verbesserte operative behandlung der mammakarzinome. *Berl Klin Wochenschr.* 1896;33:69.
15. Mahler F. Ueber die in der heidelberger klinik 1887–1897 behandelten fälle von carcinoma mammae. *Beitr Z Klin Chir.* 1900;26:681.
16. Joerss K. Ueber die beutige prognose der exstirpatio mammae carcinomatosae. *Dtsch Z F Chir.* 1897;44:101.
17. Hutchison RG. Radiation therapy in carcinoma of the breast. *Surg Gynecol Obstet.* 1936;62:653–664.
18. Bland KI, Copeland EM III. Halsted radical mastectomy. In: Bland KI, Copeland EM, eds. *The Breast: Comprehensive Management of Benign and Malignant Diseases.* 4th ed. Philadelphia, PA: Saunders Elsevier, 2010:779–802.
19. Wickerham DL, Fisher B. Surgical treatment of primary breast cancer. *Semin Surg Oncol.* 1988;4(4):226–233.
20. Largiarder F. Surgical treatment of local recurrence after mastectomy [German]. *Helv Chir Acta.* 1992;59(1):157–161.
21. Osborne MP, Borgen PI, Wong GY, et al. Salvage mastectomy for local and regional recurrence after breast-conserving operation and radiation therapy. *Surg Gynecol Obstet.* 1992;174(3):189–194.
22. Sweetland HM, Karatsis P, Rogers K. Radical surgery for advanced and recurrent breast cancer. *J R Coll Surg Edinb.* 1995;40(2):88–92.
23. Cody HS III, Laughlin EH, Trillo C, Urban JA. Have changing treatment patterns affected outcome for operable breast cancer? Ten-year follow-up in 1288 patients, 1965 to 1978. *Ann Surg.* 1991;213(4):297–307.
24. Meier P, Ferguson DJ, Karrison T. A controlled trial of extended radical versus radical mastectomy. Ten-year results. *Cancer.* 1989;63(1):188–195.
25. Noguchi M, Taniya T, Koyasaki N, Miyazaki I. A multivariate analysis of en bloc extended radical mastectomy versus conventional radical mastectomy in operable breast cancer [Japanese]. *Nippon Geka Gakkai Zasshi.* 1990;91(7):883–888.
26. Noguchi M, Taniya T, Koyasaki N, Miyazaki I. A multivariate analysis of en bloc extended radical mastectomy versus conventional radical mastectomy in operable breast cancer. *Int Surg.* 1992;77(1):48–54.
27. Wyman A, Rogers K. Radical breast surgery with a contact Nd:YAG laser scalpel. *Eur J Surg Oncol.* 1992;18(4):322–326.
28. O'Dwyer PJ, O'Higgins NJ, James AG. Effect of closing dead space on incidence of seroma after mastectomy. *Surg Gynecol Obstet.* 1991;172(1):55–56.
29. Patrizi I, Maffia L, Vitali CM, et al. Immediate reconstruction after radical mastectomy for breast carcinoma with a Becker-type expander prosthesis [Italian]. *Minerva Chir.* 1993;48(9):453–458.
30. Russell IS, Collins JP, Holmes AD, Smith JA. The use of tissue expansion for immediate breast reconstruction after mastectomy. *Med J Aust.* 1990;152(12):632–635.
31. Patel RT, Webster DJ, Mansel RE, Hughes LE. Is immediate postmastectomy reconstruction safe in the long-term? *Eur J Surg Oncol.* 1993;19(4):372–375.
32. Morrow M, Scott SK, Menck HR, et al. Factors influencing the use of breast reconstruction postmastectomy: a National Cancer Data Base study. *J Am Coll Surg.* 2001;192(1):1–8.
33. Winchester DP. Standards of care in breast cancer diagnosis and treatment. *Surg Oncol Clin North Am.* 1994;3(1):85–99.
34. Osteen RT, Cady B, Chmiel JS, et al. 1991 national survey of carcinoma of the breast by the Commission on Cancer. *J Am Coll Surg.* 1994;178(3):213–219.
35. Osteen RT, Steele GD Jr, Menck HR, Winchester DP. Regional differences in surgical management of breast cancer. *CA Cancer J Clin.* 1992;42(1):39–43.
36. Bland KI, Menck HR, Scott-Conner CE, et al. The National Cancer Data Base 10-year survey of breast carcinoma treatment at hospitals in the United States. *Cancer.* 1998;83(6):1262–1673.

21 Chest Wall Resection and Reconstruction for Advanced/Recurrent Carcinoma of the Breast

Kirby I. Bland, R. Jobe Fix, and Robert J. Cerfolio

 INDICATIONS/CONTRAINDICATIONS

The incidence of local–regional recurrence following breast conservation surgery or mastectomy varies between 5% and 40% (1). The probability of recurrence depends upon the presenting pathobiological characteristics of the primary neoplasm and/or the American Joint Committee on Cancer (AJCC) clinical tumor stage. Currently, no international standards for local recurrence have been fully defined, but, typically, the combination of surgery, radiation therapy, chemotherapy, and/or targeted immunotherapy is directed for principal control. Following local–regional recurrence that defines a clinical and radiographically resectable tumor, protocol will typically embrace resection with pathologically negative margins followed by subsequent radiation therapy; many clinics will also utilize hormone-receptor markers (ER, PR, and HER2/neu status) to assist in therapeutic guidance.

For many clinics internationally, despite curability with isolated metastases, the chest wall recurrences are left untreated. In contradistinction, while resection of chest wall *metastases* related to breast carcinoma or other primary neoplasms (e.g., melanoma and sarcoma) may be therapeutically achievable, such recurrences cannot be completed with curative intent. Previous surgical dogma suggesting that chest wall recurrences are the "harbinger of systemic disease" does not necessarily apply when the patient has been fully staged clinically and radiographically and only the isolated breast cancer recurrence is evident.

 PREOPERATIVE PLANNING

We have previously published guidelines at the University of Alabama at Birmingham for resection of the chest wall in patients presenting with recurrence/advanced disease related to breast carcinoma.

The indications for operation, as discussed, pertain only to an isolated chest wall recurrence/advanced disease that can be surgically managed with curative intent.

■ Individuals who have locally confined disease, with requirement of palliation for pain and/or nonhealing/ulcerative lesions related to postirradiation injury with pathologically negative ulcerative sites are included in this group.

■ It is incumbent upon the oncologic surgeon involved in the care of the patient to establish that there is absence of systemic disease and to exclude multifocally recurrent sites that are being considered for resection.

■ Relative contraindications that one would consider include advancing age, short disease-free interval of recurrent disease, diminished pulmonary reserve, biopsy-proven extrathoracic disease, and existing systemic comorbidities (e.g., cardiac and endocrine).

■ Contemporary radiographic imaging is essential for all patients being considered for full-thickness chest wall resection and reconstruction. To properly evaluate chest wall anatomy and extent of tumor progression, we advocate dedicated chest wall magnetic resonance imaging (MRI) and/or computed tomography (CT)-angiography as standard imaging modalities. Standard CT scanning with intravenous contrast also provides invaluable information. Many medical oncologists also consider a positron emission tomography (PET) as a definitive test, but coexisting inflammatory sites, especially ulceration, with the associated false-positive and false-negative features of PET do not allow use of this procedure as an exclusive screening modality. However, it is extremely useful in evaluating systemic disease. Evidence of extensive direct lung invasion and pleural effusion are absolute contraindications for consideration of chest wall resection.

■ The principal site of focally recurrent disease typically presents between the third and sixth rib interspaces; however, the recurrence location, as well as history of the patient's operative procedure, is paramount.

■ Review of the surgical history is essential, especially if a transverse or vertical rectus abdominis muscle (TRAM) pedicle flap is being considered with prior abdominal operations, as the same will often affect the flap choice for defect coverage.

■ The most versatile and most commonly used flap is the latissimus dorsi pedicle flap. Ideally, flaps from previously irradiated fields should be avoided when possible.

■ Resection that extends beyond four ribs will routinely require rigid chest wall reconstruction. This maneuver constitutes the creation of mesh with polypropylene that may be used as a singular sheet or with creation of a mesh "sandwich" together with methyl methacrylate. Myocutaneous flaps should be liberally used to cover these reconstructions. When defects are small and of less probability for creation of the flail defect of the chest wall, mesh alone may be sufficient with this smaller area for coverage.

■ Preoperative planning between the surgical oncologist and reconstructive surgeons, following discussion with the medical oncologist, should define the indications, relative merits, and technical approaches essential for full oncologic resection (Table 21.1).

Surgery Positioning and Incisions

Following patient intubation with a double-lumen, endotracheal tube, the patient is positioned in the supine or lateral decubitus position depending upon the planned resection of the local recurrence and flap choice. An appropriately sized double-lumen, endotracheal tube should be selected. The area for harvest of the potential skin flap and graft-donor sites should also be prepped and draped into the operative field.

Preferentially, we prefer a minimal 2-cm margin developed 360 degrees around the periphery of the planned resection area (Fig. 21.1) (2). It is critical that both the oncological surgeon and the plastic surgeon plan the operative incision prior to skin incision, estimating the maximum cephalad, caudad, medial, and lateral extent of the tumor, such that the estimate for margins of resection can be discussed with the patient

TABLE 21.1	Preoperative Considerations

- Indications for operation include isolated chest wall recurrence, curative intent, or palliation for painful, nonhealing, ulcerated lesions.
- Preoperative planning between oncologic and reconstructive surgeons should help elucidate flaps that will be available after oncologic resection.
- Absolute contraindications for resections with curative intent include systemic disease or multifocal recurrence.
- Relative contraindications include advanced age, short disease-free interval, poor pulmonary function, and high operative risk.
- Preoperative imaging and staging are essential for evaluation of chest wall anatomy, tumor invasion, metastatic disease, and preoperative planning. MRI (magnetic resonance imaging), PET (positron emission tomography), and CT (computed tomography) are standard imaging modalities. Bronchial washings may be appropriate to rule out direct lung invasion if suspicious by imaging.
- Resection extending beyond four ribs will usually require rigid chest wall reconstruction with a mesh and methyl methacrylate sandwich. Mesh alone may be sufficient for smaller defects with less risk of flail chest.
- Recurrence location, as well as patient's operative history, will affect flap choice for defect coverage. A latissimus pedicle flap is the most versatile and is usually the most readily available. Flaps from previously radiated fields should be avoided if possible.

From Howard JH, Tzeng CWD, Fix RJ, Bland KI. Chest wall resection. In: Klimberg VS, ed. *Atlas of Breast Surgical Techniques.* Philadelphia, PA: Saunders, 2010, with permission.

and family prior to the planned resection. Such estimates are simultaneously planned with radiographic imaging, if necessary.

▣ Margins should extend a minimal one intercostal space *above and below* the tumor mass inclusive of the cephalad–caudad aspect of the planned rib resections.

▣ Circumferential full-thickness skin punch biopsies (6 mm) should be sent for frozen section analysis following skin prep and induction. These biopsies will validate a

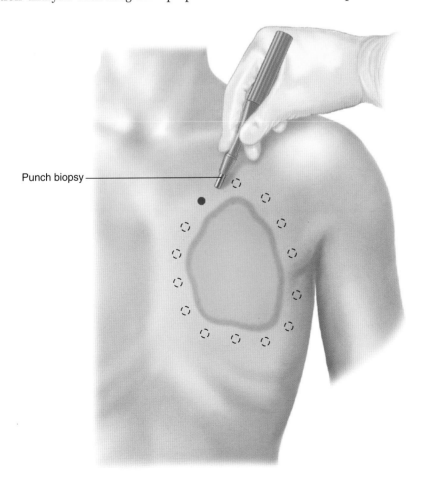

Punch biopsy

Figure 21.1 Chest wall topographic anatomy with outline of planned marginal clearance. Preferentially a minimal 2-cm margin developed 360 degrees about the periphery of the planned resection area is ideal. Use of a punch biopsy (4 to 6 mm) should be taken approximately every 1 to 2 cm about the tumor margin resection to validate a negative pathological margin before opening the chest.

Part VI: Extensive Resections

negative pathological margin prior to incision (Fig. 21.1). Once negative margins are confirmed with pathology, the extent of the incision through the skin overlying the pectoralis major muscle may be completed using cold blade and, thereafter, electrocautery for subcutaneous and muscular tissues.

Technique of Resection

The pectoralis major and minor are incised outside the tumor-bearing area to the level of the chest wall; all ribs for planned resection are medially and laterally exposed. The incision will include all previous punch biopsied areas. In the cephalad-most extent of the planned rib resection, the rib is incised on its cephalad surface, and the ipsilateral lung is deflated by the anesthesiologist at the instruction of the surgeon. The thoracotomy should be initiated via the superior margin of the planned resection (Fig. 21.2). Upon entering the thorax, previous pleural adhesions created by prior radiation therapy and/or surgery should be sharply dissected and mobilized. Attention must be directed to avoidance of injury to the parietal pleura and inadvertent damage to the pulmonary parenchyma. When dissection is incomplete or inadequate, lysis of adhesions should be completed and performed with sharp dissection to avoid the formation of an alveolar-pleural fistula. With dense adhesions related to tumor invasion of the parietal pleura of the lung, complete pleurectomy with simultaneous segmental resection of the focally involved lung segment may be necessary. Repair of any parenchymal tears may be completed by stapling or suturing with 3-0 absorbable polypropylene suture after adequate deflation of the lung without injury. The incision is thereafter extended around the peripheral margins of the tumor mass through the intercostal muscles (Figs. 21.3–21.6). The surgeon must be cognizant of ligation of the intercostal neurovascular bundles on the inferior margins of the rib with 2-0 silk suture ligatures (Fig. 21.5).

As the incision is extended around the margins of the resection, the periosteum of the rib should be elevated with a Doyen retractor followed by a periosteal elevator prior

Figure 21.2 In the usual circumstance, incision above the most cephalad rib with opening on its superior margin is preferable. Upon entering the thorax, prior pleural adhesions created by radiation therapy and/or surgery should be sharply dissected and the lung mobilized. Attention must be focused on the avoidance of injury to the visceral pleura of the lung and inadvertent damage to the pulmonary parenchyma.

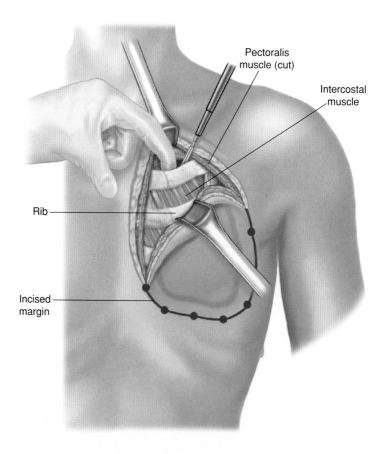

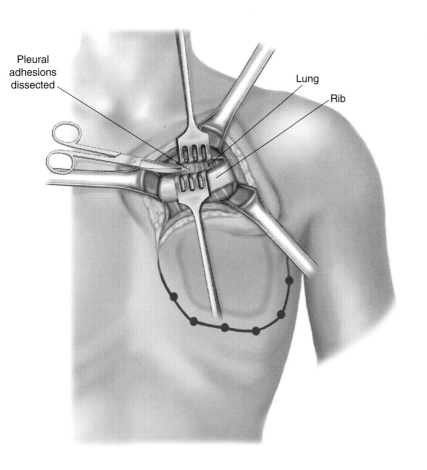

Figure 21.3 Extension of the incision around the periphery of the margins of the tumor mass through the intercostal muscles and via the outline of the punch biopsies that have been confirmed pathologically negative.

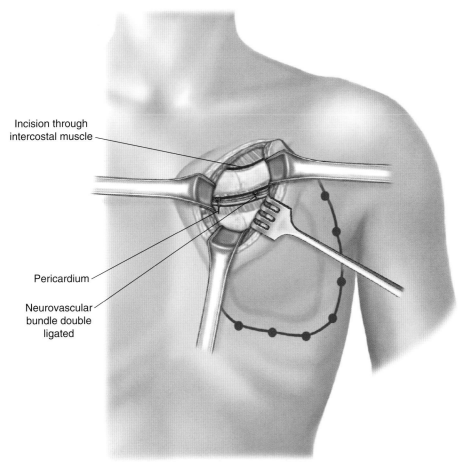

Figure 21.4 Planned line of resection of rib on cephalad most extension with division on its medial surface following ligation of the neurovascular bundle.

Part VI: Extensive Resections

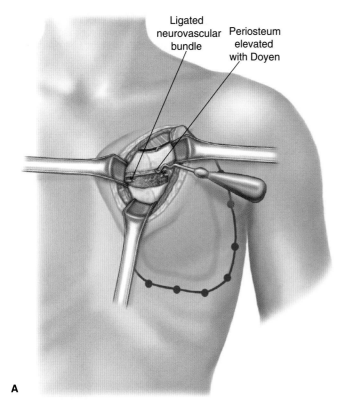

A

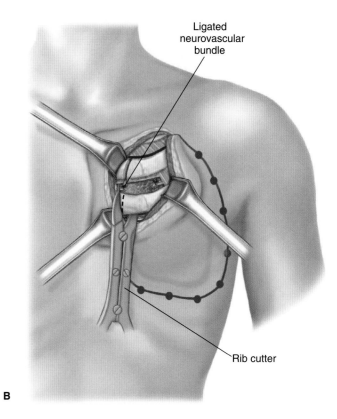

B

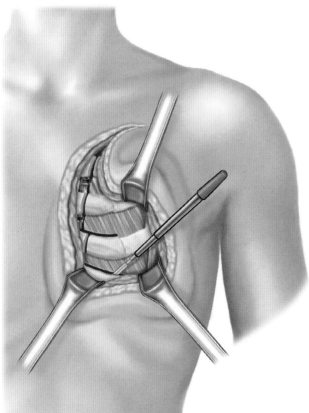

C

Figure 21.5 A. Isolation and ligation of both medial and lateral neurovascular bundles. **B.** Division of rib on its medial surface with rib cutter. **C.** Further extension of the medial cut with rib cutter to the third rib on its medial surface.

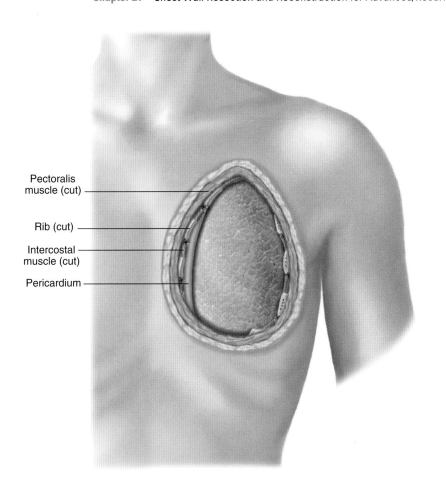

Figure 21.6 The completed resection both medially and laterally, including four ribs in the resection with exposure of the visceral pleural surface of the lung following resection of parietal pleura with chest wall.

Pectoralis muscle (cut)

Rib (cut)

Intercostal muscle (cut)

Pericardium

to initiating rib division with a rib cutter (Fig. 21.5A). Following completion of the entire incision, the surgeon should be cognizant to include all the punch biopsy sites to ensure negative surgical margin.

When the tumor margin extends medially to the sternum, it may be necessary to utilize a sternal saw or osteotome to create a partial sternotomy up to and inclusive of the biopsied skin that establishes a clear surgical margin. Moreover, the incision should be extended to the sternocostal margin where the internal mammary artery (IMA) can be palpated, ligated, and divided. The sternum thereafter may be partially resected, but diligence must be exercised to protect the pericardium, which may be centrally adherent to the investing parietal pleura of the sternum, secondary to irradiation.

In all circumstances, the specimen should be resected en bloc, thus exposing the chest wall defect with the exposed, inflated, protuberant lung. Insufflation of the underlying lung following resection of tumor invasion requires visualization of alveolar-parenchymal leak; repair must be instituted for closure of such leaks. If invasive disease is detected grossly or with biopsy, the well-exposed lung can then be managed by a wedge resection of the involved lung with a stapler. Leaking defects should again be oversewn and tested for air leaks prior to tube placement and chest closure (Fig. 21.6).

Prior to initiating chest wall reconstruction, one apical-posterior chest tube should be placed in the midaxillary line inferior to the defect. The second tube is placed posteriorly and positioned toward the lung apex for fluid and air collection. Smaller caliber tubes are generally sufficient to manage the resulting iatrogenic pneumothorax.

Flap Reconstruction

The inset of Figure 21.7 confirms the methyl methacrylate-mesh "sandwich" shaped and contoured for the chest wall defect. This reconstructive sandwich should be layered such that the methyl methacrylate is interposed between two layers of the polypropylene mesh.

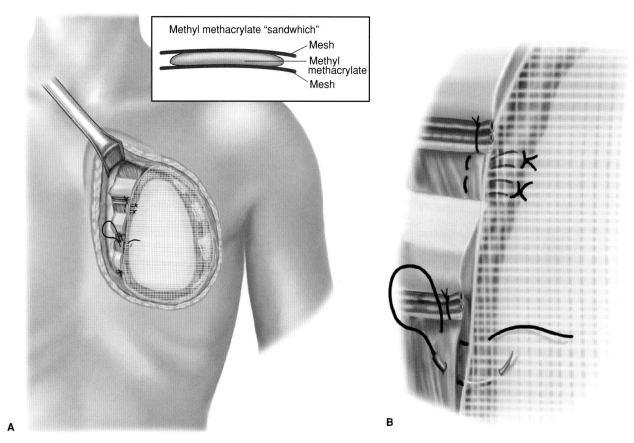

Figure 21.7 A. Inset identifies the optional creation of the methyl methacrylate "sandwich," in which methyl methacrylate interposes between two mesh surfaces of nonabsorbable polypropylene mesh. The strut of this prosthesis is created with the folding in half of a large piece of polypropylene mesh to ensure coverage of the sandwich over the defect without undue tension. **B.** Suturing of the polypropylene mesh encircling the rib margin on its superior and inferior surface of the resection with creation of the planned suture knots *external* to the mesh with full-thickness purchase through the musculature of the chest wall. Neurovascular bundle has been separately ligated.

The prosthetic strut may be created with the folding in half of a larger piece of polypropylene mesh that ensures coverage of the sandwich over the defect without undue tension.

With planning of surface area of the prosthetic strut to cover the defect, the mesh should be contoured beyond all margins of the resection such that it can be sutured to the resected rib edge. We prefer that the first layer of the mesh be sutured to the edges of the wound using nonabsorbable 0 or 1 polypropylene sutures (Fig. 21.7A). Figure 21.7B confirms that suturing should encircle ribs on the superior and inferior edges of the resection and that sutures are created external to the mesh, then full-thickness purchase through the musculature, exiting external to the musculature and incorporating the edges of the prosthetic strut, and are tied external to the mesh (Fig. 21.7A). Care must be taken to avoid entrapping the intercostal neurovascular bundle while securing the mesh. The latter neurovascular bundle should have previously been ligated in isolated fashion. All sutures are tied external (anterior) to both folded edges of the mesh.

▓ Following placement and completion of suturing of the methyl methacrylate "sandwich," reconstruction of the soft-tissue defect is initiated. Again, the most commonly utilized and versatile flap reconstruction of this area is the *pedicled latissimus dorsi flap* that is inclusive of a vascularized skin paddle. Such design and transfer of tissue is highlighted in Figure 21.8A in which the planned latissimus flap (Fig. 21.8B), together with the exposed latissimus muscle and skin paddle, has been harvested. Figure 21.8C confirms the completed inset of the flap following its in situ placement in the created defect.

▓ Figures 21.9 to 21.11A–C highlight the *omental flap*, which designates an increase in potential morbidity as it adds complexity to the chest wall defect with abdominal entry. The omental flap is based upon the right gastroepiploic artery that is utilized for tissue coverage (Fig. 21.9). With selection of this approach, the upper midline

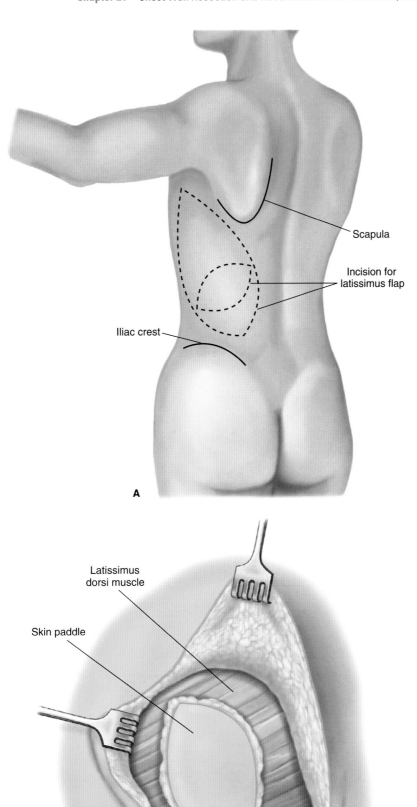

Figure 21.8 A. Design of the most commonly utilized and versatile flap reconstruction as a *pedicled latissimus dorsi flap.* Note that the flap is inclusive of a vascularized skin panel in the central inner outline, and in which the planned latissimus flap **B,** together with the exposed latissimus muscle and skin panel, has been harvested. **C.** identifies the completed inset of the vascularized latissimus dorsi pedicled flap following its *in situ* placement in the created chest wall defect. (*continued*)

Scapula

Incision for
latissimus flap

Iliac crest

Latissimus
dorsi muscle

Skin paddle

Part VI: Extensive Resections

Figure 21.8 (*Continued*)

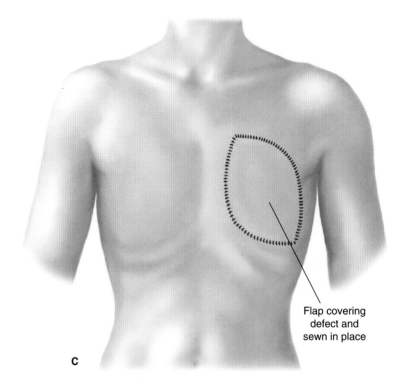

Flap covering
defect and
sewn in place

c

Figure 21.9 The intra-abdominal
vasculature of the greater omentum, in which the selection of this
approach requires upper midline
laparotomy incision for access to
the omentum. The omental flap
approach by necessity enhances
potential morbidity as it adds
complexity to the chest wall defect
with abdominal entry. Following
division of the left gastroepiploic
artery, vascular perforators (vasa
brevia) to perfuse this arcade are
ligated in continuity for revascularization purposes.

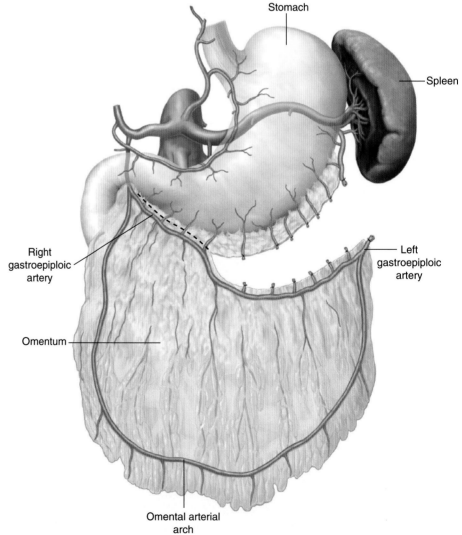

Stomach

Spleen

Right
gastroepiploic
artery

Left
gastroepiploic
artery

Omentum

Omental arterial
arch

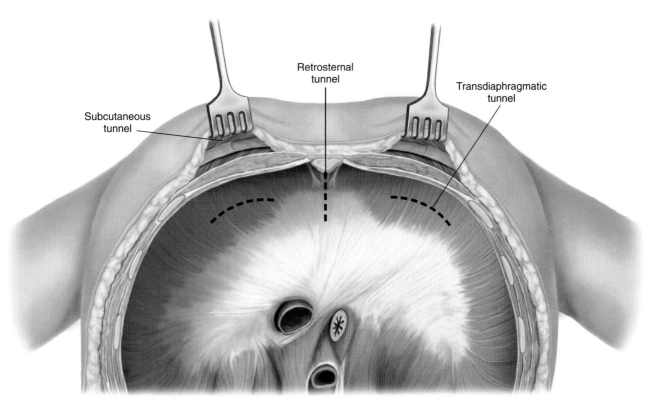

Figure 21.10 The anterior inferior diaphragmatic incisions that require hepatic mobilization and creation of the transdiaphragmatic tunnel to the created defects of each side and thereafter placement in a subcutaneous tunnel.

laparotomy incision is utilized for access to the omentum. Figure 21.11 indicates that the omentum has been transected together with the splenocolic ligament, and divided from the inferior gastric surface from the splenocolic ligament to the base of the right gastroepiploic artery. Ligation and division of the vasa recta of the anterior and posterior omental leaves is performed using 3-0 nonabsorbable sutures (Fig. 21.11).

Options exist for transfer of the vascularized omental pedicle flap. After exiting the midline abdominal incision, the omentum may be transferred to the chest wall defect via a retrosternal, transdiaphragmatic, or subcutaneous tunnel as indicated in Figure 21.10. To maintain the integrity of vascular perfusion, the surgeon must be cognizant of rotation of the omental pedicle to ensure preserved vasculature to its periphery and all the

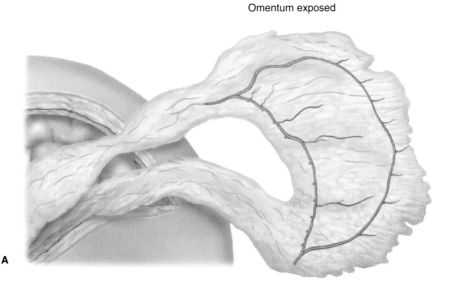

Omentum exposed

A

Figure 21.11 **A.** Mobilization of the omentum, together with the spleno-colic ligament, and division from the inferior gastric surface from the gastrocolic ligament to the base of the right gastroepiploic artery. To maintain integrity of the vascular perfusion pedicle, the surgeon must be cognizant of inadvertent rotation of the omental pedicle and avoidance of vascular injury to the peripheral and central components of the pedicle. **B.** indicates the omentum exposed and inserted into the tunneled subcutaneous space created with reconstruction of the defect. **C.** Placement of the optional split-thickness skin graft coverage of the pedicle, which has been inserted in the patient as visualized at the time of a postoperative visit. (*continued*)

Part VI: Extensive Resections

Figure 21.11 (*Continued*)

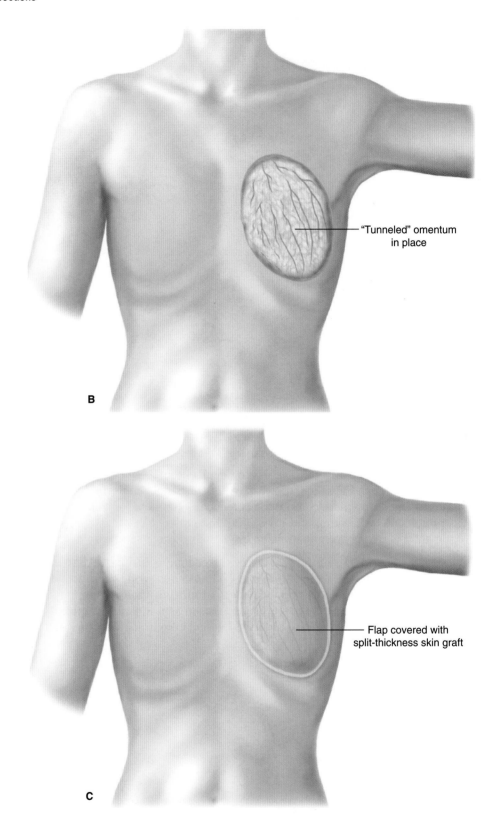

"Tunneled" omentum in place

B

Flap covered with split-thickness skin graft

C

central components of the pedicle. Figure 21.11A confirms the omentum exposed, and Figure 21.11B confirms the adequately planned coverage of the defect prior to tunneling of the omental pedicle. Figure 21.11C confirms the optional skin grafting of the pedicle that has been inset in the patient as visualized at her postoperative visits.

▪ A third option includes a *pedicled free flap* utilizing the TRAM flaps with skin paddles to bridge alternatives for covering these defects (Fig. 21.12). In addition, for

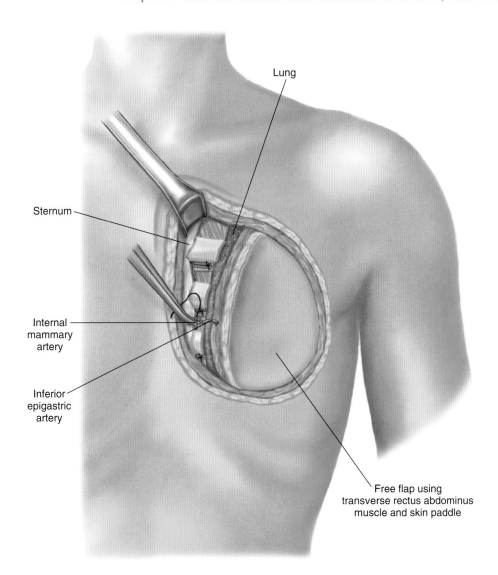

Lung

Sternum

Internal
mammary
artery

Inferior
epigastric
artery

Free flap using
transverse rectus abdominus
muscle and skin paddle

Figure 21.12 An additional option utilizing the pedicled free transverse or vertical rectus abdominis muscle (TRAM) flap as skin panels to bridge as the alternative for covering these defects. In the heavily irradiated parasternal and chest wall tissues, the pedicled free-flap TRAM represents the preferred harvested reconstruction and anastomotic technique. Anastomosis is completed of the vasculature (inferior epigastrics) of the free TRAM to the ipsilateral internal mammary artery (IMA) and provides both arterial inflow and venous outflow to the vascularized graft.

Part VI: Extensive Resections

heavily irradiated parasternal and chest wall tissues, most plastic surgeons prefer the free flap harvested as a TRAM reconstruction with anastomosis to the ipsilateral IMA that provides arterial and venous inflow/outflow to the vascularized graft.

The inset flap should be closed in two layers inclusive of a deep dermal layer that is sutured with 3-0 absorbable sutures. A running subcuticular closure with absorbable 4-0 suture is used for skin.

■ Chest tube drains are essential to evacuate the pneumothorax created with thoracotomy in these patients. In addition, we prefer large defects have subcutaneous closed-suction drains around the soft-tissue reconstruction for avoidance of hematoma and seroma. Internal Doppler probes may be placed for monitoring purposes of the flap's arterial blood supply (Fig. 21.13).

 ## POSTOPERATIVE MANAGEMENT

Immediately after operation, a chest x-ray is obtained to evaluate the potential of an existing and retained pneumothorax that is best drained by functional chest tubes. Proper suction drainage on the catheters is essential for vacuum decompression of the pneumothorax created with opening of the chest. If the patient has an air leak, water seal is the optimal chest tube setting. Pulmonary management should include preventative care for ventilator-associated pneumonia.

Figure 21.13 Depiction of the inset flap enclosure with completed closure of two layers of the deep dermal layer and a running subcuticular closure with absorbable suture. The opened thorax requires closed-suction chest tubes to evacuate the pneumothorax. In addition, the large defects require subcutaneous closed-suction drainage for evacuation of hematoma and seroma in the reconstruction site. The placement of internal Doppler probes over the vascularized free- flap arterial blood flow provides continual monitoring of the patient.

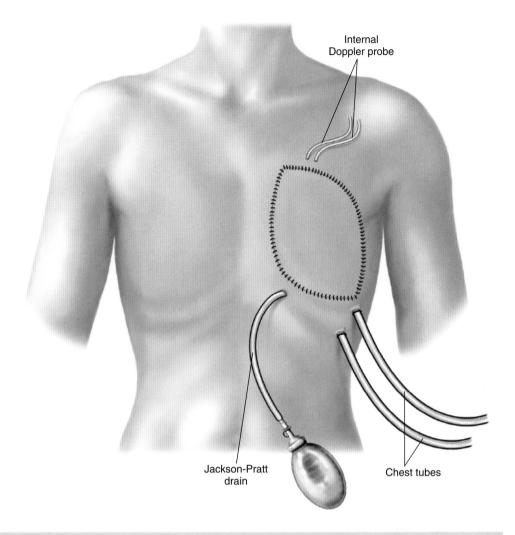

Internal Doppler probe

Jackson-Pratt drain

Chest tubes

COMPLICATIONS

Aggressive pulmonary toilet following extirpation is an essential part of care to prevent atelectasis and subsequent nosocomial pneumonia. Because of the considerable pain experienced with division of the ribs, postoperative epidural pain control should be considered, together with systemic analgesics and sedation.

Continual wound care and flap management are essential; monitoring for flap ischemia and necrosis are the requisite. Arterial supply can best be evaluated by an *internal* Doppler that is placed intraoperatively. However, the hand-held *external* Doppler is commonly utilized together with visual inspection of capillary refill. Standard criteria are utilized in the management of chest tubes for the timing of removal of these tubes and subcutaneous drains. Removal is dependent upon complete resolution of the pneumothorax and decreasing subcutaneous serous wound drainage.

Morbidity related to these wound is experienced in virtually all patients. Complications have been reported in as many as as 40% of patients(1) and vary from 5% to 40%. The most common complications relate to wound dehiscence, separation and drainage, as well as pneumonia related to deficient pulmonary toilet. Pulmonary complications also include the risk of re-intubation, flail chest, and pleural infection. Wound complications include infection, delayed wound repair, and partial flap or skin-graft necrosis. The serious complications of advanced wound infection often require debridement of portions or all of the methyl methacrylate-polypropylene mesh repair and may include major portions of the reconstruction. Despite the significant morbidity associated with the resection, mortality for the procedure is less than 5%. The surgeon must have a low threshold to evaluate and treat suspected wound and pulmonary infections.

RESULTS

The contemporary surgical literature is devoid of prospective randomized studies for selective patients undergoing full-thickness chest wall resections that are designed to eradicate locally recurrent/advanced breast carcinoma. Such procedures are regarded as highly mutilating interventions that harbor high morbidity and mortality. Moreover, the utility of plastic reconstruction of the full-thickness chest wall resection for recurrent disease is largely unknown and rarely utilized in surgical clinics. Friedel et al. (3) report the largest series to date for advanced chest wall invasion related to recurrent breast carcinoma utilizing myocutaneous flap coverage. In this series, the cumulative 5-, 10-, and 15-year survival rates were 46%, 29%, and 22%, respectively (median survival = 56 months). When an R0 resection was possible, the 5-year survival was 50.4%. Similarly, outstanding results have been reported by Hanagiri et al. (4), Hameed et al. (5), Veronesi et al. (6), Rivas et al. (7), Cordeiro et al. (8), Suryanarayana Deo et al. (9), Chagpar et al. (10), Kolodziejski et al. (11), Santillan et al. (12), and Pameijer et al. (13).

In the report by Pameijer et al. (13) from the City of Hope National Medical Center, this select group of patients had an R0 resection in 71% of patients; in this cohort, the 5-year disease-free survival was 67%. These reports suggest improvement in long-term palliation and potential cure for this select patient group with chest wall recurrence of breast carcinoma.

CONCLUSIONS

- The pathobiological character of the primary breast neoplasm and prior surgical technique with adjuvant/neoadjuvant approaches determines tumor recurrence.
- *Sine quo none* to eligibility as candidate for chest wall resection is confirmation of the absence of systemic disease following staging.
- A team approach with plastic and thoracic surgeons is essential with the oncologic surgeon to allow tissue transfer with reconstruction.
- Confirmation of absence of skin/muscle involvement with "punch" biopsy technique enhances local control.
- Resections that extend beyond four ribs will routinely require rigid chest wall reconstruction.
- Disease-free survival in properly selected patients exceeds 50% at 5 years.

References

1. Bedwinek J. Natural history and management of isolated local-regional recurrence following mastectomy. *Semin Radiat Oncol.* 1994;4:260–269.
2. Howard JH, Tzeng CWD, Fix RJ, Bland KI. Chest wall resection. In: Klimberg VS, ed. *Atlas of Breast Surgical Techniques.* Philadelphia, PA: Saunders, 2010.
3. Friedel G, Kuipers T, Dippon J, et al. Full-thickness resection with myocutaneous flap reconstruction for locally recurrent breast cancer. *Ann Thorac Surg.* 2008;85:1894–1900.
4. Hanagiri T, Nozoe T, Yoshimatsu T, et al. Surgical treatment of chest wall invasion due to the local recurrence of breast cancer. *Breast Cancer.* 2008;15:298–302.
5. Hameed A, Akhtar S, Naqvi A, Pervaiz Z. Reconstruction of complex chest wall defects by using polypropylene mesh and a pedicled latissimus dorsi flap: a 6-year experience. *J Plast Reconstr Aesthetic Surg.* 2008;61:628–635.
6. Veronesi G, Scanagatta P, Goldhirsch A, et al. Results of chest wall resection for recurrent or locally advanced breast malignancies. *Breast.* 2007;16:297–302.
7. Rivas B, Carrillo JF, Escobar G. Reconstructive management of advanced breast cancer. *Ann Plast Surg.* 2001;47(3):234–239.
8. Cordeiro PG, Sanatamaria E, Hidalgo D. The role of microsurgery in reconstruction of oncologic chest wall defects. *Plast Reconstr Surg.* 2001;108(7):1924–1930.
9. Suryanarayana Deo SV, Purkayastha J, Shukla NK, Astana S. Myocutaneous versus thoraco-abdominal flap cover for soft tissue defects following surgery for locally advanced and recurrent breast cancer. *J Surg Oncol.* 2003;83:31–35.
10. Chagpar A, Langstein HN, Kronowitz SJ, et al. Treatment and outcome of patients with chest wall recurrence after mastectomy and breast reconstruction. *Am J Surg.* 2004;187:164–169.
11. Kolodziejski LS, Wysocki WM, Komorowski AL. Full-thickness chest wall resection for recurrence of breast malignancy. *Breast J.* 2005;11(4):273–277.
12. Santillan AA, Kiluk JV, Cox JM, et al. Outcomes of locoregional recurrence after surgical chest wall resection and reconstruction for breast cancer. *Ann Surg Oncol.* 2008;15(5):1322–1329.
13. Pameijer CRJ, Smith D, McCahill LE, et al. Full-thickness chest wall resection for recurrent breast carcinoma: an institutional review and meta-analysis. *Am Surgeon.* 2005;71:711–715.

Part VI: Extensive Resections

22 Skin Flaps for Extensive Soft Tissue and Skin Resection

Jorge I. de la Torre and Luis O. Vásconez

Reconstruction following mastectomy was initially described for soft tissue coverage of the chest wall defect. During the 1940s, Meier described techniques to reconstruct the chest wall with local cutaneous flaps. Refinement of the reconstructive techniques and the implementation of multistaged procedures followed. Over the subsequent 60 years, chest wall and breast reconstruction has undergone tremendous change with regard to the variety and complexity of flaps employed to maximize efficacy and aesthetics.

Currently, chest wall defects in breast cancer patients can be divided into two subcategories—those defects that are secondary to surgical resection of the tumor and those changes that occur later as a result of radiation therapy. Before considering any option for chest wall or breast reconstruction, it is important to understand the extent to which the soft tissue is affected.

INDICATIONS/CONTRAINDICATIONS

The local skin flaps are indicated when skin coverage is required for coverage of extensive resection of the skin of the chest wall or to facilitate delayed reconstruction with an implant. It is particularly well suited in patients who have a skin deficit and who are not candidates for autologous breast reconstruction. This flap can be harvested and inset very simply and in a single stage. The thoracoepigastric flap can be combined with breast reconstruction by using an expander/implant. The donor site morbidity is limited to an area along the inframammary fold, which can be hidden within the inframammary fold and under the bra. It can be particularly useful when the patient does have excess skin in the upper abdominal region. Typically, healthy patients, with few comorbidities, are candidates for more extensive breast reconstructive options. Currently, the latissimus dorsi myocutaneous flap, with an implant or one of the variants of the rectus abdominus flaps, is preferable to local skin flaps as it offers soft tissue coverage for the chest wall and soft tissue to facilitate recreation of the breast mound. Local skin, soft tissue flaps are not indicated for patients who are candidates for immediate reconstruction.

Patients who have had prior surgical incisions in the upper abdomen may not be candidates for the medially based thoracoepigastric flap. If the scars traverse the planned flap, perfusion to the distal segment will be compromised and can result in flap loss. Similarly, patients who have undergone prior radiation therapy affecting the intended flap have a higher risk of poor perfusion and flap necrosis. In these situations, alternate local flap options would include the delayed deltopectoral flap or the contralateral upper rectus abdominus myocutaneous flap.

PREOPERATIVE PLANNING

Preoperatively, the quality of the remaining tissue and the amount of skin and soft tissue required must be considered in flap selection and design. The actual markings and measurements should be conducted with the patient in an upright position. The location of the inframammary fold is delineated on both the affected and contralateral side for comparison.

The thoracoepigastric flap is designed with either medially based or laterally based pedicles. These local skin flaps do not have a discrete vascular pedicle and depend on the distribution of the angiosome for blood supply. Therefore, it is critical to maintain the appropriate width to length ratio of 1 to 3. The width of the flap is limited by the amount of upper abdominal skin that can be mobilized to permit primary closure of the donor site.

The medially based flap is designed as a horizontal flap extending laterally to the midaxillary line. (See Fig. 22.1A and B—preoperative marking of the flap is outlined in red on the patient's left side. The red area on the patient's right side indicates a prior thoracoepigastric flap for reconstruction of a previous contralateral mastectomy.) If a longer flap is required, the flap should be delayed; incising around the planned flap and elevating the edges but leaving it in place for 2 weeks before mobilizing and insetting it.

The laterally based flap is designed as an oblique flap extending inferiorly and medially, permitting rotation without excessive kinking of the rotation point of the pedicle. It is based on the skin perforators from the external oblique muscle. The more of these perforators that are captured, the more robust the blood supply to the distal flap. Unfortunately, it may limit the length of the flap and the degree of rotation. It can be difficult to primarily close the donor defect by mobilizing the inferior skin and soft tissue; skin grafts are often used to close the remaining donor defect.

SURGERY

Relevant Anatomy

Positioning
Under general anesthesia, the patient is positioned in the supine position, with a bump or slight elevation of the surgical side. Local anesthesia (0.5% lidocaine with epinephrine) is injected along the planned incision site.

Steps of the Procedure

Elevation of Flaps
The flap is elevated from lateral to medial in a plane deep to the fascia (see Fig. 22.1C to indicate the extent of elevation obtained with the thoracoepigastric flap). Dissection proceeds medially to the lateral border of the rectus sheath, preserving the perforators from the rectus muscle to the skin paddle. As the flap is elevated medially, additional perforators from the intercostal vessels will be encountered and should be preserved if possible to augment perfusion of the flap.

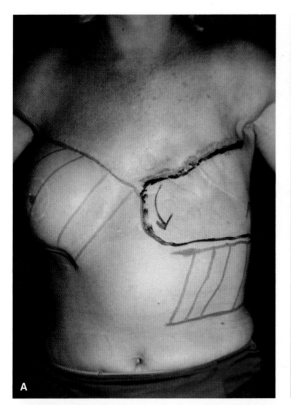

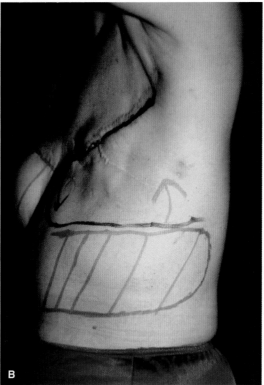

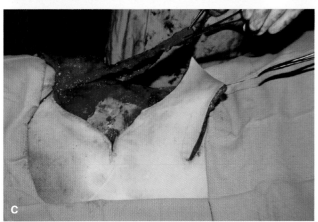

Figure 22.1 A and **B**. Preoperative views indicating preoperative markings. Note: the red marking on the patient's left indicates the planned flap. The red markings on the patient's right outline a prior thoracoepigastric flap for reconstruction of a previous mastectomy. **C**. Intraoperative image of elevation of the flap.

Donor Site Closure

The donor site is closed by aggressively undermining the upper abdominal skin (see Fig. 22.2A–C). It is often necessary to undermine the lower edge to the level of the superior iliac crest. In addition, placing the patient in a semiflexed position will facilitate donor site closure. Once the donor site is closed, the patient can be repositioned in the full supine position.

Drainage

Closed suction drains are brought out from both the flap site and the donor site, because of the wide undermining.

If skin coverage alone is desired, the thoracoepigastric flap is mobilized to cover the defect, and the edges are inset and sutured into position. If breast reconstruction is sought, an expander or small implant can be placed. Typically, an expander would be placed in the subpectoral plane to provide muscle coverage. The pectoralis major muscle is elevated off the chest wall, and the insertion along the inferior and medial aspects

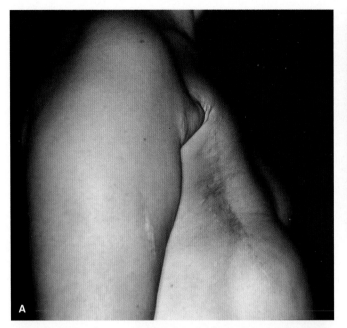

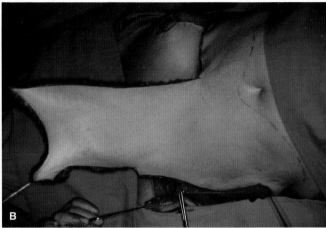

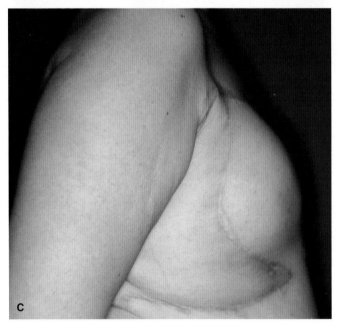

Figure 22.2 **A.** Preoperative view following mastectomy **B.** Extent of flap elevation. **C.** Primary closure of donor site even in this large flap.

are released using electrocautery. This will provide only partial coverage of the implant, so adequate soft tissue coverage with the thoracoepigastric flap is critical.

PEARLS AND PITFALLS

The use of local advancement flaps is limited in the reconstruction of the breast with extensive soft tissue and skin defects. Mastectomy procedures especially the skin-sparing approach can leave the skin flaps of variable thickness and compromise the subdermal plexus. Identification of viable skin can be difficult and surgical resection should err on the side of extra resection rather than leaving nonviable skin. In addition, the

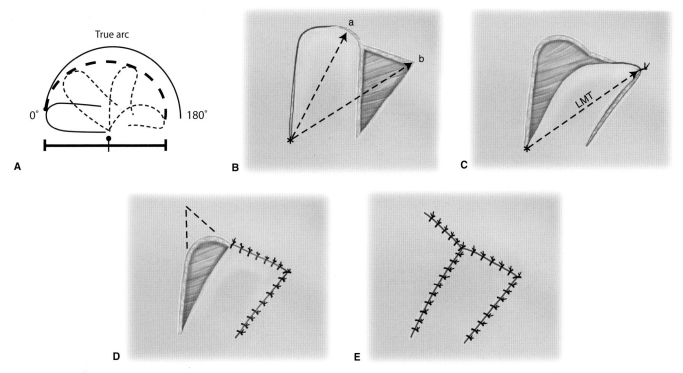

Figure 22.3 Rotational random flap. **A.** The effective length of a flap becomes shorter the farther the flap is rotated. Therefore, it should be designed larger than the defect. **B–E.** Transposition flap. LMT, line of maximal tension. Asterisk (*) indicates pivot point.

use of adjunct radiotherapy can further jeopardize thin skin flaps. Although this will necessitate a more complicated reconstruction, many are available.

For limited skin defect, techniques such as the rotational random flap or the rectangular advancement flap may be employed (Figs. 22.3 and 22.4). The V–Y flap (Fig. 22.5) can mobilize skin but would be rarely recommended for breast skin coverage. It creates an unfavorable scar line and distorts the residual tissue should recurrence require re-resection. The Z-plasty (Fig. 22.6) uses laxity in one direction to reduce the tightness

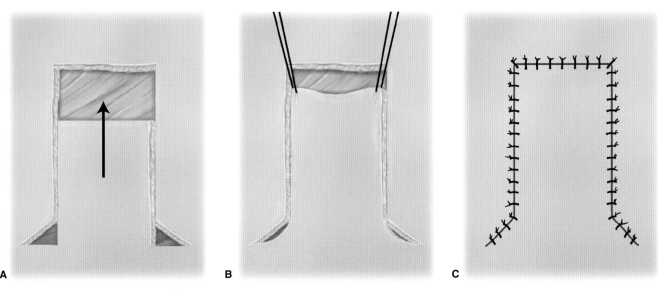

Figure 22.4 Rectangular advancement flap.

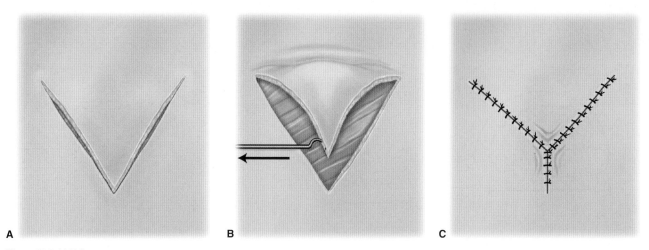

Figure 22.5 V–Y flap.

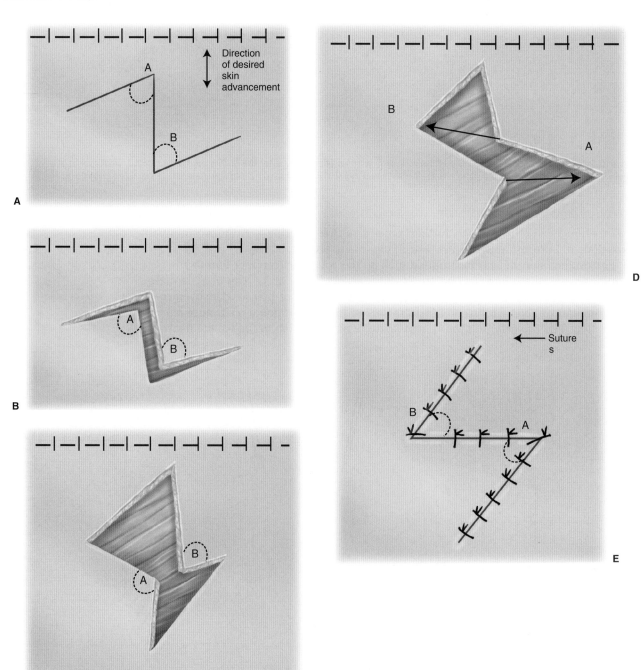

Figure 22.6 Z-plasty.

in a perpendicular vector. Like the V–Y flap, it may not be of particular value for the closure of large mastectomy defects, it is of tremendous value in the delayed breast reconstruction. Often, these patients have a tight transverse scar, which limits breast projection even with an autologous reconstruction. A Z-plasty will release the transverse tightness of the mastectomy scar, allowing the autologous flap to provide natural fullness and shape of the breast.

The use of these skin rearrangement techniques provides only limited value to address large soft tissue and skin defects because the vascular supply is dependent on the subdermal plexus. The thoracoepigastric flap, although similar in design, is based on several random perforators to the skin paddle, making it more robust. The pedicle flaps such as the transverse rectus abdominus myocutaneous (TRAM) and latissimus bring their own arterial supply, which is even more dependable and tolerant of radiation.

 POSTOPERATIVE MANAGEMENT

Management following the design and implementation of the thoracoepigastric flap is to protect and monitor the vascularity of the flap. Early recognition of ischemia is important to minimize progressive flap necrosis. Because the random skin flap does not have a major vascular pedicle, clinical observation is the best method to assess the flap. If the color of the flap is white or the capillary refill is insufficient, it indicates that arterial inflow is inadequate. This can be a result of excessive kinking or stretch on the flap and sutures should be released or the flap completely released to permit distal blood flow. A blue flap is consistent with venous congestions, and use of leeches may be indicated. In addition, the distal portion of the flap is pricked with a sterile needle to assess the quality of bleeding if there is a question on clinical examination.

In the immediate postoperative period, it is beneficially to limit activities of the ipsilateral upper extremity and torso to minimize tension on the flap. If it is healing well at 3 weeks, it is unlikely to develop an ischemia along the margins. Once the flap has fully matured, at approximately 3 months following inset, tissue expansion or implant placement can be considered. Tissue expansion can take several weeks to slowly inflate the expander under the skin flap. Once expansion is complete, the expander can be replaced with a permanent implant (see Fig. 22.7A–D). Subsequent procedures will permit fine-tuning of the flap aesthetics, nipple areolar reconstruction and tattooing of the areola.

 COMPLICATIONS

Major complications are unusual with local skin flaps. Patients may report a sensation of tightness along the area of the donor site or flap inset, but this resolves with 5 to 7 days. Seromas are not common but are a significant enough risk that drains are recommended. Flap necrosis is unusual when the flap is properly designed and elevated. If there is some necrosis at the distal tip, in most cases, it is relatively minor and can be managed with limited local wound care. The same is true for limited wound healing problems along the donor site closure.

 RESULTS

Thoracoepigastric flaps provide reliable coverage for soft tissue defects of the chest wall with robust skin flaps (see Fig. 22.8A and B). Operative time is similar to alternative breast and chest wall reconstructive options. Limitations of the procedure are that despite coverage of the chest wall, these flaps do not permit adequate soft tissue for breast reconstruction. The donor site is fairly limited and the coverage does permit reconstruction in a staged fashion.

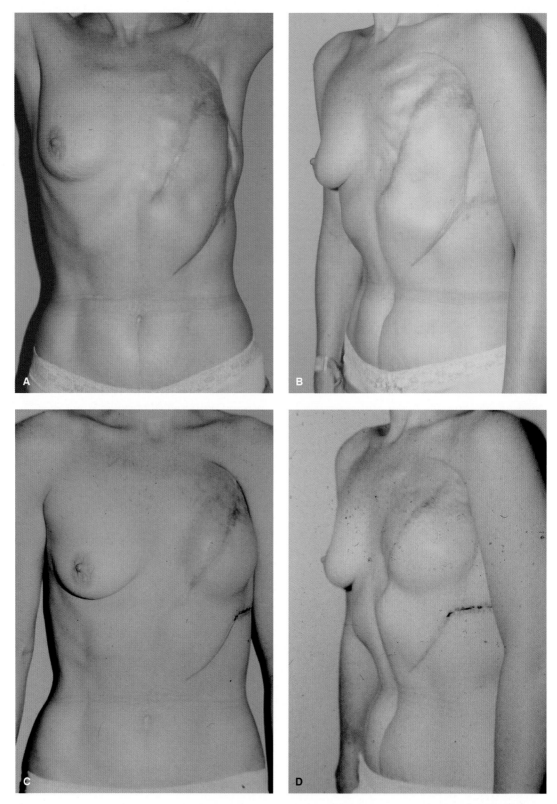

Figure 22.7 A and **B.** Postoperative views of a patient following reconstruction of chest wall with a well-healed thoracoepigastric flap. **C** and **D.** Following expansion and placement of a silicome gel implant for first stage of breast reconstruction.

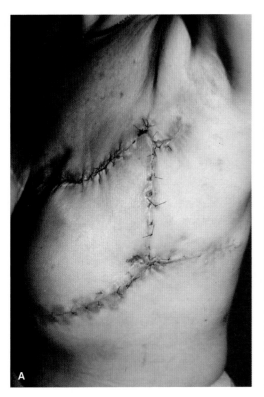
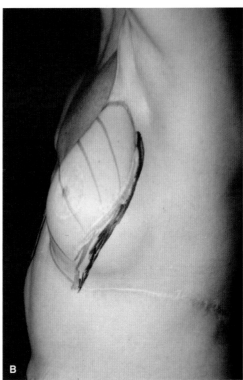

Figure 22.8 A. Early postoperative view following thoracoepigastric flap reconstruction. Note some ischemic necrosis around the margin of the flap. **B.** Late results of thoracoepigastric flap in the same patient.

Suggested Readings

Baroudi R. A transverse thoracoabdominal skin flap for closure after radical mastectomy. *Plast Reconstr Surg.* 1978;61:547–554.

Davis AM, McCraw JB, Carraway JH. Use of a direct transverse thoracoabdominal flap to close difficult wounds of the thorax and upper extremity. *Plast Reconstr Surg.* 1977;60:526.

Deo SV, Purkayastha J, Shukla NK, et al. Myocutaneous versus thoraco-abdominal flap cover for soft tissue defects following surgery for locally advanced and recurrent breast cancer. *J Surg Oncol.* 2003;83:31–35.

Hultman CS, Daiza S. Skin-sparing mastectomy flap complications after breast reconstruction: review of incidence, management, and outcome. *Ann Plast Surg.* 2003;50(3):249–255, discussion 255.

Maier HC. Surgical management of large defects of the thoracic wall. *Surgery.* 1947;22:169.

McCraw JB, Bostwick J, Horton CE. Methods of soft tissue coverage for mastectomy defect. *Clin Plast Surg.* 1979;6:57.

Newman MI, Samson MC, Tamburrino JF, et al. Intraoperative laser-assisted indocyanine green angiography for the evaluation of mastectomy flaps in immediate breast reconstruction [published online ahead of print June 10, 2010]. *Reconstr Microsurg.* doi: 10.1055/s-0030-1261701.

Skoracki RJ, Chang DW. Reconstruction of chest wall and thorax. *J Surg Oncol.* 2006;94:455–465.

Woods JE. Transposition and advancement skin flaps. In: Strauch B, Vasconez LO, Hall-Findlay EJ, eds. *Grabb's Encyclopedia of Flaps.* 2nd ed. Philadelphia, PA: Lippincott-Raven; 1998:1383–1386.

23 Forequarter Amputation

Keila E. Torres, Kelly K. Hunt, and Raphael E. Pollock

INDICATIONS/CONTRAINDICATIONS

Amputation is one of the most ancient of all surgical procedures. Because of the lack of hemostatic techniques and antibiotic therapy, amputation was previously associated with a high mortality rate. The earliest report on the use of surgical forequarter amputation, or interscapulothoracic amputation, was published by Cuming in 1829 (1). Unfortunately, the patient died of gangrene a few days following the procedure. Because of the advances in regional and systemic therapies, radical amputation procedures are rarely performed. Forequarter amputation is performed almost exclusively for tumors of the shoulder girdle or surrounding soft tissues that invade the glenohumeral joint, the brachial plexus, or the axillary vasculature, making limb salvage or shoulder disarticulation unfeasible. This radical operation has been selectively utilized in the treatment of recurrent breast cancer, specifically when there is disease in the axilla (2). Recurrent tumor in the axilla with invasion into the brachial plexus and axillary vessels can lead to significant morbidity secondary to pain, lymphedema, limb dysfunction, and ulceration. In some instances, palliative forequarter amputation has provided effective pain relief for selected patients with unresectable metastatic disease to the axilla and shoulder girdle in whom radiation therapy and/or chemotherapy have not been effective (3).

Forequarter amputation indications are as follows:

- Large fungating tumors involving the shoulder girdle, chest wall, and/or axilla (Fig. 23.1)
- Patients who have had a failed attempt at limb-sparing resection
- Involvement of the brachial plexus or axillary vasculature (Fig. 23.2)

PREOPERATIVE PLANNING

Detailed clinical and pathologic data should be obtained in the planning phase. A core needle biopsy or incisional biopsy is recommended to confirm the diagnosis prior to any surgical intervention (4). The placement of the biopsy site should be chosen carefully, as it will need to be included in the formal resection. High-quality, contrast-enhanced computed tomography (CT) scanning can define all necessary anatomical details that will be

Figure 23.1 A large fungating tumor involving the shoulder, chest wall, and axilla.

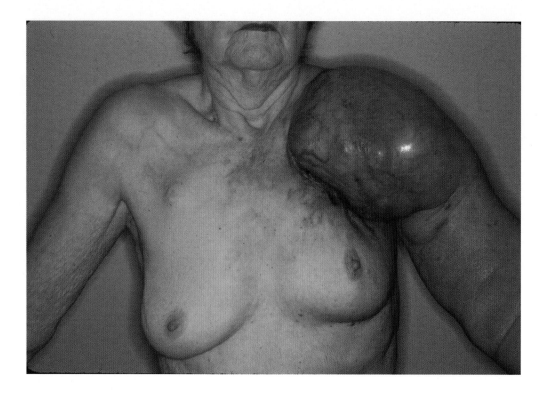

important in determining resectability (5,6). Magnetic resonance imaging (MRI) has the advantage of providing a more detailed assessment of individual muscle involvement and extent of brachial plexus involvement in selected patients (6). In equivocal cases a local exploration with intra-operative biopsies may be needed (Fig. 23.3).

The nutritional status and immunocompetence of the patient should be assessed prior to operative intervention. Malnourished or immunocompromised patients will have markedly increased rates of perioperative complications that may prevent a successful recovery. The forequarter amputation is a radical procedure that will result in a hypermetabolic state postoperatively. Significant medical comorbidities or any active infection should be addressed prior to surgery. Depending on the extent of the tumor,

Figure 23.2 A large soft-tissue tumor of the axilla arising posterior to the brachial plexus and involving the chest wall. (From Pollock RE. *American Cancer Society Atlas of Clinical Oncology: Soft Tissue Sarcomas*. 1st ed. Hamilton, BC, Canada: Decker Inc, 2002:231, with permission.)

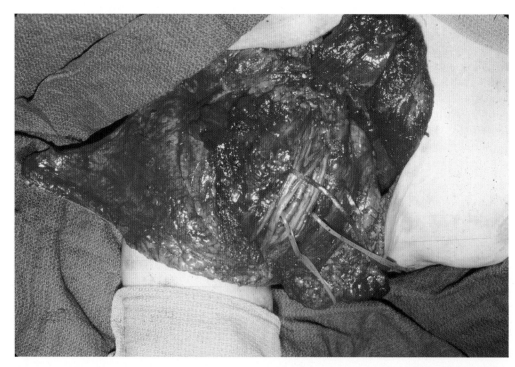

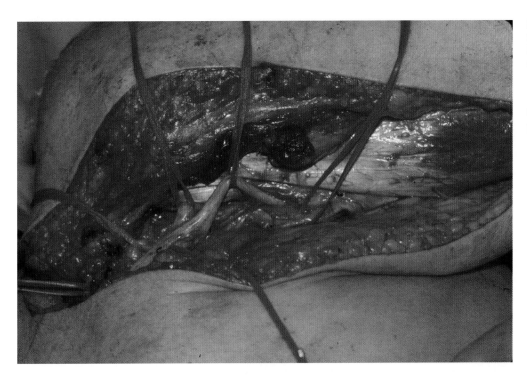

Figure 23.3 Local exploration will reveal the involvement of the brachial plexus and axillary vasculature. (From Pollock RE. *American Cancer Society Atlas of Clinical Oncology: Soft Tissue Sarcomas.* 1st ed. Hamilton, BC, Canada: Decker Inc, 2002:237, with permission.)

Part VI: Extensive Resections

this procedure can involve significant blood loss and plans for perioperative transfusion should be made.

The need for additional skin and soft-tissue coverage of the amputation site should be considered preoperatively. When the tumor involves a considerable portion of the medial aspect of the axillary skin and soft tissue, the resection defect following forequarter amputation will often necessitate the use of split thickness skin grafts or myocutaneous flaps for wound closure. A fasciocutaneous deltoid flap can be utilized when a proximal but medial tumor necessitates more skin and soft-tissue resection near the chest wall. If the resection necessitates removal of more than two ribs, coverage of the defect and stabilization of the chest wall will be needed and consultation with a plastic and reconstructive surgeon should be obtained.

Preoperative assessment includes:

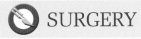 biopsy to confirm diagnosis,
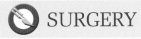 proper imaging of the proximal vasculature and neural plexus for surgical planning, and
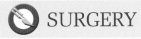 optimization of the patient's medical and nutritional status.

SURGERY

Forequarter amputation removes the entire upper extremity in the interval between the scapula and the chest wall (7–9). Resection of the chest wall may also be required (Fig. 23.4).

Three approaches to the forequarter amputation have been described:

1. Anterior approach (Berger)
2. Posterior approach (Littlewood)
3. Combination of the anterior and posterior approaches

Positioning

The patient should be placed in a lateral decubitus position with the affected side up and secured to the operating table at several points. The affected shoulder, axillary region, and upper extremity should be prepped with sterile solution and draped with a

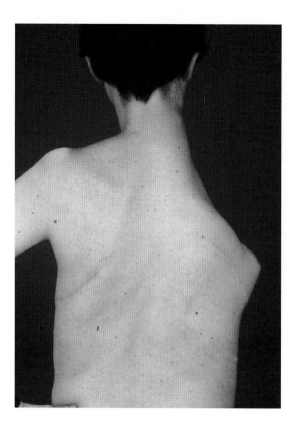

Figure 23.4 A forequarter amputation with chest wall resection. (From Pollock RE. *American Cancer Society Atlas of Clinical Oncology: Soft Tissue Sarcomas.* 1st ed. Hamilton, BC, Canada: Decker Inc, 2002:233, with permission.)

wide operative field. The upper extremity should be prepped free and covered with a stocking so that it can be manipulated to facilitate exposure during the procedure.

Operative Technique for the Posterior Approach

The posterior approach to the forequarter amputation requires two incisions: one posterior (cervicoscapular) and one anterior (pectoroaxillary) (Fig. 23.5). If a fasciocuta-

Figure 23.5 Skin incision for the posterior approach. (Redrawn from Cleveland KB. Amputations of the upper extremity. In: Canale ST, Beaty JH, eds. *Campbell's Operative Orthopaedics.* 11th ed. New York NY: Mosby, 2007:626–629, with permission.)

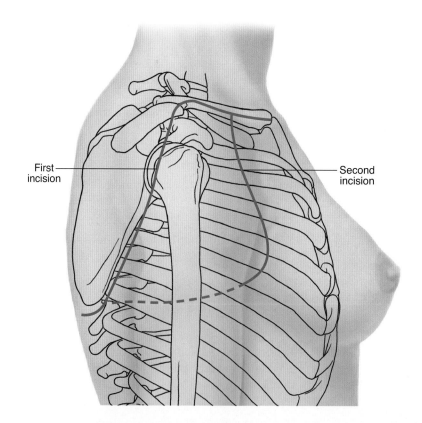

First incision

Second incision

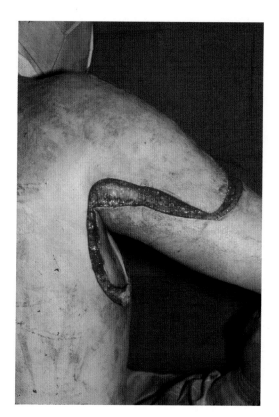

Figure 23.6 Planned incision for a forequarter amputation to include the deltoid flap. (From Pollock RE. *American Cancer Society Atlas of Clinical Oncology: Soft Tissue Sarcomas.* 1st ed. Hamilton, BC, Canada: Decker Inc, 2002:232, with permission.)

neous deltoid flap is required for closure of the wound, the incision will extend out over the shoulder following the outline of the deltoid muscle just distal to its insertion on the humerus (Fig. 23.6).

- The posterior incision is initiated at the medial end of the clavicle and extended laterally for the entire length of the bone. The incision is then extended to the acromion and the lateral border of the scapula to the inferior angle of the scapula.
- A flap of overlying skin flap and subcutaneous tissue medial to the vertebral border of the scapula is elevated, extending it from the inferior angle of the scapula to the clavicle (Fig. 23.7).
- The trapezius muscle is identified and divided near the scapula (Fig. 23.7).
- The scapula is then pulled away from the chest wall with a retractor, and the levator scapulae and rhomboideus minor and major muscles are divided (Fig. 23.8). The dissection is continued around the inferior angle of the scapula where the latissimus dorsi muscle is divided.
- Ligation of the superficial cervical and descending scapular vessels is then undertaken.
- The superior digitations of the serratus anterior muscle are divided close to the superior angle of the scapula followed by the remaining insertions of the serratus anterior muscle along the vertebral border of the scapula (Fig. 23.9).
- The clavicle and subclavius muscle are divided at the medial end of the bone, allowing the upper extremity to fall anteriorly. The neurovascular bundle will now be under tension. The neurovascular bundle is identified close to the superior digitations of the serratus anterior muscle. As the dissection is carried deeper, the brachial plexus is encountered in addition to the subclavian artery and vein. The cords of the brachial plexus are ligated and divided close to the spine with 0-silk sutures. The subclavian artery and vein should be dissected free and doubly ligated with 0-silk sutures prior to transecting the vessels. The surgeon is careful to avoid any injury to the pleural dome.
- The omohyoid muscle is divided, followed by ligation and division of the suprascapular vessels and the external jugular vein.
- The anterior incision is then created at the middle of the clavicle and extended inferiorly just lateral to but parallel with the deltopectoral groove. The anterior incision is extended to meet the posterior incision at the inferior angle of the scapula (Fig. 23.5).

Figure 23.7 Elevation of a posterior skin flap (Redrawn from Cleveland KB. Amputations of the upper extremity. In: Canale ST, Beaty JH, eds. *Campbell's Operative Orthopaedics.* 11th ed. New York NY: Mosby, 2007:626–629, with permission.)

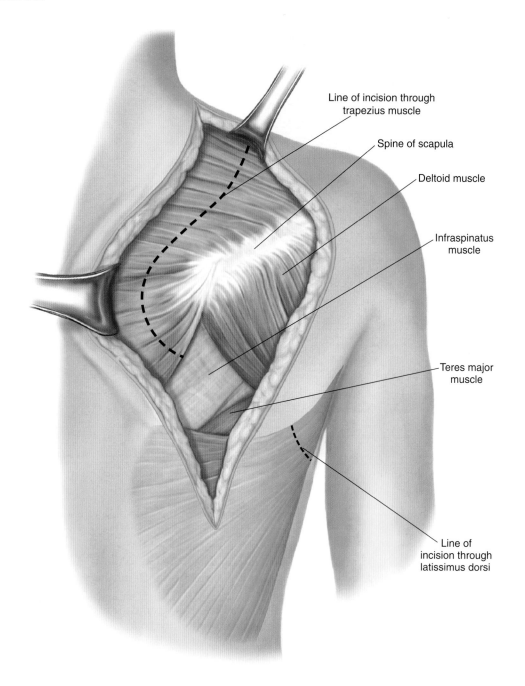

Line of incision through trapezius muscle

Spine of scapula

Deltoid muscle

Infraspinatus muscle

Teres major muscle

Line of incision through latissimus dorsi

■ The anterior dissection is continued down to the fascia of the pectoralis major muscle. The pectoralis major is divided close to its sternal and costal origins (Fig. 23.10). The pectoralis minor muscle is divided from its origin at the third to the fifth ribs. The scapula is freed all the way around approaching the area of the lower neck.

■ The skin flaps are then closed after hemostasis and placement of closed-suction drains. Any tension on the skin flaps should be avoided. Closure with a skin graft may be necessary if there is excessive tension. Care should be taken to place the skin graft over a bed of viable muscle or healthy subcutaneous tissue.

Operative Technique for the Anterior Approach

■ The upper aspect of the incision is begun at the lateral border of the sternocleidomastoid muscle and extended laterally along the anterior aspect of the clavicle, across the acromioclavicular joint, over the superior aspect of the shoulder to the spine of the scapula (Fig. 23.11). This incision should extend across the body of the scapula to the scapular angle. The lower aspect of the incision will extend inferiorly from the

Figure 23.8 Division of the levator scapule and the rhomboideus major and minor muscles. (Redrawn from Cleveland KB. Amputations of the upper extremity. In: Canale ST, Beaty JH, eds. *Campbell's Operative Orthopaedics.* 11th ed. New York NY: Mosby, 2007:626–629.)

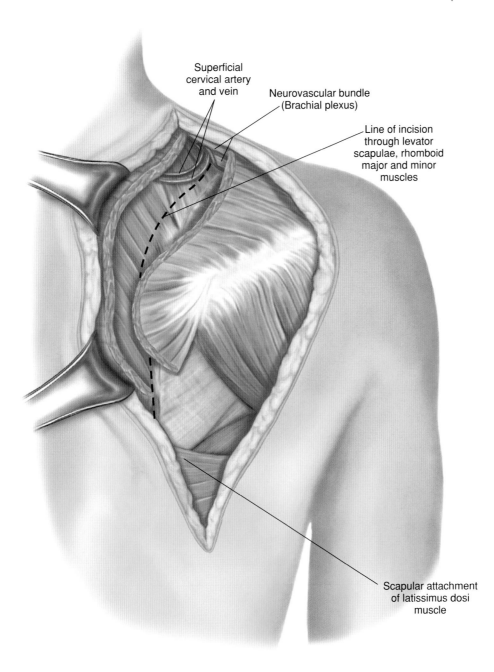

Superficial cervical artery and vein

Neurovascular bundle (Brachial plexus)

Line of incision through levator scapulae, rhomboid major and minor muscles

Scapular attachment of latissimus dosi muscle

Part VI: Extensive Resections

middle third of the clavicle, then inferiorly and laterally toward the groove between the deltoid and pectoral muscles. The incision is then extended across the axilla to join the posterior incision at the angle of the scapula (Fig. 23.11).

■ Dissection is carried toward the clavicle where the pectoralis major muscle is divided at its clavicular origin (Fig. 23.12).

■ Dissection then proceeds through the deep fascia over the superior border of the clavicle. The deep aspect of the clavicle is freed with a blunt curved dissector or the surgeon's finger. The external jugular vein should then be ligated and divided (Fig. 23.12).

■ The clavicle is divided at the lateral border of the sternocleidomastoid muscle and removed by separating the acromioclavicular joint (Fig. 23.12).

■ The insertion of the pectoralis major muscle is released from the humerus and the origin of the pectoralis minor separated from the coracoid process.

■ A 2-cm portion of the midclavicle is divided with a Gigli saw, and the bone is removed. Once this bone is removed, the subclavian artery and vein can be easily identified. The subclavian vein is identified first and is encircled, ligated, and divided. The subclavian artery is just posterior to the vein and should be encircled and ligated proximally

Figure 23.9 Division of the superior digitations of the serratus anterior muscle along the vertebral border of the scapula. (Redrawn from Cleveland KB. Amputations of the upper extremity. In: Canale ST, Beaty JH, eds. *Campbell's Operative Orthopaedics.* 11th ed. New York NY: Mosby, 2007:626–629.)

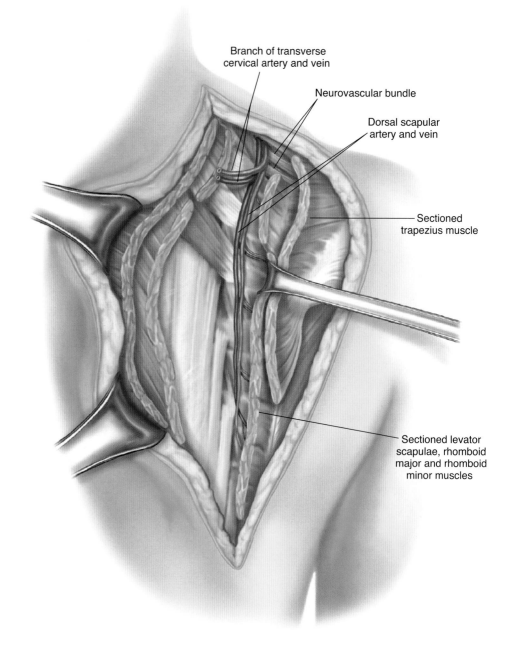

Branch of transverse cervical artery and vein

Neurovascular bundle

Dorsal scapular artery and vein

Sectioned trapezius muscle

Sectioned levator scapulae, rhomboid major and rhomboid minor muscles

with a 0-silk ligature and a 4-0 Prolene suture ligature. Distally, the artery can be divided after ligation with a single 0-silk ligature. With these two structures divided, the surgeon may proceed to division of the brachial plexus. The cords of the brachial plexus are identified in close proximity to the spine. A 0.25% Marcaine solution without epinephrine can be injected into each branch of the plexus. These are then ligated and sharply bisected at each of the plexus branches (Fig. 23.13).

■ The latissimus dorsi is then divided as well as the remaining soft tissues that bind the shoulder girdle to the anterior chest wall. This will allow the limb to fall posteriorly (Fig. 23.14).

■ The patient's arm is held across the chest and a gentle downward traction is exerted. This allows for division of the remaining muscles that fix the shoulder to the scapula.

■ Divide the muscles that hold the scapula to the thorax in addition to the trapezius muscle. Then proceed to divide the omohyoids, levator scapulae, rhomboids major and minor, and serratus anterior. Once the limb is free from these attachments, it may be removed.

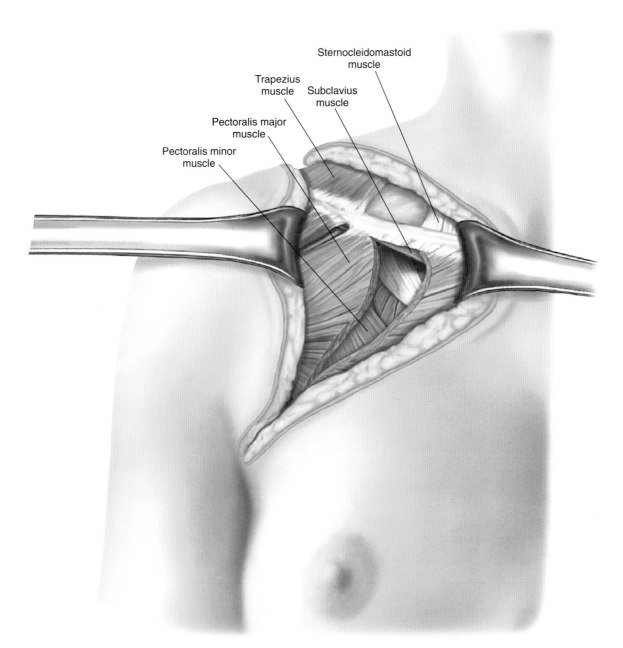

Sternocleidomastoid
muscle

Trapezius
muscle   Subclavius
muscle

Pectoralis major
muscle

Pectoralis minor
muscle

Figure 23.10 Division of the pectoralis major muscle close to its sternal and costal origins. (Redrawn from Ferrario T, Palmer P, Karakousis CP. Technique of forequarter (interscapulothoracic) amputation. *Clin Orthop Relat Res*. 2004;423:192, with permission.)

■ The pectoralis major, trapezius, and any other remaining muscular structures are secured over the lateral chest wall. The skin flaps are trimmed and then approximated to form a smooth closure. Closed-suction drains are placed beneath the skin closure. The skin edges should be closed with interrupted nonabsorbable sutures (Fig. 23.15).

Technique for the Combined Anterior and Posterior Approaches

In order to use this combined approach, the surgeon should initiate the incision similar to the one performed as described earlier for the posterior approach. After developing the posterior flap and dividing the trapezius muscle, one may proceed to create the anterior incision and divide the pectoral muscles. Mobilization of the specimen is performed prior to ligation of the subclavian vessels. Division of the vessels is the last step (4).

Part VI: Extensive Resections

Figure 23.11 Skin incision for the anterior approach. (Redrawn from Cleveland KB. Amputations of the upper extremity. In: Canale ST, Beaty JH, eds. *Campbell's Operative Orthopaedics*. 11th ed. New York, NY: Mosby, 2008:626–629, with permission.)

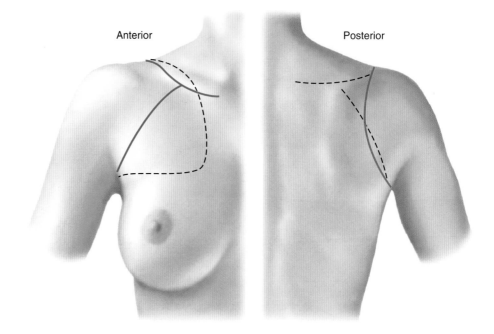

Anterior

Posterior

Figure 23.12 Division of the clavicle at the lateral border of the sternocleidomastoid muscle followed by removal of the bone by dividing the acromioclavicular joint. (Redrawn from Cleveland KB. Amputations of the upper extremity. In: Canale ST, Beaty JH, eds. *Campbell's Operative Orthopaedics*. 11th ed. New York NY: Mosby, 2007:626–629, with permission.)

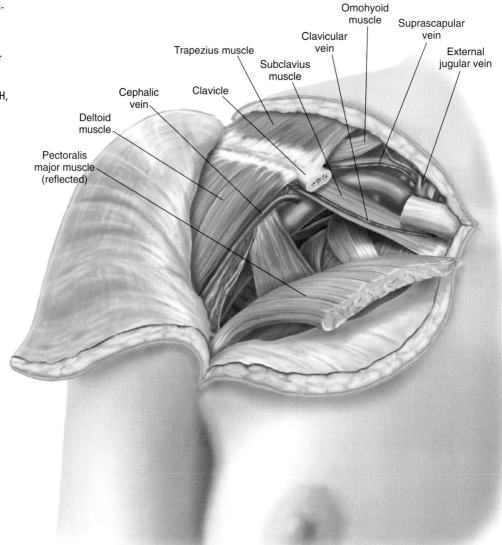

Omohyoid muscle

Clavicular vein

Suprascapular vein

Trapezius muscle

Subclavius muscle

External jugular vein

Cephalic vein

Clavicle

Deltoid muscle

Pectoralis major muscle (reflected)

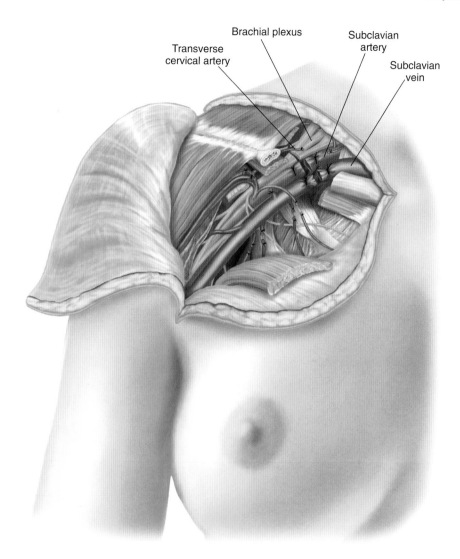

Transverse
cervical artery

Brachial plexus

Subclavian
artery

Subclavian
vein

Figure 23.13 Ligation and sharp division of each of the plexus branches. Dissection and ligation of the subclavian artery and vein. (Redrawn from Cleveland KB. Amputations of the upper extremity. In: Canale ST, Beaty JH, eds. *Campbell's Operative Orthopaedics.* 11th ed. New York NY: Mosby, 2007:626–629, with permission.)

Part VI: Extensive Resections

➡ POSTOPERATIVE MANAGEMENT

Postoperative care will require a multidisciplinary team approach. The team should include a physical medicine specialist, a physical therapist, an occupational therapist, a psychologist, and a social worker in addition to the surgeon. An internist often is required to assist in the management of postoperative medical problems. Perioperative antibiotics, deep venous thrombosis prophylaxis, and pulmonary hygiene are critical for a proper recovery. Postoperative pain should be controlled with intravenous narcotics followed by oral medication. Patients might suffer phantom pain in the postoperative period. Nerve blocks might be helpful in this situation.

Although a mechanical arm and hand is the preferred prosthesis for a forequarter amputation patient, such prosthesis is not readily available. Most patients with forequarter amputation use a shoulder pad to allow the use of normal clothes and provide a symmetrical appearance to the torso (4). Female patients who undergo radical mastectomy and forequarter amputation will require a breast-shoulder prosthesis. Considerable cosmetic improvement has been described in the literature by use of a one-piece artificial shoulder and breast device giving a more pleasing contour (10).

Consultation with physical and occupational therapy are important in the recovery process. The occupational therapist can assist in evaluating the home environment as most

Figure 23.14 Division of the latissimus dorsi muscle and the remaining soft tissues that bind the shoulder girdle to the anterior chest wall. (Redrawn from Cleveland KB. Amputations of the upper extremity. In: Canale ST, Beaty JH, eds. *Campbell's Operative Orthopaedics*. 11th ed. New York NY: Mosby, 2007:626–629, with permission.)

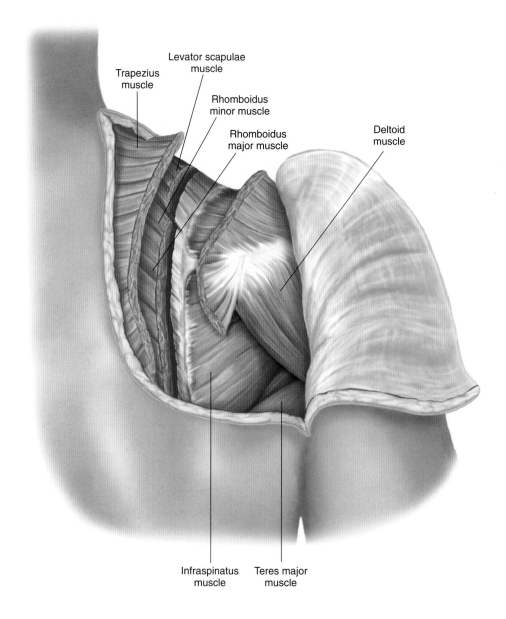

Trapezius muscle

Levator scapulae muscle

Rhomboidus minor muscle

Rhomboidus major muscle

Deltoid muscle

Infraspinatus muscle

Teres major muscle

Figure 23.15 Wound closure. (Redrawn from Cleveland KB. Amputations of the upper extremity. In: Canale ST, Beaty JH, eds. *Campbell's Operative Orthopaedics*. 11th ed. New York NY: Mosby, 2007:626–629, with permission.)

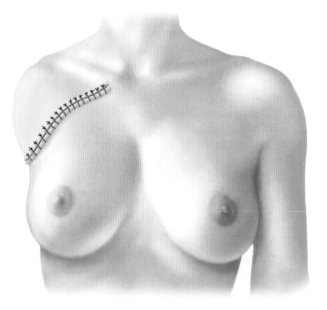

patients will need training to perform activities of daily living. Activities such as driving are not necessarily precluded in well-motivated amputees but may provide substantial challenges and require retraining of the individual. It is vital that rehabilitation should focus on both prosthetic and nonprosthetic training to achieve maximal independence. A significant number of patients will experience problems with the contralateral limb, with shoulder pain being the most common problem (45%) (11). Back and neck pain are also commonly reported. In those patients who require a substantial portion of chest wall resection as part of the procedure, proper spine stabilization should be considered. It is important to advise patients of overuse injuries early on in the rehabilitation process.

 # COMPLICATIONS

The most common complication reported is residual pain following the amputation. This pain is described as phantom limb pain. The incidence of phantom pain has been estimated to occur in 60% to 90% of amputees (12). Flap necrosis has also been reported (3,12–15).

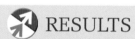 # RESULTS

The majority of forequarter amputations are performed for bone or soft-tissue sarcomas. The procedure has also been utilized to treat extensive osteomyelitis of the upper limb. Forequarter amputation has scarcely been reported for the management of patients with locally advanced or recurrent breast cancer. Most of the published studies describe the results of this technique on a small number of patients or are individual case reports (12–15). The potential for cure after this procedure is dependent on the underlying biology of the disease and the presence and extent of any evident or occult distant metastases. The use of radical amputations for control of primary tumors has better overall outcome than of amputations for locally recurrent disease (13).

CONCLUSIONS

- Forequarter amputation removes the entire upper extremity in the interval between the scapula and the chest wall. While the vast majority of forequarter amputations are performed for large bone and soft-tissue sarcomas or extensive osteomyelitis of the upper limb, these have also been used for the control of locally advanced and recurrent breast cancer.
- Indications for this procedure in the setting of recurrent breast cancer include the following:
    - Immobile unresectable tumor involving the shoulder girdle, chest wall, and/or axilla
    - Patients who have had a failed attempt at limb-sparing resection
    - Involvement of the brachial plexus or axillary vasculature
    - Severe intractable pain with loss of extremity function
    - Ulceration, fungation, sepsis, hemorrhage gangrene, severe lymphedema, and paralysis
- Thorough preoperative evaluation and preparation is critical for a successful outcome.
- Three approaches have been described:
    - Anterior approach (Berger)
    - Posterior approach (Littlewood)
    - Combination of the anterior and posterior approaches
- Postoperative care requires a multidisciplinary team approach including involvement of physical medicine and rehabilitation specialists.

References

1. Cuming R. Removal of the arm, scapula, and clavicle (after gunshot wound). Report by Dr Hutchinson. *Lond Med Gaz.* 1829;5: 273.

2. Goodman MD, Mcintyre B, Shaughnessy EA, Lowy AM, Ahmad SA. Forequarter amputation for recurrent breast cancer: a case report and review of the literature. *J Surg Oncol.* 2005;92:134–141.

3. Wittig JC, Bickels J, Kollender Y, et al. Palliative forequarter amputation for metastatic carcinoma to the shoulder girdle region: indications, preoperative evaluation, surgical technique, and results. *J Surg Oncol.* 2001;77(2):105–113.

4. Clark MA, Thomas JM. Amputation for soft-tissue sarcoma. *Lancet Oncol.* 2003;4(6):335–342.

5. Watkins RM, Thomas JM. Role of computed tomography in selecting patients for hindquarter amputation. *Br J Surg.* 1987; 74:711–714.

6. Hughes TMD, Spillane AJ. Imaging of soft tissue tumours. *Br J Surg.* 2000;87:259–260.

7. Cleveland KB. Amputations of the upper extremity. In: Canale ST, Beaty JH, eds. *Campbell's Operative Orthopaedics.* 11th ed. New York, NY: Mosby, 2007:626–629.

8. Chapman MW. *Chapman's Orthopaedic Surgery.* 3rd ed. Philadelphia, PA: Lippincott Williams & Wilkins, 2001: 3346–3359.

9. Ferrario T, Palmer P, Karakousis CP. Technique of forequarter (interscapulothoracic) amputation. *Clin Orthop Relat Res.* 2004; 423:191–195.

10. Knight NK, Setzler DM, Sabella SR. Construction of shoulder and breast prostheses. *Am J Occup Ther.* 1975;29(4):209–212.

11. Wright TW, Hagen AD, Wood MB. Prosthetic usage in major upper extremity amputations. *J Hand Surg.* 1995;20(4):619–622.

12. Katz J, Melzack R. Pain memories in phantom limbs: review and clinical observations. *Pain.* 1990;43:319–336.

13. Sakamura R, Nohira K, Shibata M, Sugihara T. Coverage of a large soft-tissue defect of the chest with a free fillet forearm and hand flap. *J Reconstr Microsurg.* 2001;17:229–231.

14. Mussey RD. Palliative forequarter amputation for recurrent breast carcinoma. *AMA Arch Surg.* 1956;73:154–156.

15. Pressman PI. Interscapulothoracic amputation for the complications of breast cancer: a new approach. *Surgery.* 1974;75: 796–801.

24 Oncoplastic Surgery: Segmental Resection for Lumpectomies

Kristine E. Calhoun and Benjamin O. Anderson

INDICATIONS/CONTRAINDICATIONS

Breast conserving therapy was first investigated as a treatment option for women affected by breast cancer beginning in the 1970s, and clinical trials have since demonstrated equivalency in terms of overall survival between lumpectomy plus radiation and mastectomy (1,2). Although there are clear contraindications to lumpectomy, such as widespread multicentric disease and persistently positive surgical margins, for the appropriately selected individual, breast conserving therapy can offer effective treatment and offer the psychological benefit of retention of the breast.

In a typical lumpectomy, the skin is opened, the tumor removed, and the wound closed without any specific effort being made to obliterate the internal resection cavity. Closing the fibroglandular tissue can result in unsightly defects if alignment of the breast tissue is suboptimal. Often times, fibroglandular tissue that is sutured and closed at middle depth in the breast while the patient is supine on the operating table results in a dimpled, irregular appearance when the patient stands up. Given this potential, most surgeons choose to only close the skin of a lumpectomy without approximation of the underlying tissue. While the simple "scoop and run" approach to lumpectomy may work well for smaller tumors, declivity of the skin and/or displacement of the nipple–areolar complex (NAC) can result at final healing if the lesion removed from the breast is sizable.

For breast conservation to be maximally effective, the cancer must be resected with adequate or wide surgical margins while simultaneously maintaining the breast's shape and appearance, goals that may prove challenging and in some settings seem to be conflicting (3,4). In 1994, Werner P. Audretsch was one of the first to advocate the use of "oncoplastic surgery" for repair of partial mastectomy defects by combining the techniques of volume reduction with immediate flap reconstruction (5). Although initially used to describe the partial mastectomy combined with large myocutaneous flap reconstruction using the latissimus dorsi or the rectus abdominis muscles, oncoplastic surgery now more commonly describes a series of surgical approaches that utilize partial mastectomy and breast-flap advancement to address tissue defects following wide resection. The most widely utilized techniques include parallelogram mastopexy lumpectomy (including the lateral segmentectomy variant), batwing mastopexy lumpectomy, donut mastopexy lumpectomy, reduction mastopexy lumpectomy, and central lumpectomy (3,6).

The use of oncoplastic surgical techniques for breast conservation allows for wider resections without subsequent tissue deformity, and thereby allows surgeons to achieve wide surgical margins while preserving the shape and appearance of the breast (7). While oncoplastic techniques are varied in type and approach, the general principle of fashioning the tissue resection to the anatomic shape of the cancer minimizes the removal of uninvolved breast tissue while ensuring that wide margins, ideally more than 1 cm, are achieved in an optimal number of patients (3,6). The indications, as well as the contraindications, for oncoplastic surgery are the same as those of traditional breast conserving surgery. Such techniques are offered only to those otherwise believed to be breast preservation candidates, including patients with single quadrant disease and individuals who can tolerate and have access to postsurgical radiation therapy.

The techniques described in this chapter are those oncological resections that use breast-flap advancement (so-called tissue displacement techniques). Compared with breast reconstruction using a myocutaneous flap, the breast flap advancement technique is easily learned and implemented by breast surgeons, even those lacking formal plastic surgery training. In a review of 84 women who underwent partial mastectomy and radiation therapy, Kronowitz and colleagues showed that immediate repair of partial mastectomy defects with local tissues results in fewer complications (23% vs. 67%) and better aesthetic outcomes (57% vs. 33%) than that with a latissimus dorsi flap, which some surgeons used for delayed reconstructions (8,9).

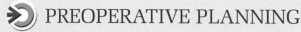

PREOPERATIVE PLANNING

General

Patients should undergo standard preoperative history and physical, with the elements of gynecologic, family, and social history including smoking emphasized. Special attention should be given to any prior breast surgical history, including the placement of breast implants. Preoperative laboratory work, such as complete blood cell count, comprehensive metabolic panel including liver function tests, and tumor markers are generally obtained as initial staging tests, as is a two-view chest radiograph. Core biopsy should be performed and conclusive proof of malignancy documented, with mandatory internal review of all external pathology slides required at our institution.

Imaging

Patients being considered for oncoplastic lumpectomy should undergo a standard preoperative breast imaging workup, which typically includes some combination of mammography, ultrasound, and in selected circumstances breast magnetic resonance imaging (MRI). Although mammography may underestimate the extent of ductal carcinoma in situ (DCIS) by as much as 1 to 2 cm, especially when the fine, granular microcalcifications generally seen with DCIS are present, it is still warranted and is often the initial diagnostic study (10).

Although controversial, the use of MRI may contribute greatly to the surgeon's ability to preoperatively determine the extent of disease present, especially for more mammographically subtle or occult cancers. Compared with mammographic and ultrasound images, the extent of disease seen on MRI may correlate best with the extent of tumor found at pathologic evaluation. In addition, MRI has the lowest false-negative rate in detecting invasive lobular carcinoma (11). Although its sensitivity for detection of invasive breast cancer is high, MRI unfortunately has a low specificity of 67.7% in the diagnosis of breast cancer before biopsy (12). Up to one-third of MRI studies will show some area of enhancement that needs further assessment that ultimately proves to be histologically benign breast tissue (3). A consensus statement from the American Society of Breast Surgeons updated in 2007 supports the use of MRI for determining ipsilateral tumor extent or the presence of contralateral disease, in patients with a proven breast cancer (especially those with invasive lobular carcinoma) when dense breast tissue precludes an accurate mammographic assessment (13). For cancers containing both invasive and noninvasive components, a combination of imaging methods (mammography with magnification views, ultrasonography, and/or MRI) may yield the best estimate of overall tumor size (14).

Preoperative Wire Localization

Once a patient commits to breast conservation, decisions regarding the use of preoperative wire localization for nonpalpable malignancies must be made. In planning oncoplastic resections, the surgeon needs to accurately identify the area requiring removal. Silverstein and colleagues (15) previously suggested the preoperative placement of 2 to 4 bracketing wires to delineate the boundaries of a single lesion. In a study by Liberman and colleagues, wire bracketing of 42 lesions allowed for complete removal of suspicious calcifications in 34 (81.0%) (16). It has been suggested that single wire localization of large breast lesions is more likely to result in positive margins, because the surgeon lacks landmarks to determine where the true boundaries of nonpalpable disease are located. For such scenarios, multiple bracketing wires may assist the surgeon in achieving complete excision at the initial intervention.

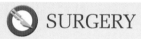 SURGERY

Relevant Anatomy

A comprehensive understanding of normal ductal anatomy, as well as its influence on the distribution of cancer in the breast, is critical to planning an oncoplastic partial mastectomy (3,6). The modern anatomic analysis of ductal anatomy suggests that the number of major ductal systems is probably fewer than 10 (17). The size of ductal segments is variable and while some ducts pass radially from the nipple to the periphery of the breast, others travel directly back from the nipple toward the chest wall (see Fig. 6.1A and B). In contrast, the well-collateralized breast vasculature allows the surgeon to remodel large amounts of fibroglandular tissue within the skin envelope without a major risk of breast devascularization and/or necrosis. The most common source of arterial blood supply in the human breast arises from the axillary and internal mammary arteries (see Fig. 25.2B). By maintaining communication with one of these two arterial connections and by limiting the degree of dissection between the fibroglandular tissue and skin, an adequate blood supply for the breast parenchyma is maintained during tissue advancement and mastopexy closure.

Preoperative Marking

Before the procedure, skin landmarks should be marked with the patient in the upright, sitting position. Relevant landmarks to be identified include the inframammary crease, the anterior axillary fold at the pectoralis major muscle, the posterior axillary fold of the latissimus dorsi muscle, the sternal border of the breast, and the periareolar circle. Identifying these entities with the patient in the upright position is very important to the final cosmetic outcome, because these anatomic sites may prove challenging to accurately locate once the patient is anesthetized and lying supine on the operating room table (Fig. 24.1A and B).

Positioning

For all oncoplastic techniques, the patient should be supine on the operating room table, with the arms abducted and secured. It is preferable to have both breasts prepped

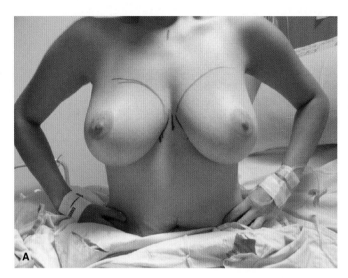
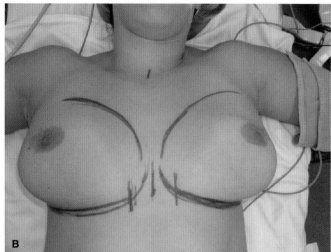

Figure 24.1 Preoperative **(A)** and intraoperative **(B)** view of breasts illustrating the value of preoperative marking with the patient in the upright position. Natural skin creases useful for planning operative incisions are easily seen with the patient upright but can be difficult to locate definitively when the patient lies supine.

and draped into the field so that visual comparison with the patient in a beach chair position is possible as the wound is closed. Such an approach allows the surgeon to identify any areas of unnecessary tugging or dimpling, which are inadvertently created so that they can be corrected.

Description of Individual Oncoplastic Techniques

Parallelogram Mastopexy Lumpectomy (Figs. 24.2 and 24.3)

This technique involves removal of the island of skin that is located directly superficial to the area of known disease. The parallelogram shape, when properly proportioned, guarantees that the two skin edges that are reapproximated at closure will be equidistant. This approach is most commonly used for superior pole or lateral cancers, with the skin incision lines designed to follow Kraissl lines, which follow the natural skin wrinkles and are generally oriented horizontally on the skin (18). The parallelogram incision allows for greater glandular exposure than the typical curvilinear incision of the traditional lumpectomy, while skin island excision avoids excessive, redundant skin from being left behind after excision. For lesions located in the upper inner quadrant, skin island excisions should be small, or the resection should be performed using a simple reapproximation of breast tissue and skin without removal of a skin island (19).

Incision

A rounded parallelogram with two equal length lines is drawn, thus marking the skin island to be excised in conjunction with the underlying target lesion and surrounding tissues (Figs. 24.2A and 24.3A). The width of the skin parallelogram can be used to estimate the distance by which the NAC will shift toward the resection after skin closure. For lesions in the upper breast, incisions should be curvilinear, following the horizontal skin creases, also called Kraissl lines (Fig. 24.2A), while for those located within the lower breast, including the 3 o'clock and 9 o'clock positions, the parallelogram is placed radially and best referred to as a "lateral segmentectomy" (Fig. 24.3). At the corner of the parallelogram, which comes closest to the nipple, the design can be positioned such that the closed incision after resection will approach the NAC tangential to the periareolar line (Fig. 24.3A). This reduces deviation of the NAC towards the lesion, a condition that can result from scar contraction. This radial approach gives more projection to the nipple, avoiding the downward-displacement that can be caused by a purely horizontal scar.

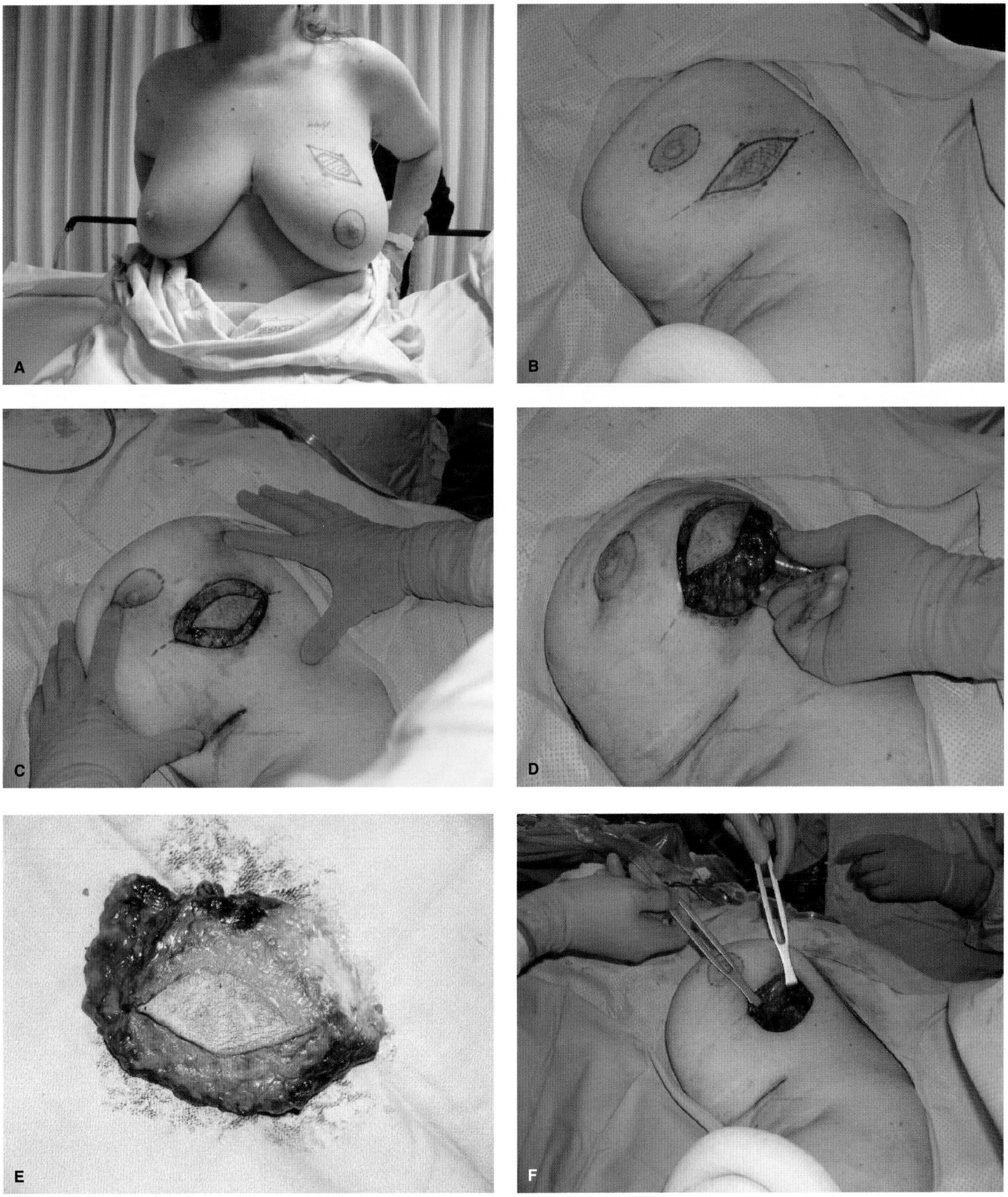

Figure 24.2 Parallelogram partial mastectomy, upper pole cancer preoperative, and intraoperative images. **A.** Preoperative target marking and placement of parallelogram. **B.** Intraoperative marking with patient in supine position. **C.** Initial skin incision revealing wide exposure over target lesion. **D.** Full-thickness dissection posteriorly to chest wall to facilitate delivery of target lesion. **E.** Inked resected specimen. **F.** Deep fibroglandular closure using mastopexy advancement technique to close breast tissue over exposed muscle. **G.** Final wound closure. (*continued*)

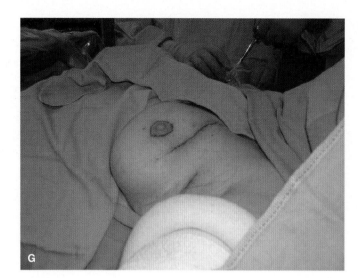

Figure 24.2 (*Continued*)

Dissection

After excision of the skin island, short-distance mastectomy-type skin flaps are raised along both sides of the wound. The dissection is carried down to the chest wall, and the breast gland is lifted off the pectoralis muscle (Fig. 24.2D), and a standard tumor resection is then performed (Figs. 24.2E and 24.3B). After full-thickness excision of the tumor, and before mastopexy closure, 4 to 6 marking clips are typically placed at the base of the defect within the surrounding fibroglandular tissue. A small drain may also be placed in the lumpectomy wound in cases where the dissection is more extensive. For adequate evaluation of margin status by the pathologist, sharp rather than cautery dissection should be considered, as sharp dissection will not alter the histological margins of the resected tissues with so-called cautery effect. Larger intraparenchymal vessels can be ligated or coagulated during the dissection and cautery can then be used on the exposed fibroglandular tissue faces to control bleeding.

Mastopexy Closure

Once all tissues are resected and hemostasis obtained, the fibroglandular tissue at the level of the pectoralis fascia is undermined so that breast tissue advancement can be performed over the muscle (Fig. 24.4). Once the fibroglandular tissues are sufficiently mobilized and hemostasis is confirmed, the margins of the residual cavity are shifted together by the advancement of breast tissue over muscle and the defect is sutured at the deepest edges by using 3-0 absorbable suture. The direction of tissue advancement can be adjusted depending on the location of the fibroglandular defect and the excess tissue that can be shifted to close it. In some cases, fatty tissue from the lateral breast can be shifted medially with relatively little tissue loss being notable postoperatively. The goal of the mastopexy is to perform as complete of a closure over the pectoralis muscle as possible to discourage communication between the anterior skin and the deeper tissues. The superficial tissue layer is next closed with interrupted subdermal 3-0 absorbable suture, whereas the skin is closed by 4-0 absorbable subcuticular sutures in routine fashion (Figs. 24.2G and 24.3C). Typically, the cavity between the deep and superficial layer will be filled by seroma, which will reabsorb during radiotherapy.

Batwing Mastopexy Lumpectomy (Fig. 24.5)

For cancers adjacent to or deep to the NAC, but without direct involvement of the nipple, lumpectomy can successfully be performed without sacrifice of the nipple itself. The batwing approach preserves the viability of the NAC while preserving the breast mound by using mastopexy closure to close the resulting fibroglandular defect of the full-thickness resection. This procedure may result in lifting of the nipple into the upper breast, and a contralateral lift may need to be performed to achieve symmetry.

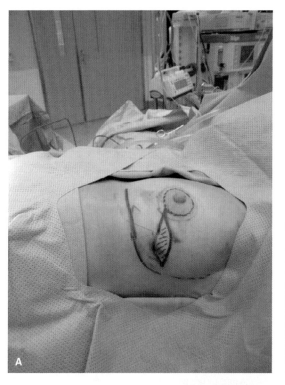

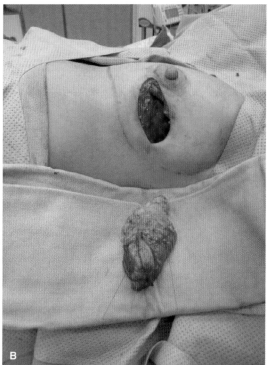

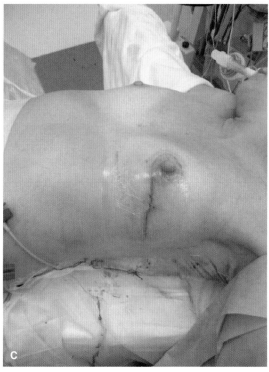

Figure 24.3 Parallelogram partial mastectomy, lateral segment ("lateral segmentectomy"), preoperative, and intraoperative images. **A.** Intraoperative marking with patient in supine position demonstrating the tangential approach of the parallelogram skin marking to the nipple–areolar complex. **B.** Full-thickness fibroglandular resection. **C.** Final skin closure.

Incision

Two similar semicircle incisions are made with angled "wings" on each side of the areola (Fig. 24.5A and B). The two half-circles are positioned so as to allow them to be reapproximated to each other at wound closure. Removal of these skin wings allows the two semicircles to be shifted together without creating redundant skin folds at closure.

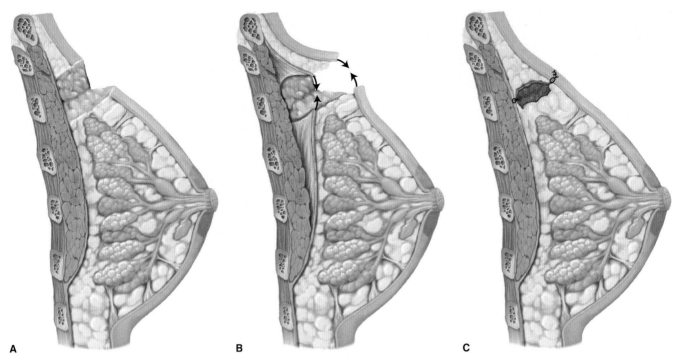

A   **B**   **C**

Figure 24.4 Mastopexy fibroglandular flap advancement closure. **A.** Full-thickness tissue resection completed. **B.** Fibroglandular tissue elevated off chest wall in preparation for mastopexy closure. **C.** Flap advancement and closure of breast tissue at chest wall and final skin closure, leaving small cavity for transient seroma formation that will resolve during radiation therapy.

Dissection

Fibroglandular tissue dissection is carried down deep to the known cancer, with the depth in relation to the chest wall dictated by the position of the lesion within the breast. In most situations, the dissection is carried down to the chest wall and the breast gland is lifted off the pectoralis muscle in a fashion similar to that for the parallelogram lumpectomy (Figs. 24.5C, also shown in Fig. 24.4A and B). The principles of sharp dissection and the placement of marking clips are the same as those of parallelogram mastopexy lumpectomy.

Mastopexy Closure

Following full-thickness resection of the target, some mobilization of the fibroglandular tissue for mastopexy closure may be required. The breast tissue is elevated off of the chest wall at the plane between the pectoralis muscle and breast gland, and the fibroglandular tissue is then advanced to close the resulting defect. The deepest parts are approximated by interrupted sutures (Fig. 24.5D). We typically secure the fibroglandular tissue to itself and do not place anchoring stitches into the chest wall, thereby allowing the approximated breast tissues to move on the chest wall and adjust to find its most natural way to settle in for final healing. The superficial layer is then closed in the same fashion as the parallelogram mastopexy lumpectomy. As this procedure can cause some lifting of the nipple, it may create asymmetry compared with the noncancerous breast. If desired, a contralateral lift can be performed afterward adjuvant radiation has been completed and the treated breast has "declared" its new size and shape to achieve symmetry.

Donut Mastopexy Lumpectomy (Fig. 24.6)

For segmentally distributed cancers that are located in the upper or lateral breast, the donut mastopexy lumpectomy can be used to achieve effective resection of long, narrow segments of breast tissue. The donut mastopexy avoids a visible long radial scar,

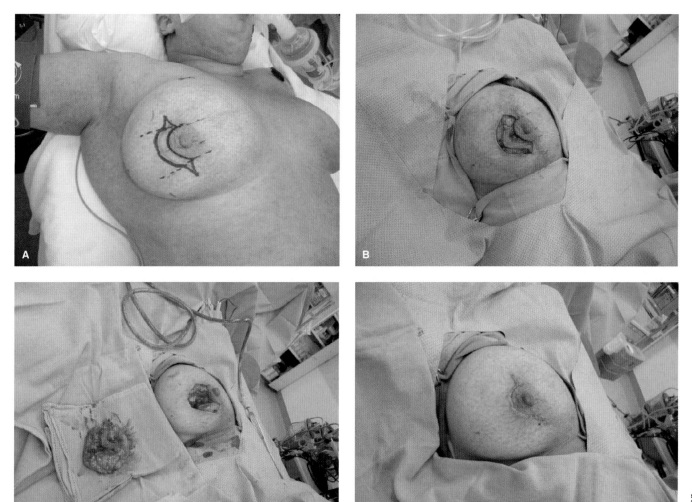

Figure 24.5 Batwing mastopexy lumpectomy for laterally oriented central (periareolar) breast cancer. **A.** Preoperative marking including placement of parallel arcs and wings. **B.** Initial skin incision. **C.** Full-thickness fibroglandular resection down to chest wall with superior-to-inferior mastopexy closure. **D.** Final skin closure.

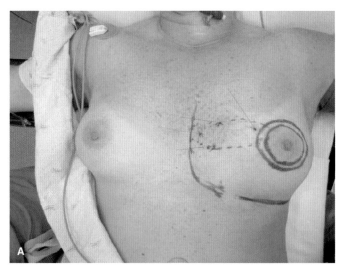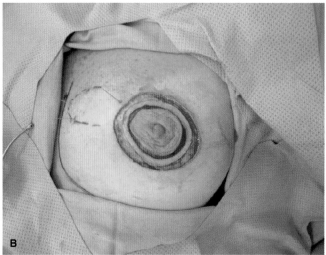

Figure 24.6 Donut mastopexy lumpectomy, medial breast lesion. **A.** Preoperative marking including marking of region to be removed based on preoperative bracketing wires and concentric circles for skin donut excision. **B.** Initial skin incision. (*continued*)

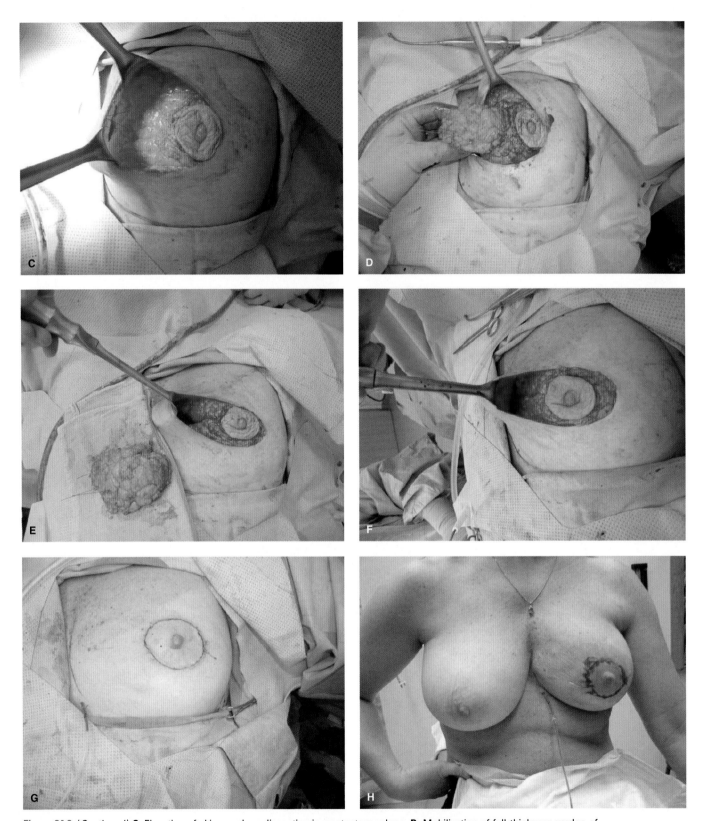

Figure 24.6 (*Continued*) **C.** Elevation of skin envelope dissecting in mastectomy plane. **D.** Mobilization of full-thickness wedge of disease-bearing fibroglandular tissue. **E.** Excised specimen and resulting fibroglandular defect. **F.** Mastopexy closure. **G.** Skin closure. **H.** Postoperative result.

which is against the Kraissl line or Langer line. In this procedure, two concentric lines are placed around the areola and a periareolar "donut" skin island is excised, with only a periareolar scar visible after this operation.

Incision

Two concentric lines are placed around the areola, and a "donut" skin island is excised (Fig. 24.6A and B). Deepithelialization by separating this skin island from the underlying tissues is done next, taking care to avoid full devascularization of the areolar skin. The width of the "donut" skin island should be approximately 1 cm but is somewhat dependant on the size of areola and expected extent of excision. Removal of this tissue ring is required, as it allows both for adequate access and exposure to the breast tissue and for closure of the skin envelope around the remaining fibroglandular tissue that will reduce tissue volume overall.

Dissection

A skin envelope is created in all directions around the NAC. The quadrant of breast tissue containing the target lesion is fully exposed utilizing the same dissection used for a skin-sparing mastectomy (Fig. 24.6C). The full-thickness breast gland is then separated from the underlying pectoralis muscle and delivered through the circumareolar incision (Fig. 24.6D). The segment of breast tissue with the tumor is resected in a wedge-shaped fashion (Fig. 24.6E), with the width of tissue excision required to achieve adequate surgical margins balanced against the difficulty that will be created by virtue of an oversized segmental defect.

Mastopexy Closure

The remaining fibroglandular tissue is returned to the skin envelope and the peripheral apical corners of the fibroglandular tissue are secured to each other and then anchored to the chest wall (Fig. 24.6F). This anchoring maintains proper orientation of the mobilized fibroglandular tissue within the skin envelope during the initial phases of healing. A purse string using absorbable 3-0 suture is placed around the areola opening and is clamped, but not tied, at a size that reapproximates the original NAC (Fig. 24.6G). Interrupted inverted 3-0 absorbable sutures are placed subdermally around the NAC, at which time the purse string suture is tied and then 4-0 subcuticular sutures are used to close the wound. Uplifting of the NAC may create mild asymmetry in comparison with the untreated breast (Fig. 24.6H). If desired, a contralateral lift can be performed to achieve symmetry.

Reduction Mastopexy Lumpectomy (Fig. 24.7)

Initially used in women with macromastia and excessive breast ptosis, this procedure is best used for resection of lesions in the lower hemisphere of the breast between the 4 o'clock to 8 o'clock positions. For cancers in the lower pole of the breast, traditional lumpectomy using circumareolar incision may result in unacceptable down-turning of the nipple due to scar contracture after radiotherapy. This unpleasant cosmetic outcome can be prevented by using the technique of reduction mastopexy lumpectomy.

Incision

A reduction mammoplasty keyhole pattern incision is made (Fig. 24.7A and B), and the skin above the areola is deepithelialized in preparation for skin closure.

Dissection

A superior pedicle flap is created by inframammary incision and undermining of the breast tissue off the pectoral fascia to mobilize the NAC and underlying tissues. Mobilization of the breast tissue allows palpation of both the deep and superficial surfaces

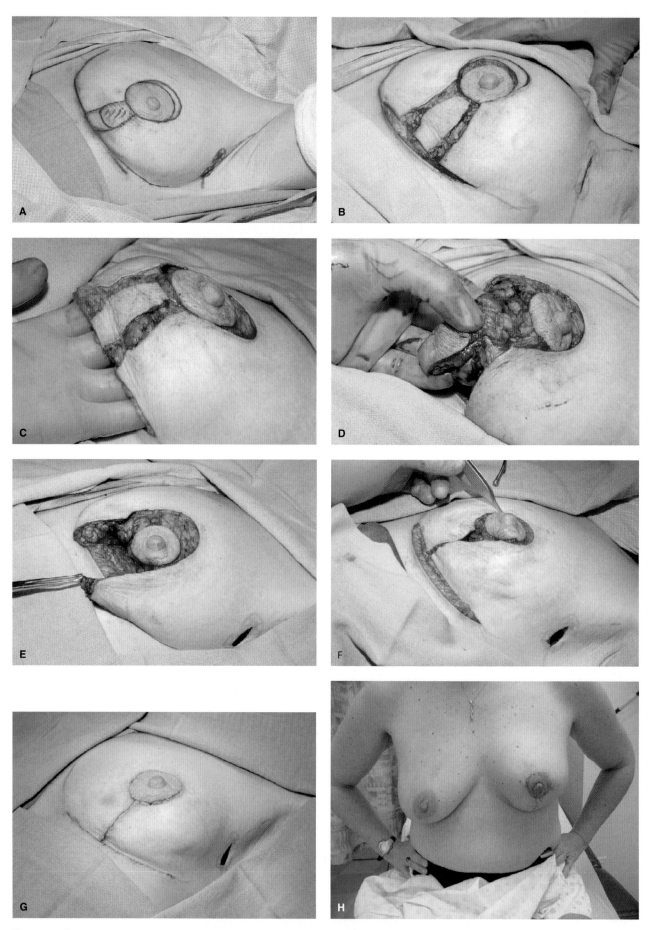

Figure 24.7 Reduction mastopexy lumpectomy. **A.** Skin incision design showing keyhole incision pattern. **B.** Initial skin incision. **C.** Manual examination of dissected tissues facilitating excision of specimen. **D.** Specimen excision. **E.** Fibroglandular defect after specimen excision. **F.** Wound approximation. **G.** Final wound closure. **H.** Postoperative result (previously published).

of the tumor, which can aid the surgeon in determining the lateral margins of excision around the target lesion (Fig. 24.7C). For cancers located in the inferolateral or inferomedial quadrants, the keyhole pattern can be rotated slightly to allow for a more lateral or medial excision, while at the same time, the NAC is moved in a direction opposite to that of the surgical defect (20). Commencing inferiorly and proceeding superiorly beneath the tumor, full-thickness excision of the lesion is completed (Fig. 24.7D and E), with at least a 1 cm macroscopic margin of normal tissue and the skin overlying the lesion being removed. The principle of sharp dissection and the placement of marking clips are the same as those of parallelogram mastopexy lumpectomy.

Mastopexy Closure

Recentralization of the NAC is performed to recreate a harmonious breast size and shape. The medial and lateral breast flaps are undermined and sutured together to fill the excision defect, leaving a typical inverted-T scar (Fig. 24.7F). Uplifting of the NAC by virtue of removal of the skin island superior to it helps restore a youthful appearance to the breast but can create mild asymmetry in comparison with the contralateral breast (Fig. 24.7G). For patients with macromastia, consistent positioning of the breast for radiotherapy may be difficult, resulting in dosing inhomogeneity and suboptimal treatment (20). These patients can benefit from reduction mastopexy lumpectomy using a unilateral or bilateral approach.

Central Lumpectomy (Fig. 24.8)

For cancers involving the NAC, or for Paget disease of the nipple, the cosmetic impact of a central lumpectomy, with concurrent nipple removal, likely accounts for the common use of mastectomy in this situation. While central lumpectomy removes the NAC

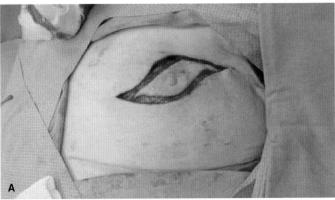

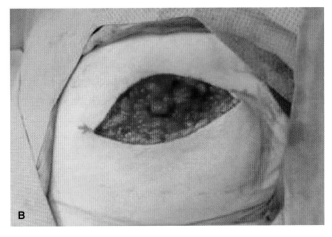

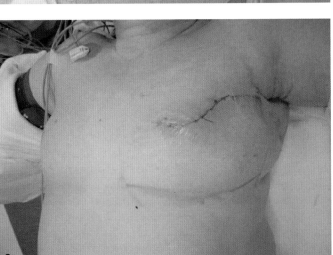

Figure 24.8 Central lumpectomy. **A.** Parallelogram incision for central mastectomy. **B.** Completed central mastectomy. **C.** Closure of central mastectomy using parallelogram incision.

Part VII: Breast Reconstruction

and underlying central tissues, it typically leaves behind a significant breast mound. The cosmetic outcome with central lumpectomy can range from good to outstanding, depending on the woman's body habitus, and is likely to be better tolerated than reconstruction of an entire breast (3). The central lumpectomy can be particularly valuable in women with large breasts where loss of the entire breast with mastectomy may create prominent asymmetry.

Incision

In central lumpectomy, the incision can be made in the pattern of a large parallelogram, which encompasses the entire NAC (Fig. 24.8A).

Dissection and Mastopexy

The operative procedures and principles are the same as those of the parallelogram mastopexy lumpectomy (Fig. 24.8B and C). Mastopexy closure is performed as needed.

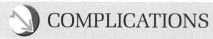

PEARLS AND PITFALLS

■ In oncoplastic surgery, very large areas of breast can be removed as long as the blood supply that enters at the level of the skin is preserved. Care should be taken especially to preserve the perforators medially as they are easily damaged as they can be quite medial (see Fig. 25.2B). Making the flap a bit thicker as one nears the chest wall is helpful.

■ A specimen radiograph is mandatory especially if one is removing calcifications to determine the success of complete removal. Although specimen radiograph is not completely accurate at accessing complete removal, it is very accurate in determining whether complete removal has not been achieved as is the case if calcification is seen on the edge of the specimen.

■ Multicolored ink should be used to label the specimen ideally before it leaves the operating field. All margins—superior, inferior, medial, lateral, anterior, and posterior—should be marked. If the pathologist prefers to perform the inking process then the surgeon should at the very least mark and orient the specimen with suture, clips, or tags.

POSTOPERATIVE MANAGEMENT

Drains are rarely required in standard partial mastectomy cases, as any seroma will generally be reabsorbed. With more extensive dissections, such as the donut mastopexy lumpectomy, fluid accumulation can become more pronounced and may require postoperative aspiration on occasion. In recent years, we have started to place small, 15-F drains overnight to avoid excessive fluid accumulation in the dissected breast that might distort the oncoplastic closure. These drains are typically removed either prior to discharge or on postoperative day one in the clinic.

COMPLICATIONS

When using oncoplastic approaches, surgeons without formal plastic surgery training must determine which procedures they are comfortable performing without plastic surgery consultation or intraoperative collaboration (3). Wound infection, fat necrosis, and delayed healing in the more advanced reduction mastopexy lumpectomy are all potential, reported complications (21). The blood supply of the external nipple arises from underlying fibroglandular tissue by using major lactiferous sinuses rather than the collateral circulation from surrounding areolar skin, so nipple necrosis may occur if dissection extends high up behind the nipple (3).

RESULTS

The main goal of oncoplastic lumpectomy remains negative surgical margin resection. Complete excision of calcified lesions and masses should be confirmed with specimen radiography during surgery (Fig. 24.9A). Additional oriented margins can be resected prior to mastopexy closure when the radiograph suggests inadequate resection may have occurred, hopefully eliminating the need for a delayed reexcision. While some centers utilize intraoperative analysis with frozen section to aid in decisions regarding the resection of additional segments of tissue, it is not our policy.

Multicolored inking can help orient the specimen and is best performed by the operating surgeon. Inking kits are now available with six colors (black, blue, yellow, green, orange, and red), which are very useful for labeling all of the surgical margins (superior, inferior, medial, lateral, superficial, and deep) (Fig. 24.9B). Clear uniformity between surgeon and pathologist in terms of what color means what margin is required.

Although the historic gold standard for negative surgical margin has been 10 mm, what constitutes a true "negative margin" varies widely from center to center, with 3 mm or greater accepted at our institution. Low local recurrence rates after breast conservation therapy, especially in the era of postlumpectomy irradiation, can be achieved with intermediate surgical margin width between 1 and 10 mm (1,2). If reexcision is needed for inadequate surgical margins following the initial resection, both the surgical approach and timing of the operation must be considered (3). In most instances, use of the same incision is feasible and preferred. When the positive margin involves a minority of the specimen, the entire biopsy cavity does not need to be reexcised. If reexcision is delayed for 3 to 4 weeks, the previous seroma cavity may be nearly reabsorbed, which leaves a fibrous biopsy cavity that can be easily located by intraoperative palpation. With noninvasive cancer, Silverstein (15) has suggested that it is feasible to delay reexcision for up to 3 months, at which point the seroma cavity has been fully reabsorbed.

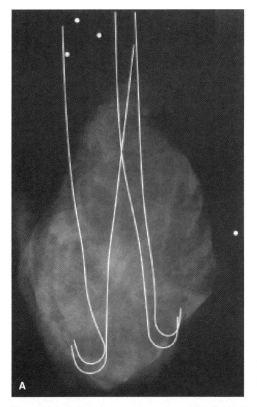
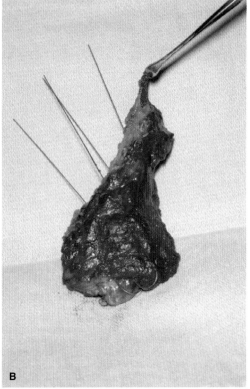

Figure 24.9 A. Specimen radiograph and **(B)** final inking illustrating the bracketing wire technique for breast cancer localization.

Part VII: Breast Reconstruction

When all the margins of resection are positive, mastectomy may be needed to attain satisfactory surgical clearance. In this instance, it may be technically challenging to include both the initial oncoplastic incision, and the NAC in a subsequent total mastectomy and consultation with the plastic surgeon in the event of immediate postmastectomy reconstruction is mandatory.

Although large studies of long-term outcomes specifically addressing oncoplastic approaches in breast conservation are lacking, the few available results are promising. One investigation from Europe followed 148 women for a median of 74 months (range 10–108 months) and only 2 were lost to follow-up. Among the 146 individuals available for analysis, there were only 5 (3%) women who suffered an ipsilateral in-breast cancer recurrence after 5 years, and all had either T2 or T3 tumors at presentation. These authors argued that recurrence rates for women with oncoplastic resections and concurrent radiation therapy were comparable to the in-breast recurrence rates reported with standard breast conservation techniques (22). While additional studies are needed, it is reasonable to presume that oncoplastic approaches, which often results in wider margins of resection than the traditional segmental mastectomy, will prove an oncologically sound option for breast conservation therapy.

CONCLUSIONS

Although shown to be a reasonable alternative to mastectomy for the appropriately selected breast cancer patient, traditional "scoop and run" lumpectomy may result in poor cosmesis. Oncoplastic techniques, including the parallelogram mastopexy lumpectomy, batwing mastopexy lumpectomy, donut mastopexy lumpectomy, reduction mastopexy lumpectomy, and central lumpectomy, have been developed to address this issue. By combining tumor removal with breast flap advancements, the oncoplastic approaches allow for wider margins of resection and better breast shape and contour preservation. Candidates are those felt to be standard lumpectomy candidates and include those with no evidence of multicentric disease.

Standard preoperative workup, including dedicated breast imaging, and preoperative wire localization are necessary to aid the surgeon in successful resection. Complications of tissue necrosis are fortunately rare, despite sometimes significant remodeling of the fibroglandular tissues due to the breast's rich blood supply. Outcomes appear at least equivalent to standard breast conservation techniques, although large case series are lacking. Despite this paucity of long-term results, oncoplastic lumpectomy can be learned by individuals familiar with breast surgical techniques and generally results in better cosmesis and equivalent oncologic outcomes.

References

1. Veronesi U, Cascinelli N, Mariani L, et al. Twenty-year follow-up of a randomized study comparing breast-conserving surgery with radical mastectomy for early breast cancer. *N Engl J Med.* 2002;347(16):1227–1232.
2. Fisher B, Anderson S, Bryant J, et al. Twenty-year follow-up of a randomized trial comparing total mastectomy, lumpectomy, and lumpectomy plus irradiation for the treatment of invasive breast cancer. *N Engl J Med.* 2002;347(16):1233–1241.
3. Anderson BO, Masetti R, Silverstein MJ. Oncoplastic approaches to partial mastectomy: an overview of volume-displacement techniques. *Lancet Oncol.* 2005;6(3):145–157.
4. Masetti R, Pirulli PG, Magno S, et al. Oncoplastic techniques in the conservative surgical treatment of breast cancer. *Breast Cancer.* 2000;7(4):276–280.
5. Audretsch WP. Reconstruction of the partial mastectomy defect: classification and method. In: Spear SL, ed. *Surgery of the Breast: Principle and Art.* 2nd ed. Philadelphia, PA: Lippincott Williams & Wilkins; 2006:179–216.
6. Chen CY, Calhoun KE, Masetti R, et al. Oncoplastic breast conserving surgery: a renaissance of anatomically-based surgical technique. *Minerva Chir.* 2006;61(5):421–434.
7. Silverstein MJ. An argument against routine use of radiotherapy for ductal carcinoma in situ. *Oncology (Huntingt).* 2003;17(11):1511–1533, discussion 1533–1534, 1539, 1542 passim.
8. Kronowitz SJ, Feledy JA, Hunt KK, et al. Determining the optimal approach to breast reconstruction after partial mastectomy. *Plast Reconstr Surg.* 2006;117(1):1–11.
9. Nahabedian MY. Determining the optimal approach to breast reconstruction after partial mastectomy: discussion. *Plast Reconstr Surg.* 2006;117(1):12–14.
10. Holland R, Faverly DRG. The local distribution of ductal carcinoma in situ of the breast: whole-organ studies. In: Silverstein MJ, ed. *Ductal Carcinoma in Situ of the Breast.* 2nd ed. Philadelphia, PA: Lippincott Williams & Wilkins; 2002:240–254.
11. Boetes C, Veltman J, van Die L, et al. The role of MRI in invasive lobular carcinoma. *Breast Cancer Res Treat.* 2004;86(1):31–37.
12. Bluemke DA, Gatsonis CA, Chen MH, et al. Magnetic resonance imaging of the breast prior to biopsy. *JAMA.* 2004;292(22):2735–2742.
13. The American Society of Breast Surgeons Consensus Statement: the use of magnetic resonance imaging in breast oncology. Published May 6, 2007. Available at: http://www.breastsurgeons.org/statements.

14. Silverstein MJ, Lagios MD, Recht A, et al. Image-detected breast cancer: state of the art diagnosis and treatment. *J Am Coll Surg.* 2005;201(4):586–597.

15. Silverstein MJ, Larson L, Soni R, et al. Breast biopsy and oncoplastic surgery for the patient with ductal carcinoma in situ: surgical, pathologic, and radiologic issues. In: Silverstein MJ, ed. *Ductal Carcinoma in Situ of the Breast.* 2nd ed. Philadelphia, PA: Lippincott Williams & Wilkins; 2002: 185–204.

16. Liberman L, Kaplan J, Van Zee KJ, et al. Bracketing wires for preoperative breast needle localization. *AJR Am J Roentgenol.* 2001;177(3):565–572.

17. Love SM, Barsky SH. Anatomy of the nipple and breast ducts revisited. *Cancer.* 2004;101(9):1947–1957.

18. Kraissl CJ. The selection of appropriate lines for elective surgical incisions. *Plast Reconstr Surg.* 1951;8(1):1–28.

19. Grisotti A. Conservation treatment of breast cancer: reconstructive problems. In: Spear SL, ed. *Surgery of the Breast: Principles and Art.* Philadelphia, PA: Lippincott-Raven Publishers; 1998:137–153.

20. Masetti R, Di Leone A, Franceschini G, et al. Oncoplastic techniques in the conservative surgical treatment of breast cancer: an overview. *Breast J.* 2006;12(5)(suppl 2):S174–S180.

21. Iwuagwu OC. Additional considerations in the application of oncoplastic approaches. *Lancet Oncol.* 2005;6(6):356.

22. Rietjens M, Urban CA, Rey PC, et al. Long-term oncological results of breast conservation treatment with oncoplastic surgery. *J Breast.* 2007:16;387–395.

Part VII: Breast Reconstruction

25 Total Skin-Sparing Mastectomy

V. Suzanne Klimberg

Introduction

Preservation of the native skin envelope facilitates immediate breast reconstruction (IBR) and has begun a new era in breast reconstruction. The skin-sparing mastectomy (SSM) removes the breast, nipple–areola complex (NAC), previous biopsy incisions, and skin overlying superficial tumors. Toth and Lappert (1) in 1991 were the first to describe the SSM followed by IBR. The most apparent advantage of SSM followed by IBR is the superior aesthetic and cost-effective result compared with either simple mastectomy with IBR or delayed reconstruction (2,3). In addition, this surgical technique is also psychologically beneficial to the patient (4,5).

Gerber and colleagues (6) described the SSM with conservation of the NAC (a subcutaneous mastectomy) to leave a woman with a natural-appearing breast. Petit and colleagues (7) have described technique what is basically a subcutaneous mastectomy followed by intraoperative radiation to the preserved NAC with a very low recurrence rate (1.4%) none of which were in the NAC. The NAC necrosed totally in 3.5% and partially in 5.5% or was removed in 5% of 1,001 reported cases. Twenty-month follow-up demonstrates 96% disease-free survival rate.

The term *total skin-sparing mastectomy (TSSM)* was described by Margulies et al. to denote that the NAC proper was removed but the skin overlying the NAC was spared (8). Other authors describe the procedure as nipple-sparing mastectomy (9). This is a confusing term in that only the skin overlying the nipple proper has been retained. This is considered safe as the cuboidal-lined ducts begin only at approximately 7 mm from the surface of the nipple (10).

There is no long-term follow-up after TSSM. A few small series with short follow-up show the expected safety of TSSM with approximately a 5% partial or full-thickness loss of the NAC skin but a much higher rate (17%–20%) of NAC involvement and elective removal dependent on selection criteria (11).

Sakamoto and colleagues (12) described an endoscopic technique for TSSM. A 52-month follow-up showed no local recurrences in a series of 87 patients. The rate of nipple necrosis among the procedures with nipple coring was statistically higher than that among those without nipple coring (7 of 17, 41% vs. 9 of 72, 13%).

INDICATIONS/CONTRAINDICATIONS

The indications for a TSSM include the following:

- Can include any indication that a simple mastectomy can be performed for (see Simple Mastectomy chapter) as long as the pathological entity does not involve the NAC. This most commonly would involve ductal carcinoma in situ that by review of the pathology and imaging studies does not appear to involve the NAC. In-house review of pathology is important to rule out an invasive component or a significant risk of such a component (high-grade, >2 cm, multicentric) as to warrant a sentinel lymph node. A cytologic diagnosis is not considered sufficient to proceed with mastectomy.
- Prophylactic contralateral simple mastectomy (SM) is indicated for those patients with a high risk of bilaterality (lobular pathology, locally advanced or inflammatory invasive breast cancer, and especially multicentricity).
- Prophylactic bilateral mastectomy can be performed in those with atypia and lobular carcinoma in situ who cannot reliably be screened (difficult mammogram or examination) or in those with a known genetic predisposition to breast cancer.
- Completion mastectomy after a conservative surgery with positive margins
- Completion mastectomy after a local recurrence although prior radiation if administered can cause sufficient skin damage to significantly increase the complication rate and impair the cosmetic result.

Contraindications/Relative Contraindications

Many patient-related risk factors such as smoking, previous irradiation, diabetes, increased body mass index, and large ptotic breast have been found to associate with an increased risk of skin necrosis in SSM.

PREOPERATIVE PLANNING

Preoperative planning of TSSM should include consideration of preexisting incisions, need or risk of resection of the NAC, and removal of the entire breast parenchyma.

Order of Procedures

The radiopharmaceutical is injected into the breast first and blue dye is injected into the arm for axillary reverse mapping (ARM) (see Axillary Reverse Mapping chapter). Blue dye should be avoided in the skin or around the areola in TSSM as it may cause a higher incidence of skin loss when doing so. The sentinel lymph node biopsy is then performed (see Sentinel Lymph Node Biopsy chapter) first but if one wants to avoid, a separate incision can be done through the same incision as the TSSM but with much greater difficulty and delay in the results of the SLN intraoperatively and whether or not the patient requires an ALND (Fig. 25.1).

SURGERY

Relevant Anatomy

Figure 25.2A demonstrates the limits of a simple mastectomy that run from the second to third rib superiorly down to the insertion of the rectus and medially to the sternum and lateral to the mid axillary line. Figure 2B demonstrates the blood supply to the skin of the breast. Superiorly the skin is feed by the superficial cervical artery, laterally by the lateral thoracic vessels, medially by the perforators from the internal mammary vessels, and inferiorly from branches of the superficial epigastric and vessels extending from the medial and lateral blood supply.

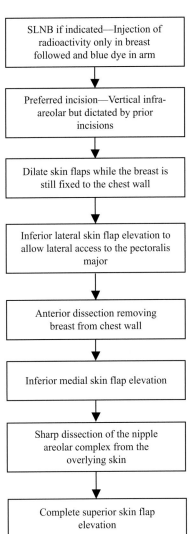

SLNB if indicated—Injection of radioactivity only in breast followed and blue dye in arm

↓

Preferred incision—Vertical infra-areolar but dictated by prior incisions

↓

Dilate skin flaps while the breast is still fixed to the chest wall

↓

Inferior lateral skin flap elevation to allow lateral access to the pectoralis major

↓

Anterior dissection removing breast from chest wall

↓

Inferior medial skin flap elevation

↓

Sharp dissection of the nipple areolar complex from the overlying skin

↓

Complete superior skin flap elevation

Figure 25.1 Order of procedure for total skin-sparing mastectomy (TSSM).

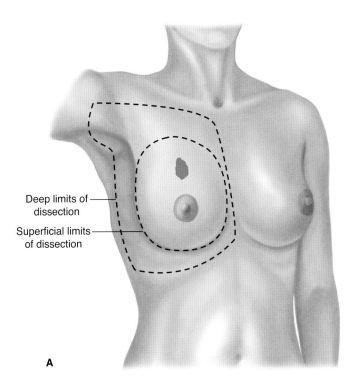

Figure 25.2 A. Borders of breast and limits of dissection for total skin-sparing mastectomy. **B.** Blood supply of the skin of the breast. (*continued*)

Deep limits of dissection

Superficial limits of dissection

A

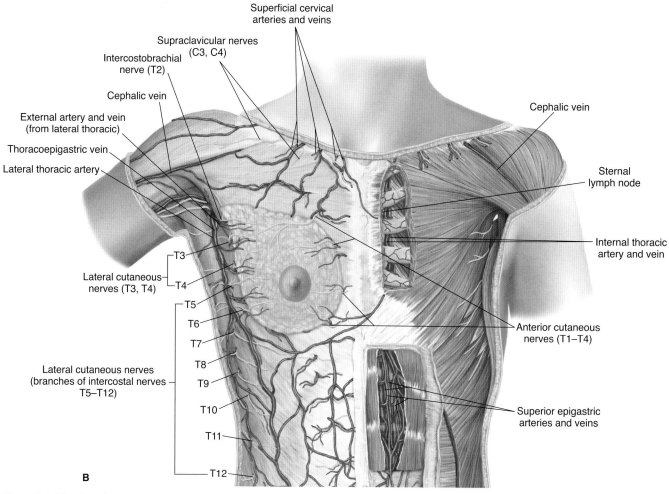

Superficial cervical
arteries and veins

Supraclavicular nerves
(C3, C4)

Intercostobrachial
nerve (T2)

Cephalic vein

External artery and vein
(from lateral thoracic)

Thoracoepigastric vein

Lateral thoracic artery

Lateral cutaneous
nerves (T3, T4)

Lateral cutaneous nerves
(branches of intercostal nerves
T5–T12)

Cephalic vein

Sternal
lymph node

Internal thoracic
artery and vein

Anterior cutaneous
nerves (T1–T4)

Superior epigastric
arteries and veins

T3
T4
T5
T6
T7
T8
T9
T10
T11
T12

B

Figure 25.2 (*Continued*)

Figure 25.3 Anatomy of the breast
and chest wall.

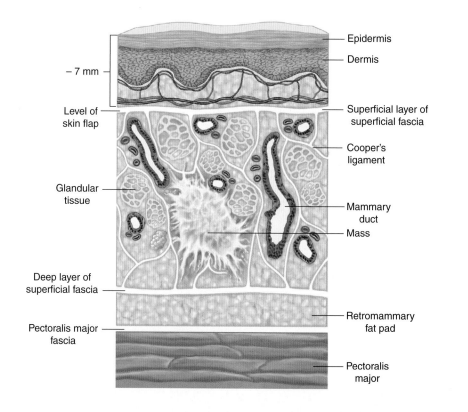

Epidermis

Dermis

– 7 mm

Level of
skin flap

Superficial layer of
superficial fascia

Cooper's
ligament

Glandular
tissue

Mammary
duct

Mass

Deep layer of
superficial fascia

Retromammary
fat pad

Pectoralis major
fascia

Pectoralis
major

Figure 25.3 demonstrates the relevant anatomy of the overlying breast. The cosmetic result of any lumpectomy depends on the depth of the subcutaneous tissue underneath the incision. Thus, if only thin flaps remain after the resection of a superficial tumor and breast, it is best to resect an overlying ellipse of skin. A simple mastectomy also removes the fascia overlying the muscle because the fascia of the breast melds with the fascia of the pectoralis major. Removal of the pectoralis major fascia facilitates as much removal of breast tissue as possible. Complete removal is impossible as some breast tissue intercollates into the muscle itself. If the tumor is deep, muscle may be removed.

The ducts of the breast proper begin approximately 7 mm from the skin surface, thus making it safe to leave the thin skin overlying the nipple proper (10). Rusby et al. have tried to develop a model to predict the risk of nipple areolar involvement and thus recurrence. The percentage of NAC involvement appears to be dependent on the distance from the NAC but also proportional to the depth at which one defines the NAC (13,14) (Fig. 25.4).

Surgical Technique

Anesthesia
Although a simple mastectomy can be performed under local anesthesia, it is rarely if ever necessary and should be performed under general anesthesia. Some have advocated spinal or vertebral block for anesthesia. Significant time preoperatively should be allocated to this endeavor not only by the patient but for coordination of the team effort. The preoperative pain experienced by the patient for the necessary block is the trade-off for avoidance of general anesthesia.

Positioning
The patient is placed supine with the arm extended at right angle with the body positioned as with lumpectomy juxtaposed to the edge of the table for a unilateral mastectomy such that the surgeon and assistant can stand on opposing sides of the arm and assist in surgery. Both breasts should be prepped in the field as a TSSM is almost always done with follow-up reconstruction. The patient should be positioned in the middle of the table for bilateral mastectomies. The arm board should be padded, so the arm is at the level of the body. Too much or too little padding can lead to nerve praxis. For a simple mastectomy, there is no need to drape the lower arm into the field (Fig. 25.5).

Figure 25.4 Anatomy of the nipple. NAC, nipple–areola complex.

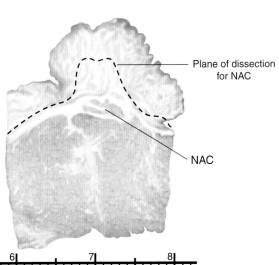

Plane of dissection for NAC

NAC

6   7   8

Part VII: Breast Reconstruction

Figure 25.5 Positioning of the patient for surgeon access above and below the arm.

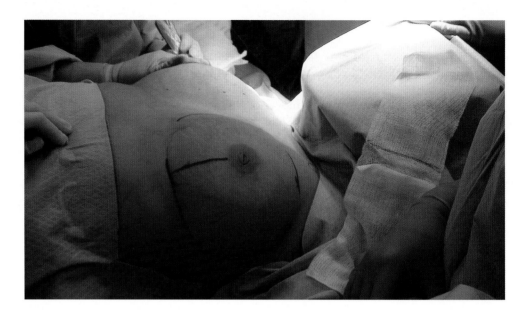

Incision

There is no long-term follow-up on local recurrence after TSSM or comparison or clear consensus in the literature on what is the best incision for TSSM. Several incisions have been described, such as the mastopexy incision, incisions crossing the NAC, radial and the inframammary, (15) axillary approach, and from the previous scar. Figure 25.6A demonstrates the numerous incisions that can be made. Our data demonstrates that the infraareolar vertical incision gives the best cosmetic result and with the least skin flap complications as it retains the most collateral blood supply. At times, other incisions are prudent such as when there is a large preexisting lumpectomy incision. Some surgeons prefer an areolar incision but the loss of the nipple areolar increases with the use of more circumference of the areolar. Figure 25.6B demonstrates the circumference of the breast tissue and a vertical incision to be made, and Figure 25.6C demonstrates the incision down to the level of the subcutaneous tissue.

Dilation of Skin Flaps

Because the plain of dilation of the skin flap can be difficult to effect from a 4 to 6 cm incision, a process of successive dilation has been developed to guide the dissection. Beginning with a 16-F dilator and going as large as a 44-F dilator, this process finds the plain that may differ considerable in thickness dependent on body habitus (Fig. 25.7A–C).

Inferior Lateral Skin Flap Elevation

To gain access to the pectoralis major muscle, the inferior lateral skin flap is elevated first (Fig. 25.8A).

In the average patient, there is approximately 7 mm plane of relatively avascular fat between the skin and the glandular tissue, which is the plane you want to use to develop a flap (Fig. 25.8B). Holes left by the dilation help to guide the plain of dissection. S-retractors are useful to facilitate the initial dissection (Fig. 25.9A, B). The dissection is most easily completed with cutting electrocautery as the heat generated is much less damaging to the flap than that generated by the coagulation mode. Harmonic scalpel may also be used to minimize generated heat and damage but is a slower process. Alternatively, a blade or Mayo scissors may be used. As one approaches the chest wall, the flaps are made a bit thicker to avoid injury to the feeding vessels.

Anterior Dissection

The anterior dissection encompasses removal of the breast from the pectoralis major in continuity with the fascia. Figure 25.10A and B demonstrate the beginning dissection starting from identifying the pectoralis major muscle medially and inferiorly (Fig. 25.10A)

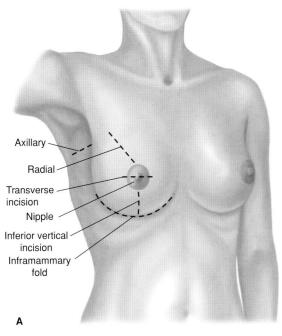

Axillary

Radial

Transverse
incision

Nipple

Inferior vertical
incision
Inframammary
fold

A

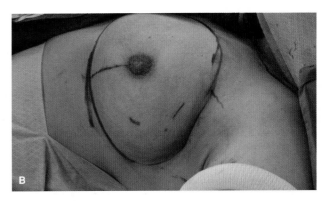

B

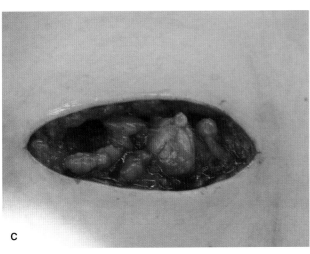

C

Figure 25.6 A. Potential incisions for total skin-sparing mastectomy. **B.** Extent of breast tissue in a patient and where a vertical incision would be made. **C.** Vertical incision in the breast.

and carrying it up superiorly and medially (Fig. 25.10B). As the pectoralis muscle is divested of the breast and its overlying fascia, a C-Strang retractor is ideal to hold up the breast (Fig. 25.11A–C).

Inferior Medial Skin Flap Elevation
The inferior medial skin flap is elevated next (Fig. 25.12A) in a fashion similar to the inferior lateral skin flap, taking care to avoid the medially located internal mammary perforators (Fig. 25.12B).

Dissection of NAC from Overlying Skin
The NAC is removed from its overlying skin next (Fig. 25.13A). A blind blade in the plane of dissection is fast and easy and provides the least trauma (Fig. 25.13B). Figure 25.13C demonstrates the dermis of the undersurface of the nipple.

Superior Skin Flap Elevation
Once the lower hemisphere of the skin flap is free, the skin flap is elevated superiorly to the level of the palpable breast, which is usually the second or third clavicle (Fig. 25.14). A St. Marks retractor can be helpful in reaching the superior pole of the breast in a long thorax.

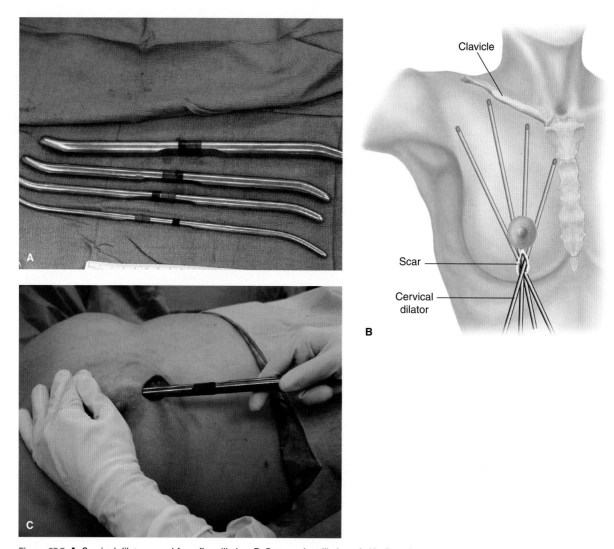

Figure 25.7 **A.** Cervical dilators used from flap dilation. **B.** Progressive dilation of skin flaps for total skin-sparing mastectomy. **C.** Dilation of skin flap with cervical dilator.

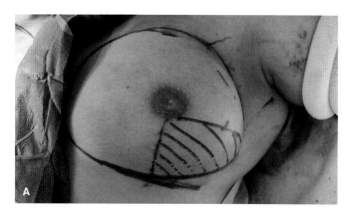

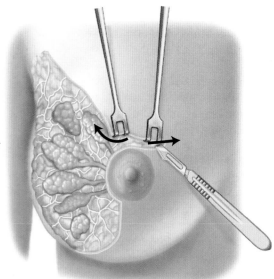

Figure 25.8 **A.** Extent of inferior lateral skin flap. **B.** Plane of skin flap elevation.

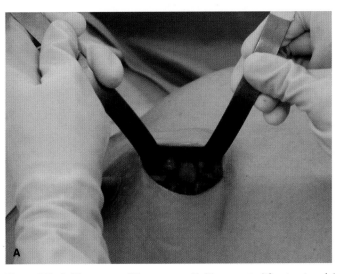

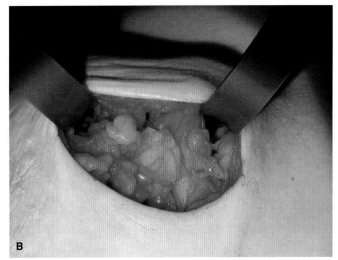

Figure 25.9 **A.** Placement of S-retractors. **B.** Placement of S-retractors (close-up of holes left by dilators).

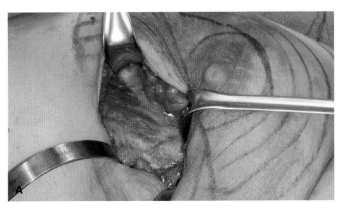

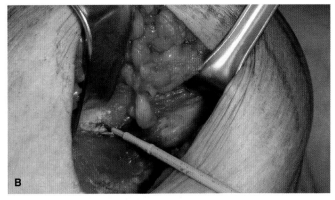

Figure 25.10 **A.** Finding the pectoralis major muscle inferiorly and medially to begin the formal anterior dissection. **B.** Deeper into the anterior dissection removing the breast from the chest wall.

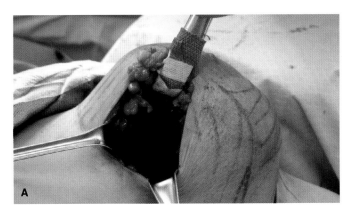

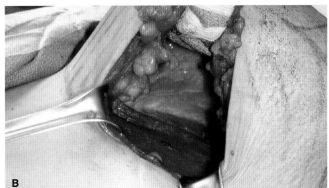

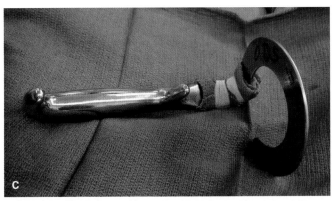

Figure 25.11 **A.** C-Strang retractor to hold up the breast as it is being removed with the addition of appendiceal retractors. **B.** View as anterior dissection is completed added by C-Strang. **C.** C-Strang retractor used for elevation of breast and skin flaps.

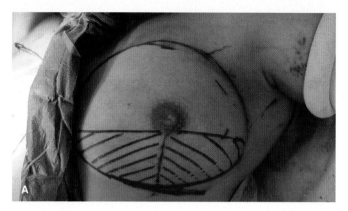

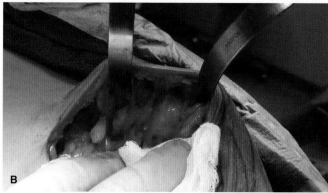

Figure 25.12 **A.** Skin marking demonstrating the plane of the inferior medial skin flap to be elevated. **B.** Elevation of inferior medial skin flap with S-retractors inserted in the holes left by the dilators to guide the plane of dissection.

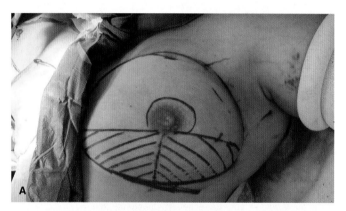

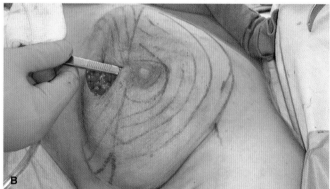

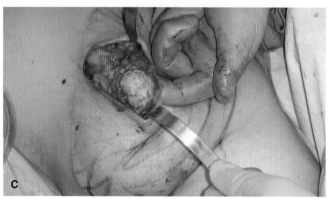

Figure 25.13 **A.** Skin marking demonstrating area to be dissected under the nipple–areola complex (NAC). **B.** Demonstration of sharp dissection of the NAC from the overlying skin. **C.** Everted skin that was overlying the NAC demonstrating complete removal of the NAC.

Figure 25.14 Skin marking demonstrating completion of superior pole skin flaps.

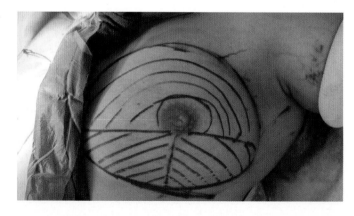

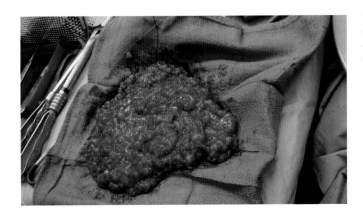

Figure 25.15 Total skin-sparing mastectomy removed specimen demonstrating pathological marking.

Removal of Breast and Pathological Marking

The breast should be oriented for pathology with at least two markings with suture, clips, or tags (Fig. 25.15).

Core of Skin of Nipple Areola

Figure 25.16 demonstrates intraoperative removal of underlying dermis of the nipple to be sent for frozen section intraoperatively. In approximately 20% of all patients, there is involvement of the NAC. In the carefully chosen patient, there is less than 5% involvement.

Completed Dissection

Inspection of this removed breast demonstrates the intact NAC that has been successfully removed from the overlying skin (Fig. 25.17A). Reexcision of the previous scar demonstrates the site of the prior cancer after failed lumpectomy. Figure 25.17B demonstrates the healthy viable freed skin envelope after removal of the breast and NAC (Fig. 25.17B).

One should reexcise scars where positive margins have exited, also margins of tissue superficial to the tumor location and blind margins around the cavity are at times helpful but not mandatory.

Irrigation/Packing of Wound

The wound is thoroughly irrigated to remove devascularized fatty tissue. Water and hydrogen peroxide are used for irrigation reasoning that tumor cells, if present, will be removed or osmotically lysed. The wound is then packed with hot laps to promote hemostasis.

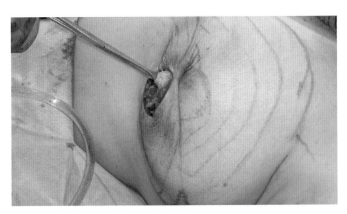

Figure 25.16 Removal of core of nipple to be sent for margin evaluation.

Part VII: Breast Reconstruction

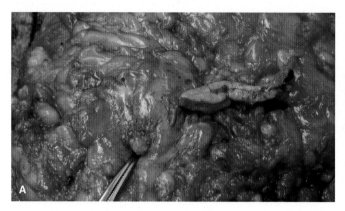 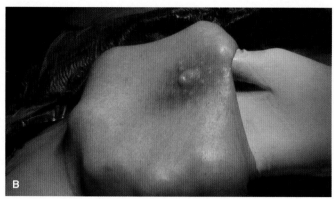

Figure 25.17 A. Delivered mastectomy specimen with visible nipple–areola complex. Pick-ups point to removed nipple. **B.** Viable intact skin envelope after total skin-sparing mastectomy.

Clean Field

Gloves and instruments are changed and the surgical field is completely broken down and redraped. It is thought that blood soaked towels or instruments can possibly seed tumor cells. The wounds are then irrigated again to reduce the risk of infection that for a patient with an implant would mean removal of the device.

Hemostasis

Perfect hemostasis should be achieved especially when using implants to reduce the risk of hematoma. The key in breast surgery is to inspect the wound for cut or torn vessels that are not necessarily bleeding. These vessels will later dilate and potentially cause significant problems.

Procedure with Reconstruction

The pectoralis major muscle is elevated and a two-stage reconstruction is begun via the insertion of an expander, and the muscle is subsequently slowly expanded into the skin envelope. A single-stage reconstruction can be performed by covering an inflated implant medially with pectoralis major muscle and using a lateral "sling" of allodermal or other dermal product (Fig. 25.18) (see Chapter 26, Implant Reconstruction).

Drain Placement

Two drains are used—one in the inferior sulcus and another superiorly lateral.

Closure

Any number of closures are acceptable, so long as a seal is maintained so that the drain will work. A 3.0 running polydioxanone (PDS) with a 4.0 subcuticular stitch is sufficient and fast.

Dressing

Closure of the wound with skin glue allows the patient to shower immediately after surgery and allows complete inspection of the wound for any signs of infection (Fig. 25.19A, B). Pressure dressings or bras do not prevent seromas and can put undue pressure on the skin and cause skin flap compromise.

PEARLS AND PITFALLS

- Attention to a consistent flap—not too thin or too thick is key—the dilation method helps keep this consistency.
- Take care to keep the base of the flaps circumferential a little thicker to avoid removing the blood supply to the flap at the base.

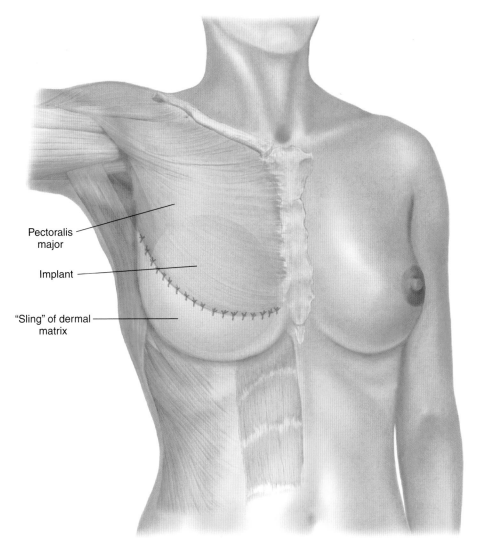

Pectoralis
major

Implant

"Sling" of dermal
matrix

Figure 25.18 Implant under pectoralis major facilitated with a dermal matrix closure.

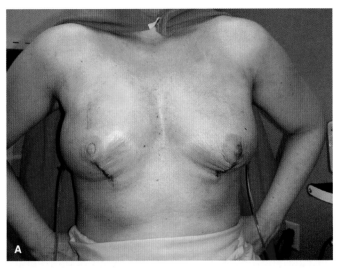

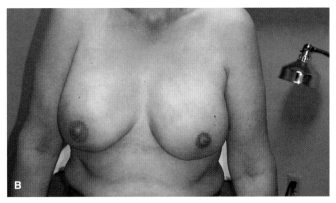

Figure 25.19 A. Total skin-sparing mastectomy (TSSM) with immediate implant reconstruction 1 week postoperation. **B.** Example of long-term result of TSSM with immediate implant reconstruction.

■ The cosmetic result can be decreased by too aggressive removal of fat versus breast tissue, especially superiorly and medially, causing a scalloping of the upper part of the chest and of reducing the cleavage medially.

 # POSTOPERATIVE MANAGEMENT

Postoperative management is identical to that of any partial mastectomy. With the skin glue, patients may shower. There is no need for a pressure dressing, and bras should be avoided in the first postoperative week to avoid undue pressure on the skin flaps and potential for necrosis. Oxygen (2L) is usually continued for the length of the hospital stay, patients are encouraged to use an incentive spirometer, and the hematocrit is kept in the 30 range. All of this is designed to promote the best oxygen tension in the flap.

Patients are usually kept overnight to manage initial pain and hydration until they are able to take food and oral medication. During this time, patients are taught to care for their drains and keep a log of output. Drains are removed when output is less than 30 cc but not before 7 days and not left for more than 10 days. This maintains the lowest seroma rate and the lowest risk of infection. Patients are sent home on oral antibiotics that cover *Staphylococcus* in a particular hospital setting as the risk of infection is low but mandates implant removal most of the time.

 # COMPLICATIONS

Skin Loss

Skin loss is one of the most common complications for a TSSM. The TSSM skin flap should be dissected as thin as possible to remove all glandular breast tissue and avoid residual disease while at the same time, the blood supply to the skin should not be compromised and the perforating arteries should be preserved whenever possible. Dilation helps guide this difficult dissection and helps the operator stay in the correct plane. One can check on the viability of the skin flap by using fluorescein (after a test dose to avoid allergic reaction). A Wood black light lamp intraoperatively should show green viable skin in sharp contrast to dark necrotic areas. The test is not completely reliable but can add information to the decision-making process. If flap necrosis is evident intraoperatively, immediate resection may be best. Postoperatively, allowing the area of necrosis to demarcate may be best, and then remove only the tissue necessary. If the wound is not dry and the potential for infection is high, immediate resection may be best.

Infection

Risk of infection has not been increased in the limited experience with this procedure. Attention to hemostasis, thorough irrigation, and prophylactic antibiotics are critical as an infection in a reconstructed patient often leads to explant of the device.

Hematomas

Hematomas occur less than 1% of the time. A small next-day stable hematoma can be watched but if expanding—the patient should be taken back to the operating room, the hematoma removed, the source subdued, and the wound thoroughly irrigated.

Pneumothorax

This complication is rare but occurs slightly more often when reconstruction is involved.

Positive Margins on Pathology

If margins are close and not in an area where resection is possible, another option would be to add irradiation.

Seroma

Seromas occurs in approximately 30% of patients and feels like ballotable fluid. This may occur secondary to premature removal of the drain or a drain that is not working properly. First, check that the drain has not been sutured in too tightly and obstructed. Strip the drain to make sure a clot has not obstructed the drain. If the drain is not working at all, it should be removed. An ultrasound should be used to detect the seroma, and a 20-gauge butterfly on a 30 to 50 cc syringe is used to drain. The needle is placed at an angle and under ultrasound guidance. The patient will need drainage every 3 to 4 days or at shorter intervals if the accumulation is too rapid. Unaddressed seromas can cause undue tension and flap necrosis. Excessive aspirations in the face of an implant lead to a higher rate of infection and cellulitis. A chronic seroma may need to be opened and the capsule excised or if small left alone.

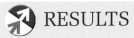 RESULTS

There is limited but favorable reports with TSSM. There is approximately a 10% rate of partial or full-thickness skin loss, especially of the skin overlying the NAC. In the carefully chosen patient, another 5% require removal of the nipple areolar skin because of involvement (6,9,11–13,15,16). Recurrent tumor in the NAC skin is extremely low as most recurrence are near the site of the original tumor. Cosmetic results, when tested, scored on average 8 of 10 for TSSM but surprisingly not that much higher than with SSM or delayed reconstruction (4). Psychological benefits are obvious especially when immediate one-stage reconstruction is performed (4,5).

CONCLUSIONS

TSSM appears to be oncologically safe in patients with disease distant to the NAC and may give superior cosmetic results to traditional skin-sparing incisions.

References

1. Toth BA, Lappert P. Modified skin incisions for mastectomy: the need for plastic surgical input in preoperative planning. *Plast Reconstr Surg.* 1991;87:1048–1053.
2. Elkovitz A, Colen S, Slavin S, et al. Various methods of breast reconstruction after mastectomy: an economic comparison. *Plast Reconstr Surg.* 1993;92(I):77–83.
3. Khoo A, Kroll SS, Reece GP, et al. A comparison of resource costs of immediate and delayed breast reconstruction. *Plast Reconstr Surg.* 1998;101(4):964–968.
4. Rosenqvist S, Sandelin K, Wickman M. Patients' psychological and cosmetic experience after immediate breast reconstruction. *Eur J Surg Oncol.* 1996;22(3):262–266.
5. Al-Ghazal SK, Sully L, Fallowfield L, et al. The psychological impact of immediate rather than delayed reconstruction. *Eur J Surg Oncol.* 2000;26(I):17–19.
6. Gerber B, Krause A, Reimer T, et al. Skin-sparing mastectomy with conservation of the nipple-areola complex and autologous reconstruction is an oncologically safe procedure. *Ann Surg.* 2003;238:120–127.
7. Petit JY, Veronesi U, Orecchia R, et al. Nipple sparing mastectomy with nipple areola intraoperative radiotherapy: one thousand and one cases of a five years experience at the European institute of oncology of Milan (EIO). *Breast Cancer Res Treat.* 2009;117(2):333–338.
8. Margulies AG, Hochberg J, Kepple J, et al. Total skin-sparing mastectomy without preservation of the nipple-areola complex. *Am J Surg.* 2005;190(6):907–912.
9. Crowe JP, Kim JA, Yetman R, et al. Nipple-sparing mastectomy: technique and results of 54 procedures. *Arch Surg.* 2004;139:148–150.
10. Love SM, Barsky SH. Anatomy of the nipple and breast ducts revisited. *Cancer.* 2004;101:1947–1957.

11. Garcia-Etienne CA, Cody Iii HS III, Disa JJ, et al. Nipple-sparing mastectomy: initial experience at the Memorial Sloan-Kettering Cancer Center and a comprehensive review of literature. *Breast J.* 2009;15(4):440–449.

12. Sakamoto N, Fukuma E, Higa K, et al. Early results of an endoscopic nipple-sparing mastectomy for breast cancer. A*nn Surg Oncol.* 2009;16(12):3406–3413.

13. Rusby JE, Brachtel EF, Othus M, et al. Development and validation of a model predictive of occult nipple involvement in women undergoing mastectomy. *Br J Surg.* 2008;95(11):1356–1361.

14. Rusby JE, Brachtel EF, Michaelson JS, et al. Breast duct anatomy in the human nipple: three-dimensional patterns and clinical implications. *Breast Cancer Res Treat.* 2007;106(2): 171–179.

15. Wijayanayagam A, Kumar AS, Foster RD, et al. Optimizing the total skin-sparing mastectomy. *Arch Surg.* 2008;143(1): 38–45.

16. Stolier A, Sullivan S, Dellacroce F. Technical considerations in nipple-sparing mastectomy: 82 consecutive cases without necrosis. *Ann Surg Oncol.* 2008;15:1341–1347.

26 Implant-Based Reconstruction

James C. Yuen

INDICATIONS/CONTRAINDICATIONS

After Standard and Modified Radical Mastectomy

Implant-based breast reconstruction is currently the most common method for breast reconstruction. Implantation of a breast implant under the available soft-tissue is technically the simplest method. However, in most cases of standard mastectomy, this is not appropriate if local soft-tissue coverage is inadequate to allow placement of a permanent implant large enough to match the size of the contralateral breast. With placement of a tissue expander (Fig. 26.1), the soft-tissue envelope can be expanded until the desired volume is reached to match the opposite breast, or in bilateral cases, until the volume is reached to match the patient's desired size. At a second procedure, the expander is exchanged for a permanent implant, saline or gel (currently available cohesive gel implant).

The advantages of implant-based breast reconstruction, especially with a single-stage implant insertion, are obvious. The surgery is localized to the same area, thus avoiding major surgical trauma, complications, and scars to other areas. The surgery does not eliminate the chance for autologous reconstruction if deemed necessary in the future. In a single-stage reconstruction, the procedure and process is relatively simple and completed in a single step, not including any need for nipple reconstruction. In the case of tissue expansion, the procedure is also relatively simple compared with the complexity of autologous reconstruction using pedicled or microvascular flaps. However, in addition to the need for a second operation, there is a major commitment for multiple office visits and a long delay of 3 to 6 months between the two operations. On the other hand, for bilateral cases, the patients can choose to reconstruct neo breasts that are larger than their preexisting breasts. These patients also can decide, to a certain extent, on their final breast size. Therefore, they gain the advantage of a sense of control when their femininity and normal health have been threatened by cancer.

Implant-based reconstruction obviously is much less invasive compared with autologous reconstruction; however, a host of potential immediate and delayed complications are present. In ipsilateral cases, the natural breast will descend with age while the recon-

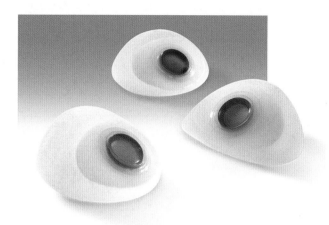

Figure 26.1 Representative samples of tissue expanders. This set is from Mentor: low-height, medium height, and tall height.

structed side remains resistant to gravitational ptosis. In addition, it is generally more difficult to achieve a natural result compared with autologous tissue. After simple mastectomy in a patient with a remaining large breast, the expanded soft tissue may have difficulty producing a well-defined inframammary crease or significant ptosis. Despite these advantages, many patients still choose to undergo implant-based reconstruction for various reasons. This decision may be influenced by surgeon's choice. The patient may wish to avoid major flap reconstruction for concerns of associated complications and longer recovery time. She may not have enough donor tissue, which is more commonly true in bilateral cases.

In the case of the standard mastectomy, especially modified radical mastectomy, insertion of a tissue expander is routinely needed to recruit additional soft tissue by expansion, unless that patient's contralateral breast in relatively small and there is not significant ptosis or atrophy. Expansion is normally performed 2 to 4 weeks after expander insertion and continued serially 1 to 2 weeks apart until desired size, at which point overexpansion is performed up to 20% extra. After an additional waiting period of at least 2 months, the expander is then exchanged for a permanent breast implant (Fig. 26.2). For immediate reconstruction, traditionally, the tissue expander is inserted with elevation of the pectoralis major and origins of the serratus anterior muscles in order to provide complete or near coverage of the prosthetic device. Muscle coverage helps protect the tissue expander under the thin mastectomy skin flap and prevent implant extrusion or exposure in the event of mastectomy skin necrosis or ischemic suture line dehiscence. Muscle turnover flaps and abdominal fasciocutaneous flap advancement have been described for implant coverage and enhanced development of the inferior pole. Single-

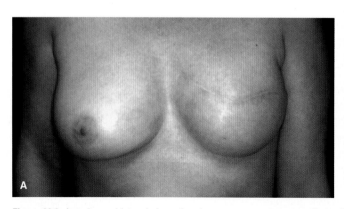
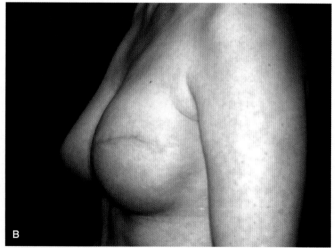

Figure 26.2 Anterior and lateral view of patient status post two-stage immediate reconstruction after left simple mastectomy with initial placement of anatomical tissue expander followed by exchange of expander to permanent saline-filled textured anatomical implant.

stage reconstruction with this modification has been described. The use of the latissimus flap with an implant is not included in this discussion, since this is considered a hybrid technique between autologous and implant-based reconstruction.

For two-stage reconstruction, because of the difficulty in expanding the inferior pole with complete muscle coverage, the technique was modified later to a dual-plane coverage in which only the pectoralis major muscle was raised to cover the upper aspect of the expander. Subpectoral positioning, and not complete muscle coverage, allowed for quicker and less painful surgery and gave rise to better inframammary fold definition. However, the limitations of the dual-plane positioning include less secure coverage of the implant's inferior pole by the mastectomy skin flap. There is also less control over the position of the inframammary fold and possible superior retraction of the pectoralis major muscle postoperatively.

Use of Human Acellular Dermal Matrix

Over the past decade, simultaneously in a multitude of centers, the use of human acellular dermal matrix (HADM) in implant reconstruction emerged seemingly as a revolutionary promising augmentation in nonautologous breast reconstruction. This matrix is used to cover the lower and lower lateral part of the breast implant or tissue expander, while the pectoralis covers the respective upper portion. Several products of human acellular dermal tissue matrix are available: Alloderm (LifeCell Corp., Branching, NJ); AlloMax (CR Bard/Davol Inc., Cranston, RI); DermaMatrix (Synthes Inc., West Chester, PA); FlexHD (Musculoskeletal Transplant Foundation/Ethicon Inc., Somerville, NJ); and NeoForm (Mentor Corp., Santa Barbara, CA). These products are biologically prepared human dermis in which components causing rejection are removed and viral, bacterial, and fungal organisms are tested and removed. Alloderm was the first HADM used, which has been shown to revascularize rapidly with high retention rates. The HADM suspends and stabilizes the implant, while allowing high-volume fill within the implant. The tissue expander is no longer restricted by the tightness of complete muscle coverage. Since the pectoralis major is released along the inframammary crease and there is preservation of natural skin envelope with skin-sparing mastectomy (SSM) or total skin sparing mastectomy (TSSM, also referred to as nipple-sparing mastectomy or NSM), there is greater inferior pole and inframammary crease definition, which is usually difficult to achieve in traditional tissue expansion reconstruction following conventional mastectomy. The HADM provides some support between the implant and the mastectomy skin flap. In the case of SSM or TSSM, because of extra surface area of preserved skin compared with standard mastectomy, there is an associated higher rate of ischemic changes and skin necrosis. When not accompanied by secondary infection, the HADM provides coverage of the underlying prosthetic device, thus increasing the chance of implant retention. The advantages of the acellular dermal allograft are the following:

- Creates a large pocket, confluent with the pectoralis major muscle to accommodate a full permanent implant or a substantially inflated tissue expander
- Allows definition of inframammary and lateral mammary fold
- Provides suspensory support of the implant at the lower pole
- Establishes a protective interface between the prosthetic device and the mastectomy skin flap
- Contributes to thickness of soft tissue over the prosthetic device
- Minimizes or even obviates the need for serial expansion
- Decreases periprosthetic changes, such as soft-tissue atrophy and chest-wall deformity
- By attachment to the lower cut edge of the muscle, it prevents cephalad displacement of pectoralis major muscle

In summary, implant-based reconstruction is indicated for the patient who does not wish to undergo lengthy and complicated autologous reconstruction, who does not wish to take the risks of donor site morbidity, and who will not tolerate prolonged recovery time. However, for implant-based reconstruction to be indicated, the patient has to accept the host of potential complications associated with implantation and she has to accept the staged procedures. In ipsilateral cases, implant reconstruction is indicated only if the patient accepts the potential inherent asymmetry and the need for a contralateral procedure, such as mastopexy or reduction mammoplasty. If the patient cannot accept the implant-related complications and the limitations of asymmetry in ipsilateral cases, or if she will not accept a contralateral procedure to improve symmetry, then implant-based reconstruction is relatively contraindicated, especially if the patient is a candidate for autologous reconstruction. In bilateral or even ipsilateral mastectomy, if the patient does not possess large enough volume of donor tissue for the breast size desired, then implant-based reconstruction is also indicated.

Single-Stage Versus Two-Stage with Tissue Expansion

Indications for single-stage versus tissue expander reconstruction depend on a multitude of variables. With the one-stage procedure in ipsilateral cases of standard mastectomy, the contralateral breast has to be small and cannot exhibit significant ptosis. In bilateral cases of standard mastectomy, if the patient desires small neo breasts, then single-stage reconstruction may be indicated. In moderate-sized breasts, traditional reconstruction using tissue expander with complete muscle coverage or dual-plane positioning would be indicated. With the utilization of HADM, single-stage reconstruction with permanent breast implant insertion has found wider applications, even in the presence of large and ptotic breasts.

After Skin-Sparing and Total Skin-Sparing Mastectomy

Especially, in the case of skin-sparing and nipple-sparing mastectomy, single-stage reconstruction with a permanent breast implant is a viable option. However, if larger breasts are desired, insertion of tissue expanders with HADM would still be indicated. If the patient has large breasts, for example "D" cup, and wishes to maintain a large size, tissue expander reconstruction would afford more control in the final breast size in the patient who does not wish to downsize. Keep in mind that for the patient with massively large breasts (above "D" cup), a skin reduction procedure would likely be indicated. Nipple-sparing (or total skin-sparing mastectomy) would be relatively contraindicated in face of mammary gigantism because the excessively redundant mastectomy skin, void of perforator perfusion from the breast, would be destined for major skin ischemia and necrosis. In addition, the volume of mastectomy skin flap would supersede the sizes of available tissue expanders, leading to unacceptable overhang and wrinkling of skin.

When skin-sparing or nipple-sparing mastectomy is performed, especially in moderate size or large-breasted patients there is a need to fill this empty space beneath the preserved skin flap. Insertion of a large-volume prosthetic device is needed to minimize wrinkling of the overlying skin. The use of HADM is indicated for coverage and stabilization of this large-volume prosthetic device. Alternatively, partial muscle coverage by the pectoralis major only or the addition of a turnover muscle flap are also options in place of HADM. Partial muscle coverage does have its limitations as described earlier, especially in immediate reconstruction where the mastectomy skin flap has inherent ischemia. Muscle turnover flaps require major dissection below the inframammary, which, in skin-sparing or nipple-sparing mastectomy, can render more ischemia to the mastectomy skin flap.

Contraindications for Implant-Based Reconstruction

A definite contraindication for implant reconstruction, as in any type of reconstruction, is advanced local disease and the presence of metastatic disease. Relative contraindications include a history of radiation with this becoming a definite contraindication when there is associated significantly adverse skin damage. Preoperatively, anticipated radiation therapy may be viewed as a relative contraindication for implant-based reconstruction. However, some centers advocate initiation of the required radiation therapy after completion of implant-based reconstruction.

PREOPERATIVE PLANNING

The most important part of preoperative planning is to decide the operation of choice for the patient. First, the surgeon needs to ascertain whether the patient has chosen immediate or delayed reconstruction. The type of mastectomy chosen by the surgical oncologist has to be determined:

- Modified radical mastectomy
- Standard mastectomy (conventional mastectomy)
- Skin-sparing mastectomy
- Total skin-sparing mastectomy (also known as nipple-sparing mastectomy).

If the patient is not highly motivated and undecided with regard to reconstruction, then delayed reconstruction is recommended as a possibility. If the patient is undergoing a nipple-sparing mastectomy with moderate-sized or large breasts, then immediate reconstruction is more favorable to avoid contour irregularities from skin contracture with delayed reconstruction. If the patient is capable of tolerating implant reconstruction from the risk factor standpoint, the surgeon has to decide whether she can emotionally accept the staged procedures, including a delay of 4 to 6 months, or more, between the two operations from tissue expander insertion to exchange.

The patient must be informed of the relatively high rate of potential complications: bleeding, seroma, infection, dehiscence, skin necrosis, implant exposure, explantation, deflation or leak of the implant, migration of implant, capsular contracture, contour irregularities, asymmetry, and pain. The patient needs to be informed that body's response to implantation is quite variable from person to person. While one person may suffer very little pain with the tissue expander in place, another person may have significant discomfort or pain. The process of tissue expansion can be quite uncomfortable for some but less for others. While most patients would accept the prosthetic device without significant contracture, a small subset of the population may develop significant capsular contracture. In the event the patient requires postoperative radiation, the potential untoward effects of radiation on the reconstructed breast needs to be discussed with the patient ahead of time.

If the patient undergoes a standard mastectomy, then there is a higher chance that a tissue expander would provide a better result. If the mastectomy is skin-sparing or nipple-sparing, then there is relatively higher change that a single-stage reconstruction with a breast implant would be favorable. The surgeon has to ascertain whether the patient would like to have reconstructed a slightly smaller breast size or to maintain her current breast size. The patient may choose to have smaller or even larger breast size. The surgeon may favor selection of tissue expansion for the individual who adamantly desires to maintain the same or larger breast size.

The surgeon has to ascertain the patient's view of quality of life with or without reconstruction and the patient's tolerance to complications. If the patient feels that having breast reconstruction is not a high priority, then relative to her intolerance to potential complications, reconstruction is not recommended.

Once the decision is made to proceed, the size and type of the implant or tissue expander is chosen. This is determined by measuring the width and height of the breast mound. The goal is to maximize the width of the prosthetic device, whether it would be a permanent breast implant or a tissue expander. The author uses the Mentor textured (Siltex®) Contour Profile®, integrated-valve expanders (Mentor Corporation, Santa Barbara, CA). This is an anatomically shaped expander. The maximum width of prosthesis aids in defining the mammary fold laterally and the cleavage medially. For ipsilateral cases, the base diameter of the contralateral breast is the critical measurement. Other factors to consider are the height and projection of the breast. The majority of patients are amenable to the medium height expander, style 6200. For the obese patient with low chest height the low-height expander, style 6100, is used. In the thin, tall patient with firm breast without much ptosis the tall-height expander is chosen, that is, style 6300.

A multitude of expander products can be used, depending on surgeon's preference from previous experience. Inamed tissue expanders and permanent breast implants (Allergan, Santa Barbara, CA) have comparable anatomically shaped tissue expanders and implants (BioDIMENSIONAL® System). Other available brands include PMT (Permark Corporation, Chanhassen, MN) and SSP (Specialty Surgical Products, Inc., Victor, MN). For completeness, it should be noted that an adjustable permanent implant with a remote port can also be used for implant reconstruction, especially, if a high-volume permanent implant cannot be employed at the time of the mastectomy.

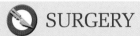 SURGERY

Surgical Prep and Positioning

It is crucial to reprep and redrape the patient to minimize contamination from the mastectomy surgical field. The old draping from the mastectomy is taken down without disturbing the surgical wound. The patient's arms are positioned on arm boards and secured with slight flexion at the elbow. The operating table is checked to make sure that the back can be elevated to a sitting position during the surgery. Fresh prepping and draping are then performed, and the use of a new set of instruments is implemented.

Immediate Reconstruction

Inspection and Hemostasis

The skin is evaluated for its circulatory status. Any areas of obvious loss of perfusion within the mastectomy skin flap would need to be resected, which can change the plan for a single-stage implant reconstruction. In rare cases, in nipple-sparing or skin-sparing mastectomy, if significant portion of the mastectomy skin flap is compromised, initial plan for a single-stage implant insertion would need to be converted to a two-stage reconstruction with tissue expander. After copious irrigation, meticulous hemostasis utilizing electrocautery and bipolar cautery is performed.

Dissection of the Prosthesis Pocket

Generally, the mastectomy incision is not enlarged to complete the reconstruction. In the case of nipple-sparing mastectomy, this incision can be quite small and can be

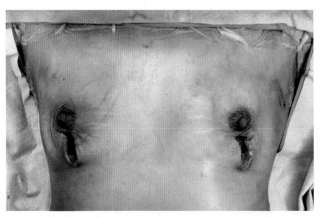

Figure 26.3 Bilateral total skin-sparing (also known as nipple-sparing) mastectomy via a vertical incision between the nipple and the inframammary crease.

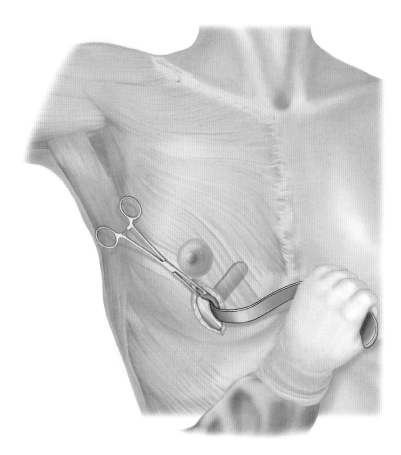

Figure 26.4 Dissection of the pocket beneath the pectoralis major muscle. The Allis clamp helps to stabilize the muscle under tension during dissection. The pocket outside of the pectoralis major muscle does not require dissection, since this is the space after the mastectomy in immediate reconstruction.

located in a number of possible locations depending on the oncological surgeon and previous biopsy incisions. The preferred mastectomy incision for nipple-sparing mastectomy at our center is a vertical incision centered on the breast meridian (6 0'clock) between the areola and the inframammary crease (Fig. 26.3). Through this incision, the lateral border of the pectoralis major muscle is controlled by an Allis clamp and dissection is performed using electrocautery (Figs. 26.4 and 26.5). In combination with digital blunt dissection, a plane is established beneath the pectoralis major muscle proper (Fig. 26.6). The pectoralis major is separated from the pectoralis minor muscle. The origin of the pectoralis major is separated off the entire width of the inframammary

Part VII: Breast Reconstruction

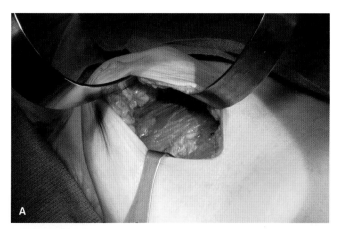
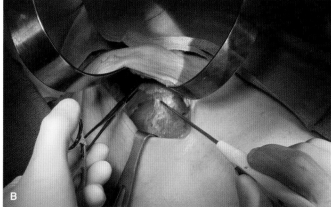

Figure 26.5 **A.** The pectoralis major muscle via the vertical mastectomy incision after total skin-sparing mastectomy on a large patient who previously wore D-cup brassieres (same patient as in Fig. 26.13). **B.** Elevation of the pectoralis major muscle toward the sternal border.

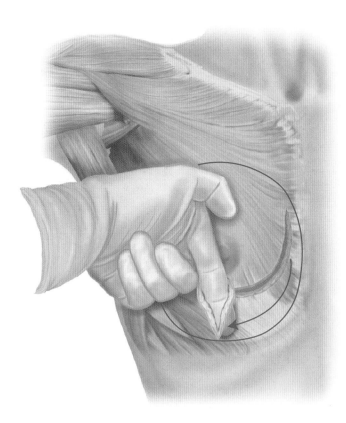

Figure 26.6 The use of blunt dissection in creating much of the submuscular pocket beneath the pectoralis major muscle.

crease and partially up along the border of the sternum (Fig. 26.7). Depending on patient's existing cleavage, the more medial the breast mount desired, the more releasing is required of the pectoralis major origin along the sternum, even up as high as the second intercostals space. Attention is paid to avoid vigorous dissection here with the electrocautery to prevent creating a button hole of the skin or creating a plane too close to the opposite side, which would lead to symmastia. Depending on the extent of space needed, some of the most medial pectoralis major muscle fibers along the sternum may be maintained along its line of release. Hemoclips are required as necessary for parasternal perforators, which can be clipped and divided with impunity if they are no longer contributing to the mastectomy skin flap circulation.

At this point the procedure is different depending on whether it is a conventional tissue expansion reconstruction with complete muscle coverage or an acellular dermis-assisted reconstruction following a skin-sparing and nipple-sparing mastectomy.

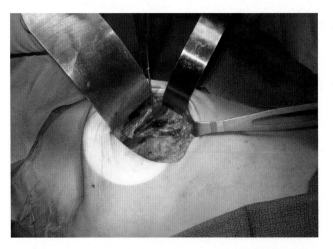

Figure 26.7 Separation of the pectoralis major muscle off the inferior border and also up along the lateral border of the sternum. Note the cauterized tissue for absolute hemostasis in difficult-to-control areas.

Two-Stage Reconstruction after Conventional Mastectomy–Complete Muscle Coverage over the Expander

The pectoralis major muscle origin inframammary crease is not divided, but elevated, if possible, in continuity with the anterior rectus fascia to maintain total prosthesis coverage. The serratus muscle origin is elevated off the chest wall up the midaxillary line to provide coverage of the lateral and lower lateral portion of the tissue expander. When the pectoralis major lateral border is sutured to the serratus muscle, there would be complete prosthesis coverage (Fig. 26.8). It is important to note that the submuscular pocket should be large enough for the tissue expander without potential space for prosthesis to slide around. Incomplete muscle coverage at the junction of the pectoralis major and rectus sheath is likely due to patient's anatomy and loss of tissue from the mastectomy.

Two-Stage Reconstruction with an Expander or Single-Stage Implant Insertion Using Human Acellular Dermal Matrix

The HADM is prepared according to packaging guidelines (Fig. 26.9). The common dimension of HADM is 8 cm by 16 cm (Alloderm dimension). The thickness of 0.79 to 2.03 mm is considered thick for the product Alloderm graft. The X-thick may also be used for breast reconstruction. If a larger dimension is required, then two pieces can be utilized with the creation of a seam between the two pieces of HADM without overlap. A 16 cm by 20 cm piece is available for the large ("D" cup) reconstruction. Using forceps, this material is inserted through the incision with minimal contact to the skin or surgeon's gloves. The corner of the HADM is sutured to the most medial extent of the

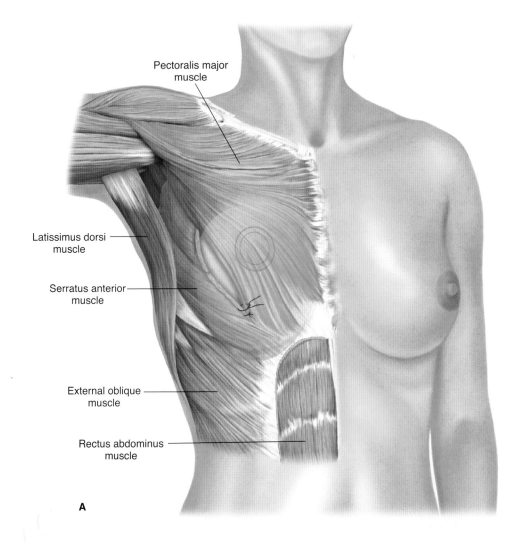

Figure 26.8 **A and B.** Tissue expander inserted beneath the pectoralis major muscle and the serratus muscle for complete muscle coverage in reconstruction after standard mastectomy (A); skin closure of mastectomy incision over site of reconstruction (B). (*continued*)

Pectoralis major muscle

Latissimus dorsi muscle

Serratus anterior muscle

External oblique muscle

Rectus abdominus muscle

A

Part VII: Breast Reconstruction

Figure 26.8 (*Continued*)

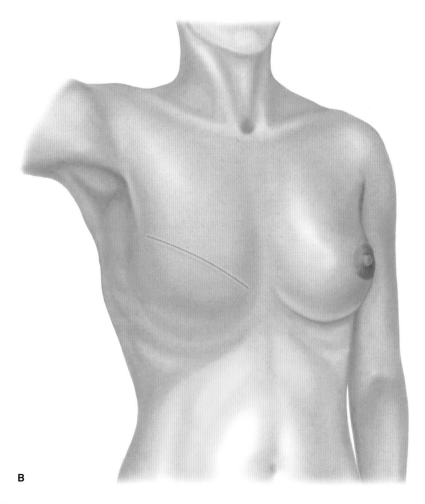

B

pectoralis major lower edge. The author prefers using monofilament absorbable sutures, 3-0 Monocryl (Poliglecaprone 25, Ethicon, Somerville, NJ), in a through-and-through vertical compression fashion. Instead or in combination, a longer-lasting absorbable suture may be desirable, such as PDS (Polydioxanone, Ethicon, Somerville, NJ). Approximation to the pectoralis major muscle is pants-over-vest with the HADM sliding under it (Fig. 26.10). For the boundary below the pectoralis major, the HADM is sutured in a pants-over-vest fashion to the cephalad extent of the rectus fascia. When there is no fascial edge to which to suture, the myofascia is used to anchor the HADM (Fig. 26.11). Along the serratus muscle the edge of the HADM is folded away from the mastectomy skin flap with mattress and figure-of-eight sutures placed until the most lateral and cephalad extent of the pectoralis major muscle edge is reached. At this point, the HADM is once again sutured to the pectoralis major muscle in a pants-over-vest fashion. Any seam between the pieces of HADM is then completed with a running suture. After the breast device insertion, the center portion of the pectoralis pocket is now closed at this time to provide complete coverage of prosthesis (Fig. 26.12).

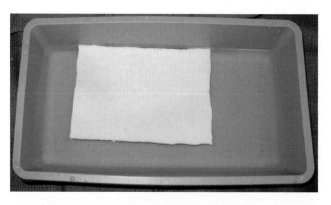

Figure 26.9 Alloderm (a brand of human acellular dermal matrix) is being soaked in normal saline prior to insertion.

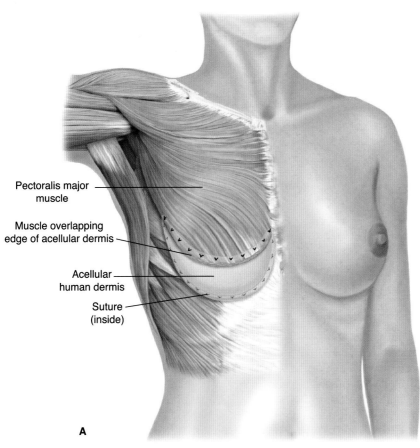

Pectoralis major
muscle

Muscle overlapping
edge of acellular dermis

Acellular
human dermis

Suture
(inside)

A

Figure 26.10 The human acellular dermal matrix (HADM) partially sutured in place along the lower border of the pectoralis major and along the fascia along the infra-mammary crease.

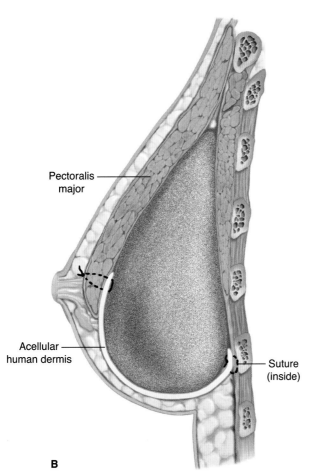

Pectoralis
major

Acellular
human dermis

Suture
(inside)

B

Part VII: Breast Reconstruction

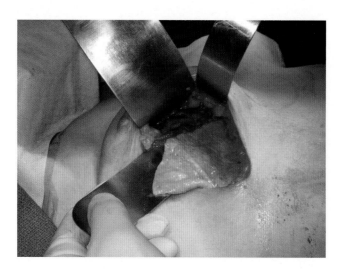

Figure 26.11 Alloderm partially sutured in place.

Single or Two-Stage Reconstruction: Insertion of the Prosthesis

Drains are placed prior to prosthesis insertion. Routinely, two drains are placed with one positioned above and one beneath the muscle-HADM pocket. For smaller individuals and patients with excellent inherent hemostasis, a single drain can be used with the tip passed under the edge of the HADM inside the pocket. The drains are brought out immediately above the lateral inframammary crease and secured with suture.

For both the tissue expander and permanent saline implant, the prosthesis is evacuated of air and primed with a small volume (several to 50 cc) of sterile normal saline. A sterile intravenous (IV) tubing connected to a bag of injectable normal saline is used for this process. A closed system using a three-way stopcock and 60 cc Luer-Lok syringe is used to avoid exposing the saline with each injection into the prosthesis. A new pair of gloves are employed when preparing the prosthesis. The surgeon should change to a new pair of sterile gloves when inserting the prosthesis with minimal contact to the skin edges.

At this time the prosthesis is filled with injectable saline, at the port via a needle in the case of the tissue expander or adjustable implant and via the fill tube in the case of a permanent saline implant. In the case of the tissue expander, as much saline is filled as necessary without placing undue tension to the mastectomy skin flap.

In the case of single-stage reconstruction with saline-filled or silicone cohesive gel implants, a temporary sizer implant can be inserted instead of the permanent one if the size of the implant to be employed is uncertain. The sizer can also be used as a tem-

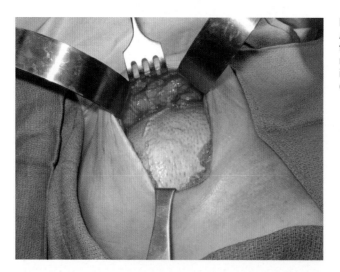

Figure 26.12 Two large pieces of Alloderm inset in place and sutured to each other to provide complete muscle-HADM coverage of saline implant. HADM, human acellular dermal matrix.

plate as the HADM is sutured in and contoured in place. Once the HADM is tailored and secured, but incompletely closed, the sizer is removed, and then the permanent implant is inserted.

Following a nipple-sparing or skin-sparing mastectomy, it is vital to replace the loss of volume vacated by the mastectomy to minimize wrinkling and redundancy of skin. In patients with gigantomastia, additional skin from the mastectomy may need to be resected to avoid an awkward appearance. A discussion of resection pattern of redundant skin is beyond the scope of this chapter, but it is vital to note that this needs to be performed with careful attention to skin circulation. With the insertion of a permanent saline implant in a single-stage reconstruction, the preoperatively desired breast mound size should be reached without excessive tension on the overlying soft-tissue envelope. The remaining approximation of the HADM to the pectoralis major muscle is then commenced for complete coverage of the prosthesis (Fig. 26.12).

Assessing Symmetry

Before final closure of the muscle pocket, the patient is placed in the almost sitting position by elevation of the back of the operating table for assessment of symmetry. For bilateral reconstruction with expanders using the integral port, the port finder is used to mark the position of the injection port. This landmark is used to measure its distance from the sternum and sternal notch. The distances on one side are compared with those on the opposite side. A sterile measuring tape is used to drape across the chest from one portal mark to the other for an additional visual cue in assessing symmetry. The expander or expanders can then be repositioned if necessary. When the surgeon is satisfied with symmetry, the patient is then placed back in the flat position for placement of remaining sutures between the HADM and the pectoralis major.

Skin Closure

Surgical trauma to the mastectomy incision is anticipated, especially when utilizing a small incision, which may be only 5 to 6 cm. This is the time to incise and remove any devitalized or heavily damaged skin edges, which would allow skin closure with relatively healthier dermis. After further irrigation, the skin is closed with simple interrupted inverted dermal sutures of 3-0 and 4-0 Monocryl, followed by a continuous buried subcuticular suture of 4-0 or 5-0 Monocryl. I prefer two layers of Dermabond (Ethicon, Somerville, NJ) to seal the suture line. See Fig. 26.13A–F for the preoperative and postoperative photos of the same patient as described in the surgical dissection illustrated by Figures 26.5, 26.7, 26.11, and 26.12.

Delayed Reconstruction (Tissue Expander Placement)

The steps during delayed reconstruction are similar once the planes of dissection are established. Preoperative markings are made for the incision and position of the prosthesis (Fig. 26.14). If a remote port is used, this site is marked and it should be assessable through the conventional mastectomy incision to avoid an additional scar. The inframammary crease is delineated and the pocket dissection should be 2 to 3 cm below this; pocket size should be marked as wide as the opposite breast's lateral limits in ipsilateral cases. Keep in mind that the expander is selected on the basis of its base dimension, and its width should match that of the opposite or desired breast mound. Attention should also be placed on expander projection since different brands and different volume sizes within the same brand have different levels of projection. As in immediate reconstruction, the pocket size should not exceed significantly over the space required for the expander.

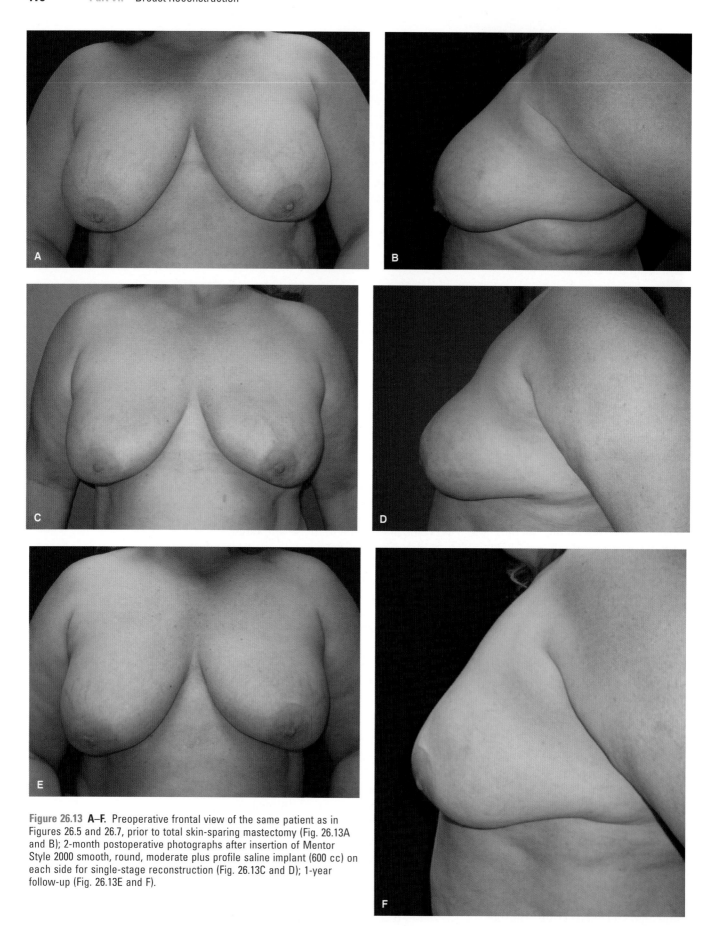

Figure 26.13 A–F. Preoperative frontal view of the same patient as in Figures 26.5 and 26.7, prior to total skin-sparing mastectomy (Fig. 26.13A and B); 2-month postoperative photographs after insertion of Mentor Style 2000 smooth, round, moderate plus profile saline implant (600 cc) on each side for single-stage reconstruction (Fig. 26.13C and D); 1-year follow-up (Fig. 26.13E and F).

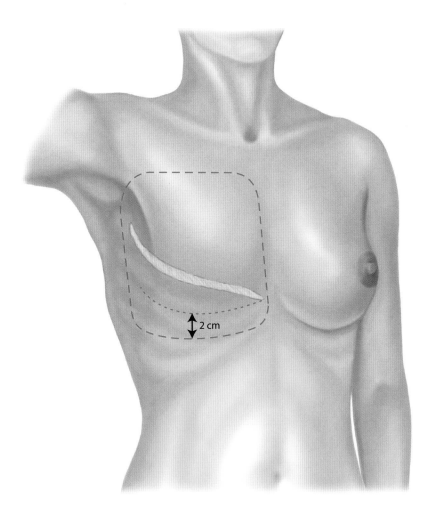

Figure 26.14 Preoperative markings in delayed reconstruction. The lower limit of the dissection is outlined 2 to 3 cm below the inframammary crease on the contralateral side.

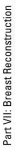

The lateral part of the standard mastectomy scar is chosen for the approach. The lateral border of the pectorals major is delineated with a combination of sharp and electrocautery dissection, after which the underlying attachments are lifted with blunt finger dissection and electrocautery. Perforators are hemoclipped and divided. The origin of the pectoralis major muscle is divided and freed as high along the sternum as necessary for anticipated cleavage development. Inferior dissection has to free up any constricting band that may limit expansion. The serratus muscle is elevated as described before for complete muscle coverage. Alternatively, HADM may be employed instead, which would be inserted, tailored, and secured as described in immediate reconstruction. Another option, especially for patients with thick, healthy, and well-healed mastectomy skin flaps, would be to insert the tissue expander in a "dual-plane" position where the lower part of the prosthesis is subcutaneous and uncovered by muscle (Fig. 26-15). This technique was described by Spear and Spittler. External sutures are passed through the skin and back out, capturing the lower edge of the pectoralis major muscle to maintain its position over the upper portion of the implant (these marionette sutures are removed near postoperative day 10). A single Silastic drain is inserted and brought out via the existing drain scar. As described in immediate reconstruction, the tissue expander is prepared, tested for leaks, primed with injectable sterile normal saline, and then inserted in the submuscular pocket. In case of the need for complete or near-complete muscle coverage, the serratus muscle is sutured to the lateral border of the pectoralis major with absorbable sutures. In case of human acellular dermal support, the graft is then sutured to the lateral and inferior borders of the pectoralis major. Symmetry is assessed with the head of operating table elevated and then skin is closed. Unlike immediate reconstruction, a postoperative bra is applied immediately with ample fluffs for snug compression to minimize bleeding and expander movement.

Figure 26.15 A and B. The dual-plane technique is illustrated for insertion of tissue expander after standard mastectomy, leaving the lower third or more of the prosthesis uncovered by muscle, except for the overlying skin and subcutaneous layer of the mastectomy skin flap.

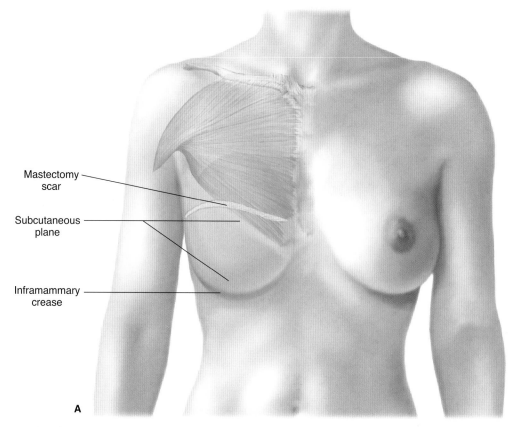

Mastectomy scar

Subcutaneous plane

Inframammary crease

A

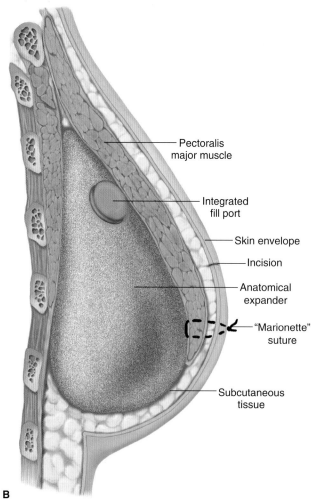

Pectoralis major muscle

Integrated fill port

Skin envelope

Incision

Anatomical expander

"Marionette" suture

Subcutaneous tissue

B

POSTOPERATIVE MANAGEMENT

Immediate Reconstruction

The Dermabond applied serves as the dressing for the mastectomy incision, and no compressive dressing is applied to avoid compression to the mastectomy skin flap. The type of dressing employed should be a mutual decision between the oncological surgeon and reconstructive surgeon. A dressing with Xeroform (Covidien, Mansfield, MA) and dry gauze is used around each drain site. The Xeroform helps to protect the entry point around the drain tube.

The mastectomy skin is examined for circulation and hematoma. The patient is maintained in the hospital until nausea and pain is controlled, typical for the standard mastectomy patients, which is 1 to 2 days. Because of the presence of foreign material inserted, judicious postoperative antibiotic therapy is recommended.

Daily activities utilizing the upper extremity in elevation above the shoulder level are avoided for 3 to 4 weeks postoperatively. Driving is also avoided until soreness is minimal and full control of upper extremity is regained.

Delayed Reconstruction

In delayed reconstruction, there is likely less postoperative pain, and hospitalization usually can be completed within a 24-hour observation. In addition, the use of the postoperative garment can be initiated immediately to stabilize the internal prosthesis. Unlike immediate reconstruction, the mastectomy skin flap has secured perfusion, and a compression garment is well tolerated.

Tissue Expansion

The mastectomy skin flaps need to recover good perfusion before tissue expansion is begun for patients with tissue expanders. This usually occurs around 3 to 4 weeks after insertion. The incision should be healing well before subjecting it to expansion. The location of the port is identified by a port finder, which matches the expander used depending on the manufacturer. The Mentor tissue expander requires a locator with a magnetic pendulum that becomes perpendicular at the center of the port. In thin patients, this port is actually palpable, but the port locator is still recommended for confirmation (Fig. 26.16).

Part VII: Breast Reconstruction

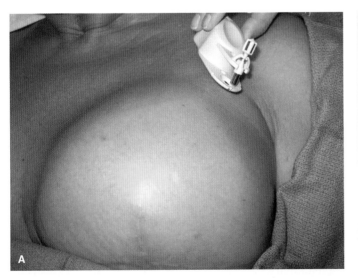 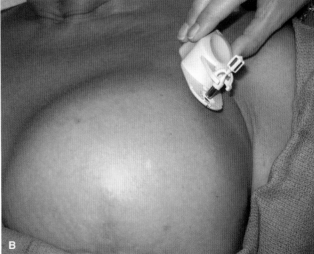

Figure 26.16 **A and B**. When the magnetic pendulum is perpendicular, the port is localized underneath.

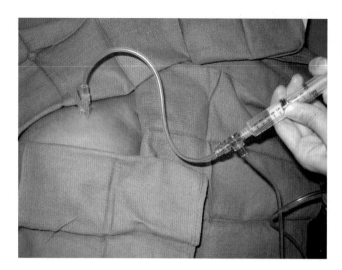

Figure 26.17 Filling of the tissue expander is performed using a closed tubing system via one-way valves (provided by Mentor).

The injection site is prepped out with Betadine and then alcohol wipe or with antiseptic solution of choice. A sterile towel is placed over each breast to allow palpation in assessing skin tightness during filling. Usually, the volume of each fill is judged by patient's tolerance and skin tightness. This volume can be 30 to 50 cc for the small patient and up to 80 cc or more for the larger patient. Sterile injectable saline is delivered via a 21-gauge needle at a perpendicular direction (Fig. 26.17). Each expansion session is spaced 1 week apart but may be extended longer because of difficulty with travel or other issues. The expansion process is continued until the desired volume is reached, chosen by the patient with recommendation by the surgeon. This should be 10% to 20% above the actual desired size of the breast mound in order to allow natural retraction of the skin.

Postoperative Garment

Following mastectomy, especially skin-sparing or nipple-sparing mastectomy, the skin flap has inherently poor perfusion. A tight dressing or compressive garment is avoided for the first 2 to 3 weeks to avoid further compromising mastectomy skin flap circulation. After this period, when the skin flap has much improved circulation, the patient is fitted with a postoperative bra or garment to assist in soft-tissue redraping and stabilizing the position of the prosthesis, whether it is an expander or a permanent implant. For adequate medialization of the implant to create more natural cleavage, additional padding can be applied laterally under the garment. The garment is worn for the next 2 to 3 months while the implant capsule is forming. If tolerated, it should be worn at nighttime as well.

For Tissue Expander Exchange to Permanent Breast Implant

For patients undergoing two-stage reconstruction with tissue expanders, the exchange to a permanent implant is performed a minimum of 2 months after completion of tissue expansion. This waiting period helps to minimize soft-tissue retraction after expander removal. During this surgery, the subaxillary and lateral adiposity can be addressed with direct excision with or without suction-assisted lipectomy. These folds of fat become prominent and uncomfortable to the patient after mastectomy despite reconstruction since the prosthesis, unlike the mammary gland, is not confluent with the adiposity. It

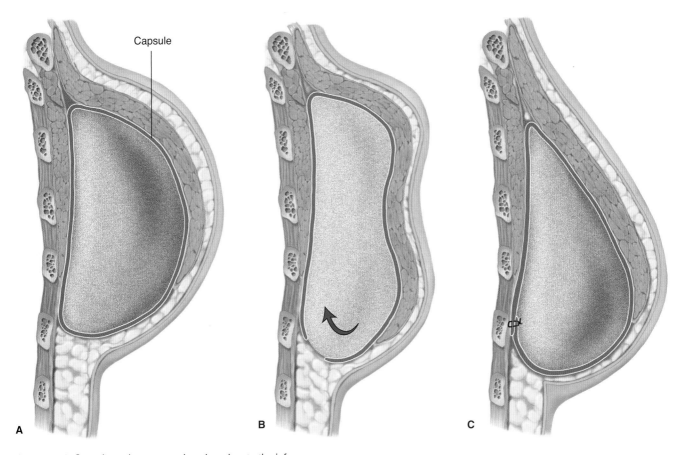

Capsule

A   B   C

Figure 26.18 Capsulorraphy sutures placed to elevate the inframammary crease.

should be noted that in most cases, some element of capsular contracture develops around the tissue expander.

The original mastectomy incision is used for exposure. Usually this incision is only 5 to 6 cm. A headlight is used with or without lighted retractor to facilitate visualization through a small incision. An 18-gauge needle is placed percutaneously into the port and the expander fluid is withdrawn while dissection is carried out to expose the prosthesis. If at all possible, some undermining is performed of the mastectomy skin flap so that the expander capsule is entered along the lateral edge of the pectoralis major muscle and in a different line to the original mastectomy incision. This avoids exposing the inner layer suture line if any skin incision healing problem was to develop. When the fluid is evacuated through continuous suction, the expander is then removed intact and the pocket copiously irrigated.

Some degree of capsulotomy using electrocautery is required to soften the appearance and feel of the final reconstruction. Standard release of the capsule is performed at the base of the capsule along the level of the inframammary crease, along the sternum, and along the lateral mammary fold. For the expander that has migrated laterally, extensive capsulotomy and soft-tissue elevation is required to medialize the position of the final implant. Sometimes for the tighter capsules, radial cuts in the capsule are performed with the electrocautery. For significant displacement of the tissue expander, such unnecessary capsular space can be closed with capsulorraphy sutures using figure-of-eight 3-0 Monocryl or similar sutures. This is commonly required in the lateral or inferior locations of the capsule (Fig. 26.18).

During the second stage for expander exchange to permanent implant, if the inframammary crease needs to be well defined to enhance symmetry, an upper abdominal advancement flap is transferred (Fig. 26.19). After opening the lower portion of the

Figure 26.19 Elevation of abdominal advancement flap to define the inframammary crease if indicated. (*continued*)

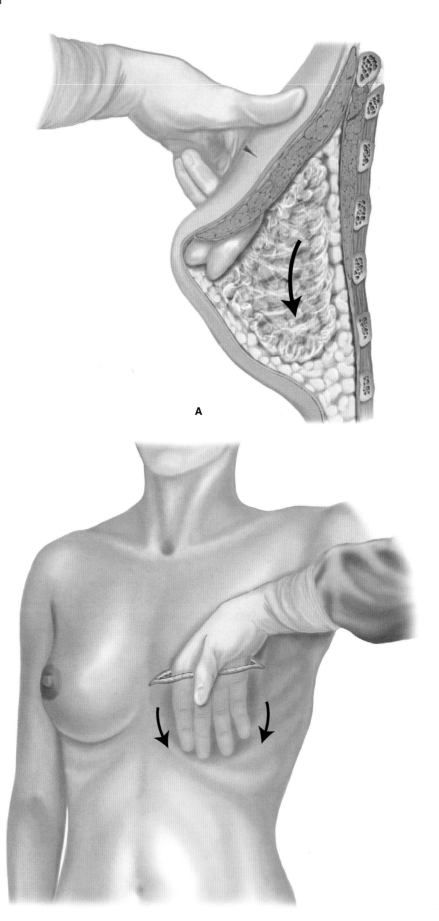

A

B

Figure 26.19 (*Continued*)

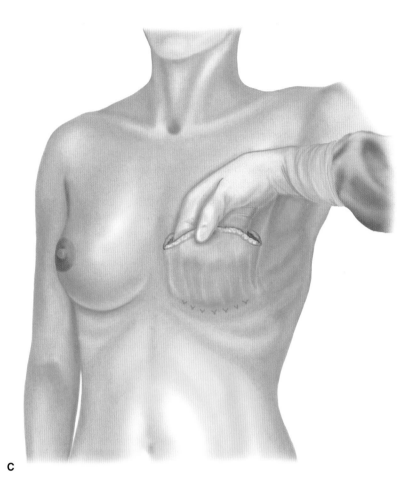

c

capsule, the skin is undermined as far down as the level of the umbilicus, if necessary, to advance the skin in a cephalad direction with deep sutures placed underneath between the subcutaneous tissue and dermis and costal periosteum. This aids in gaining ptosis and defining the inframammary fold. Depression in the skin at the neo inframammary crease will resolve as the suture material is absorbed.

Insertion of Permanent Implant (Second-Stage Reconstruction)

Various types and styles can be used depending on surgeon's preference. Saline-filled or silicone cohesive gel implants are options based on the preferences of surgeon and patient (Fig. 26.20). Smooth and textured implants are available options. Round and anatomical implants are available options, keeping in mind that if the anatomical

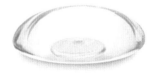 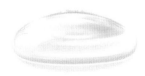

Figure 26.20 Silicone cohesive gel and saline-filled smooth implants.

implant rotates, the shape of the breast mound would change. Round implants from Mentor come in different projection levels: moderate, moderate plus, and high. Also available is a postoperative adjustable implant that comes with a remote port. For ipsilateral cases, the different levels are especially important to match the breast mound to the opposite side.

The patient may also have a special request for a certain type of implant, cohesive gel versus saline-filled. For insertion of the gel implant, the incision would need to be larger to accommodate the implant during insertion. For the saline implant, the incision is small, since the implant is inserted deflated. The implant is prepared similar to a tissue expander, making sure that all major air bubbles are removed. Once inserted, via the fill tube, sterile injectable normal saline is injected with the patient in the sitting position to assess for proper positioning and symmetry. It is not uncommon to place additional capsulorraphy sutures at this juncture. In many cases, especially in ipsilateral reconstruction, if the final implant size is uncertain, an implant sizer can be initially inserted. With this temporary implant in place, capsulorraphy can be readjusted without concern for damaging the permanent implant. Once the permanent implant is in place, the opening in the capsule is reapproximated with a running 3-0 Monocryl or other absorbable suture. Skin closure is similar to that during the first operation. However, a drain is not required. Unlike the first stage, a postoperative bra is employed with ample fluffed gauze placed diffusely and also laterally to compress the soft tissue and medialize the implant. This helps to stabilize the implant and prevent bleeding. Patients are usually discharged on the same day with by mouth (PO) antibiotics for 7 days and PO analgesics.

COMPLICATIONS

Immediate complications include skin necrosis, implant exposure, seroma, and infection. Reported rates of infection exceed routine elective surgery infection rates, partly because of the relative ischemic tissues after mastectomy in combination with the insertion of foreign material. Infection ranges from low-grade cellulitis treatable with antibiotics to wound sepsis requiring explantation. In skin-sparing or nipple-sparing mastectomy, complications of ischemic changes and necrosis of the mastectomy skin flap are higher than that of conventional mastectomy. The addition of HADM may also increase the risk of infection slightly, although some authors have found this risk to be negligible. Delayed complications include asymmetry, implant deflation, capsular contracture, implant migration, chronic pain or discomfort, and contour irregularities, such as rippling of the implant visualized through the skin. The reader is advised to go over the risks carefully with the patient. Implant package inserts contain details pertaining to the risks and percentages of complications.

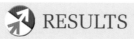 RESULTS

With immediate reconstruction, it has been shown that patients have improved body image with retention of the breast mound. In general, conventional reconstruction with complete muscle coverage has been shown in various studies to achieve a patient satisfaction rate in the 80% range or higher. Preliminary studies with nipple-sparing and skin-sparing mastectomy immediate alloplastic reconstruction with human acellular dermis are promising with majority of patients achieving good or excellent results and complication rates being relatively low (Figs. 26.21–26.27). The lower pole of the breast mound created by the HADM allows for less tension and improved projection. Although the reconstructive surgeon is usually not involved in the selection process for the type of mastectomy chosen, he or she needs to be cognizant of the oncological safety of the skin-sparing techniques. Especially in case of total skin-sparing (nipple-sparing) mastectomy, the oncological safety of this operation remains to be established with extended long-term results of recurrence rate. Follow-up studies of skin-sparing and nipple-sparing mastectomy or total skin sparing lack randomized trials. A single prospective study of 121 patients undergoing nipple-sparing subcutaneous mastectomy with median follow-up of 13 years showed that the disease-free survival rates of 51.3% and overall survival rates of 76.4% were comparable to that of conventional mastectomy performed in other trials (Benediktsson and Perbeck). With preservation of the nipple-areola skin only, the oncological safety is felt to be secured and there is no question that the aesthetic results of alloplastic reconstruction are improved compared with the reconstruction that follows conventional mastectomy.

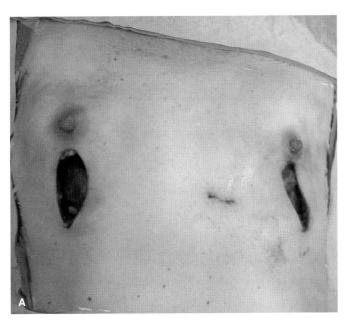

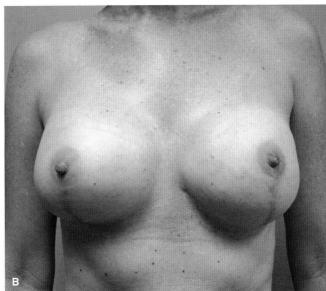

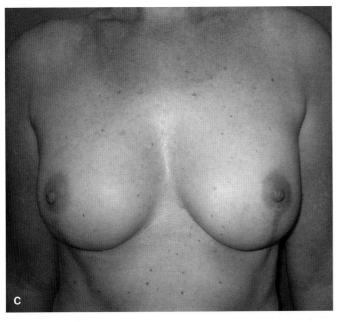

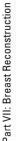

Figure 26.21 **A–E.** Intraoperative photograph after bilateral total skin-sparing mastectomy in a 48-year-old with right-sided breast cancer (Fig. 26.21A); immediate reconstruction was performed with placement of Alloderm and tissue expanders (Mentor Style 6200 medium height Contour Profile with 450 cc capacity at 12.7 cm width). Initial fill was 220 cc of saline followed by serial expansion to 420 cc as depicted in photograph 4 months after mastectomy (Fig. 26.21B); 6 months after tissue expander exchange to saline-filled implants (Mentor Style 3000 smooth, round, high profile with 420 to 500 cc capacity at 12 cm width [normal and midrange fill]). Final normal saline fill was 420 cc (Fig. 26.21C–E). (*continued*)

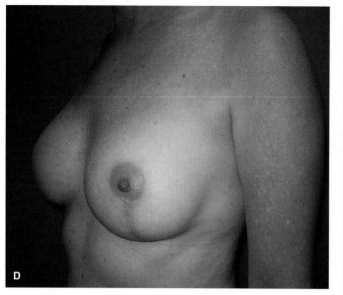

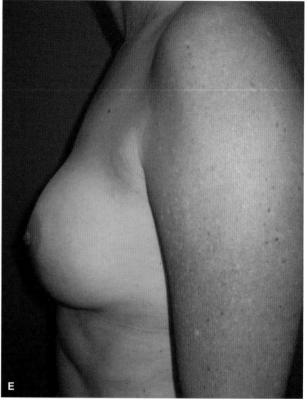

Figure 26.21 (*Continued*)

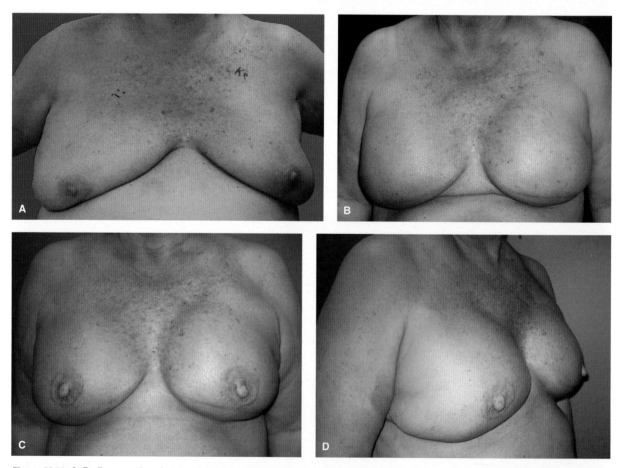

Figure 26.22 A–D. Preoperative photograph prior to bilateral skin-sparing mastectomy in a 54-year-old with right-sided lobular breast cancer (Fig. 26.22A); immediate reconstruction was performed with placement of Alloderm and tissue expanders (Mentor style 6100 low height contour profile with 750 cc capacity). Initial fill was 450 cc of saline followed by serial expansion to 990 cc as depicted in photographs 6 months after mastectomy (Fig. 26.22B); 7 months after tissue expander exchange to saline-filled implants (Mentor style 2000 smooth, round, moderate plus profile with 800 to 960 cc capacity). Final normal saline fill was 950 cc. She is also 5 weeks after bilateral nipple reconstruction with skate flap and full-thickness skin graft from subaxillary lipectomy skin (Fig. 26.22C and D).

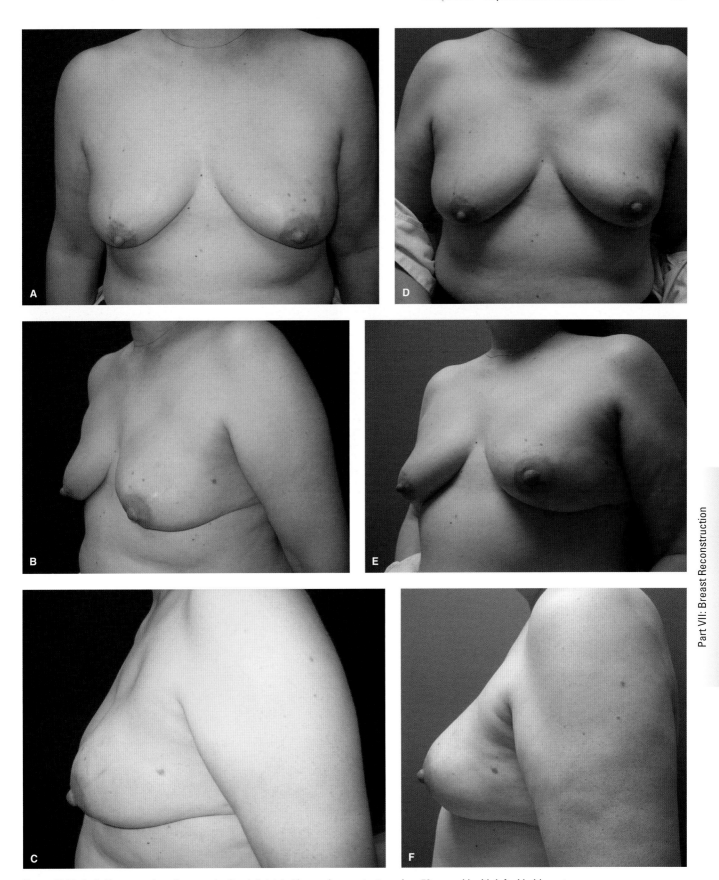

Figure 26.23 A–F. Postoperative photograph after left total skin-sparing mastectomy in a 50-year-old with left-sided breast cancer. Immediate reconstruction was performed on the left with placement of Alloderm and tissue expander (Mentor style 6100 low height contour profile with 550 cc capacity at 15 cm width). Initial fill in the operating room was 420 cc of saline followed by serial expansion to 550 cc as depicted in photograph 3.5 months after mastectomy (Fig. 26.23A–C); 8 months after tissue expander exchange to saline-filled implants (Mentor style 2000 smooth, round, moderate profile with 525 to 570 cc capacity at 15 cm width. Final normal saline fill was 525 cc (Fig. 26.23D–F).

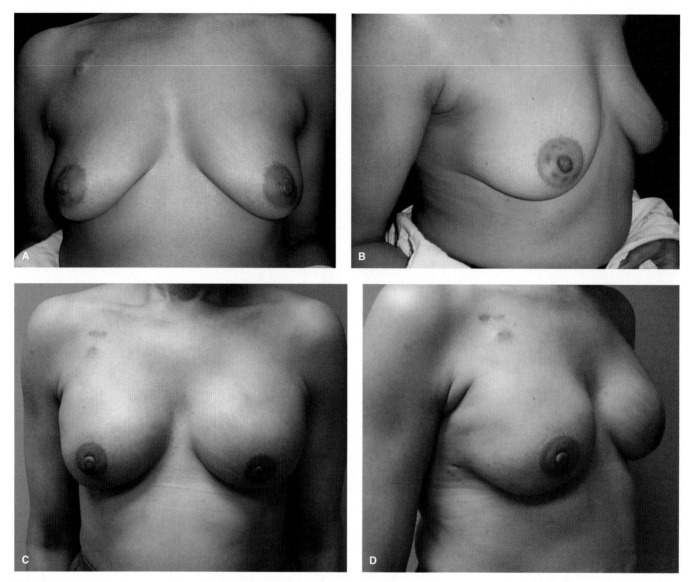

Figure 26.24 A–D. Fifty-four-year-old female, planning to undergo bilateral total skin-sparing mastectomy for right breast cancer, desired single-stage reconstruction with saline implant and Alloderm. Preoperative photographs (Fig. 26.24A and B); for intraoperative photograph after total skin-sparing mastectomy, see Figure 26.3 (same patient); 5 months after single-stage reconstruction with Mentor smooth, round, high-profile saline implants (420 to 500 capacity) filled to 440 cc (Fig. 26.24C and D). Note that the left nipple is displaced slightly lower compared with the right. Patient did not desire any revision.

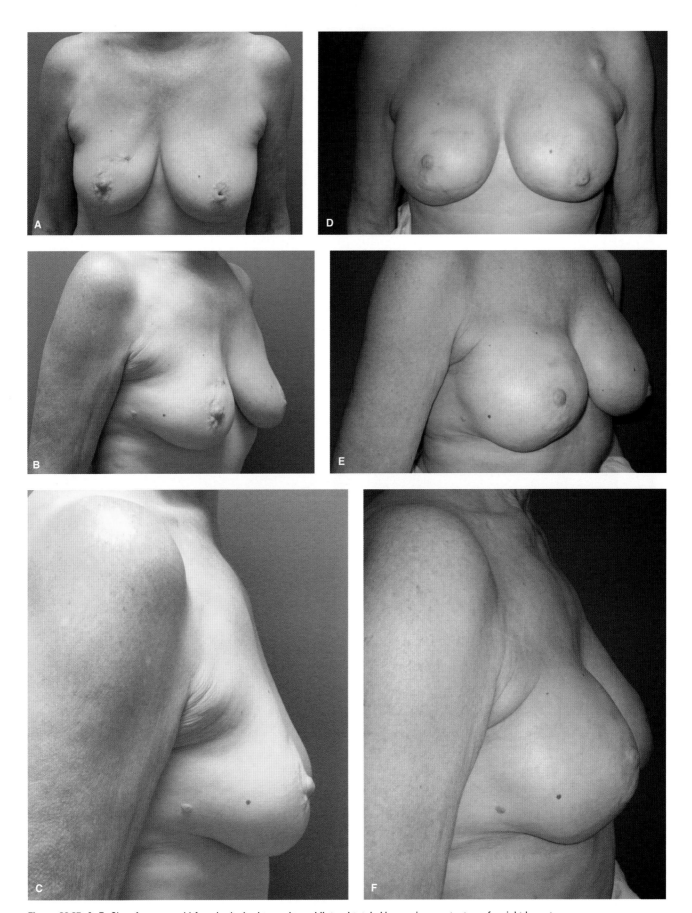

Figure 26.25 A–F. Sixty-four-year-old female desired to undergo bilateral total skin-sparing mastectomy for right breast cancer underwent immediate, single-stage reconstruction with saline implant and Alloderm. Preoperative photographs (Fig. 26.25A–C); 6 months after single-stage reconstruction with Mentor smooth, round, moderate plus profile saline implants (375 to 450 capacity) filled to 395 cc on the right and 385 cc on the left. On each side, a single 8 × 16 cm piece of Alloderm (1.04- to 2.28-mm thick) was utilized. Note that the left nipple is positioned slightly lower compared with the right, which was not significant to the patient (Fig. 26.25D–F).

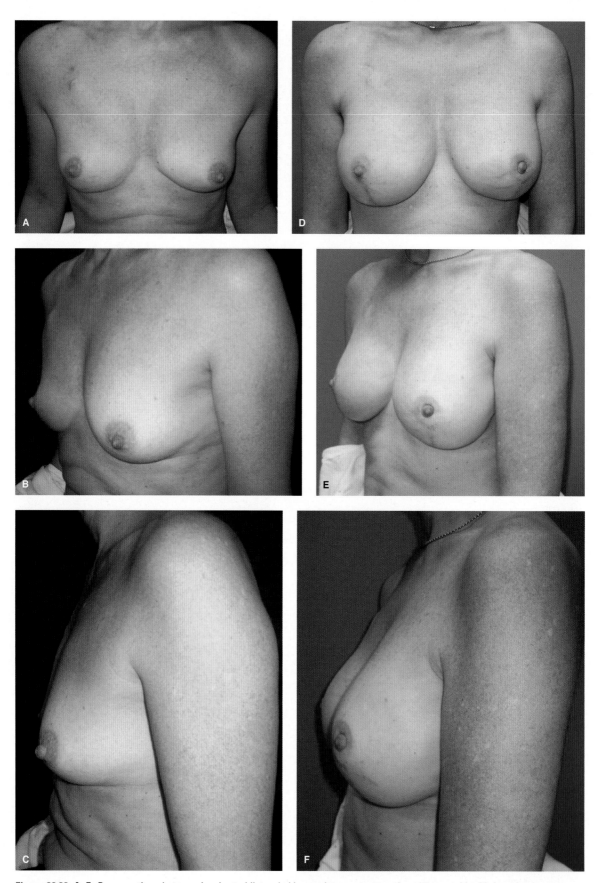

Figure 26.26 A–F. Preoperative photograph prior to bilateral skin-sparing mastectomy in a 49-year-old with invasive breast cancer who had completed neoadjuvant chemotherapy 2 months earlier (Fig. 26.26A–C). Immediate reconstruction was performed with placement of Alloderm and tissue expanders (Mentor style 6200 medium-height contour profile with 450 cc capacity). Initial fill was 180 of saline followed by serial expansion to 400 cc. Alloderm dimension used on each side was 8 × 12 cm with thickness of 1.04 to 2.28 mm). Six months after first-stage reconstruction, she underwent tissue expander exchange to saline-filled implants (Mentor Style 2000 smooth, round, moderate plus profile with 375 to 450 cc capacity). Final normal saline fill was 420 cc on the right and 405 cc on the left. Two-month postoperative photographs (Fig. 26.22D–F).

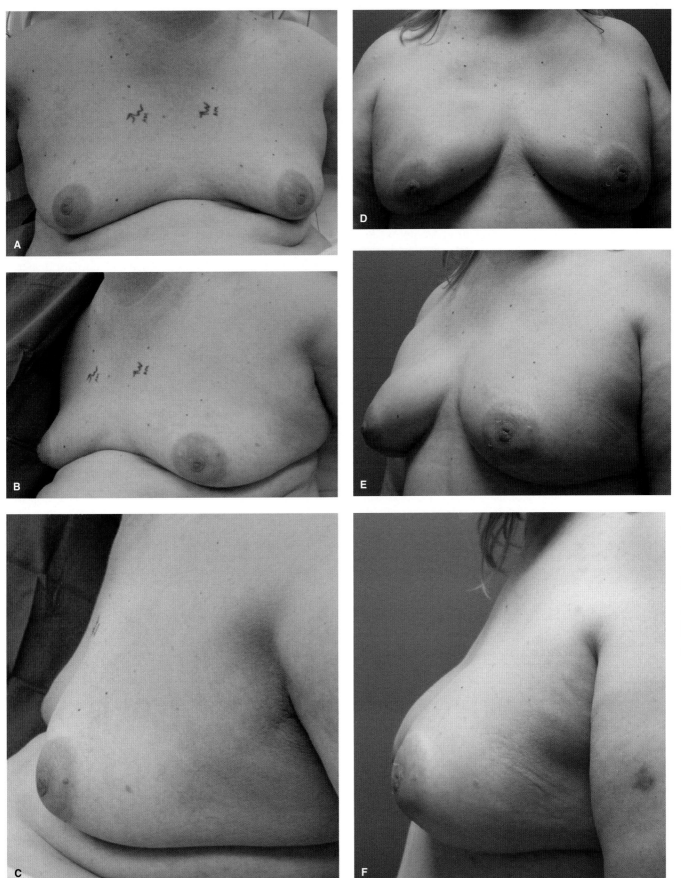

Figure 26.27 A–F. Fifty-nine-year-old female desired to undergo bilateral total skin-sparing mastectomy for right breast cancer followed by immediate, single-stage reconstruction with saline implant and Alloderm. Preoperative photographs (Fig. 26.27A–C); 2 months after single-stage reconstruction with Mentor smooth, round, moderate plus profile saline implants (500 to 600 capacity) filled to 550 cc on each side (Fig. 26.27D–F). On each side, 8 × 12 cm and 6 × 16 cm pieces of Alloderm (1.04 to 2.28 mm thick) were utilized.

⊛ CONCLUSIONS

The recommendation for implant-based reconstruction is formulated after consideration of a multitude of variables, including patient's risk factors, anatomy, expectations, tolerance of potential complications, and acceptance of postoperative course. In addition, size of existing breast(s), conditions of the opposite breast, and mastectomy types have a major influence on the type of implant reconstruction to be recommended. With the advent of skin-sparing and nipple-sparing or total skin-sparing mastectomy, the use of HADM has allowed completion of implant-based reconstruction in a single or two-stage procedure with excellent results and acceptable complication rates. The preservation of natural skin followed by immediate filling of the mastectomy space using a permanent implant or tissue expander, stabilized by HADM, allows for reconstruction of the lateral and inframammary folds and a very natural appearance. Implant-based reconstruction has many variations and requires a repertoire of techniques and implant designs, depending on the defect at hand.

Suggested Readings

Benediktsson KP, Perbeck L. Survival in breast cancer after nipple-sparing subcutaneous mastectomy and immediate reconstruction with implants: a prospective trial with 13 years median follow-up in 216 patients. *Euro J Surg Oncol.* 2008;34(2):143–148.

Bindingnavele V, Gaon M, Ota KS, et al. Use of acellular cadaveric dermis and tissue expansion in postmastectomy breast reconstruction. *J Plast Reconstr Aesthet Surg.* 2007;60:1214–1218.

Breuing KH, Warren SM. Immediate bilateral breast reconstruction with implants and inferolateral Alloderm slings. *Ann Plast Surg.* 2005;55:232–239.

Chun YS, Verma K, Rosen H, et al. Implant-based breast reconstruction using acellular dermal matrix and the risk of postoperative complications. *Plast Reconstr Surg.* 2010;125(2):429–436.

Chung AP, Sacchini V. Nipple-sparing mastectomy: where are we now? *Surg Oncol.* 2008;17:261–266.

Garwood ER, Moore D, Ewing C, et al. Total skin-sparing mastectomy, complications and local recurrence rates in 2 cohorts of patients. *Ann Surg.* 2009;249(1):26–32.

Gerber B, Krause A, Dietrich M, et al. The oncological safety of skin sparing mastectomy with conservation of the nipple-areola complex and autologous reconstruction: an extended follow up study. *Ann Surg.* 2009;249(3):461–468.

Gui GPH, Tan S, Faliakou EC, et al. Immediate breast reconstruction using biodimensional anatomical permanent expander implants: a prospective analysis of outcome and patient satisfaction. *Plast Reconstr Surg.* 2003;111:125–138.

Hochberg J, Margulies A, Yuen JC, et al. Alloderm (acellular human dermis) in breast reconstruction with tissue expansion. *Plast Reconstr Surg.* 2005;116(3):126–128.

Margulies AG, Hochberg J, Kepple J, et al. Total skin-sparing mastectomy without preservation of the nipple-areola complex. *Am J Surg.* 2005;190(6):907–912.

Meretoja TJ, von Smitten KAJ, Leidenius MHK, et al. Local recurrence of stage 1 and 2 breast cancer after skin-sparing mastectomy and immediate breast reconstruction in a 15-year series. *Euro J Surg Oncol.* 2007;33:1142–1145.

Salzberg CA. Nonexpansive immediate breast reconstruction using human acellular tissue matrix graft (Alloderm). *Ann Plast Surg.* 2006;57:1–5.

Sookman N, Boughey JC, Walsh MF, Degnim AC. Nipple-sparing mastectomy: initial experience at a tertiary center. *Am J Surg.* 2008;196:575–577.

Spear SL, Hannan CM, Willey SC, Cocilovo C. Nipple-sparing mastectomy. *Plast Reconstr Surg.* 2009;123:1665–1673.

Spear SL, Parikh PM, Reisin E, Menon NG. Acellular dermis-assisted breast reconstruction. *Aesth Plast Surg.* 2008;32:418–425.

Spear SL, Pelletiere CV. Immediate breast reconstruction in two stages using textured, integrated-valve tissue expanders and breast implants. *Plast Reconstr Surg.* 2003;113(7):2098–2103.

Spear SL, Spittler CJ. Breast Reconstruction with implants and expanders. *Plast Reconstr Surg.* 2001;107(1):177–187.

Topol BM, Dalton EF, Ponn T, Campbell CJ. Immediate single-stage breast reconstruction using implants and human acellular dermal tissue matrix with adjustment of the lower pole of the breast to reduce unwanted lift. *Ann Plast Surg.* 2008;61(5):494–499.

Zienowicz RJ, Karacaoglu E. Implant-based breast reconstruction with allograft. *Plast Reconstr Surg.* 2007;120:373–381.

27 Free Fat Grafting Techniques for Correction of Residual Contour Deformities after Breast Reconstruction

Michael S. Wong and Lee L. Q. Pu

Introduction

It is not uncommon to have residual contour irregularities or asymmetries between breasts after breast reconstruction, whether implant or autologous. As refinements in breast reconstruction techniques have occurred over the years, the aesthetic goals of our patients have risen. Rippling following implant reconstructions may be improved by converting a saline implant to silicone or camouflaged by use of capsular augmentation or acellular dermis. Autologous fat grafting is another technique that can improve upon these contour deformities and increase patient satisfaction with their breast reconstructions.

Background

The first use of autologous fat to replace a breast deformity was reported in 1895, when Czerny transplanted a back lipoma to replace breast tissue removed in an adenoma resection. Experience with fat injection through cannulas was described by Charles C. Miller in 1926 and liposuction in the 1980s aided in the popularization of fat as an injectable. Despite mixed results in the hands of a variety of surgeons, autologous fat grafting has grown in popularity as the demand for injectable fillers has increased.

We have adopted the Coleman technique, believing smaller amounts of fat grafts placed in multiple tunnels in multiple planes achieve the best results. We have successfully used autologous fat grafting for the correction of contour deformities of the face, upper and lower extremities, and residual deformities associated with breast reconstruction. In this chapter, we will focus on the latter, discussing preoperative planning, informed consent, surgical technique, postoperative care, and results.

INDICATIONS/CONTRAINDICATIONS

There are numerous irregularities that may occur after total breast reconstruction, including both autologous and implant. Volume excess occasionally seen after autologous reconstructions can be successfully addressed with focused liposuction or direct excisional techniques. Irregularities secondary to volume deficiency are often improved with autologous fat grafting. The most common area of contour deformities occurs at the periphery of the reconstructed breast mound. In autologous reconstructions, this is often seen at the superior chest wall and breast mound junction, manifesting as a concavity or "shelf." It may also occur in the areas of skin closure or flap inset. Implant reconstructions may have similar concavities amenable to improvement with fat grafting. Those women interested in a more natural appearing implant reconstruction will often desire additional volume at the superior pole to create a more gentle transition between the chest wall and the implant.

Controversy arises when one considers the use of autologous fat grafting to reconstruct the postlumpectomy deformity. Because there is a known recurrence rate associated with breast conservation therapy, any necrosis of autologous fat grafts may elicit anxiety surrounding the possibility of a recurrence. Although the spectrum of fat necrosis and postoperative changes mimicking carcinoma has been documented mammographically, the natural history of autologous fat grafts injected into the breast has not been as clearly delineated. Despite early data suggesting that calcifications following fat injection into the breast can be distinguished from carcinoma, biopsy may still be prompted by either a palpable mass or a mammographic calcification combined with patient and surgeon anxiety. Until stronger data are available and because varying degrees of calcification in breast parenchyma after autologous fat grafting is expected, our current opinion is that lumpectomy defects should generally not be reconstructed with autologous fat injections.

PREOPERATIVE PLANNING

Timing

Because graft take is reliant on an adequate wound bed, timing is an important consideration. We prefer to wait at least 3 months after the most recent breast surgery before proceeding with any autologous fat injections. This allows sufficient time for edema dissipation, revascularization, and stabilization of the contour deficit. Complete photographic documentation is beneficial in characterizing the three-dimensionality of the contour irregularity. We currently wait 4 to 6 months between subsequent fat injections to allow for dissipation of edema and inflammation, graft revascularization, and stabilization. We have found a three-dimensional camera to be particularly helpful in defining the volume deficit to both the patient and the surgeon.

Informed Consent

Although autologous fat grafting has been used for at least 20 years for the correction of deformities in the face, trunk, and extremities, its use in the breast has been shrouded in controversy. Much of this is based on theoretical concerns that areas of fat necrosis may mimic or conceal a breast cancer recurrence. Because of this, informed consent for autologous fat grafting to contour irregularities of the breast must be taken with particular care. Most radiologists are able to distinguish fat necrosis and postoperative changes from cancer recurrence. If there are any questions regarding the appearance of a mass after fat grafting, this should be treated as a cancer, until proven otherwise. Thus, patients must be counseled in the possibility of biopsies to rule out breast cancer recurrence. In addition, patients must understand that fat grafting is a process often involving additional grafting procedures. Again, if patients desire additional fat grafting into a previously injected area, we currently wait for 4 to 6 months between injections. This allows sufficient time for the resolution of edema and inflammation, revascularization of graft, and the stabilization of any fat resorption.

Donor Sites

Consideration must also be given to the best donor sites. Coleman preferentially harvests from the lower abdomen and the inner thighs, believing these areas to have the easiest graft harvest. Interestingly, there is evidence that these areas have higher concentration of adipose-derived stem cells than do other areas. For patients reconstructed with implants, the lower abdomen is often available. However, for those who have had transverse rectus abdominis myocutaneous (TRAM) flap reconstructions, this is no longer available, and we then elect to harvest the inner thighs. If these areas will yield inadequate graft material, then alternate sites, such as flanks, are chosen on the basis of availability.

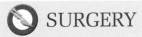 SURGERY

Fat Graft Harvesting and Processing

Patients who elect to undergo fat grafting should not have any major systemic metabolic diseases or lipid disorders. Our preferred donor site of fat grafting is the abdomen although each inner thigh can also be selected if more fat grafts are needed (Fig. 27.1). We prefer to use the Coleman technique with some modifications for fat graft harvesting and processing because this technique is a well-described and standardized method and is used by many surgeons worldwide. Briefly, through a small incision, a mixed solution (0.5% lidocaine with 1:200,000 of epinephrine in Lactated Ringer's solution) was infiltrated into the lower abdominal donor site or inner thigh using a blunt Lamis infiltrator (Byron Medical, Inc., Tucson, Arizona) (Fig. 27.2). The solutions are infiltrated in a ratio of 1 cc of solution per cubic centimeter of fat grafts to be harvested. The fat grafts are harvested through the same incisions made previously. The harvesting canula is 3 mm in diameter and 15 or 23 cm in length with a blunt tip (Byron Medical, Inc., Tucson, Arizona). It is connected to a 10-cc Luer-Lok syringe. Gently pulling back on the plunger of a 10-cc syringe provided a light negative pressure while the cannula is advanced and retracted through the harvested site (Fig. 27.3). After filling the syringe with harvested tissue, the cannula is removed from the syringe. A Luer-Lok plug is twisted onto the syringe to seal the Luer-Lok aperture and the plunger is removed from the barrel of the syringe and the body of the filled syringe is placed into a centrifuge (Byron Medical, Inc., Tucson, Arizona) and spun at 3000 rpm for 3 minutes (Fig. 27.4). After centrifugation, the aqueous layer (lower level) is also drained out of the syringe (Fig. 27.5) and the oil layer (upper level) is decanted off (Fig. 27.6). The

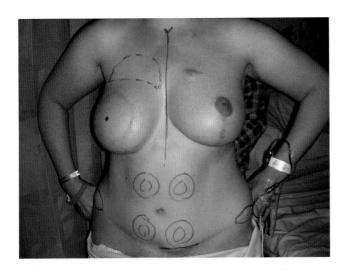

Figure 27.1 A preoperative photo shows the soft-tissue contour depression in the patient's right upper chest after a pedicled transverse rectus abdominis myocutaneous (TRAM) flap reconstruction. Her lower abdomen and bilateral hips have served as donor sites for fat graft harvest.

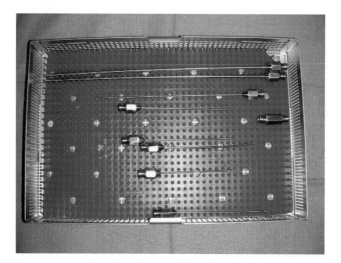

Figure 27.2 An intraoperative photo shows a complete set of the Coleman's instrument including infiltrating canula, harvesting canula, and various injection cannulae.

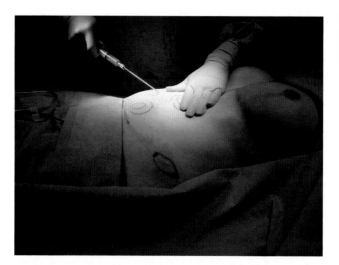

Figure 27.3 An intraoperative photo shows the Coleman technique of fat graft harvest from the abdomen of a patient.

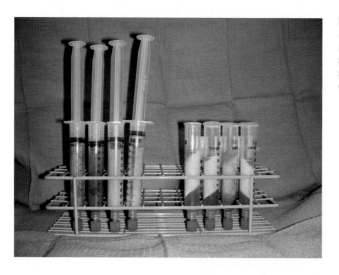

Figure 27.4 Syringes on the left await centrifugation and syringes on the right have been centrifuged for 3 minutes at 3000 rpm, resulting in separation into three layers: oil, fat graft, and aqueous.

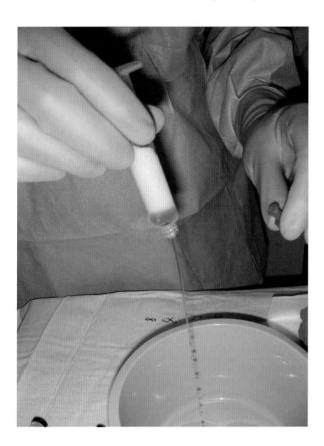

Figure 27.5 After centrifugation, the aqueous layer is discarded.

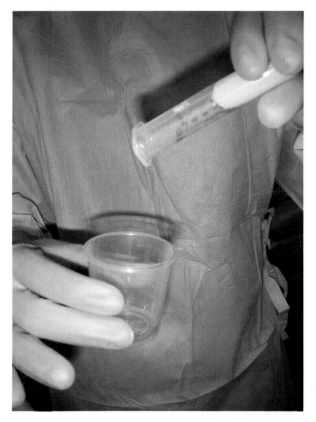

Figure 27.6 The oil layer is poured off.

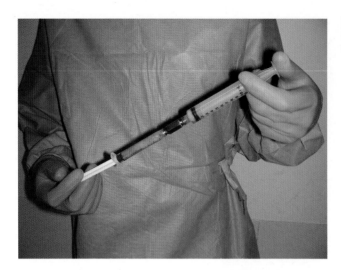

Figure 27.7 Fat graft is then transferred from 10-cc syringes into 1-cc syringes.

middle layer, composed of predominantly fat grafts, is then transferred to multiple 1-cc syringes (Fig. 27.7) for subsequent placement of fat grafts to the area with a residual deformity (Fig. 27.8).

Placement of Fat Grafts

The contour deformity of a reconstructed breast is marked preoperatively while the patient is in a standing position. The amount of fat grafts needed is estimated by the surgeon. To determine the appropriate incision locations for placement of the fat grafts, the periphery of the concavity needs to be carefully delineated. Incisions should be placed a minimum of 1 to 2 cm away from the concavity to allow sufficient room for

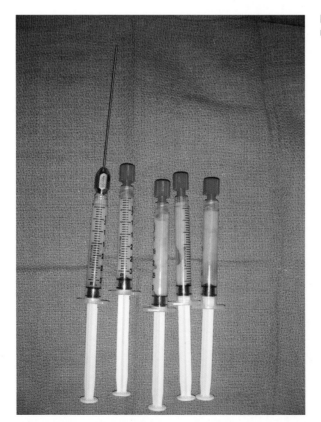

Figure 27.8 Fat grafts in 1-cc syringes are ready for injection.

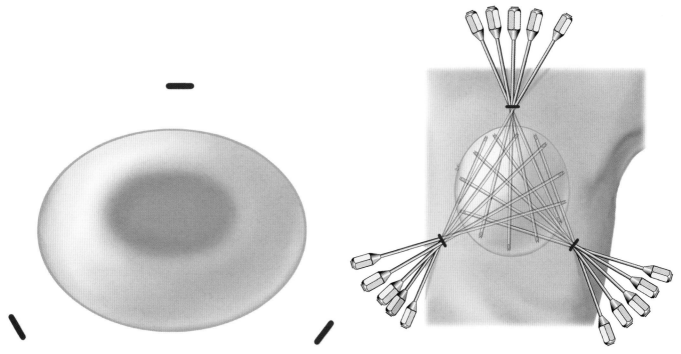

Figure 27.9 Schematic diagrams show crisscrossing of tunnels created for fat graft placement.

feathering and blending of the transition between the depression and the surrounding soft tissue. Attention should be paid to placing incisions strategically around the volume deficit to allow for maximal crisscrossing of tunnels created for graft placement (Fig. 27.9). To maximize the survivability, stability, and integration of grafts, we place 0.1 cc of the fat grafts each pass while the canula is being withdrawn in a fan-like pattern, in multiple layers or planes, in multiple tunnels, making multiple passes (Fig. 27.10 and 27.11). All effort is made to avoid the creation of pockets within the subcutaneous tissue. All grafts should fit securely within individually created tunnels. Although it is tempting to inject large volumes to immediately correct the defect, it is more prudent to fill only to the extent the recipient bed will allow, and plan on returning for subsequent grafting when this tissue bed has greater capacity. We do not perform overcorrection, preferring to return for subsequent grafting procedures.

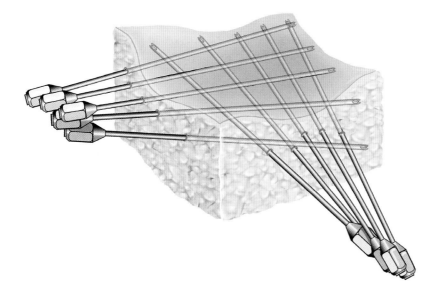

Figure 27.10 Schematic diagram shows placement of fat grafts in a fan-like patten with multiple passes in multiple tunnels and tissue planes.

Part VII: Breast Reconstruction

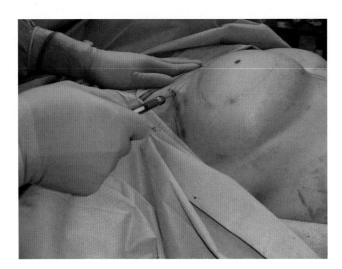

Figure 27.11 An intraoperative photo shows the placement of fat grafts in the subcutaneous tissue while the canula is being withdrawn. Only 0.1 cc of fat grafts is placed in each pass.

 POSTOPERATIVE CARE

Access incisions are closed with a single, buried dermal absorbable suture. A Reston foam or Microfoam tape is applied to the fat grafted areas for protection. Patients are instructed not to manipulate or massage the grafted area for a minimum of 2 weeks. The donor abdomen and thighs may be placed in compression garments for comfort and edema control.

 COMPLICATIONS

The most common complication is volume loss over time. In general, the majority of volume change is noted within the first 3 months. Whether this is due to resolution of edema or actual graft resorption is unclear. In our early experience, it does appear that volume remains stable beyond 3 months. Although fat necrosis with nodularity and firmness has been described, we have not yet encountered this, perhaps because of the small volumes of injection in multiple tunnels and planes as recommended by Coleman and others.

 RESULTS

All patients who underwent free fat grafting for correction of residual contour deformity after breast reconstruction have showed noticeable or substantial improvement of the contour deformity and asymmetry between the breasts in either autogenous or implant-reconstructed breasts in our series (Figs. 27.12–27.14). Subsequent fat grafting procedures are often necessary to achieve additional improvement of contour or asymmetry after 4 to 6 months. Most patients state the improvement after free fat grafting has met or exceeded their expectations and are willing to have subsequent procedures for additional correction of their residual contour deformities.

 PEARLS AND PITFALLS

Autologous fat grafting has been considered a valid option for soft-tissue augmentation for many years. However, it has often been criticized for its poor or unpredictable results, often considered largely surgeon dependant. It is the authors' opinion that less desirable outcomes after fat grafting are most commonly due to suboptimal surgical technique.

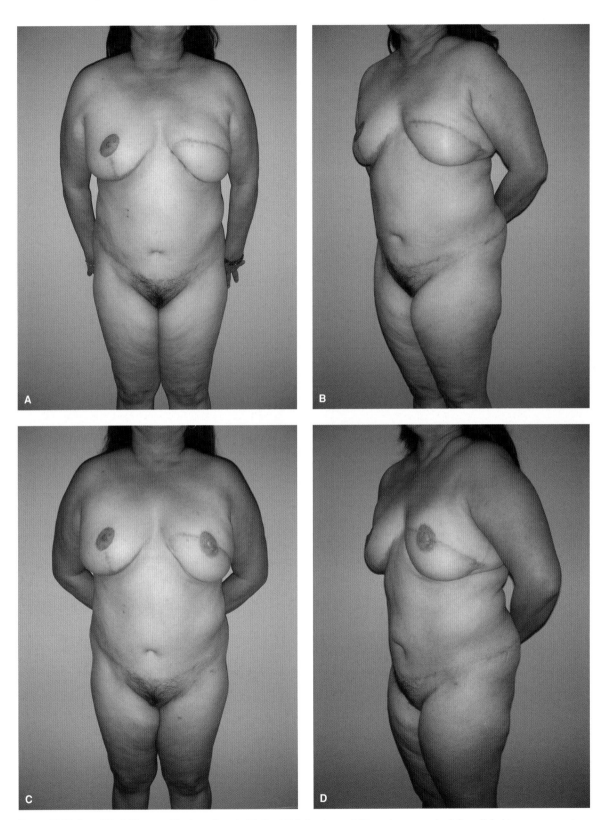

Figure 27.12 A and B. A 55-year-old, obese female (Patient 1) following a right mastopexy and a left pedicled transverse rectus abdominis myocutaneous (TRAM) breast reconstruction with noted upper pole contour irregularities at the junction of the TRAM flap and the chest wall. There are also some dimples noted in the medial inframammary fold. **C and D.** Same patient at 7 months following 68 cc fat grafting from inner thigh to the junction of the left TRAM flap and the left chest wall and nipple reconstruction using C-V flap technique and full-thickness skin graft from inner thigh.

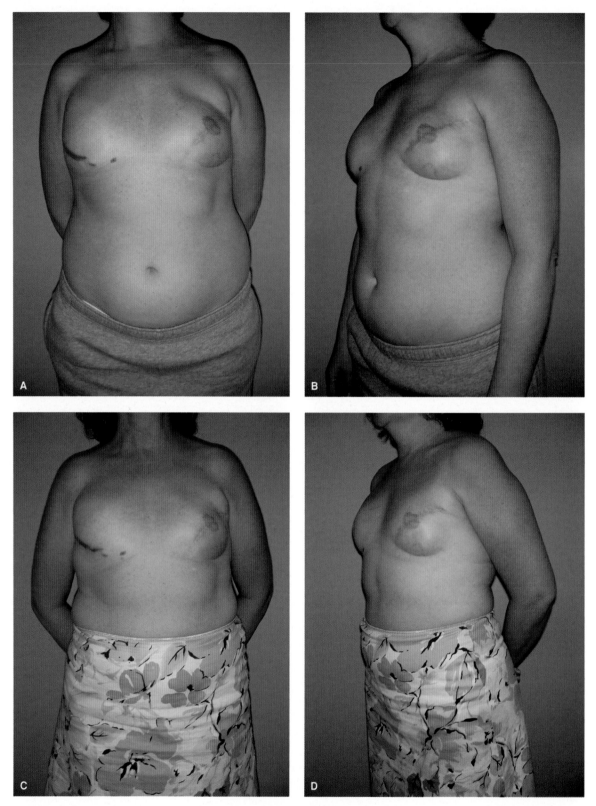

Figure 27.13 A and B. A 48-year-old women (Patient 2) who initially underwent breast conservation therapy for left breast cancer and subsequently had a recurrence and was treated with bilateral tissue expanders and implant reconstruction. During tissue expansion on the left, she was noted to have more chest wall depression than soft-tissue expansion. She elected to discontinue expansion and accept smaller implants. Upon placing the final saline implants, she was noted to have a severe upper pole depression on the left, remnants of her depressed thoracic rib cage. **C and D.** Same patient at 6 month postoperatively following 36 cc of fat grafting harvested from lower abdomen and inner thighs to the upper pole of the left implant reconstructed breast.

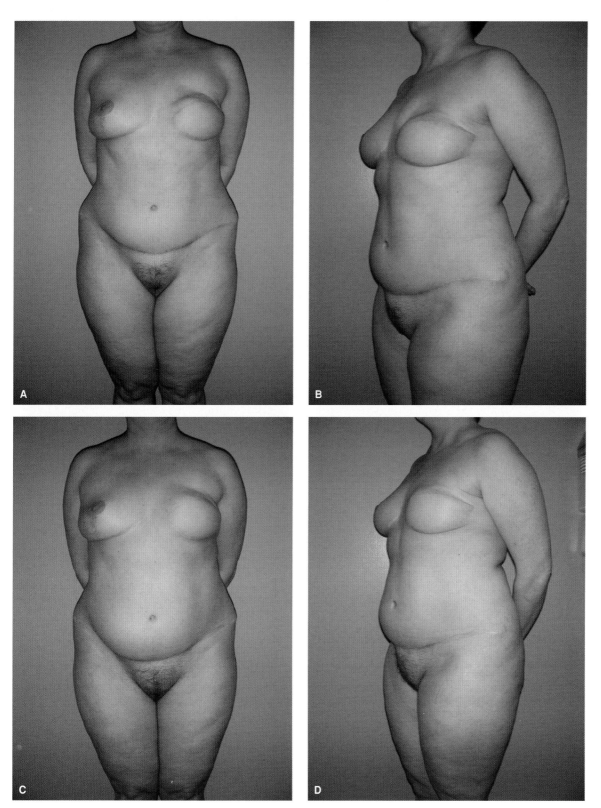

Figure 27.14 A and B. A 44-year-old female (Patient 3) treated with a mastopexy on the right and a left pedicled transverse rectus abdominis myocutaneous (TRAM) breast reconstruction after a failed attempt at a tissue expander-implant reconstruction with noticeable upper pole volume deficiency secondary to inadequate TRAM volume and tissue expander chest wall deformity. **C and D**. Same patient at 6 months postoperatively following 58 cc of fat grafting harvested from inner thighs to the upper portion of the left TRAM flap.

For those considering incorporating autologous fat grafting into their surgical armamentarium, we recommend the Coleman technique. As one gains experience, personal modifications are acceptable as long as the basic tenants of the technique are observed. Most surgeons appreciate the importance of "atraumatic" fat graft harvest. Conventional liposuction should not be used as this has been shown to have negative effects on fat graft viability. When a large volume of the fat grafts is needed, a closed fat graft harvest and transfer system has been developed with reasonably good success. Once the fat graft is harvested with a syringe using an atraumatic technique, fat graft viability can be optimized by centrifugation at 3000 rpm for 3 minutes. In order to achieve better graft survival, there should be a maximal amount of contact of the fat grafts with the vascularized tissue in the grafted site. This requires that fat grafts be placed in small amounts with each pass. We call this the 3 "M" technique, emphasizing the importance for grafts to be placed using multiple passes creating multiple tunnels in multiple tissue levels. It is critical to place fat grafts in such a fashion to ensure the optimal graft take. The surgeon should take his or her time to precisely place fat grafts in small amounts and avoid the temptation of placing "too much" fat graft within each tunnel. Consequences of ignoring these principles can lead to less reliable engraftment, fat necrosis, and graft loss.

✳ CONCLUSIONS

As breast reconstruction techniques have been refined over the years, expectations of many women opting for breast reconstruction after mastectomy have risen. Women who desire more than simply "looking better in clothes" now have the opportunity to further refine their reconstructions with the use of fat grafting. This safe and reliable technique can be used to improve on the many contour irregularities and asymmetries seen after implant-based or autologous breast reconstruction techniques. As surgeons and radiologists gain more experience and understanding about the natural history of fat grafts into breast parenchyma, autologous fat grafting to reconstruct the postlumpectomy defect may become a more widely accepted technique. Until this time, fat grafting for the reconstruction of lumpectomy defects remains controversial and should be done only in the context of a well-designed, interdisciplinary study involving breast surgeons, plastic surgeons, radiologists, and oncologists or according to the guideline published by the American Society of Plastic Surgeons. Nevertheless, free fat grafting as an effective option can be performed by the "experienced" plastic surgeons with satisfactory outcome. Such an approach should be considered with enthusiasm for correction of residual contour deformity after either autologous or implant breast reconstruction.

Suggested Readings

Bucky LP, Percec I. The science of autologous fat grafting: views on current and future approaches to neoadipogenesis. *Aesthetic Surg J.* 2008;28:313–321.

Carvajal J, Patiño JH. Mammographic findings after breast augmentation with autologous fat injection. *Aesthet Surg J.* 2008;28:153–162.

Coleman SR, Saboeiro AP. Fat grafting to the breast revisited: safety and efficacy. *Plast Reconstr Surg.* 2007;119:775–785.

Coleman SR. Hand rejuvenation with structural fat grafting. *Plast Reconstr Surg.* 2002;11:1731–1744.

Coleman SR. Structural fat grafting. In: *The Art of Aesthetic Surgery: Principles & Techniques.* St. Louis, MO: Quality Medical Publishing, Inc., 2005:290–363.

Coleman SR. Structural fat grafting: more than a permanent filler. *Plast Reconstr Surg.* 2006;118(suppl 3):108S–120S.

Hyakusoku H, Ogawa R, Ono S, et al. Complications after autologous fat injection to the breast. *Plast Reconstr Surg.* 2009;123:360–370.

Gutowski KA; ASPS Fat Graft Task Force. Current applications and safety of autologous fat grafts: a report of the ASPS Fat Graft Task Force. *Plast Reconstr Surg.* 2009;124:272–280.

Padoin AV, Braga-Silva J, Martins P, et al. Sources of processed lipoaspirates cells: influence of donor site on cell concentration. *Plast Reconstr Surg.* 2008;122:614–618.

Pu LL, Coleman SR, Ferguson REH, et al. Autologous fat grafts harvested and refined by the Coleman technique: a comparative study. *Plast Reconstr Surg.* 2008;122:932–937.

Pu LL. Invited Discussion. Sources of processed lipoaspirate cells: influence of donor site on cell concentration. *Plast Reconstr Surg.* 2008;122:619–620.

Spear SL, Bulan EJ, Venturi ML. Breast augmentation. *Plast Reconstr Surg.* 2006;118(suppl 3):188S–196S.

Spear SL, Wilson HB, Locjwood MD. Fat injection to correct contour deformities in the reconstructed breast. *Plast Reconstr Surg.* 2005;116:1300–1305.

Wang H, Jiang Y, Meng H, et al. Sonographic assessment on breast augmentation after autologous fat graft. *Plast Reconstr Surg.* 2008;122:36e–38e.

Yie Y, Zheng D, Li QF, et al. An integrated fat grafting technique for cosmetic facial contouring. *J Plast Reconstr Aesthet Surg.* 2010; 63(2):270–276.

28 Autologous Reconstruction: TRAM Flap

Luis O. Vásconez and Dean R. Cerio

Introduction

Breast reconstruction has evolved considerably. Initially, reconstructive efforts created an imperfect product, consisting only of a breast mound with an implant. This has now developed into a most satisfactory and acceptable method, where following the extirpation of either one or both breasts, the reconstructed breast is soft, pliable, symmetric, and often more aesthetically pleasing than the original breast. This is particularly true with the use of autologous tissue in the form of the TRAM flap. In addition, experience has demonstrated that as the years progress, patient satisfaction increases with an autologous reconstruction, which is different from the experience of patients who undergo reconstruction with expanders or implants (1).

Patients who develop breast cancer, have had previous pregnancies, and have an abdominal convexity are excellent candidates for autologous breast reconstruction. The procedure is very well accepted by the patient because of the additional benefit of an improved body contour with the abdominoplasty effect. Whenever one uses an implant for reconstruction of the breast, be this preceded by an expander or even with the use of the latissimus dorsi myocutaneous flap for the additional padding, over a period of time, the implant is subject to a number of changes that interfere with the aesthetic result of the reconstruction. These changes consist of capsular contracture, which brings the implant upward; rupture of the implant, be this saline, or silicone; or malposition of the implant, usually in a position more lateral than one would wish, which may interfere with the proper movement of the arm. Moreover, it is impossible to recreate the teardrop shape of the breast, even despite the use of so-called anatomically shaped implants. This is so because implants have a tendency to become rounded, creating an unattractive convexity in the infraclavicular area. To avert this potential distorted appearance, whenever reconstruction is done with implants, it is advisable that one consider a symmetry procedure with an implant for the opposite normal breast.

Advantages and Disadvantages of TRAM Reconstruction

Autologous reconstruction has both advantages and disadvantages. The advantages are clear. The reconstructed breast is usually lasting, staying soft and symmetric, and the same size over time (except for weight changes). The disadvantages include a longer operating time, longer hospitalization, and a new breast mound that is devoid of sensibility. A TRAM reconstruction creates an additional scar in the lower abdomen, although this is compensated for by the abdominoplasty effect, and there is the rare possibility of flap loss.

Autologous breast reconstruction can be performed with the "conventional method," which maintains its vascular attachment through the superior epigastric vessels, or by the "free TRAM," which divides all attachments of the flap. The deep inferior epigastric vessels are then anastamosed with the use of the microscope to the internal mammary artery and vein.

We will emphasize the conventional TRAM flap, but we will also mention the microvascular methods.

Immediate Versus Delayed Breast Reconstruction

At our Breast Center, it is our experience that when patients are offered immediate reconstruction following a skin-sparing mastectomy, they accept it readily and are very pleased with the decision and eventual results. There is a considerable amount of literature indicating the positive and beneficial psychological effects of immediate breast reconstruction, particularly when it is done with safety and results in a symmetric and aesthetically pleasing breast (2). Presently, it is not unusual for patients to request a prophylactic skin-sparing mastectomy on the opposite unaffected side at the same operative setting (3). A bilateral breast reconstruction with autologous tissue is then performed.

Questions that patients and oncologists often ask include the following:

1. "Will reconstruction hide or delay the detection of recurrent breast cancer?"
2. "Will reconstruction delay the beginning of adjuvant chemotherapy?"
3. "Is radiation therapy precluded in the reconstructed TRAM flap?"

The answers to these questions are clear and factual. Breast reconstruction with the TRAM flap does not interfere with the detection of possible cancer recurrence in a palpable postoperative mass (4). A recurrence, if it occurs, usually appears at the subcutaneous tissue level along the scar, in a similar location to the primary tumor (5). This is easily detectable by palpation, although a number of breast centers are performing postoperative magnetic resonance examinations. What may occur in 14% of reconstructions is the development of a palpable lump due to fat necrosis (6). This can be easily distinguished from cancer recurrence because it appears shortly after the operation. It can be confirmed very easily by the use of fine needle aspiration. The answer to the second question is also clear. Chemotherapy is instituted within 8 weeks following breast reconstruction, which is the timing followed by most breast centers. Reconstruction should, therefore, not delay the start of adjuvant chemotherapy. Although a wound problem could develop and persist long enough to delay the start of adjuvant chemotherapy beyond this time frame, the literature shows no difference in survival between patients given chemotherapy at 3 weeks and those given chemotherapy at 12 weeks (7). As far as radiotherapy, the answer is also clear, but not totally satisfactory. If one knows beforehand that the patient is to receive postmastectomy radiotherapy, it is best to delay the reconstruction until at least 3 months following completion of the radiotherapy. This is because radiotherapy will usually shrink and produce a certain amount of fibrosis of the reconstructed breast, thus diminishing any symmetry obtained. If the oncologic surgeon indicates intraoperatively that because of the proximity of the tumor to the pectoralis major fascia, he or she is going to advise radiotherapy, and the reconstructive surgery has already begun by elevating the TRAM flap, it is advisable that the reconstructed breast be made larger than the opposite breast in anticipation of a certain amount of shrinkage that may occur (in our breast unit, the mastectomy and reconstruction is begun simultaneously with two sets of instruments and two separate operating teams). It should be noted that with newer methods of radiotherapy, fibrosis and shrinkage of the breast have decreased considerably.

INDICATIONS/CONTRAINDICATIONS

Immediate reconstruction is not indicated for patients with systemic diseases that would make reconstruction more hazardous, such as those on steroids or with uncontrolled diabetes.

In patients with large tumors who receive preoperative chemotherapy to shrink the tumor, immediate reconstruction is appropriate, although it is performed with caution, with the expectation of wound healing problems in both the reconstructed breast and the abdominal wound. In patients with postlumpectomy, postradiation, persistent or recurrent tumors, immediate reconstruction is essential, with either a latissimus dorsi or a TRAM flap, because delayed healing of the postradiation wound is likely to occur in any alternative reconstructive effort other than bringing fresh tissue with its own blood supply.

Delayed reconstruction is also a satisfactory option, although it has the obvious disadvantages of an additional operative procedure and a second hospitalization. Nonetheless, the safety and the aesthetic result is similar to the one obtained with immediate reconstruction (8). It does require additional expertise on the part of the reconstructive surgeon to shape the flap to obtain symmetry with the opposite breast. This is also true if one is doing a bilateral reconstruction, because the mastectomy, which usually has been done through a transverse incision, and the contralateral prophylactic mastectomy, which is usually a skin-sparing mastectomy, have differing incisions that make it more challenging to achieve symmetry.

PREOPERATIVE PLANNING

Conventional TRAM Flap

The transverse abdominal myocutaneous (TRAM flap) is the most commonly used method of autologous reconstruction of the breast. It remains the standard, although in more sophisticated breast centers, it is being replaced by the microvascular free TRAM or the DIEP flap. Regardless of how it is done, autologous reconstruction produces the most natural result with symmetry of the contralateral breast in most cases. However, it does require an operating time of approximately 4 to 5 hours and a hospitalization as long as 3 to 5 days.

Conventional TRAM: Blood Supply

The superficial and deep epigastric vessels and the segmental intercostal vessels form the blood supply to the abdominal wall. The deep system is formed by the epigastric arcade, which is vertically oriented at the deep portion of the rectus abdominis muscle, between the superior epigastric and the deep inferior epigastric vessels. In addition, we have the segmental intercostal vessels, which are more horizontally oriented and travel deep to the internal oblique muscle and fascia to anastomoses with the epigastric arcade on the deep portion of the rectus muscle. The nerve supply travels in a segmental fashion with the intercostal vessels. The epigastric arcade branches into segmental perforators that pierce the muscle and the overlying anterior rectus sheath. For the conventional TRAM, the most important perforator is in the periumbilical area, approximately 2 cm below the umbilicus. In this operation, one divides the deep inferior epigastric vessels and the periumbilical perforator, supplied by the superior epigastric vessel via the epigastric arcade, the flap (see Fig. 25.2B). Obviously,

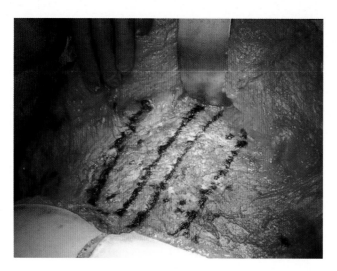

Figure 28.1 Upper abdominal flap has been elevated. The tunnel will be in the midline. The two central lines are 1 cm from the midline. The lateral lines mark the amount of anterior rectus sheath to be included with the entire rectus muscle. Note the ink dots indicating the location of the perforators.

the segmental intercostal vessels and nerves to the rectus abdominis muscle are divided as one elevates the flap. It is easy to see the perforator vessels on the anterior rectus sheath. In fact, they should be noted so that they can serve as a guide to the underlying vessels, which have to be preserved in the elevation of the TRAM flap (Fig. 28.1). The superficial and the deep venous system have valves that prevent the reflux of blood (except in patients with cirrhosis, in which one sees the caput medusa due to the incompetence of the venous system) (9).

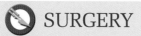 SURGERY

Elevation of the TRAM Flap

The upper incision is placed at the umbilicus to include the very important periumbilical perforator. The lower incision is made suprapubically as for an aesthetic abdominoplasty, which then gently curves upward and extends as far laterally as necessary (Figs. 28.2 and 28.3). Variations of the incision include a higher placement of the flap, particularly in very obese patients who may have an abdominal panniculus that extends below the suprapubic region. The outline should never be placed below the umbilicus in an effort to maintain the scar at the lowest possible level. Such a low outline may result in the exclusion of the periumbilical perforator, which may lead to flap necrosis.

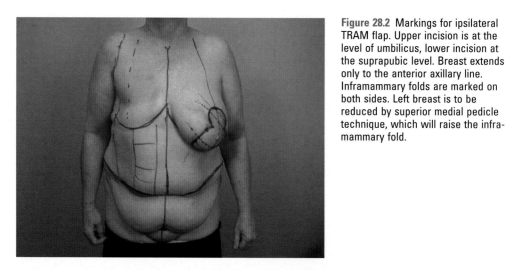

Figure 28.2 Markings for ipsilateral TRAM flap. Upper incision is at the level of umbilicus, lower incision at the suprapubic level. Breast extends only to the anterior axillary line. Inframammary folds are marked on both sides. Left breast is to be reduced by superior medial pedicle technique, which will raise the inframammary fold.

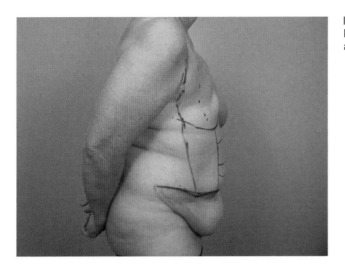

Figure 28.3 Lateral view of patient. Note the lateral extension of the abdominal flap.

The upper incision is performed first after one circumscribes the umbilicus and maintains it in place (Fig. 28.4). It is not necessary to bevel the incision. Dissection extends down to the anterior rectus sheath and the external oblique aponeurosis. The upper abdominal flap is elevated at the fascial level toward the costal margins and xiphoid. As the flap is elevated, segmental perforators from the epigastric arcade are identified and divided with hemoclips or electrocautery. We use Xylocaine with epinephrine along the incisions to decrease the amount of blood loss. Some surgeons will tumesce the upper abdominal flap with a dilute solution of Xylocaine with epinephrine. If this is done, the use of the electrocautery is less effective because of the fluid in the tissues.

According to preoperative markings, the abdominal flap is elevated and brought down to the intended lower incision to ensure that it is at a satisfactory level to allow for closure of the abdominal wound. Although some surgeons feel that traction of the abdominal flap will lower the inframammary fold, we have not found this to be the case.

The lower incision is then made all the way across the abdomen and deepened through scarpa's fascia, dividing the superficial epigastric vessels and proceeding down to the anterior rectus sheath and the external oblique aponeurosis.

The flap is designed with the intention of using the ipsilateral hemiabdomen. This has the advantages of a shorter rotation and avoids the bulge over the epigastrium as long as the tunnel to pass the flap is made along the midline. The inframammary fold should not be completely released as this serves the most helpful guiding role throughout the reconstruction. The abdominal flap is elevated from lateral toward the midline.

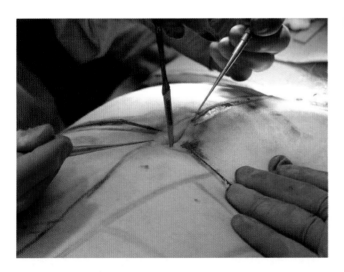

Figure 28.4 The procedure is begun by circumscribing the umbilicus. The upper abdominal flap is elevated first. The patient had a previous lower midline incision. We will utilize only the hemiflap, which increases the safety.

Part VII: Breast Reconstruction

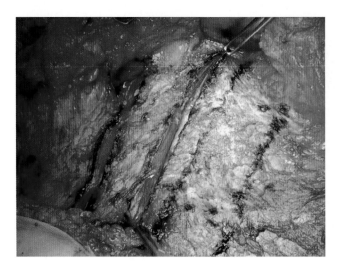

Figure 28.5 The medial and lateral fascial incisions have been made. The rectus muscle will be separated bluntly from the posterior sheath.

Please refer to Figures 28.5 through 28.9 for the following discussion. Fascial incisions cephalad to the abdominal flap are then made to dissect free the rectus abdominis pedicle. It is essential to maintain a 4- to 5-cm segment of the anterior rectus sheath, extending from just inside the midline to a point just lateral to the emergence of the epigastric perforators. This has two advantages.

1. It will help in calculating how much fascia to save at the level of the abdominal flap, which will include and maintain the perforator supplying the flap.
2. It avoids the need to dissect the fascia off the intersectiones tendineae, which is usually a bloody procedure.

The lateral aspect of the fascial incision, which was saved over the rectus muscle and maintains the perforators, has previously been identified and is continued in a caudal direction toward the pubis.

If a bilateral reconstruction is being performed, the flap may be divided in the midline from the umbilicus down to the pubis. The fascia may also be divided, saving at least 1 cm on each side of the midline.

If a unilateral flap is planned, the flap is elevated, beginning on the contralateral side of the flap and moving toward the midline. The medial endpoint corresponds to the medial incision in the anterior rectus fascia that was saved over the rectus muscle more proximally. Thereafter, division of the anterior rectus sheath is continued toward the pubis.

Once the fascia has been divided on both sides, the rectus muscle is dissected free circumferentially and the deep inferior epigastric vessels are identified on the lateral

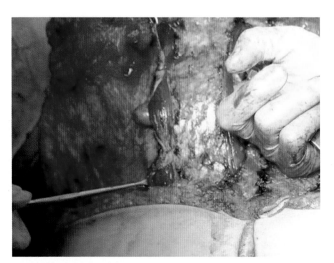

Figure 28.6 The muscle and overlying fascia have been freed up. There is need only for a sharp dissection at the level of the intersectiones tendineae.

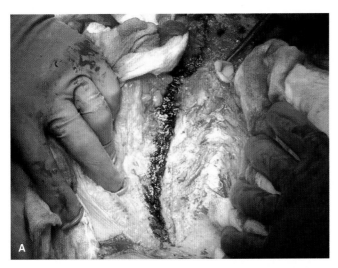
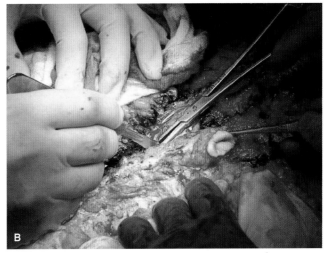

Figure 28.7 A. The fascial incisions are continued laterally and medially down to the pubis. **B.** Having the superior fascial incisions as guidelines, one can do this safely.

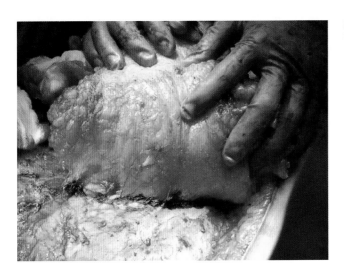

Figure 28.8 Close-up view of the lateral incision over the rectus muscle.

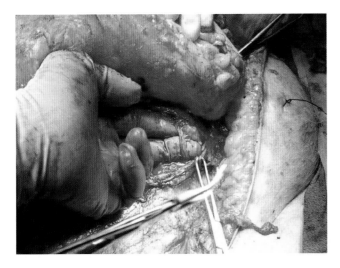

Figure 28.9 The deep inferior epigastric vessels are isolated and divided in between the hemoclips. The vessels are always surrounded by fat.

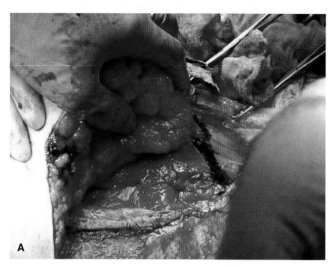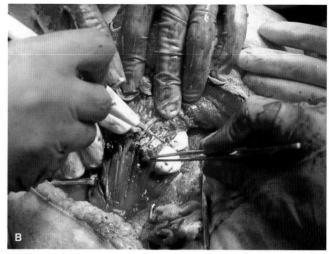

Figure 28.10 A. The rectus muscle is marked for division with electrocautery at approximately the semicircular line. **B.** The muscle is divided with electrocautery.

and deep aspects of the muscle. The vessels are usually surrounded by fat. This dissection can be done bluntly with a finger. The deep inferior epigastric vessels are isolated and divided between hemoclips. The rectus muscle is then divided at the level of the semicircular line. Attention is constantly paid to the entrance of the deep inferior epigastric vessel on the under surface of the rectus muscle (see Fig. 28.10).

The isolated muscle and the skin flap are then elevated by dividing the segmental intercostal perforators. The 12th intercostal vessels should be divided to avoid a bothersome contraction of that portion of the rectus muscle.

Following the elevation of the flap, it is returned to its anatomical position and supported temporarily with staples. Attention is then redirected toward the chest and the creation of the tunnel for passage of the flap.

If a skin-sparing mastectomy has been performed with sentinel node dissection, the oncologic surgeon usually extends the dissection toward the anterior border of the latissimus dorsi muscle, which corresponds to the posterior axillary line. The breast itself extends only to the anterior axillary line; consequently, the first maneuver is to close the posterior dissection to the anterior axillary line by approximating the chest skin flap to the chest wall with sutures at the level of the anterior axillary line. A suction catheter is placed to collapse this cavity. The second maneuver is to create a midline tunnel superficial to the anterior rectus sheath, performed by simultaneously working from both the abdominal and mastectomy incision sites (Fig. 28.11). The tunnel should be in the midline and large enough to allow for safe passage of the flap.

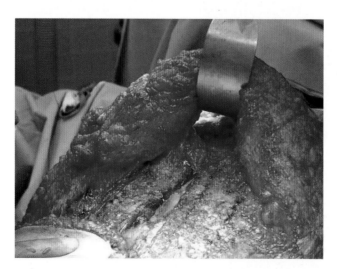

Figure 28.11 By working from the chest and abdominal incisions, a midline tunnel has been opened. A large Deaver shows the tunnel through which the flap will pass.

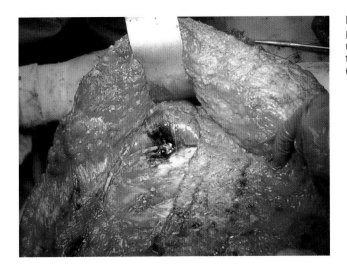

Figure 28.12 The flap has been passed into the chest. The blue marking indicates the location of the superior epigastric vessels (confirmed by Doppler).

The flap is now ready to be passed to the chest. A large Deaver retractor is placed in the tunnel and elevated by the assistant. The flap is wetted with saline solution, and two Allis clamps are placed on the contralateral tip of the flap to pull the flap to the chest. The surgeon and the assistant pull or push the flap toward the chest. If excessive traction or pushing is required, the tunnel is not large enough and the flap is returned to the abdomen to allow further tunnel dissection. Once the flap is passed to the chest, the skin side is usually toward the ribs and the flap is checked to make sure that there is no twisting of the pedicle (Figs. 28.12 and 28.13). It should be noted that if the tip of the flap needs additional length to reach the clavicle, a measurement that predicts the flap's ability to reconstruct the axillary tail of the breast, it may be necessary to divide the 12th intercostal vessels, as well as the rectus muscle that lies on the ribs, so that additional length can be obtained. Dividing the muscle over the ribs is a very safe maneuver, although there is a vessel that usually bleeds and needs to be controlled with electrocautery. One should remember that the superior deep epigastric vessels emerge from under the ribs at approximately the junction of the medial and mid-third of the muscle.

Molding of the Breast

In a skin-sparing mastectomy, the molding is relatively straightforward. The inframammary fold is marked preoperatively, as most oncologic surgeons will allow the reconstructive surgeon to place sutures or staples just below the inframammary fold. It should be noted that the inframammary fold corresponds to the lower portion of the breast and

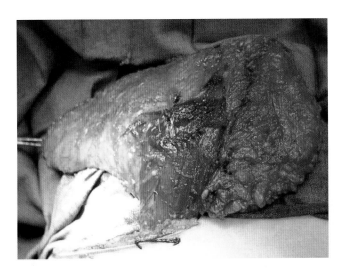

Figure 28.13 The flap on the chest wall. Note the skin side is down. There is no twisting of the muscular pedicle.

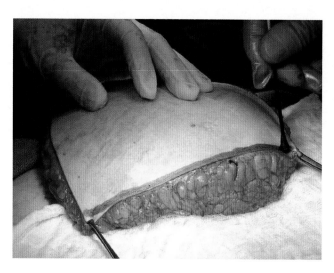

Figure 28.14 The flap has been turned so that the skin side is now apparent.

is replaced by the lower portion of the TRAM flap for the reconstruction. The flap itself can be folded in many ways, but the usual way is to position the flap so that the tip or tail corresponds to the axillary portion of the breast (Figs. 28.14 and 28.15). The flap is then allowed to fill in the skin envelope of the skin-sparing mastectomy, and in doing so, it begins to acquire a symmetry and projection closely resembling the opposite breast. The flap is then de-epithelialized except for the skin island that is to be saved to fill the periareolar incision. One suture can be used to anchor the tail of the flap. Finally, the dermis of the skin-sparing mastectomy flap is sutured to the dermis of the skin island of the TRAM flap (Figs. 28.16–28.18).

Variations on the Molding and of the Excess Skin of the Skin-Sparing Mastectomy

If the removed breast is large and/or pendulous and the patient wants to have a more youthful and a smaller breast, it is necessary to decrease the excess skin envelope from the skin-sparing mastectomy. Circumferentially excising skin around the periareolar incision and then performing a purse-string or circlage to decrease the diameter to 5.5 cm, a skin island diameter that is usually left on the TRAM flap, is one method of achieving this goal. Very rarely, a vertical incision is employed to resect an ellipse of skin. If more projection of the reconstructed breast is desired, one can decrease the width of the flap by placing it slightly more anterior to the anterior axillary line and closing the midline dissection over the lateral aspect of the sternum. This accordion effect gives the flap more projection. No additional drain is necessary in the reconstructed breast other than the one placed along the midaxillary line.

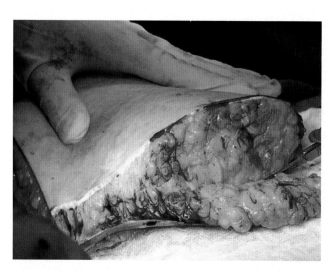

Figure 28.15 The medial aspect of the flap is incised to check its vascularity. Note the bright red bleeding (indicative of a well-vascularized flap). If the bleeding were dark or venous-like, the flap is not healthy and needs to be resected further.

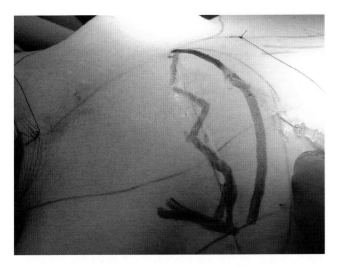

Figure 28.16 Chest incisions for insetting of the flap. Note the zigzag marking, which allows for projection of the breast mound. The skin bridge between the upper and lower incisions will be resected (the lower incision marks the inframammary fold).

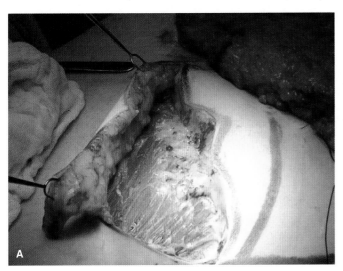

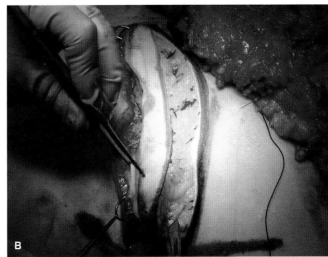

Figure 28.17 A. The upper chest flap is elevated above the pectoralis major muscle. **B.** The skin bridge is resected.

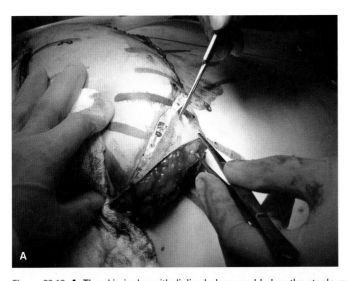

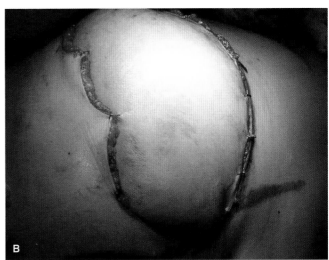

Figure 28.18 A. The skin is de-epithelialized above and below the staple marks. **B.** The flap is molded and temporarily inset with staples. The projection is less than on the opposite side. To increase it, we should have decreased the width of the flap, which is easily done by stopping the incision 5 cm from the lateral border of the sternum.

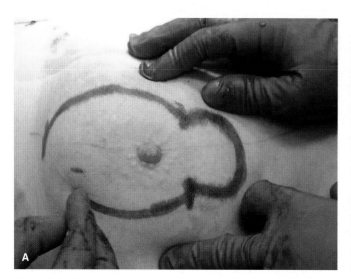 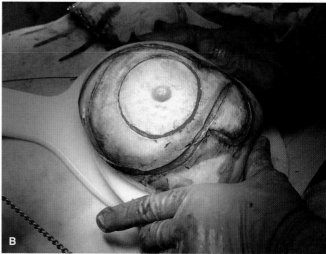

Figure 28.19 **A.** The opposite breast is to undergo a small reduction and mastopexy. **B.** Superior medial pedicle is used (Hall–Findlay).

The Opposite Breast

The decision to modify the opposite breast is usually made preoperatively. This may be in the form of a mastopexy or a reduction mammoplasty (Figs. 28.19–28.22). The markings are made ahead of time, and our preferred method of reduction is via a superior medial pedicle, which includes a resection excess breast tissue from the lateral, inferior, and superior portions of the breast (10). Again, it is noteworthy that the inframammary fold is the lowest portion of the breast. If a superior medial pedicle breast reduction is chosen, the inferior pole of the breast is resected, and the inframammary fold will be elevated on the side that is reduced. Consequently, in the attempt to achieve symmetry, sutures must be placed on the reconstructed side as well to elevate the inframammary fold. This is done by approximating the inferior portion of the skin envelope breast flap to the chest wall for whatever distance is necessary to equalize the folds.

During the superior medial pedicle technique, breast parenchyma is excised on the superior, lateral, and inferior aspects of the breast. Following the resection, the pedicle is transposed superiorly, suspended temporarily with staples, and the keyhole skin resection design is recreated with a single suture at its base. This temporarily reapproximates

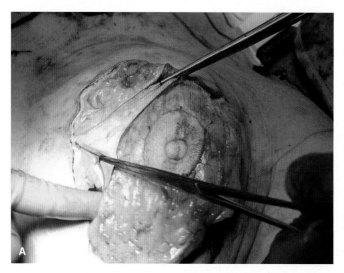 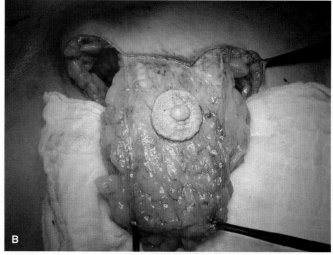

Figure 28.20 **A.** The breast resection is from inferior, lateral, and superior. **B.** The pedicle is ready to be transposed.

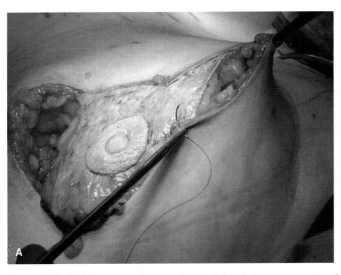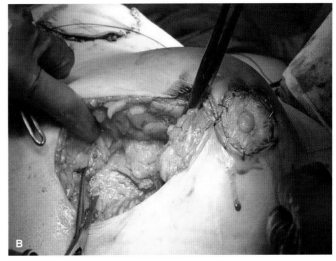

Figure 28.21 **A.** To transpose the superior medial pedicle, one recreates the key role with a suture. **B.** The pedicle with the nipple and areola are transposed and the areola temporally anchored with staples.

the shape and expected diameter of the intended nipple–areola complex. We then maintain the superior medial pedicle elevated the medial and lateral columns of the remaining breast tissue are approximated with interrupted sutures to give projection and fullness to the upper portion of the breast. The excess skin is then resected, and we usually end up with a vertical scar. To shorten the vertical scar, one has the choice either to "T" it off at the inframammary fold or to wrinkle it up in the lower portion to take up the excess skin. We advise to "T" it off at the inframammary fold because the wrinkling may be of concern to the patient and a secondary revision may be necessary.

Evaluation of the Reconstructed Breast and the Opposite Breast for Symmetry

Following the molding of the reconstructed breast, which is anchored temporarily with staples, and the reduction of the opposite breast, which is also temporarily closed with staples, the patient is sat up with the help of anesthesia, and the symmetry is evaluated. The major points to keep in mind during this period of evaluation are the following:

1. Ensure the inframammary folds are at the same level, and if not, the inframammary fold on the reconstructed side will most likely need to be raised.

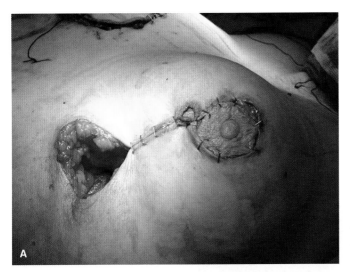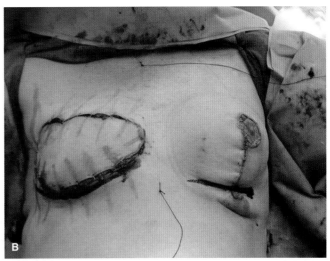

Figure 28.22 **A.** The reduced breast has been molded. **B.** The inframammary fold is marked at the same level as the opposite side.

Part VII: Breast Reconstruction

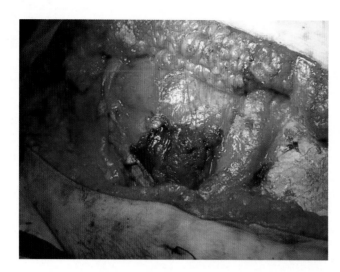

Figure 28.23 The first step of abdominal closure is to resuture the remnant of the rectus abdominus muscle to the semicircular line (see text).

2. Assess the projection of each breast.
3. Adequately evaluate the fullness at the upper pole of the breasts. Fullness in the upper portion is the most difficult aspect to correct because the height of the abdominal flap may not extend as high as the takeoff of the breast on the normal side. If this were the case, the surgeon would be wise to accept some flattening in the infraclavicular area to be filled up subsequently with fat grafting.

When satisfied with these points, and with the appropriate markings made for any planned adjustments, the patient is returned to the recumbent position and the final closure and corrections are performed.

Closure of the Abdominal Wall

In unilateral cases, primary closure is always possible. We advise the following method of closure. First, one approximates the remnants of the rectus muscle to the semicircular line with 3–0 nylon sutures. Since the muscle will tear if sutured alone, it is necessary to include an edge of the remnant of the anterior rectus sheath (Fig. 28.23). Next, we approximate the fascial layers. Anatomically, the external and the internal oblique are fused and then separated into two distinct layers somewhere at the midpoint between the umbilicus and the pubis (Fig. 28.24). We advise identifying these two layers and completing the division of the internal and external oblique toward the costal margin. Once this has been done and the patient is completely paralyzed by the anesthesiologist, the internal oblique layer is advanced toward the midline and approximated with

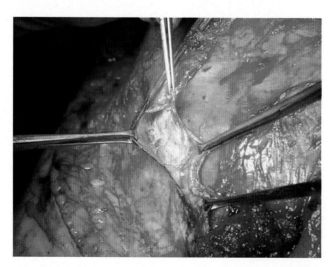

Figure 28.24 Separating the internal and the external oblique layers. The internal oblique is distinct and separate below the umbilicus. The two layers need to be separated all the way to the costal margin.

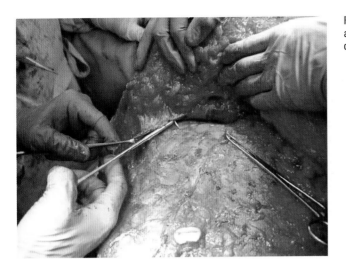

Figure 28.25 The internal oblique is approximated toward the midline (it does not reach the midline).

0-prolene sutures. It should be noted that the internal oblique will not reach the midline fascia except at the lower portion of the dissection (below the semilunar line) (Fig. 28.25). The external oblique fascia will reach the midline. This is accomplished by first placing three retention sutures: one at the level of the umbilicus from the remnants of the midline fascia to approximately 1 centimeter beyond the edges of the external oblique fascia; a second one, superiorly, near the costal margin; and a third at the lower portion of the incision. Following the retention sutures, it is a simple matter to take a running suture from the costal margin at the takeoff of the muscle right down to the pubis (Figs. 28.26–28.29). We emphasize that the internal oblique fascia and the external oblique fascia have to be approximated to the midline in the lower abdomen, from the pubis to the semilunar line. Otherwise, the internal oblique fascia will retract, and closing only the external oblique will result in a bulge in the lower abdomen, which the patient will correlate with a hernia. This is true because below the semilunar line, the transversalis fascia is much attenuated or even nonexistent. After approximating the fascial layers, the umbilicus is now eccentric, having been moved 2 or 3 cm from the midline. To centralize the umbilicus, the opposite normal anterior rectus sheath must be plicated by approximately 3 to 4 cm. In addition, if the stalk of the umbilicus is long, it can be used to push the umbilicus toward the midline. Both maneuvers are usually necessary in each case (Fig. 28.30).

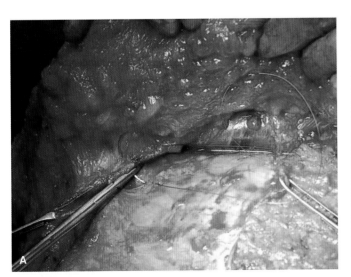
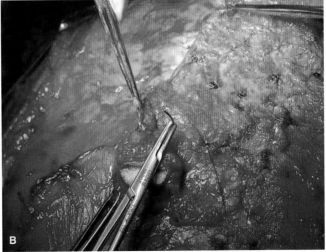

Figure 28.26 A. Retention sutures of 0-prolene are placed. **B.** One at the level of the umbilicus and a second one near the rectus muscle superiorly.

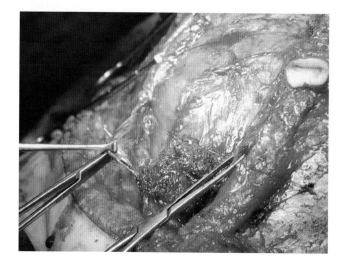

Figure 28.27 A third retention suture is placed near the pubis. It is essential that one approximates the internal and the external oblique layers at this level because the transversalis fascia is attenuated or nonexistent at this level. Otherwise, a bulge will occur, which the patient attributes to a hernia.

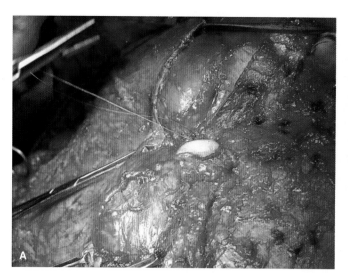
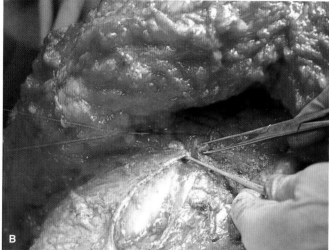

Figure 28.28 A–B. The three retention sutures are tied.

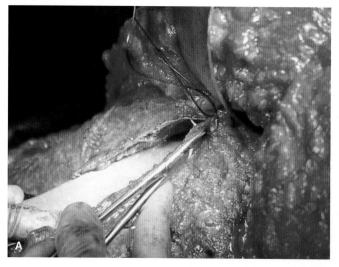
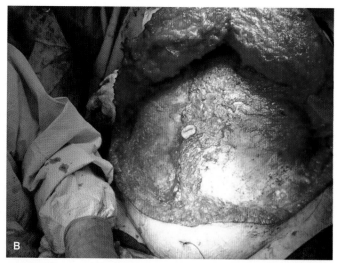

Figure 28.29 A. Following the fascial approximation with the retention sutures, one then runs a continuous suture of 0-prolene from costal margin to the pubis. **B.** Final closure. Note that the umbilicus has been moved to the right (the side of the TRAM flap).

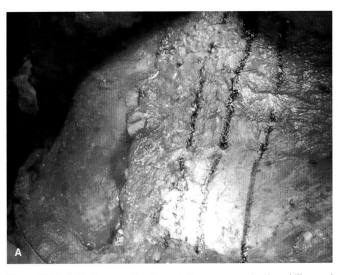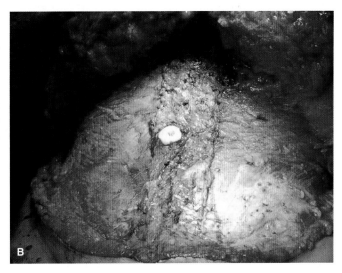

Figure 28.30 A–B. To centralize the umbilicus, one marks the midline and plicates the opposite anterior rectus sheath.

The patient is placed in the slight sitting position to allow for satisfactory and tension-free closure of the abdomen. The closure is performed from lateral toward the midline, first with staples from both sides to make sure the closure is satisfactory and to locate the point where the umbilicus will be exteriorized.

Exteriorization of the Umbilicus

With the abdominal wound temporarily closed, one identifies the location of the umbilicus by placing an Allis clamp on the umbilicus and projecting it toward the abdominal wall. A full-thickness, rhomboid-shaped piece of skin is removed. The midline temporary staples are then removed, and approximately 5 cm of fat is resected from the undersurface of the intended umbilical position on the abdominal flap. This creates a nice concavity in which the umbilicus will reside. The umbilicus is then exteriorized and approximated to the abdominal wall with mattress sutures. The abdominal wound is then closed in layers with fine monocryl sutures, and two suction catheters are brought out through the lateral edges of the incision (Figs. 28.31–28.35).

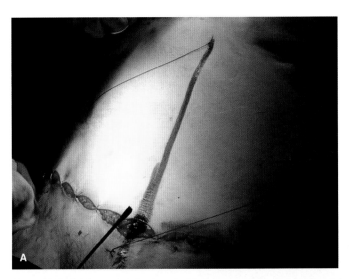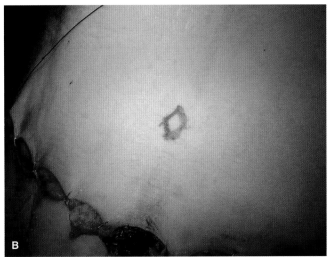

Figure 28.31 A. The patient is placed with the torso elevated, and the abdominal flap is approximated temporarily with staples.
B. The midline and the correct position of the umbilicus is marked (the umbilicus is located approximately 2 cm above the anterior iliac spines).

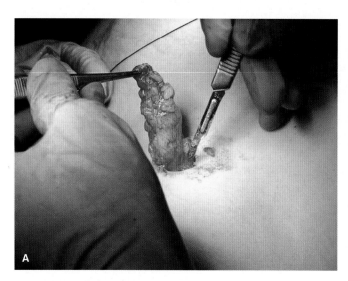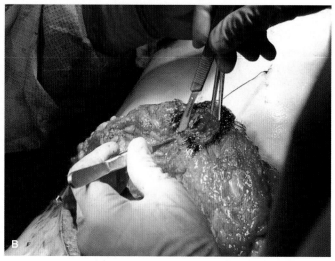

Figure 28.32 **A.** The umbilicus should be concave. A core of skin and fat is removed from the skin side. **B.** Additional fat is resected from the undersurface of the flap in a 5-cm-diameter circumference.

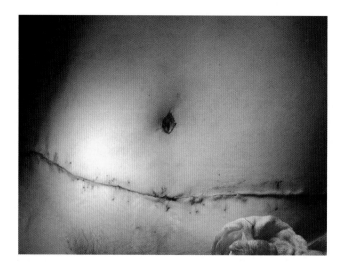

Figure 28.33 Final closure of the abdominal flap.

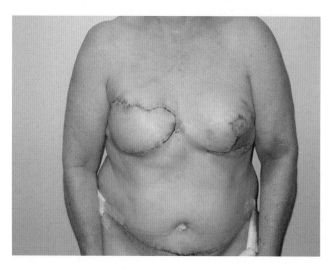

Figure 28.34 Early postoperative result. Note the decreased projection on the reconstructed breast. The width of breast should be decreased to increase the projection (see text).

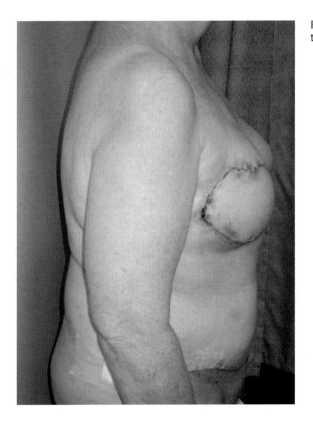

Figure 28.35 Lateral view of early postoperative result.

Bilateral Breast Reconstruction

In bilateral cases, bilateral ipsilateral flaps are utilized. The dissection is similarly done as with the unilateral flap and, again, a midline fascial strip is saved, extending off the midline by at least 1 cm on each side, from the xiphoid to the pubis. The lateral and internal oblique fascia and the anterior rectus sheath are preserved as much as possible on each side, making sure that the periumbilical perforators are included. The passage of the flap, again, is through a midline tunnel. One flap is passed at a time, and the molding procedure is similar to the ipsilateral method. Once the temporary molding has been performed, the patient is sat up for evaluation of symmetry, including a critical analysis of the inframammary folds, the projection, and the fullness of each breast. It is often the case that the prophylactic side will have more skin than the treatment side. This can be resected in a circular fashion at the periareolar level as previously described, and the approximation, de-epithelialization, and inset of the flaps is similar to the unilateral cases.

Closure of the Abdominal Wall in Bilateral Cases

Closure of the abdominal wall is more complicated in bilateral cases because more fascia has been resected. Nonetheless, unless the patient is obese, primary closure can be performed. The closure is done by first dividing the internal from the external oblique aponeurosis after one has approximated the remnants of the rectus muscle to the semicircular line. With the patient completely paralyzed and with surgeon and assistant working simultaneously, the internal oblique is approximated as far to the midline as possible on each side. We emphasize the point that simultaneous closure on both sides has to be performed. When done one side at a time, the opposite side will be difficult or impossible to close because of tearing of the fascia. Once the internal oblique has been approximated as close to the midline as possible on each side, the external oblique aponeurosis is approximated to the midline by three retention sutures—one at the level of the umbilicus, one superiorly, and one inferiorly—on both sides. Again, two surgeons tie retention sutures simultaneously to obtain the same tension. Once the retention sutures have been approximated, simultaneous closure of the external oblique fascia is performed with a running suture of 0-prolene from the takeoff of the muscle near the xiphoid toward the pubis. It is not necessary to put an onlay of polypropylene mesh, but we have no objection to surgeons who elect to do so.

Use of Mesh in Bilateral Closure

If one feels that there is excessive tension on the primary closure of the fascia, it is no problem to place mesh to bridge the defect. We prefer the use of polypropylene mesh folded twice, or even 4 times, and extending from the takeoff of the muscle at the epigastrium toward the pubis. Again, simultaneous closure of both sides is advised.

The use of three retention-type sutures is helpful: one at the umbilicus, the second superiorly, and the third inferior to the umbilicus. The internal and external oblique fascia on each side must be incorporated together with the mesh. Once the retention sutures have been placed, it is relatively easy to run a suture, simultaneously, from the epigastrium toward the pubis. A very secure closure is thus obtained.

The wound is irrigated, and the closure and exteriorization of the umbilicus are similarly performed.

Reconstruction in Postlumpectomy, Postradiation, Persistent or Recurrent Breast Cancer

Presently, we are seeing a considerable increase in the number of patients who have persistent and/or recurrent breast cancer following conservation therapy with lumpectomy and irradiation. Most of these patients, at least in our medical center, elect to have bilateral mastectomies since they no longer want to go through the possibility of additional chemotherapy or radiotherapy, if cancer were to appear in the opposite breast.

Managing the irradiated skin is the primary concern during the reconstruction of this patient population. Even though the oncologic surgeon may have performed a skin-sparing mastectomy, the blood supply to the irradiated skin cannot be trusted, and additional skin may need to be sacrificed. Attention must be paid to the inframammary fold because the irradiated breast, most likely, will have already contracted, and the inframammary fold will be higher than the contralateral normal side. Conversely, the projection will be much better on the prophylactic side. To manage the underprojection from irradiated contraction of the skin envelope on the treatment side, one may excise more skin and actually fold the flap additionally or utilize a slightly bigger flap. Nonetheless, the irradiated skin is inelastic and leather-like. Although some surgeons favor folding of the flap underneath to give more projection, we usually do not find it helpful and instead prefer to decrease the pocket size to attain the additional projection. On certain occasions, if additional projection is not possible, the patient should be informed that during a secondary procedure, that is, the nipple reconstruction, a small implant could be placed for additional projection. The implant may be placed over the pectoralis major muscle, but occasionally, the submuscular implant is sufficient, although not as effective.

 COMPLICATIONS

Partial necrosis of the flap is possible, although if one utilizes the hemiflap, it is almost always safe. The partial necrosis of the flap may occur when one utilizes additional flap beyond the midline. Although the safety of that flap beyond the midline is generally acceptable in patients 45 years or younger, it is less so in older patients and much less so in patients who are diabetic or elderly. If partial flap necrosis occurs, it needs to be debrided, and we prefer to do it in stages by first placing Betadine ointment, which penetrates through the eschar and maintains the wound quite clean. The debridement is then done every 2 to 3 days in the office, allowing the wound to granulate. If a considerable wound has developed, the use of the VAC is advised, although it is rarely necessary in our experience.

Lack of Symmetry

This is the most common disappointment in breast reconstruction. At the second operation, when one is performing the nipple reconstruction, adjustments for symmetry can be done according to what is necessary. This usually consists of raising the inframammary fold, decreasing some bulging on the lateral aspect of the reconstructed breast, which can be done with liposuction, or filling a hollow area in the infraclavicular region by fat injection. The fat is usually obtained by syringe from the lower abdomen, particularly at the level of the hips where dog-ears are most often present. Wound dehiscence of the abdominal incision is relatively infrequent, but if it happens, it needs debridement and usually the use of the VAC or frequent dressing changes. Fortunately, in most cases, spontaneous healing is obtained, although, rarely, one may need to skin graft the area.

Hernia

The incidence of hernia or bulging is at least 4% to 5%, and this is comparable to the microvascular free TRAM (11). The most common cause is the inattention to approximation of the internal oblique to the midline. If this is not done, there will be a bulge in the lower abdomen, and correction will require reoperation. At that time, approximation of the internal oblique or the use of mesh can be used.

One should keep in mind that for a true hernia to be present, one has to have a defect in the transversalis fascia. The transversalis fascia is usually weak or not present below the semicircular line. There may be a bulge along the epigastrium or above the umbilicus, but this is not a true hernia because the transversalis fascia and the posterior sheath are usually intact.

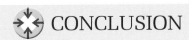 CONCLUSION

Although microvascular methods of breast reconstruction are at the forefront of reconstructive efforts in most major breast cancer centers, the pedicled TRAM is safe, is reliable, and has upheld a definitive and invaluable role as a reconstructive option for women. Overall, satisfaction, psychological burden alleviation, and morbidity are similar between the two methods, and the conventional TRAM should be a part of every plastic surgeon's surgical armamentarium.

References

1. Yueh JH, Slavin SA, Adesiyun T, et al. Patient satisfaction in postmastectomy breast reconstruction: a comparative evaluation of DIEP, TRAM, latissimus flap, and implant techniques. *Plast Reconstr Surg.* 2010;125(6):1585–1595.
2. Wilkins EG, Cederna PS, Lowery JC, et al. Prospective analysis of psychosocial outcomes in breast reconstruction: one-year postoperative results from the Michigan Breast Reconstruction Outcome Study. *Plast Reconstr Surg.* 2000;106(5):1014–1025, discussion 1026–1027.
3. Yao K, Stewart AK, Winchester DJ, et al. Trends in contralateral prophylactic mastectomy for unilateral cancer: a report from the National Cancer Data Base, 1998–2007 [published online ahead of print May 12, 2010]. *Ann Surg Oncol.*
4. Lee JM, Georgian-Smith D, Gazelle GS, et al. Detecting nonpalpable recurrent breast cancer: the role of routine mammographic screening of transverse rectus abdominis myocutaneous flap reconstructions. *Radiology.* 2008;248(2):398–405.
5. Howard MA, Polo K, Pusic AL, et al. Breast cancer local recurrence after mastectomy and TRAM flap reconstruction: incidence and treatment options. *Plast Reconstr Surg.* 2006;117(5):1381–1386.
6. Kim EK, Eom JS, Ahn SH, et al. Evolution of the pedicled TRAM flap: a prospective study of 500 consecutive cases by a single surgeon in Asian patients. *Ann Plast Surg.* 2009;63(4):378–382.
7. Lohrisch C, Paltiel C, Gelmon K, et al. Impact on survival of time from definitive surgery to initiation of adjuvant chemotherapy for early-stage breast cancer. *J Clin Oncol.* 2006;24:4888–4894.
8. Wellisch DK, Schain WS, Noone RB, et al. Psychosocial correlates of immediate versus delayed reconstruction of the breast. *Plast Reconstr Surg.* 1985;76(5):713–718.
9. Senior Author's Editorial Observation, Luis O. Vasconez.
10. Hall-Findlay EJ. A simplified vertical reduction mammaplasty: shortening the learning curve. *Plast Reconstr Surg.* 1999;104(3): 748–759, discussion 760–763.
11. Serletti JM, Moran SL. Free versus the pedicled TRAM flap: a cost comparison and outcome analysis. *Plast Reconstr Surg.* 1997;100(6):1418–1424, discussion 1425–1427.

29 Autologous Reconstruction: Microvascular TRAM and DIEP Flap

David W. Chang and Geoffrey L. Robb

Since it was first described in 1979, the free transverse rectus abdominis myocutaneous (TRAM) flap has become one of the most popular and reliable methods of microsurgical breast reconstruction. Over the years, the free TRAM flap has evolved to the muscle-sparing (MS) TRAM flap and the deep inferior epigastric perforator (DIEP) flap to minimize donor site morbidity by harvesting less muscle and less anterior rectus fascia. Each flap transfers the same lower abdominal skin and subcutaneous tissue to provide an aesthetically pleasing breast reconstruction.

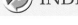 INDICATIONS/CONTRAINDICATIONS

Indications

A free TRAM/DIEP flap can be used for breast reconstruction in the overwhelming majority of mastectomy patients. A possible candidate for breast reconstruction with a free TRAM/DIEP flap is a healthy patient with moderate amounts of abdominal skin laxity and fat and a minimal to moderate volume requirement for breast reconstruction. The patient must be willing to undergo the long, complex procedure and accept the possibility of a prolonged postoperative recovery. She must also understand and accept that she will have an additional scar in the abdomen and potential donor site morbidities.

Contraindications

A patient is not a candidate for a free TRAM/DIEP flap if she

- is unwilling to accept an additional donor site scar and potential donor site morbidities;
- is unwilling to undergo the long, complex procedure with a prolonged postoperative recovery;

■ has an abdominal donor site that cannot be closed primarily because she is too thin or has a potbelly habitus;

■ has had a previous TRAM flap or abdominoplasty;

■ has had a previous abdominal surgery in which the deep inferior epigastric vessels were divided or damaged; or

■ has significant medical comorbidities that make her a poor surgical candidate.

High-Risk Patients

Smokers

Because of the free TRAM flap's excellent blood supply, a patient's history of smoking, by itself, is not an absolute contraindication for use of a free TRAM flap. In our experience, free TRAM flap breast reconstruction in tobacco smokers is not associated with a significant increase in the rates of vessel thrombosis, flap loss, or fat necrosis compared with rates in nonsmokers. However, smokers are at significantly higher risk for mastectomy skin flap necrosis, abdominal flap necrosis, and abdominal hernia compared with nonsmokers. These smoking-related complications can be significantly reduced when the patient stops smoking at least 4 weeks before surgery.

However, for free MS-TRAM flaps and DIEP flaps, where only selected few perforators are included and the perfusion of the flap is not as robust as in free TRAM flaps, we recommend a more cautious approach. For smokers, a safer approach is to optimize the perfusion to the flap by incorporating multiple perforators, thus minimizing fat necrosis and other flap-related complications. Therefore, a free TRAM or free MS-TRAM flap is recommended for smokers, and it is safer to avoid a DIEP flap.

Obese Patients

The decision about whether to use a free TRAM flap for breast reconstruction in an obese patient should be individualized. In our experience, obese patients have significantly higher flap and donor site complications than normal-weight patients. Specifically, compared with normal-weight patients, obese patients have significantly higher rates of total flap loss, flap seroma, mastectomy skin flap necrosis, abdominal hernia, donor site infection, and donor site seroma. In fact, there appears to be an almost linear relationship between complications of all kinds and body weight. Thus, for morbidly obese patients (body mass index of ≥40), TRAM flap breast reconstruction probably should be avoided, if possible. For patients who are obese but not morbidly obese (body mass index of ≥30 but <40), free TRAM flap reconstruction may be considered if a patient is in otherwise good health and is well informed about the increased risk of complications. An obese patient undergoing delayed breast reconstruction should be encouraged to reduce her risk by losing weight prior to the surgery.

As in smokers, the use of DIEP flaps where only selected few perforators are included and the perfusion of the flap is not as robust as in free TRAM flaps, a more cautious approach is recommended for obese patients. A safer approach for these patients is to optimize the perfusion to the flap by incorporating multiple perforators with use of a free TRAM or free MS-TRAM flap, thus minimizing fat necrosis and other flap-related complications.

Previous Abdominal Suction-Assisted Lipectomy

There is debate about whether a free TRAM flap can be reliably used following abdominal liposuction. The obvious concern is that the perforating vessels to the flap and the microvasculature to the flap may have been damaged by the prior suction-assisted lipectomy (SAL) procedure, which could compromise the viability of the flap. However, a few cases of free TRAM flap breast reconstruction following SAL of the abdomen have been reported. When this is being considered, preoperative Doppler ultrasonography can be used to confirm the presence and the patency of the perforating vessels of the abdominal wall. In addition, the surgeon should consider incorporating a maximum number of perforators into the flap to render it more robust for transfer.

PREOPERATIVE PLANNING

Patient Evaluation

Free flap procedures impose major surgical stress on the patient. Two simultaneous operative sites cause considerable fluid loss, and patients tend to become hypothermic because of the lengthy nature of these procedures. Thus, candidates for free flap reconstruction must have their cardiac, pulmonary, and renal statuses carefully evaluated preoperatively.

Patients must be advised to abstain from smoking preoperatively for at least 4 weeks prior to surgery to reduce the risks of anesthetic complications and wound healing problems. Avoiding aspirin-containing products for 2 weeks before surgery is also important so that the baseline coagulation status is normal.

The patient's abdomen should be evaluated to make sure she is a good candidate for a TRAM flap. In particular, the abdomen should be examined for scarring. If there are scars, their location, length, duration, and cause must be considered to determine whether a free TRAM flap can be performed safely. The abdomen should be examined with the patient in a supine position, with the knees flexed to ensure that the abdomen can be closed primarily after harvest of the TRAM flap. In addition, the integrity of the abdominal wall must be examined for the presence of hernias and for potbelly habitus.

Once it is determined that the patient is a good candidate for a free TRAM flap, the design of the flap is marked with the patient standing. The inframammary folds are marked bilaterally. The TRAM flap is designed in the lower abdomen with a transverse skin flap. The upper marking is usually just at or above the umbilicus, and the lower marking is just above the pubis, generally following the natural skin fold there. The design of the flap is then tapered to the anterior superior iliac spine so that closure of the donor site will not result in a dog-ear (Fig. 29.1).

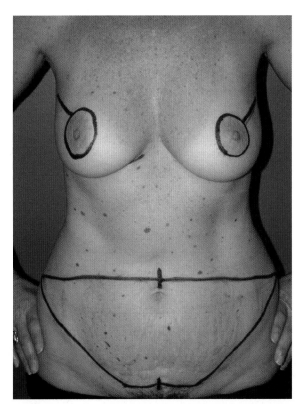

Figure 29.1 The transverse rectus abdominis myocutaneous flap is designed in the lower abdomen with a transverse skin flap. The upper marking is usually just at or above the umbilicus, and the lower marking is just above the pubis, generally following the natural skin fold there. The design of the flap is then tapered to the anterior superior iliac spine so that closure of the donor site will not result in a dog-ear.

Adjuvant Therapy

Advances in adjuvant therapies for patients with breast cancer have significantly reduced the disease's recurrence rate and associated mortality rate. Adjuvant therapies may include systemic therapy (including cytotoxic, endocrine, or biologic modulators) and/or localized treatment (such as radiation therapy). When considering breast reconstruction for patients who need adjuvant therapy, surgeons must take into account the potential effects of breast reconstruction on adjuvant therapy, and vice versa. The safety, efficacy, and timing of breast reconstruction in patients who require adjuvant therapy must be evaluated to ensure that reconstruction does not delay adjuvant therapy or negatively affect disease-free interval or overall survival. Thus, the impact of adjuvant treatment on the approach and overall outcome of breast reconstruction merits clarification.

Chemotherapy

Many studies have shown that neoadjuvant chemotherapy followed by mastectomy and immediate breast reconstruction is safe and viable, does not delay other adjuvant treatment, and can be used to identify patients who do not respond to chemotherapy, which enables oncologists to modify postsurgical treatment. Generally, neoadjuvant chemotherapy is not a contraindication to immediate breast reconstruction and does not increase the complication rate or significantly delay further adjuvant therapy. At our institution, we recommend delaying reconstruction for 3 to 4 weeks following neoadjuvant chemotherapy to allow the immunosuppressive effects of the chemotherapy to resolve.

Although whether delaying adjuvant chemotherapy affects cancer-related outcomes is not yet definitively known, most oncologists prefer to initiate therapy 4 to 6 weeks after mastectomy or breast-conservation surgery because of concerns that longer periods may increase recurrence or diminish survival. Immediate breast reconstruction may increase the risk of complications as a result of the additional surgical procedures performed, but it does not seem to delay adjuvant chemotherapy or affect overall survival and recurrence rates.

Hormone Therapy

Despite its benefits, 1% to 2% of patients on tamoxifen may experience thromboembolic events, such as deep vein thromboses, pulmonary embolisms, and cerebrovascular thrombi. Because tamoxifen presents a theoretical risk of thrombosis, it may be appropriate to have the patient stop tamoxifen therapy 10 to 14 days before undergoing free flap reconstruction and restart the therapy after breast reconstruction. However, we recommend consulting with the patient's medical and surgical oncologists to confirm that tamoxifen therapy can be stopped safely without negatively affecting the patient's cancer treatment.

Biological Therapy

Trastuzumab, a humanized monoclonal antibody directed against the human epidermal growth receptor, has been shown to significantly improve survival rates in metastatic breast cancer patients when used alone or in combination with chemotherapy. Patients who receive trastuzumab alone or in combination with other chemotherapy may experience neutropenia and an increased incidence of infections. An increase in the incidence of thrombotic events has also been reported. Because of these potential complications, we recommend that patients complete trastuzumab therapy and undergo immune status evaluation before undergoing breast reconstruction. As always, we recommend consulting with the patient's medical and surgical oncologists before making a final decision.

Radiotherapy

Given reports of the increased risk of capsular contracture associated with radiotherapy and implant reconstruction and the need for removal or reoperation despite reported acceptable cosmetic results, we recommend autologous tissue-based reconstruction instead of implant reconstruction in patients who have received or will receive radiotherapy.

For some surgeons, immediate reconstruction with autologous tissue remains the preferred approach in patients who require adjuvant radiotherapy. However, many feel that irradiating a reconstructed breast may diminish the aesthetic outcome and thus advocate delaying reconstruction in patients who require adjuvant radiotherapy. Also, delaying reconstruction until after radiotherapy decreases the risk of fat necrosis, volume loss, and the need for additional flaps. Furthermore, immediate reconstruction may cause technical problems when designing the radiation fields necessary to deliver adjuvant radiotherapy.

Relevant Anatomy

Rectus Abdominis Muscle

The rectus abdominis muscles are a pair of long, straight muscles that flex the spine and tighten the intraabdominal wall. They arise from the symphysis pubis and the pubic crest and insert on the linea alba and at the fifth, sixth, and seventh costal cartilages. Each rectus abdominis muscle is subdivided by two to five tendinous inscriptions, with the most caudal one at the level of the umbilicus. The tendinous inscriptions are adherent to the overlying anterior rectus sheath but not to the posterior sheath. The inscriptions do not usually extend completely through the muscle and may pass only halfway across it.

Rectus Sheath

The rectus abdominis muscles are enclosed by a thick sheath, except for the posterior part below the arcuate line. The rectus sheath is attached to the anterior aspect of the muscles by fusion to the tendinous inscriptions. The aponeurotic extensions of the muscles of the intraabdominal wall merge to form the anterior portion of the rectus sheath fascia.

An important transition is in the posterior sheath at the arcuate line (semicircular line, or arc of Douglas). The arcuate line is generally located halfway between the umbilicus and symphysis pubis, although this is variable. The arcuate line marks the transition point where the internal oblique aponeurosis ceases to split and the aponeuroses of all three muscles pass ventral to the rectus abdominis. The transversalis fascia is the only layer present below the arcuate line and is thus a region of weakness and potential herniation after flap dissection.

The linea alba represents the decussation of the fused aponeuroses in the midline. The linea alba is wider in the region of the xiphoid process and narrows to a fine line below the umbilicus. The lateral border of the rectus sheath is often discernable externally and is referred to as the linea semilunaris.

Blood Supply

The rectus abdominis muscle has two vascular pedicles, one composed of the deep superior epigastric artery (DSEA) and the other of the deep inferior epigastric artery (DIEA) (Fig. 29.2). The DSEA and DIEA pedicles arborize as they approach each other under the surface of the rectus abdominis. These two systems connect above the umbilicus through a system of small-caliber vessels that Taylor and Palmer refer to as "choke" vessels.

The DSEA arises from the internal mammary artery at the level of the sixth intercostal space. It generally has two venae comitantes. There is a small branch of the DSEA that courses along the costal margin to join the intercostal artery lateral to the rectus sheath.

The DIEA usually originates 1 cm above the inguinal ligament from the medial aspect of the external iliac artery, directly opposite the deep circumflex iliac artery. The main DIEA pierces the transversalis fascia and enters the rectus sheath just below the arcuate line. It then ascends obliquely and medially between the rectus abdominis muscle and the posterior wall of the sheath. Generally, the DIEA divides into two or three large branches below the level of the umbilicus. Through cadaveric studies, the degree

Figure 29.2 The rectus abdominis muscle has two vascular pedicles, one composed of the deep superior epigastric artery and the other of the deep inferior epigastric artery.

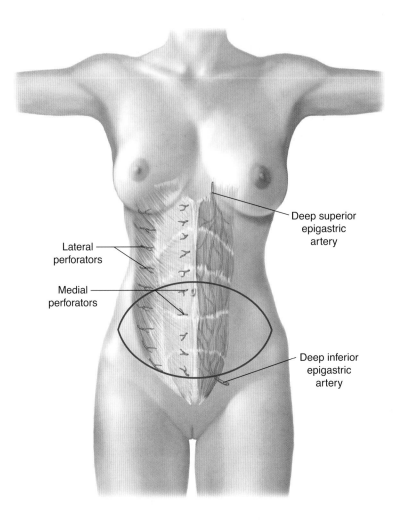

of arborization of the DIEA has been classified into three different types. In type 1, the DIEA does not divide and remains as a single vessel as it courses under the surface of the rectus abdominis (29%). Type 2 refers to a DIEA that divides into two dominant branches (57%). The type 3 pattern is a trifurcation of the DIEA (14%).

The DIEA has two venae comitantes, which usually join to form a single vein prior to their junction with the external iliac vein. In the study by Boyd et al., the deep inferior epigastric veins (DIEVs) entered the external iliac vein as a single trunk in 68% of cases and as a double trunk in 32%.

Perforators

The deep arteries supply the TRAM flap's overlying abdominal skin by a system of perforators. These vessels are terminal branches of the DIEA and DIEV. Cadaveric studies by Taylor and Palmer demonstrated a rich connection between the DIEA system and the abdominal wall skin. Many perforating arteries emerge through the anterior rectus sheath, but the highest concentration is in the periumbilical area. The fewest number of perforators is found in the suprapubic area. The branches of the periumbilical perforators have the appearance of the radiating spokes of a wheel whose hub is located at the umbilicus. Thus, incorporation of the periumbilical perforators permits the harvesting of a skin flap with virtually any orientation from the midline.

The perforators communicate with the other regional superficial vessels through a system of choke vessels that link these territories and allow the design of large skin islands based on the DIEA. The dominant connections between these systems occur within the subdermal plexus.

TRAM Flap

The blood supply to the TRAM flap is a two-tiered arrangement of muscular and subcutaneous networks. The superior and inferior epigastric artery systems form a deep longitudinal blood supply that is linked to the lower six intercostal vessels and the ascending branch of the deep circumflex iliac artery within the muscles of the abdominal wall. The DIEA is the dominant vessel of the rectus abdominis muscle and the TRAM flap. Injection of this vessel with dye will stain the abdominal wall as high as midway between the umbilicus and xiphoid process, whereas injection of the DSEA with dye rarely results in staining below the umbilicus. The subcutaneous network consists of branches of the superficial epigastric artery, superficial circumflex iliac artery, external iliac artery, superficial superior epigastric artery, and the intercostal arteries. The subcutaneous and deep systems are connected by perforators that traverse the rectus abdominis muscles.

Extensive studies of the venous circulation of the TRAM flap have revealed both superficial and deep systems. The veins of the superficial system are above Scarpa fascia and communicate extensively across the midline. The superficial veins drain into the deep venous system by way of the veins accompanying the musculocutaneous arterial perforators. Valves located in the connecting veins regulate the direction of blood flow from the superficial toward the deep system.

A TRAM flap incorporates skin from the entire lower abdomen. Four different skin zones can be included in a TRAM flap (Fig. 29.3). Zone 1 refers to the skin overlying each lateral rectus abdominis muscle. Zone 2 denotes skin of the contralateral lower abdomen overlying the opposite rectus abdominis muscle. The skin territory on each side of the abdomen lateral to the linea semilunaris is referred to as zone 3, and the skin lateral to the opposite linea semilunaris is zone 4. The blood supply to zone 4 is the most tenuous.

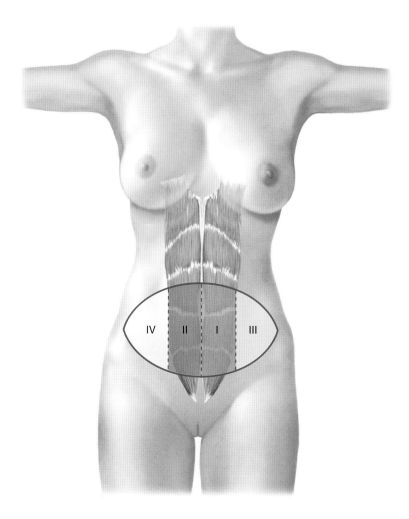

Figure 29.3 A transverse rectus abdominis myocutaneous (TRAM) flap incorporates skin from the entire lower abdomen. Four different skin zones can be included in a TRAM flap.

Innervations

The rectus abdominis muscles are innervated in a segmental fashion from the lower six intercostal nerves, derived from T7–T12, which traverse the plane between the transversus abdominis and the internal oblique muscles. These mixed motor and sensory nerves provide innervation to the rectus abdominis muscles and sensory supply to the overlying skin. The intercostal nerves enter the mid-portion of the rectus muscles at the posterior surface.

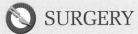

SURGERY

Positioning

The patient should be placed in a supine position, lying symmetrically and straight on the table. Her waist should be at the proper bend of the table so that she can be placed in a sitting position during flap insetting and shaping. With most operating tables, to place the patient in a sitting position, the table needs to be reversed so that the patient's head is at the foot of the table. The patient's arms are extended out and placed on arm boards with ample foam padding at the elbows and wrists. Both arms are then secured to the arm boards with gauze rolls. This allows the breast surgeons to have access to the axilla for lymph node dissection if needed.

For immediate reconstruction, the flap harvest and the breast resection are accomplished simultaneously to reduce operating time. For delayed reconstruction, the recipient site preparation and the flap harvest can be performed simultaneously by two teams of surgeons.

Flap Harvesting Technique

All flap and recipient site dissection is done under loupe magnification, and we recommend a headlight for optimal visualization of the operative field. The first step of flap harvest is to dissect out the umbilicus. It helps to make four small stab incisions with a #11 blade at the 12, 3, 6, and 9 o'clock positions. Skin hooks are then placed into the stab incisions to provide retraction, while incisions are made to connect the stab incisions. Using a tenotomy scissors, the umbilical stalk is dissected down to its base. There is no need to make the umbilical stalk overly thin or thick. A marking stitch is placed at the 12 o'clock position of the umbilicus for use as a guide during the insetting of the umbilicus and to prevent twisting of the umbilical stalk.

The border of the skin island is incised down to the abdominal wall. The superficial inferior epigastric vein (SIEV) and superficial inferior epigastric artery (SIEA) are identified and preserved (Fig. 29.4). If the SIEA is significant in size and the patient is

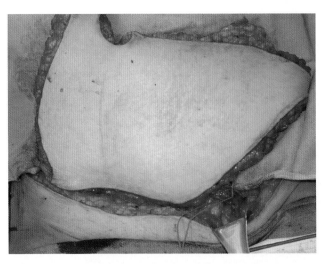

Figure 29.4 The superficial inferior epigastric vein and superficial inferior epigastric artery are identified and preserved.

a good candidate, a SIEA flap can be used for breast reconstruction (discussed in another chapter). Even if a SIEA flap is not planned, it is important to preserve and dissect out the SIEV for approximately 4 to 5 cm in length. With the increasing use of DIEP and free MS-TRAM flaps with fewer and smaller perforators being included with the flap, occasionally the SIEV needs to be used as a secondary means of venous drainage if deep venous drainage alone is not adequate.

Free TRAM Flap

For patients with high-risk factors such as smoking and obesity, optimizing perfusion to the flap by including as many major perforators as possible is a priority. In these instances, a full-muscle TRAM flap may be the best choice.

The TRAM flap is carefully dissected off of the rectus sheath, preserving all major perforators on the preferred side (Fig. 29.5). A fascia-sparing technique is used to open the rectus sheath fascia, incorporating only a small cuff of fascia around the perforators and then connecting these islands of fascia to each other (Fig. 29.6). When the fascia is opened in this manner, only a minimal amount of fascia is sacrificed, facilitating primary closure of the fascia without tension or use of synthetic mesh. The rectus sheath incision is extended inferiorly and laterally to expose the underlying rectus abdominis muscle.

The anterior rectus sheath fascia is dissected off the underlying rectus abdominis muscle and its tendinous inscriptions. The rectus sheath attachments are divided to the medial and lateral borders of the muscle. Care must be taken when separating the inscriptions to the anterior rectus sheath, where they are densely adherent. Several intercostal nerves and vessels will be seen on the surface of the posterior rectus sheath. The intercostal branches are isolated and ligated. The lateral border of the muscle is identified and dissected inferiorly, where the DIEA pedicle is found at the lateral border of the lower part of the muscle above the pubic tubercle. The rectus abdominis muscle is separated from the posterior sheath.

The rectus abdominis muscle is then gently retracted to expose the deep inferior epigastric vessels that course beneath it. Once the vascular pedicle has been identified and isolated, the inferior muscle attachment at the symphysis pubis and pubic crest is detached to facilitate exposure and dissection of the deep inferior epigastric pedicle. The deep inferior

Figure 29.5 A–B. The transverse rectus abdominis myocutaneous flap is carefully dissected off of the rectus sheath, preserving all major perforators on the preferred side. (*continued*)

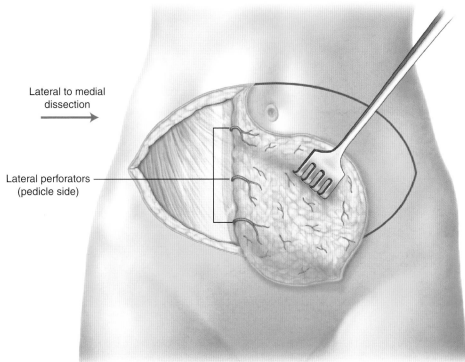

Lateral to medial dissection

Lateral perforators (pedicle side)

A

Figure 29.5 (*Continued*)

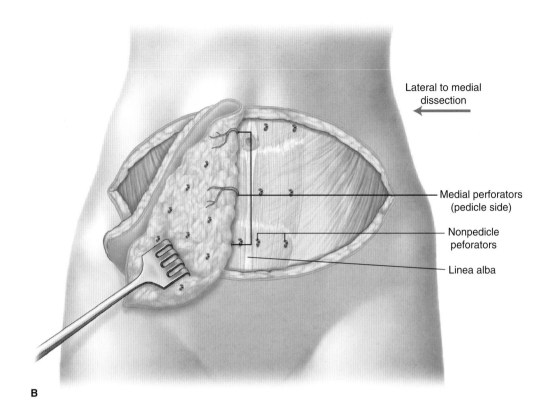

Lateral to medial
dissection

Medial perforators
(pedicle side)

Nonpedicle
peforators

Linea alba

B

Figure 29.6 A fascia-sparing technique is used to open the rectus sheath fascia, incorporating only a small cuff of fascia around the perforators and then connecting these islands of fascia to each other.

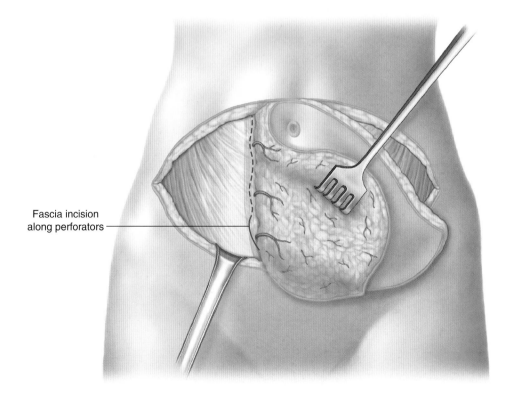

Fascia incision
along perforators

epigastric pedicle is traced toward its origin at the external iliac vessels to obtain optimal vascular pedicle length. The upper muscle attachment is divided, and the superior epigastric artery and vein are ligated. Superiorly, the muscle can be divided at any level above the perforators to the flap, even at its insertion at the costal margin if necessary. The deep inferior epigastric pedicle is left intact until the recipient site is prepared.

Once the recipient vessels are dissected and the mastectomy pocket is prepared, the TRAM flap harvesting is completed by individually ligating the DIEA and DIEVs by using either hemoclips or suture ligatures. After the flap is harvested, the muscle is secured to the overlying flap with several sutures to minimize any undue tension or twisting of perforators.

MS-TRAM Flap

The skin and subcutaneous tissues are elevated off the anterior rectus sheath from lateral to medial until the lateral perforators are seen. At this time, lateral perforators from both the right and the left side are evaluated, and the decision is made as to which perforators will be kept. The size, number, and orientation of the perforators should be considered when making this evaluation. The lateral row of perforators on the side that will not be used are hemoclipped and divided, and then the flap is elevated to expose the medial row of perforators. Once again, perforators on both sides are evaluated and the preferred perforators are kept, and the others are hemoclipped and divided. This maneuver is continued until two or more of the best perforators remain and have been selected for inclusion in the flap. With all things being equal, authors prefer medially located perforators on the contralateral side of the abdomen from the breast defect. Medial perforators provide longer pedicles, and their harvest results in less functional damage to the remaining rectus muscle since the muscle is innervated from lateral to medial. Also, compared with the laterally located perforators, more medially located perforators may provide better perfusion to the tissues across the midline of the flap. Generally, two or three moderate to large perforators will provide sufficient circulation to the TRAM flap.

The anterior rectus sheath fascia is dissected off the underlying rectus abdominis muscle and its inscriptions, and the orientation and course of the perforators within the rectus muscle are evaluated. The decision to perform an MS-TRAM or a DIEP flap is made on the basis of the number, caliber, and location of perforators as well as their orientation and course within the rectus muscle. If the perforators are located in different intramuscular layers, the muscle fibers between the perforators would need to be divided for a DIEP flap; under these circumstances, a small cuff of muscle fibers between and around the perforators is incorporated, and a free MS-TRAM flap is performed (Figs. 29.7–29.9).

Three types of free MS-TRAM flaps can be performed (Fig. 29.10). The medial portion of the rectus abdominis muscle can be preserved and a lateral portion of the rectus

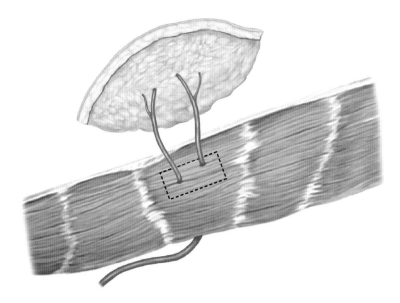

Figure 29.7 The decision to perform an muscle-sparing transverse rectus abdominis myocutaneous or a deep inferior epigastric perforator flap is made on the basis of the number, caliber, and location of perforators as well as their orientation and course within the rectus muscle.

Part VII: Breast Reconstruction

Figure 29.8 If the perforators are located in different intramuscular layers, a small cuff of muscle fibers between and around the perforators is incorporated, and a free muscle-sparing transverse rectus abdominis flap is performed.

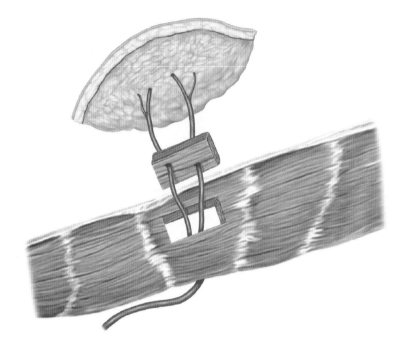

Figure 29.9 A free muscle-sparing transverse rectus abdominis flap.

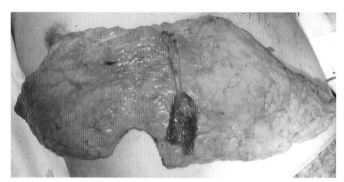

Figure 29.10 Three types of free muscle-sparing transverse rectus abdominis flaps can be performed. The medial portion of the rectus abdominis muscle can be preserved and a lateral portion of the rectus muscle harvested with the flap (MS-1M). A lateral portion of the muscle can be preserved and the medial portion of the rectus muscle harvested with the flap (MS-1L). Finally, a small cuff of muscle around the perforators can be harvested with the flap, leaving the majority of the muscles intact (MS-2).

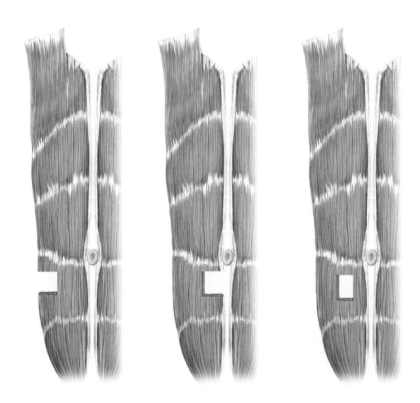

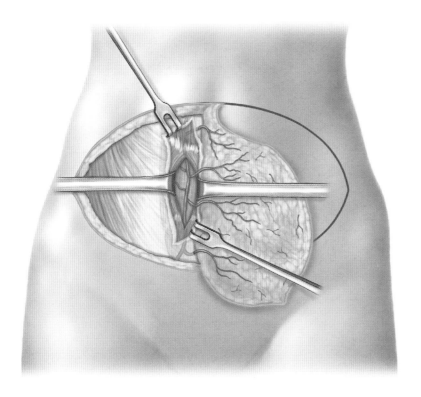

Part VII: Breast Reconstruction

Figure 29.11 Once the extent of the muscle that needs to be taken with the flap is decided, the muscle is split in the direction of the muscle fibers within the intramuscular septum medially and laterally down to the posterior rectus sheath.

muscle harvested with the flap (MS-1M). A lateral portion of the muscle can be preserved and the medial portion of the rectus muscle harvested with the flap (MS-1 L). Finally, a small cuff of muscle around the perforators can be harvested with the flap, leaving the majority of the muscles intact (MS-2).

The type of free MS-TRAM flap harvested is, for the most part, dependent on the location and orientation of the perforators. If the perforators are located very medially, then the MS-1 L is usually used. If the perforators are located in the middle of the muscle, usually the MS-2 is used. If the perforators are located laterally, then the MS-1M can be harvested. Also, the orientation of the perforators within the rectus muscle is a determining factor in how much of the rectus abdominis muscle will be taken with the perforators. If the perforators are coming directly up through the muscle, then only a small amount of muscle needs to be sacrificed. However, if the perforators are coursing obliquely through the muscle, then more muscle will need to be sacrificed.

Once the extent of the muscle that needs to be taken with the flap is decided, the muscle is split in the direction of the muscle fibers within the intramuscular septum medially and laterally down to the posterior rectus sheath (Fig. 29.11). Under the rectus abdominis muscle, the main branch to the perforators can usually be visualized at this time. Inferior to the most inferior perforator, the muscle fibers between the lateral and medial dissected plane are then divided. A bipolar device is preferred for dividing the muscles to minimize bleeding. All vascular branches should be either hemoclipped or cauterized with the bipolar device. It is important to maintain a hemostatic, clean operative field to optimize visualization and exposure. Once the inferior portion of the muscle is divided, the main pedicle should be exposed. The rectus muscle fibers are then split inferiorly to further expose and dissect out the main pedicle. With a free MS-TRAM or a DIEP flap, usually the pedicle does not need to be dissected all the way down to the origin as the pedicle is already fairly long. Finally, the muscle fibers at the superior aspect of the perforators are divided between the medially and laterally dissected plane of the rectus muscle. At this time, the superior blood supply to the rectus muscle is seen and ligated.

Once the recipient vessels are dissected and the mastectomy pocket is prepared, the flap harvesting is completed by individually ligating the DIEA and DIEVs by using either hemoclips or suture ligatures. After the flap is harvested, the muscle is secured to the overlying flap with several sutures to minimize any undue tension or twisting of perforators.

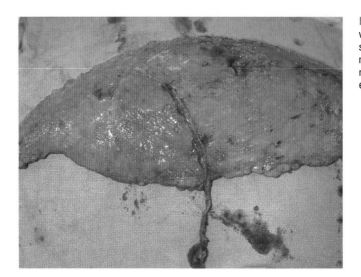

Figure 29.12 If the perforating vessels alone are harvested, sparing the entire rectus abdominis muscle, the resulting flap is referred to as a deep inferior epigastric perforator flap.

DIEP Flap

If the perforating vessels alone are harvested, sparing the entire rectus abdominis muscle, the resulting flap is referred to as a *DIEP flap* (Fig. 29.12). Sparing the entire muscle potentially reduces donor site morbidity, including abdominal bulge and weakness. However, whether DIEP flaps reduce these complications significantly more than free MS-TRAM flaps has not been clearly established.

The flap is elevated as described for the free MS-TRAM flap. A DIEP flap is selected when there is a single large perforator or when two or more perforators are located within the same intramuscular septum (Figs. 29.13 and 29.14). The optimal situation for a DIEP flap is when it can be harvested without significant damage to the rectus abdominis muscle.

Once the perforators are identified, each perforator is followed down into the intramuscular septum. The muscle is then split bluntly and sharply and the perforators are dissected to the main branch. The main branch is then followed until the deep inferior epigastric pedicle is visualized. In an ideal condition for a DIEP flap, there is a minimal need for cutting or resecting the rectus muscle. The remainder of the flap dissection is as described for free MS-TRAM flap.

Because a DIEP flap has fewer perforators than a free TRAM flap, there is concern that the reconstructed breast mound might have an insufficient blood supply, causing fat necrosis in the breast mound. Patient selection and intraoperative decision making

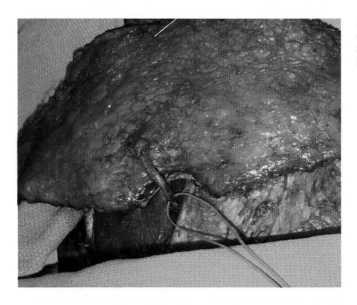

Figure 29.13 A deep inferior epigastric perforator flap is selected when there is a single large perforator.

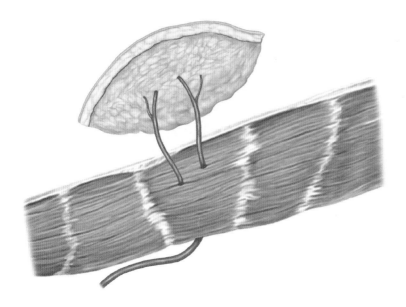

Figure 29.14 A deep inferior epigastric perforator flap is selected when two or more perforators are located within the same intramuscular septum.

is crucial to maximize the potential benefit of DIEP flap breast reconstruction. The surgeon's goal should be to perform a reconstruction that will leave the patient with the least morbidity possible while at the same time providing her with the greatest chance at a successful reconstruction.

Preparation of the Recipient Site

For immediate reconstruction, after the mastectomy is completed, the mastectomy skin flap and the mastectomy defect are carefully evaluated before the recipient vessels are dissected. For delayed reconstruction, the previous mastectomy scar is excised and sent for pathologic evaluation. The skin flap is then elevated off the pectoralis major muscle superiorly and inferiorly to recreate the mastectomy defect. Inferiorly, careful attention is paid to avoid excessive dissection, which would create a low inframammary fold.

Currently, authors use the internal mammary vessels as the primary recipient vessels of choice. The intercostal spaces are palpated to find an optimal space that is wide and readily accessible for comfortable microvascular anastomoses. This is usually at the second or third intercostal space. Then, the region above the pectoralis muscle is scanned to identify any perforator vessels that may be usable as recipient vessels. Occasionally, fairly large perforator vessels can be seen medially coming out of the pectoralis muscle fibers (Fig. 29.15). Usually, perforating veins are large with a very thin wall, and

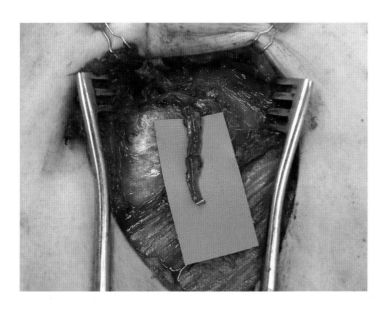

Figure 29.15 Occasionally, fairly large perforator vessels can be seen medially coming out of the pectoralis muscle fibers.

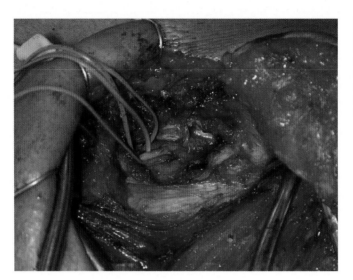

Figure 29.16 To expose the internal mammary vessels, the overlying intercostal muscle fibers are carefully divided layer by layer with a bipolar device. Usually, within 1 to 3 cm from the sternal edge, the internal mammary vein and artery are identified.

perforating arteries are small. Furthermore, most perforators will pose a size mismatch with the main DIEA and DIEV, making anastomoses challenging. Only experienced microsurgeons who are comfortable with these types of anastomoses should use perforators as recipient vessels.

If no suitable perforators are noted above the pectoralis major muscle, then the pectoralis muscle at the desired intercostal space is split in the direction of its fibers to expose the intercostal space. There is no need to detach the pectoralis muscle from the sternum. Usually, more perforators can be seen underneath the pectoralis muscle, coming out of the intercostal muscles. Again, the perforators are evaluated for their suitability, and if the surgeon feels they are large enough, then they can be used as recipient vessels.

To expose the internal mammary vessels, the overlying intercostal muscle fibers are carefully divided layer by layer with a bipolar device. Usually, within 1 to 3 cm from the sternal edge, the internal mammary vein and artery are identified (Fig. 29.16). If there is a single vein, it is medial to the artery. If there are two veins, then the artery is between the veins. It is critical to keep the operative field hemostatic for optimal exposure. Extreme care must be taken to control bleeding from all small branches. Adjacent cartilage does not need to be routinely removed; however, if the intercostal space is narrow or deep, making anastomoses difficult, then the overlying cartilage should be removed to provide better exposure of the vessels. Either the cartilage above or below can be resected. To accomplish this, the perichondrium is incised and dissected off of the cartilage, 2 to 3 cm of cartilage is removed directly over the internal mammary vessels using a rib dissector or rongeur, and then the perichondrium is carefully dissected off the internal mammary vessels. Once again, extreme care must be taken to control bleeding from all small branches. Final preparation of the recipient vessels is best performed under a microscope.

Microvascular Anastomoses

The flap is secured to the chest wall with sutures or staples with the vascular pedicle aligned for anastomoses. It is important to ensure that the vascular pedicle is not twisted before performing the microvascular anastomoses. Usually one arterial and one venous anastomoses are sufficient. Anastomoses are usually performed end to end with a coupler or with microsutures.

Flap Insetting and Shaping

The overall goal of autologous tissue breast reconstruction is to transfer well-vascularized tissue to the mastectomy site and create a breast mound that appears as anatomically and aesthetically normal as possible.

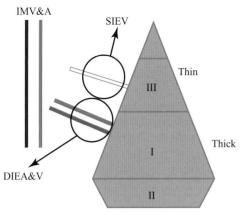

IMV&A

SIEV

DIEA&V

Thin

Thick

III

I

II

Left breast reconstruction

Figure 29.17 The flap is inset vertically on the chest with the vascular pedicle oriented medially, in an anatomically natural position, toward the internal mammary recipient vessels. IMV&A, internal mammary vein and artery; SIEV, superficial inferior epigastric vein; DIEA&V, deep inferior epigastric artery and vein.

Authors prefer to place the TRAM/DIEP flap in a vertical fashion for breast reconstruction. This is best done by using a flap from the contralateral side of the abdomen. That way, the flap lies vertically on the chest with the vascular pedicle oriented medially, in an anatomically natural position, toward the internal mammary recipient vessels (Fig. 29.17). The SIEV will also be oriented medially, so if a second source of venous drainage is needed the SIEV can be anastomosed to an internal mammary perforator vein or to a second internal mammary vein. The thin zone 3 tissue is inset in the superior region, and the tissue of zone 1 and zone 2, the thickest portion of the flap, is at the mound of the reconstructed breast. The corner of the flap from zone 3 is usually discarded, and zone 4 is always discarded. In certain situations, zone 2 (i.e., the flap across the midline) can be folded to increase the flap's projection or to create a ptotic-appearing breast.

During the insetting and the shaping of the flap, the surgeon must always be aware of the tension, the rotation, and the status of the vascular pedicle. Some surgeons like to secure the flap to the chest wall, but it is unnecessary in most cases and that the sutures create an unnatural contour of the reconstructed breast. Usually, the mastectomy skin flap alone will provide good support for the TRAM/DIEP flap. However, when the flap is significantly smaller than the mastectomy defect, the flap needs to be secured medially and superiorly so it does not fall down within the pocket, which can also cause excessive tension on the vascular pedicle.

The TRAM/DIEP flap is temporarily placed into the mastectomy defect, and the mastectomy skin flap is draped over the TRAM/DIEP flap. The mastectomy skin flap is then temporarily secured over the TRAM/DIEP flap with skin staples. The patient is placed in a sitting position, and the shaping of the TRAM/DIEP flap into a breast is performed (Fig. 29.18).

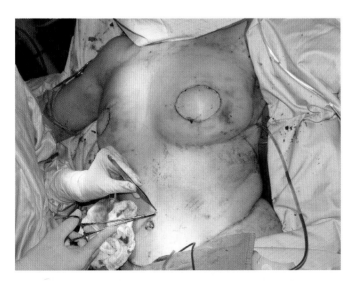

Figure 29.18 The patient is placed in a sitting position, and the shaping of the transverse rectus abdominis myocutaneous/deep inferior epigastric perforator flap into a breast is performed.

Part VII: Breast Reconstruction

When shaping a TRAM/DIEP flap for breast reconstruction, it is important to focus on the superior and medial areas of the breast to ensure adequate cleavage volume. A slightly overcorrected cleavage region can be easily revised with SAL. However, under-corrected cleavage, resulting from deficient tissue volume in the superior and medial portions of the breast, can be difficult to correct; usually, the flap needs to be reelevated and advanced to fill the hollow area, which can be a major procedure.

It is better to make the initial breast mound volume slightly larger than the contralateral breast. In most instances, mild shrinkage of the reconstructed breast will occur. Furthermore, a slightly too-large breast can usually be readily revised with SAL or direct excision. However, an overzealous attempt at achieving a "perfect" volume match at the time of initial breast reconstruction can sometimes result in a breast that is smaller than desired. If the initial reconstructed breast is significantly smaller than the opposite breast, this can be corrected only with an augmentation of the reconstructed breast or reduction of the opposite native breast. Attention also needs to be paid to ensure the inframammary fold is placed in the correct location since it is very difficult to adjust later on.

Once the optimal size and shape have been achieved compared with the contralateral breast, the skin paddle is marked. The patient is then placed back into a supine position, and the buried portion of the skin is deepithelialized. One drain is placed underneath the flap.

In unilateral breast reconstruction, the contralateral native breast is used as a guide to achieve volume and shape symmetry for the reconstructed breast. When immediate reconstruction is performed following skin-sparing mastectomy, the remaining mastectomy skin envelope can facilitate the shaping of the flap for breast reconstruction.

In delayed breast reconstruction, the surgeon must decide how to manage the inferior portion of the mastectomy skin flap. If the skin flap is abundant and soft, authors prefer to preserve it and use it for the breast reconstruction, as this allows for a more "natural" shape and appearance. If the skin flap is fibrotic from irradiation, it may be better to discard the flap and replace that area with TRAM/DIEP flap skin.

One of the most difficult parts of delayed breast reconstruction is achieving an optimal inframammary fold. A careful and accurate preoperative marking with the patient in a standing position is essential in creating an inframammary fold in the proper location. An inframammary fold that is created too high or too low during the initial reconstructive procedure is often difficult to correct. However, if one is to err, it is better to err on the side of making the fold slightly too high than too low. Authors personally find it easier to lower an inframammary fold that is too high than to move up an inframammary fold that is too low.

Management of the Donor Site

Meticulous closure of the donor site defect is required to prevent weakening or herniation of the anterior abdominal wall. If the fascia was harvested by using a fascia-sparing technique, the medial and lateral cuffs of the anterior rectus sheath can be closed primarily where it was split longitudinally without creating any tension, even in cases of bilateral flap harvest. The rectus fascia sheath is closed primarily with nonabsorbable sutures using an interrupted and running technique (Fig. 29.19). However, if the overlying fascia integrity is poor or if a significant amount of fascia was harvested and tension-free primary closure is difficult, synthetic mesh is used to reinforce the closure. Synthetic mesh can be placed using an in-lay or on-lay technique, depending on the surgeon's preference. The anterior rectus sheath should be carefully repaired below the level of the arcuate line where herniation is more likely to occur since the posterior rectus sheath is deficient in this area. Closed-suction drains are placed above the fascia closure in the subcutaneous tissue.

After the abdomen is closed, the umbilicus is brought out through an incision made in the midline of the abdominal flap and secured with sutures. Care should be taken to ensure that the umbilicus is in the correct anatomic location in the midline and that the umbilicus is not twisted at its stalk. There are many different ways to inset the umbilicus. I prefer to make a "frown" incision and to resect a small wedge from the inferior portion of the umbilicus for a more youthful-appearing umbilicus.

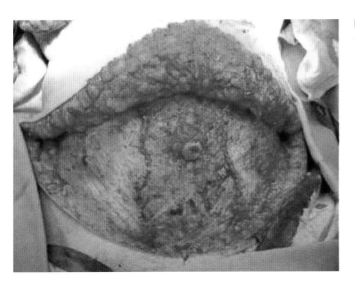

Figure 29.19 The rectus fascia sheath is closed primarily with nonabsorbable sutures by using an interrupted and running technique

 POSTOPERATIVE MANAGEMENT

Recovery

For most cases, no special vasodilators or anticoagulation agents are needed after surgery. A support bra is placed to help support and maintain the position of the reconstructed breast medially. The patient is placed in a flexed position to minimize tension at the abdominal donor site, and the flap is checked every hour by the nursing and/or surgical staff. The patient must refrain from oral intake on the day of surgery. The next morning, if the flap is doing well, the diet is advanced as tolerated. Early postoperative ambulation is encouraged. Exercise that involves the abdomen may be resumed approximately 6 weeks following surgery.

Revisions

After creation of the breast mound, a second-stage surgery may be needed to revise the reconstructed breast to achieve the final desired size and shape. Occasionally, surgical intervention on the opposite breast will be needed as well. Other procedures that may be done during this second stage include excision of fat necrosis, correction of inframammary fold asymmetry, scar revisions, minor touch-ups to the abdominal donor area, and nipple-areola reconstruction.

During the initial breast reconstruction, it is often not possible to make a breast that exactly matches the size and shape of the opposite breast. One reason for this is the position of the patient. Even if the breast is shaped with the patient in a sitting position (as much as possible), the full effect of gravity when the patient is standing cannot be duplicated on the operating table. Also, there are limitations as to how much shaping can be performed without jeopardizing the blood supply and the viability of the flap. Finally, the initial reconstructed breast rarely, if ever, completely retains its original shape or size. Thus, it is reasonable to expect that the final product will need some touch-ups in many, or even most, cases. As the flap and the surgical site heal together, the reconstructed breast's size and shape continue to evolve. For these reasons, some revision of the reconstructed breast is often necessary.

The extent of revision surgery needed can vary from minor outpatient surgery with local anesthesia to major intervention requiring general anesthesia. Often the type and extent of the revision can be planned during the initial breast reconstruction. That is, during the initial breast reconstructive surgery, insetting and shaping of the flap can be done in such a way that the second-stage revision surgery, if needed, will be minor.

Part VII: Breast Reconstruction

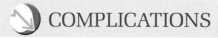
COMPLICATIONS

Flap Loss

The success of even the most elegantly designed free TRAM flap breast reconstruction is ultimately dependent on the success of the arterial and venous anastomoses. The most common cause of vessel thromboses leading to flap loss is probably technical error during the microvascular anastomoses. Thus, it is critical that the surgeon have a thorough understanding of the physiologic factors that affect anastomotic patency, technical competence, and sound clinical judgment gained from experience.

Fat Necrosis/Partial Flap Loss

Fat necrosis and partial flap loss result from inadequate perfusion to a portion of the flap. The best ways to minimize fat necrosis and partial flap loss are to ensure that the perfusion to the flap is optimal and that any poorly perfused area of the flap is discarded. This includes any areas of the flap that do not have bright red bleeding. In almost all cases, zone 4 tissue should be discarded. Usually, a small portion from the corner of zone 3 is also discarded.

As many perforators as necessary should be included to provide optimal perfusion to the flap. In many cases, only two or three perforators, and occasionally even a single large perforator, provide sufficient perfusion to a flap. However, in high-risk patients, such as those who smoke or are obese, the surgeon should consider including more perforators to reduce the risk of significant fat necrosis or partial flap loss.

Proper selection of recipient vessels is also important to ensure optimal blood inflow and outflow. It is elegant to use perforators as recipient vessels, but the surgeon must be careful to consider the vessel size match and the size of the flap being used for breast reconstruction to minimize complications.

Abdominal Bulge/Hernia

The driving force behind the development of free TRAM flap variants, such as the MS-TRAM and DIEP flaps, has been the desire to reduce abdominal donor site morbidity. One way to minimize abdominal donor site morbidity, particularly hernia or bulge, is to ensure optimal tension-free fascial closure. I prefer to use a fascia-sparing technique for harvesting most free TRAM flaps, regardless of how much rectus abdominis muscle is sacrificed. Thus, even in bilateral cases, the rectus fascia sheath can be closed primarily with minimal tension. However, if the overlying fascia integrity is poor or if tension-free primary closure is difficult, synthetic mesh can be used to reinforce the closure.

PEARLS AND PITFALLS

- A careful patient selection
  - Understand patient's goals and expectations of breast reconstruction
  - Evaluate and address patient's risk factors
- A precise and meticulous surgical technique
  - Atraumatic dissection of recipient and donor vessels, including perforators
  - Minimal sacrifice of rectus fascia
  - Minimal dissection of rectus muscle
  - Maximize preservation of innervations to the remaining rectus muscle
  - Preserve and dissect out SIEV as a potential secondary venous drainage
  - Preserve and dissect out internal mammary (IM) perforators as a potential second recipient vessel

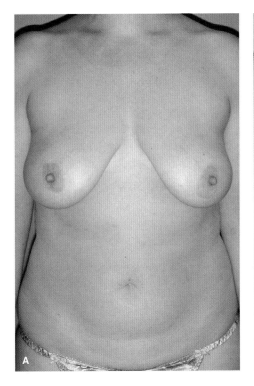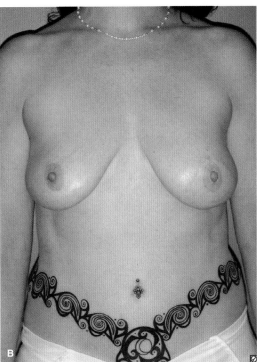

Figure 29.20 A. Preoperative photo. **B.** A patient following left skin-sparing mastectomy with immediate reconstruction with free deep inferior epigastric perforator flap.

- Use only well-vascularized portion of the flap for breast reconstruction
  - Discard zone 4
- Ensure optimal and error free microvascular anastomoses
  - Focus on proper set up so that microvascular anastomoses can be performed in a comfortable position
  - Ensure that the vascular pedicle is not twisted or kinked
  - Use atraumatic and precise microsurgical technique
- Optimal donor site closure
  - The fascia repair should be tension free
  - Do not leave dog-ears
  - Pay attention to details such as the size, the location, and the type of an umbilical repair
- Attempt to create a breast that is aesthetically optimal and natural, yet easy to revise if needed
  - Focus on creating an adequate cleavage volume
  - Better to create a breast that is slightly larger than too small

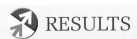 RESULTS

The free TRAM flap has many features that make it well suited for breast reconstruction. Most patients have adequate lower abdominal skin and subcutaneous tissue available for incorporation into the flap to reconstruct a breast. Its vascular pedicle is large, long, constant, and reliable. The robust blood supply of the free TRAM flap reduces the risk of fat necrosis and also enables aggressive folding, trimming, and shaping of the flap for breast reconstruction to optimize the aesthetic outcome (Fig. 29.20). In addition, the free TRAM flap requires minimal donor site sacrifice in most cases. And finally, the free TRAM flap can be harvested with the patient in a supine position while a mastectomy is being performed.

CONCLUSIONS

The free TRAM flap is one of the most popular and reliable methods of microsurgical autologous tissue breast reconstruction and has spawned several variations, including the free MS-TRAM flap, free DIEP flap, and free SIEA flap (discussed in another chapter). With proper patient selection and safe surgical technique, each of these flaps can transfer the lower abdominal skin and subcutaneous tissue to provide an aesthetically pleasing breast reconstruction with minimal donor site morbidity.

Suggested Readings

Bajaj AK, Chevray P, Chang DW. Comparison of donor site complications and functional outcomes in free muscle-sparing TRAM flap and free DIEP flap breast reconstruction. *Plast Reconstr Surg.* 2006;117(3):737–746.

Boyd JB, Taylor GI, Corlett R. The vascular territories of the superior and deep inferior epigastric systems. *Plast Reconstr Surg.* 1984;73:1.

Chang DW, Reece G, Wang B, et al. Effect of smoking on complications in patients undergoing free TRAM flap breast reconstruction. *Plast Reconstr Surg.* 2000;105(7):2374–2380.

Chang DW, Wang B, Robb G, et al. The effect of obesity on flap and donor site complications in free TRAM flap breast reconstruction. *Plast Reconstr Surg.* 2000;105(5):1640–1648.

Grotting JC. Immediate breast reconstruction using the free TRAM flap. *Clin Plast Surg.* 1994;21:207.

Holmstrom H. The free abdominoplasty flap and its use in breast reconstruction. *Scand J Plast Reconstr Surg.* 1979;13(3):423–427.

Kim JYS, Chang DW, Temple C, et al. Free TRAM flap breast reconstruction in patients with prior abdominal suction-assisted lipectomy. *Plast Reconstr Surg.* 2004;113(3):28e.

Lipa JE, Youssef AA, Kuerer HM, et al. Breast reconstruction in older women: advantages of autogenous tissue. *Plast Reconstr Surg.* 2003;111(3):1110–1121.

Moon H, Taylor GI. the vascular anatomy of the rectus abdominis musculocutaneous flaps based on the deep superior epigastric system. *Plast Reconstr Surg.* 1988;82:815.

Nahabedian MY, Momen B, Galdino G, et al. Breast reconstruction with the free TRAM or DIEP flap: patient selection, choice of flap, and outcome. *Plast Reconstr Surg.* 2002;110(2):466–475.

Schusterman MA, Kroll SS, Weldon ME. Immediate breast reconstruction: why the free TRAM over the conventional TRAM flap? *Plast Reconstr Surg.* 1992;90:255–261.

Taylor G, Palmer J. The vascular territories (angiosomes) of the body: experimental and clinical applications. *Br J Plast Surg.* 1987; 40:113.

30 Autologous Reconstruction: Latissimus Dorsi Flap

Justin M. Sacks and Steven J. Kronowitz

 INDICATIONS/CONTRAINDICATIONS

The goal of breast reconstruction is to recreate a normal-appearing breast with appropriate contour and volume. In addition, balancing inframammary folds and concealing scars is critical to any breast reconstruction. The breast mound that is created must be one that aesthetically matches that of the opposite breast in terms of shape, size, and volume. With these ideals in mind, the field of breast reconstruction has advanced through the optimization and use of both autologous and prosthetic devices.

Breast reconstruction can be performed with autologous tissue, implants, or a combination of both. Autologous tissue from the abdomen such as the transverse rectus abdominus myocutaneous (TRAM) flap and its derivatives—the muscle-sparing TRAM (msTRAM), deep inferior epigastric perforator artery flap, and the superficial inferior epigastric artery flap—are all surgical options for achieving excellent aesthetic reconstructions. In addition, autologous tissues from the buttocks using the superior and inferior gluteal artery perforator flaps along with the latissimus dorsi myocutaneous flap (LDMF) and latissimus dorsi (LD) muscle flap allow reconstructive surgeons the ability to reconstruct the breast following both complete and partial mastectomy. Prosthetic devices such as tissue expanders (TEs), postoperative adjustable implants, and permanent implants alone or in combination with autologous tissue constructs allow the reconstructive surgeon the ability to construct a breast that appears almost equal to that of the normal opposite breast, or in the case of bilateral reconstructions, to create symmetrically appearing breasts. Although there are many different ways to attain an aesthetically pleasing and natural breast reconstruction utilizing autologous tissue, prosthetic devices, or a combination of both, there are no true "gold" standards. Each patient requiring breast reconstruction represents a unique reconstructive candidate with requirements that can often be satisfied with several options.

The pedicled LD muscle flap was one of the first autologous tissue constructs used for breast reconstruction following mastectomy. Originally described and popularized by Tansini in Europe during the early 1900s, it eventually fell out of use and did not regain its popularity until the 1970s as the main flap for the reconstruction of radical mastectomy defects. With the advent of more conservative oncological approaches to breast surgery followed by immediate and delayed reconstruction using autologous tissue, specifically the TRAM flap as described by Hartrampf in 1976, the popularity of this flap has waxed and waned. The pendulum has once again shifted as newer breast implants have been created that allow the LDMF to be used in combination with these prosthetic devices for patients who require additional volume and who do not have or are not willing to spare the abdominal wall or buttock donor tissue.

Breast reconstruction with TE alone and permanent implants is often suboptimal for patients undergoing mastectomies due to a paucity of soft tissue along with a restricted skin envelope on the chest wall. Invariably these women do not have the appropriate soft tissue alone using only the pectoralis major muscle flap along with their mastectomy flaps to appropriately cover the implant. For these women, the LDMF allows additional soft tissue coverage of the prosthetic devices to create natural breast contours and volume. Recapitulating the skin envelope and ptosis of the natural breast is the key to producing excellent results. The LDMF allows the native skin to be expanded immediately allowing, at times, a permanent implant to be placed submuscularly. Furthermore, the ability to harvest the LDMF with added subcutaneous tissue or fat in an extended form allows immediate and delayed breast reconstruction to occur for women who have chosen this type of reconstruction with or without prosthetic breast implants.

Use of the LDMF in breast reconstruction offers the ability to create a natural-appearing breast for both partial and complete mastectomy defects. The soft tissue of the LDMF, which includes skin, adipose tissue, fascia, and muscle, can be utilized to fill in the contours for partial mastectomy defects with or without the use of prosthetic devices. The use of a skin island centered over the LD muscle, taking advantage of its musculocutaneous perforators, allows the breast to be reconstructed in an immediate or delayed fashion. This skin island, with its thick dermis from the back, can also be used for nipple areola reconstruction in an immediate or delayed fashion.

There are several indications for the use of the LDMF in breast reconstruction. However, since there are other excellent choices for breast reconstruction, it is important to clearly define what we feel are the optimal indications for the use of the LDMF. The LDMF still remains a distant option for most breast reconstructive surgeons secondary to the need for simultaneous implant insertion along with donor site morbidity in terms of aesthetic and sometimes functional deficits. With the advent of newer and more anatomically shaped prosthetic devices, there has been resurgence in the use of the LDMF combined with prosthetic implant devices, which in many cases may allow comparable reconstructions to that of either autologous tissue or prosthetic reconstruction alone.

Indications for the use of a LDMF in partial or complete breast reconstruction include the following:

- Mastectomy flaps not sufficient to provide appropriate contour and shaping of the reconstructed breast with TEs alone, and the patient defers the use of autologous tissue from the abdomen.
- Mastectomy flaps not sufficient to provide appropriate contour and shaping of the reconstructed breast with TEs alone and the abdominal donor site is not appropriate for use. These patients who are often thin and do not have available abdominal wall tissue. In addition, these patients may have abdominal scars such as transverse subcostal incisions or midline longitudinal incisions, which preclude the appropriate use of the abdominal wall tissue.
- Obese patients with TE and permanent implants alone will not have the appropriate breast projection. In addition, in this patient population, harvest of the LDMF is often safer with respect to donor site morbidity of using the abdominal wall where wound dehiscence, seroma, infection, bulge, and hernia rates are more common.
- Partial mastectomy defects that require soft tissue volume replacement. The nipple–areola complex (NAC) is often in a nonanatomical position secondary to scar and radiation fibrosis. In addition, if it is known that a patient will have a significant soft tissue loss from a partial mastectomy defect, it is helpful to fill the dead space with the LD muscle with or without a skin paddle.

- Poland syndrome is a congenital disorder affecting the chest wall and the ipsilateral upper extremity. The LDMF can be used to reconstruct the missing pectoralis major muscle and redefine the anterior axillary line, infraclavicular area, and breast area. Prosthetic devices can be used at the initial time of surgery or in a delayed fashion to augment volume deficits.
- The LD muscle can be used to augment the superior pole in women who have undergone autologous tissue reconstruction using TRAM flaps or their derivatives. In these women, there is a paucity of superior pole fullness, and the LD muscle allows the soft tissue deficiency to be corrected.
- Women who have thin skin overlying a potential TE reconstruction. The LD muscle is placed caudally to the pectoralis major muscle and sutured to the lower mastectomy flap just above the inframammary fold. This provides contour and coverage for the TE and ultimate permanent implant.
- Women who have excess or redundant lateral back tissue and who are not candidates for abdominal autologous tissue.
- Patients who request the use of autologous tissue but are not willing to undergo the extended recovery time of a TRAM-type reconstruction from the abdomen. These are patients who want to return to normal activities of daily living sooner and are not willing to undergo the potential for a prolonged recovery, which is often the case in breast reconstructions using the abdominal wall.

Contraindications

The LDMF is contraindicated in women who have large skin requirements for immediate or delayed breast reconstruction. In these situations, abdominal wall tissue is preferred. The LDMF can be used for chest wall coverage in cases of inflammatory breast cancer in which the mastectomy flaps are unable to be closed, and the patient will receive adjuvant radiotherapy. However, in standard breast reconstruction, this flap should not be used if the skin requirements are greater than the proposed dimensions of the LD skin paddle.

The LDMF is relatively contraindicated in patients who have previously undergone axillary lymph node dissections followed by radiation therapy. It can be extremely difficult to perform an appropriate dissection of the neurovascular pedicle in these situations. Vascular injury or insufficiency can result from a previously dissected axilla. There are certain situations when it is known that the thoracodorsal pedicle has been previously transected. Although the LDMF can potentially be harvested on the serratus branch, this has been shown to result in an increased incidence of flap necrosis.

Additional relative contraindications to using the LDMF are patients who have undergone posterior thoracotomies where the LD muscle has been transected. In addition, patients who have a known preexisting shoulder dysfunction or athletes who require the use of this muscle should not be considered candidates for this pedicle transfer.

In order for the LDMF to be utilized for breast reconstruction, certain patients must be willing to undergo the insertion of a prosthetic device. The volume of the standard LDMF is most often not sufficient to create an appropriate reconstructed breast. The extended LDMF can be considered to replicate the shape and volume; however, donor site seromas are higher in the flap technique. Patients must be clearly advised of this.

🌀 PREOPERATIVE PLANNING

Anatomy and Function

The LD muscle is responsible for extension, adduction, and internal rotation of the shoulder joint. It also plays a role in assisting with extension and lateral flexion of the lumbar spine. The LD muscle has a type V Mathes and Nahai vascular supply classification, meaning it has a dominant blood supply from the thoracodorsal artery and vein, a branch of the subscapular vessels, and secondary blood supply belonging to perforators

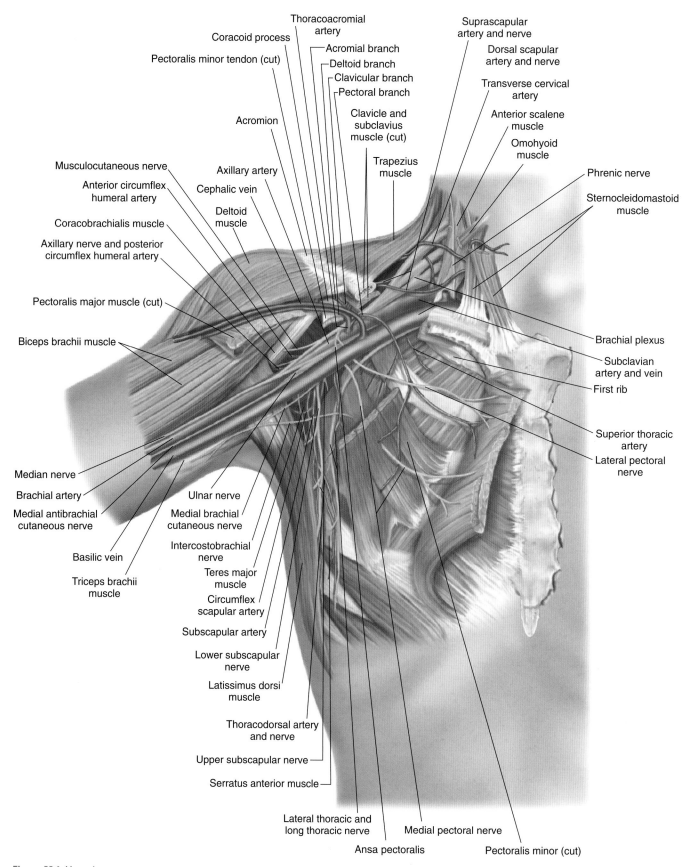

Figure 30.1 Vascular anatomy.

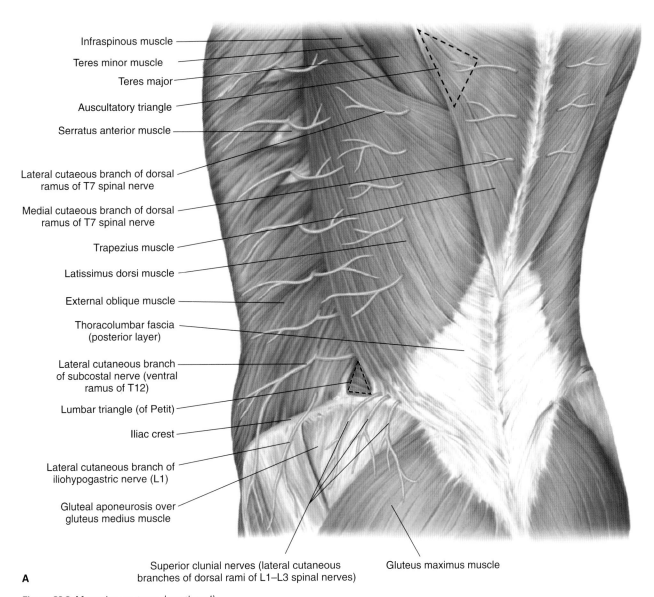

Infraspinous muscle

Teres minor muscle

Teres major

Auscultatory triangle

Serratus anterior muscle

Lateral cutaeous branch of dorsal ramus of T7 spinal nerve

Medial cutaeous branch of dorsal ramus of T7 spinal nerve

Trapezius muscle

Latissimus dorsi muscle

External oblique muscle

Thoracolumbar fascia (posterior layer)

Lateral cutaneous branch of subcostal nerve (ventral ramus of T12)

Lumbar triangle (of Petit)

Iliac crest

Lateral cutaneous branch of iliohypogastric nerve (L1)

Gluteal aponeurosis over gluteus medius muscle

Superior clunial nerves (lateral cutaneous branches of dorsal rami of L1–L3 spinal nerves)

Gluteus maximus muscle

A

Figure 30.2 Muscular anatomy. (*continued*)

from the posterior paraspinal system. The axillary vessels give rise to the subscapular vessels that give rise to the thoracodorsal vessels (Fig. 30.1). The serratus branch splits from the thoracodorsal vessels as it enters the LD muscle. The thoracodorsal pedicle enters the deep surface of the LD muscle approximately 10 cm below the axillary vessels and 2 to 3 cm inside the lateral edge of the this muscle. This vessel then splits into two terminal vessels within the LD muscle. By taking advantage of this vascular pattern, the LD muscle can be harvested separately on these branches to potentially limit the use of the muscle and move these segments independently, especially when a skin paddle is not required. Several musculocutaneous perforators supply the skin paddle, which is usually centered over the muscle. As long as the skin paddle is centered over the muscle, there is typically no concern that it will not capture a musculocutaneous perforator and have an adequate blood supply.

Nerve supply to the LD muscle is the thoracodorsal nerve. The nerve is a branch of the posterior cord of the brachial plexus, deriving its fibers from C6, C7, and C8. The nerve follows the course of the subscapular artery where it can be traced along the lower border of the muscle. The nerve is typically found in a medial position relative to the vascular bundle. The nerve is typically transected to prevent postoperative contraction of the muscle. Some surgeons do not transect the nerve because of concern that

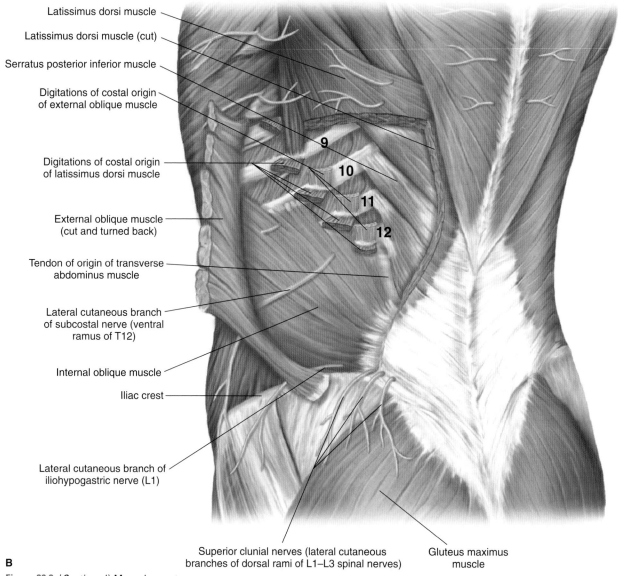

Latissimus dorsi muscle

Latissimus dorsi muscle (cut)

Serratus posterior inferior muscle

Digitations of costal origin of external oblique muscle

Digitations of costal origin of latissimus dorsi muscle

External oblique muscle (cut and turned back)

Tendon of origin of transverse abdominus muscle

Lateral cutaneous branch of subcostal nerve (ventral ramus of T12)

Internal oblique muscle

Iliac crest

Lateral cutaneous branch of iliohypogastric nerve (L1)

Superior clunial nerves (lateral cutaneous branches of dorsal rami of L1–L3 spinal nerves)

Gluteus maximus muscle

B

Figure 30.2 (*Continued*) Muscular anatomy.

the muscle will atrophy and the resultant effect of transferring the muscle to the chest wall or mastectomy site will be ameliorated. We prefer transaction of both the insertion (floor of intertubercular groove of the humerus) and its origin (spinous processes of thoracic T7–T12, thoracolumbar fascia, iliac crest, and inferior three or four ribs) but sparing the nerve creates a clinical situation that does not lead to postoperative muscle contraction and does not cause significant atrophy (Fig. 30.2).

Clinical Assessment

Determining the status of the thoracodorsal pedicle to the LD muscle must be confirmed prior to surgery. Information can be readily attained by reading prior operative notes if the patient has previously undergone an axillary lymph node dissection. The status of the pedicle is typically discussed, and this information can often be useful. However, there is no substitute for clinical evaluation. In the preoperative setting, patients are asked to place their hands at their sides and push inward. If the patient has a denervated LD, the scapula will pull upward and outward, appearing almost "winged." This is secondary to the anatomical orientation of the LD in how it drapes across the tip of the scapula, keeping it fixed to the chest wall. In addition, having patients abduct their arm and push against resistance while the LD muscle is palpated can reveal functional status. If there has been a history of a prior axillary lymph node dissection, it is critical to consider that the pedicle to the LD flap has been compromised. If this is the case, the vascular branch to the serratus muscle can be used in a retrograde fashion for blood supply to the muscle. However, in this situation, there are reported incidences of flap necrosis when the LDMF is solely based on the serratus pedicle. It is, therefore, critical that the LD muscle be assessed intraoperatively. If there is evidence of atrophy, then the neurovascular pedicle was most probably compromised during the lymph node dissection or has intimal damage from radiotherapy. In this instance, even though it can be harvested on the serratus anterior branch, the volume of the LD muscle and integrity of the skin paddle can be affected. Another autologous flap would be recommended in this situation.

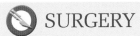

SURGERY

Marking

The patient is marked in a well-lit room in the standing position at both the recipient (mastectomy) and the donor (LDMF) sites. First, the breast markings are made, which include the sternal notch, midline, bilateral inframammary folds, and the superior borders of the breast. In the operating room, the inframammary folds are reinforced with a sterile marker as often these marks become faded following surgical preparations or from the mastectomy procedure.

The patient's back and lateral chest wall is marked to delineate the LD muscle, the skin paddle used for breast reconstruction and the pathway for which the LDMF will be placed under the axilla and into the partial or complete mastectomy defect (Fig. 30.3 A and B).

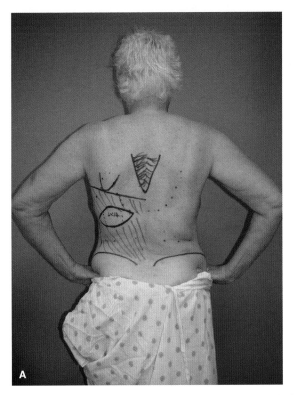
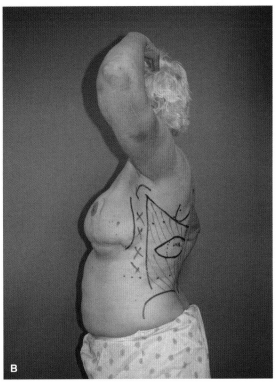

Figure 30.3 A. Anatomical landmarks are marked preoperatively. The tip of the scapula and iliac crest are marked in a standing position. The skin paddle of the latissimus dorsi muscle is centered over the muscle and placed in the bra line. The trapezius muscle is sketched as a reminder to leave this muscle down during dissection. **B.** The lateral breast fold is marked along with the anterior axillary line. The *arrow* in the upper axilla represents the subcutaneous tunnel, which the LDMF will be placed into. The *Xs* represent a zone of adherence, which should not be violated during both mastectomy, and elevation of the LDMF. If violated, the flap or prosthetic implant will migrate laterally.

Part VII: Breast Reconstruction

First, the tip of the scapula is marked, along with the iliac crest and the posterior midline. These are critical marks and should be performed only in the standing position to allow proper delineation of anatomical landmarks. It is helpful to have the patient abduct and adduct the shoulder complex to appropriately confirm the tip of the scapula. In obese patients, it is often difficult to palpate this key anatomical landmark. If this landmark is not established, the potential for inappropriately setting the skin paddle on the LD muscle becomes greater. Next, the anterior lateral and inferior borders of the LD muscle are marked. Having patients adduct their arm against resistance to feel the anterolateral edge of the LD muscle is extremely helpful when marking this border. The upper border of the muscle is marked as it extends from the axilla across the tip of the scapula. The trapezius muscle is then marked as it overlaps the upper medial portion of the LD muscle. This marking is meant to be a reminder during surgical dissection of this critical landmark. Often times, the trapezius muscle can be elevated inadvertently during the LD muscle harvest, and this anatomical boundary should not be violated.

After the LD muscle is marked along with other critical landmarks, it is then time to mark the skin paddle for appropriate breast reconstruction with or without a prosthetic implant. The skin defect from the partial or complete mastectomy defect is estimated. The potential dimensions of the defect are templated to the back over the LD muscle in the bra line. The cranial portion of the skin paddle is placed below the scapula tip while the caudal portion of the skin paddle is placed at least 10 cm superior to the posterior superior iliac line. The skin paddle is further oriented, obliquely or transversely, to allow for an adequate arc of rotation into the mastectomy defect. If the partial mastectomy defect is on the medial portion of the breast, the skin paddle is centered more posterior on the LD muscle in the back to allow for an appropriate arc of rotation.

The skin paddle dimensions typically correlate to the type of breast reconstruction required. In an immediate setting, the more common type of mastectomy is a skin-sparing mastectomy and the skin paddle requirements are rather minimal. The role of the skin paddle in this instance will be for eventual NAC reconstruction as the back dermis is rather thick and allows for optimal NAC reconstruction. In delayed breast reconstruction, the skin paddle requirements are larger secondary to potential loss of native skin from the chest wall due to radiation changes and contracture. In most patients, the skin paddle width in the craniocaudal direction should not exceed 8 to 10 cm. The length of the skin paddle can be as long as 25 to 30 cm. The skin island should be tapered off medially and laterally to limit the amount of standing cone (dog-ear) deformities. Some surgeons prefer to place the skin paddle in an oblique direction with the relaxed skin tension lines (RSTLs) to increase the potential for more aesthetically pleasing scar healing. We prefer placing the skin paddle in the transverse bra-line position, which allows the scar to be its most inconspicuous when wearing apparel.

Finally, the zone of attachment between the lateral breast and the anterolateral portion of the LD muscle is clearly marked preoperatively and needs to be reinforced in the operating room (Fig. 30.4). These marks represent a clear reminder for both the oncologic and reconstructive surgeon that this zone of attachment should not be elevated. Leaving this area intact allows the lateral border of the breast to retain its natural contour during reconstruction. This is especially critical for implant-based reconstruction with the LD muscle because any type of prosthetic device such as a TE or permanent implant can migrate laterally and potentially into the back. If compromised, this zone of attachment is extremely difficult to reconstruct with sutures. The LD muscle or LDMF must be passed high in the axilla from the back to the chest wall, and these preoperative markings help to facilitate the appropriate transfer of this muscle.

Positioning

For unilateral LD muscle and LDMF harvest, the patient is positioned in the lateral decubitus position and placed on a "beanbag" for secure positioning. The axilla and all other appropriate pressure points (hips, knees, and feet) should be well padded. The ipsilateral arm is prepped and draped and positioned to allow shoulder manipulation to help expose the neurovascular structures. The arm should not be abducted more than

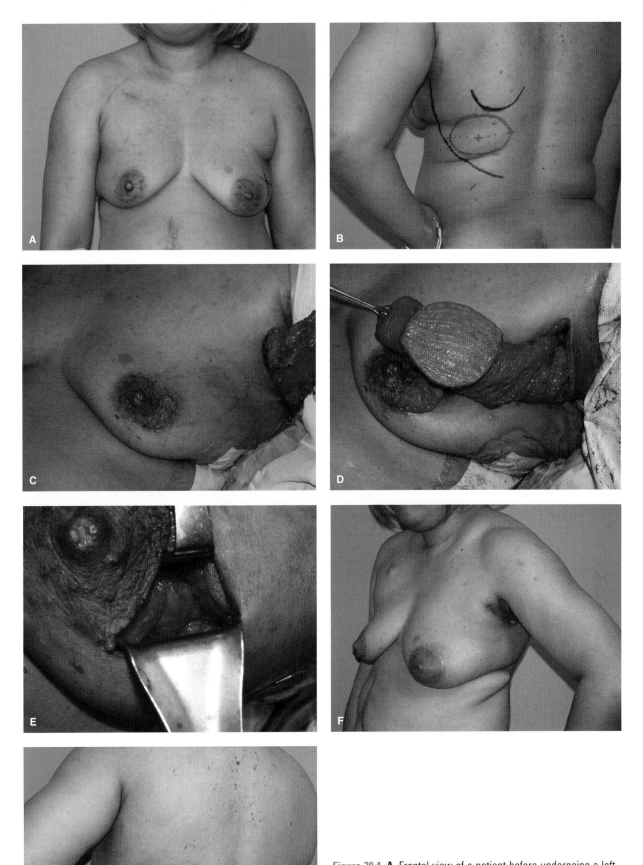

Figure 30.4 **A.** Frontal view of a patient before undergoing a left partial mastectomy. **B.** The tip of the scapula and the LD skin paddle are marked. **C.** The partial mastectomy has been performed and the LDMF has been tunneled into the axilla. **D.** The LDMF has been deepithelialized since there is no skin requirement for the lumpectomy defect. **E.** The LDMF is inset into the lumpectomy defect and sutured to the base of the wound with absorbable sutures. **F–G.** Postoperative result show well-healed scars with restoration of breast volume.

90 degrees to prevent injury to the brachial plexus and shoulder joint. The patient's donor site can be closed in this position. Preparation of the anterior chest wall or mastectomy site can be prepared in the same position. Once the back donor site is closed and the muscle flap is transferred high in the axilla into the anterior chest wall, the patient can be placed in the supine position, and the LD muscle or LDMF can be inset along with any potential prosthetic device.

For bilateral LD muscle and LDMF harvest, the patient is positioned in the prone position. Extreme care is taken to protect the patient's face and protect the airway. The arms are placed on armboards with the elbows bent at 90 degrees and the wrists in the prone position. The LD muscle or LDMF is harvested in the prone position, with the flaps being tunneled high into the axilla. Once the donor back sites are closed, simultaneously an occlusive sterile dressing is placed and the patient is turned to the supine position. The muscle flaps are then inset in the standard fashion. Care must be taken to protect the patient's head and endotracheal tube in preparation for sitting the patient up on the operating table. Typically the head of the bed is elevated to almost 90 degrees to attain unilateral and bilateral symmetrical reconstructions.

Flap Dissection for Partial Mastectomy Defect or Complete Mastectomy

Flap Elevation

The partial or complete mastectomy defect is evaluated and a template is created. We prefer to use an Esmarch bandage cut to fit into the defect as a template. Once the template is completed, it is placed in betadine and then used to design the skin island flap on the back donor site. The oncological defect in the breast is created with the patient supine. In this position, the reconstructive surgeon is able to begin the harvesting of the LD muscle. The anterior border of the LD muscle is identified and the thoracodorsal neurovascular bundle is identified. From this vantage point, the thoracodorsal nerve may be ligated here. If stimulated, it will clearly show the LD muscle contracting and will eliminate any concern as to the identity of the nerve.

Once the neurovascular bundle to the LD muscle is identified, it is now time to place the patient in the lateral decubitus position for a unilateral reconstruction or the prone position for a bilateral reconstruction. The mastectomy site is temporarily closed with a surgical stapler or interrupted nonabsorbable sutures and covered with an occlusive dressing. Once the patient is repositioned, the skin paddle design is then assessed using the previously created template.

The skin paddle preoperative markings are assessed, and the template is used to refine those that were previously drawn with the patient in the standing position. It is our belief that the best surgical position for the skin paddle is one placed in the bra line for the harvest of the LDMF. The skin paddle can be oriented obliquely in parallel to the LD muscle fibers or within the RSTLs. The critical tenet is to make sure the skin paddle is centered over the LD muscle and in the correct anatomical orientation when the LD muscle is transposed through the axilla into the mastectomy defect.

The skin island is then incised in a circumferential pattern down to the fascia of the LD muscle. Some authors recommend leaving a layer of deep adipose tissue below the superficial fascia. This technique is helpful for adding volume to the LDMF or for softening the contours of an implant-based reconstruction. Dissection proceeds at the level of the LD fascia, as we believe the muscle provides excellent coverage of any implant-based reconstruction and softens the contour of the reconstruction. The dissection then proceeds along the margins of the LD muscle, which are superiorly and lateral to the teres major muscle and superior and medial to the trapezius muscle. Anterolaterally, the LD muscle is adjacent to the serratus anterior muscle and inferior the muscle tapers and originates off of the thoracolumbar fascia along the iliac crest. At the level of the thoracolumbar fascia, the LD muscle is transected using the unipolar or bipolar cautery to help limit thermal injury. Once the superficial dissection is completed and the LD muscle is delineated, dissection off the back must be performed in the deep plane.

Thoracolumbar perforators are visualized and ligated as the LD muscle is lifted from a caudal to cranial approach. Care is taken not to lift the subscapular fat pad or serratus posterior muscle with the LD muscle harvest. At all times, the thoracodorsal pedicle must be visualized during this dissection. Typically, the pedicle runs with a small of amount of adipose tissue, which can be observed on the undersurface of the LD muscle. Once the scapula tip is reached, it is often necessary to release some attachments to the teres major muscles. At this point, the skin paddle is checked for capillary refill. It is helpful to suture the dermis of the skin paddle to the LD muscle fascia, preventing any potential shearing of the skin paddle off of the muscle during the tunneling through the axilla into the mastectomy defect. The LD muscle is dissected to its insertion in the bicepital groove. Some authors recommend leaving this insertion, transecting partially or completely. If transecting the insertion completely, the surgeon must be aware not to twist the pedicle upon transfer through the axilla into the chest. This becomes easier to do once the tendon is transected. We prefer complete transection of the tendon because it allows us to transfer the LD muscle without having to transect the thoracodorsal nerve, thus potentially limiting muscle atrophy. It also allows more medial coverage of the chest wall in the case of larger breast implants. Since there is a concern of the thoracodorsal pedicle from experiencing tension or torsion, we recommend suturing the LD tendon to the lateral edge of the pectoralis major muscle. This will also help create the anterior axillary fold and lead to a more pleasing aesthetic result.

Closure of Donor Site

The donor site is typically closed after the LDMF is harvested and prior to transposition. With patient placement in either a lateral decubitus or a prone position, the donor site is closed over suction drains. We utilize 15-F Blake drain tubes brought out the lateral caudal portion of the wound. Scarpa's fascia is closed with interrupted 3-0 absorbable sutures along with the dermis in a separate layer. A running 4-0 absorbable suture is placed in the subcuticular layer. A sterile occlusive dressing is applied.

Transposition and Inset

A subcutaneous tunnel is created from the back through the upper portion of the axilla and into the anterior chest wall. This subcutaneous tunnel should be wide enough to permit the passage of the LDMF but not too narrow to constrict the pedicle or muscle flap. Once the LDMF is transposed through the axillary tunnel and into the partial or complete mastectomy defect, it is now appropriate to inset the flap for reconstructive breast reconstruction.

Inset

The contralateral breast is used as a template for what would be considered appropriate volume and shape. The breast has three components that are critical to examine when performing reconstruction: (1) the skin envelope, (2) the volume of tissue, and (3) how these two variables interact and create levels of breast ptosis. The LDMF for partial mastectomy defects can be tunneled subcutaneously into almost any portion of the breast for skin and parenchymal volume reconstruction. Lateral defects of the breast are relatively easier to reconstruct than medial defects, but the latter can be performed as well. Excess skin from the skin paddle can be deepithelialized, and the subcutaneous tissue along with the muscle can be used to reconstruct partial mastectomy defects. For skin-sparing mastectomies or standard mastectomies the LDMF can be used to create small- to medium-sized breasts on the basis of the amount of subcutaneous adipose tissue that is transferred with the LDMF. Typically, a prosthetic implant in the form of a TE or postoperative adjustable implant is recommended, but for some patients, this is not an option based on personal preference. The flap is then inset, using absorbable stitches to tack the muscle into the defect, and the skin paddle is then "tailor-tacked" into the partial mastectomy defect. Next, the perfusion to the skin paddle is assessed. If there is any evidence of venous congestion or increased capillary refill, it is important to make sure that the axillary tunnel is wide enough to permit the transposition of the LDMF or that the vascular pedicle is not under any tension or twisted. The patient is then placed in the sitting position almost to 90 degrees to recreate normal anatomical landmarks. Once this is done, the symmetry and the volume of the reconstructed breast can be compared with that of the contralateral native breast. Final adjustments are then made between the skin paddle and the partial mastectomy defect. For defects that do not require skin reconstruction, the skin paddle can be deepithelialized and then the dermis and muscle can be buried into the defect. In the situation where the LDMF is used to close a mastectomy defect without an implant, the LD muscle is typically inset over the pectoralis major muscle and fixed into place by using absorbable sutures. LDMF breast reconstruction without a prosthetic device is typically reserved for very small-breasted women, women who chose not to undergo prosthetic reconstruction, or situations where all that is required is chest wall coverage. The latter clinical situations arise in the instance of inflammatory breast cancer where the adjuvant radiation therapy will be required. The partial or complete mastectomy skin flaps are then closed primarily or to the skin paddle under no tension. Typically one closed-suction drain is placed below the LDMF and brought out high in the axilla for optimal cosmesis.

Flap Dissection for Complete Mastectomy Defects with Insertion of Prosthesis (TE or Permanent Implant)

An LDMF with a prosthetic device represents an ideal reconstruction for a thin female not requiring adjuvant radiotherapy. In addition, the LDMF is an excellent choice for obese patients where implants alone will not supply appropriate projection or where donor site morbidity from the abdomen can become problematic. The markings, positioning, transposition, and inset are essentially the same for the patient who is to undergo a LDMF for breast reconstruction with the addition of a prosthetic device. However, there are some subtle points to be outlined. In immediate breast reconstruction a skin-sparing mastectomy represents the ideal situation to minimize donor site morbidity with an LDMF. The skin paddle of this flap is ideally suited to help reconstruct the NAC in an immediate or delayed fashion. For a mastectomy that requires larger skin coverage based on resected skin flaps, the LDMF can create a problem as far as donor site closure is concerned. Typically, an 8 to 10 cm skin paddle is used from the back, and as this becomes wider, more tension is placed on the donor site, possibly resulting in a widened scar.

Once the LDMF is elevated and transposed into the mastectomy defect, it is then time to insert the prosthesis and suture the LD muscle into its proper position based on the potential size of the reconstructed breast. For patients with larger breasts (size C–D), the pectoralis major muscle is raised off its origin along the inframammary fold and 1 to 2 cm on the sternum. The LD muscle is then sutured to the lower mastectomy flaps and to the caudal portion of the pectoralis major muscle. Elevating the pectoralis major muscle and having this muscle cover the implant creates a smooth contour in the upper pole, minimizing the prominence of the prosthetic device. The LD muscle is then sutured to the lower mastectomy flap to create the appropriate pocket for the prosthetic device. It is not sutured to the inframammary fold, as this will create an inappropriate muscle pocket for the prosthetic device. The superior border of the LD muscle is inset into the lateral chest wall to define the lateral edge of the reconstructed breast. An implant sizer is placed into this submuscular pocket, and then the patient is placed in the sitting position. The contour, shape, and volume of the reconstructed breast are then compared with that of the opposite breast. Once the appropriate volume is determined and implant device is chosen and inserted, the submuscular pocket is then closed with interrupted 3-0 absorbable sutures. The skin paddle of the LDMF is then inset with 3-0 absorbable sutures, and a running 4-0 absorbable suture is placed in the subcuticular layer.

The prosthetic device used for breast reconstruction can be a TE or a permanent or postoperative adjustable implant and is then placed in a submuscular position. Surgeon preference here typically will dictate the type of prosthesis used. We prefer a permanent implant to be placed immediately at the time of LDMF breast reconstruction as long as there are no vascularity issues with mastectomy flaps at the time of immediate reconstruction. A TE will require another procedure; however, adjustments to the reconstructed breast, specifically the skin envelope, can be made at that time. A postoperative adjustable implant allows the ability to tailor the size of the implant after the operation is completed; however, a procedure is required to remove the port. These three types of prosthetic devices all have their own inherent benefits and risk.

 # POSTOPERATIVE MANAGEMENT

The patient is placed in a surgical support bra. The ipsilateral arm is abducted to 30 degrees by using a cushion or pillow. This avoids compression of the vascular pedicle along its transaxillary course. The skin paddle capillary refill, color, and temperature are assessed, as it will be a direct indicator of the overall flap perfusion. If there is any question of flap vascularity, a return to the operating room to assess the course of vascular pedicle is mandated. In this situation, compression or kinking of the pedicle can be assessed. If the skin paddle is properly oriented over the LD muscle, there is typically no concern that a musculocutaneous perforator has not been captured.

On postoperative day 1, the patients diet is advanced and early ambulation is encouraged. Ambulation in these patients is not a problem as core abdominal muscle are not affected and getting in and out of bed is not prohibitive. Typical hospital stay is 2 to 4 days on the basis of control of postoperative pain with oral analgesics. Drains are removed once drainage has decreased to an appropriate amount.

NAC reconstruction is performed in a delayed fashion to optimize symmetry with the contralateral breast. We prefer not to perform nipple reconstruction at the initial surgery due to potential atrophy of soft tissue and settling of the prosthetic device. In unilateral breast reconstruction, this is critical as matching of the contralateral breast must always be considered. We counsel the patient appropriately in the preoperative setting about this. Balancing procedures for ipsilateral breast reconstruction are usually performed at 3 months following the primary reconstruction. Nipple reconstruction is often performed in an office-based setting 1 month later along with tattooing, unless full-thickness skin graft (FTSG) will be used for areola; in this case, it is preformed in the operating room (see chapter 33 for secondary reconstruction of nipple).

 # COMPLICATIONS

Breast reconstruction using the LDMF plus the insertion of a prosthetic device is a reliable and safe procedure with a relatively low complication rate. When complications occur, they originate either from the back donor site or at the site of the breast reconstruction site.

Donor Site Complications

1. Seroma—this is a late complication that is initially managed with appropriate drain placement. Drains can remain up to 4 to 6 weeks after flap harvest. If the collection of serous fluid persists during routine postoperative visit, aspiration of the collection can be performed under sterile conditions. Interventional radiology can be helpful here for the proper placement of seroma drainage catheters. A chronic seroma can lead to a serous cavity, in a small percentage of times requiring operative intervention to ameliorate.
2. Widened scars can occur at the donor site secondary to increased tension on the healing dermis. Appropriate maneuvers must be taken to not close the wound under tension. Placing the skin paddle in an oblique orientation parallel to Langer lines can lessen the tension on the closure of the wound.
3. Poor wound healing can occur at the donor incision site if too much soft tissue, that is (autologous) extended LD, is harvested by placing undue tension at the incision line. In addition, in this situation, the potential for seroma formation is higher.

Recipient Site Complications

1. Arterial or venous insufficiency of the skin paddle—the only way to monitor the vascularity of the LDMF is by clinically examining the skin paddle of the LD muscle. If the flap shows evidence of decreased inflow or compromised outflow, this situation must be acutely interrogated. Often times, the arm must be abducted as not to put pressure on an already swollen axillary tunnel. If positioning the patient does not improve the vascularity of the skin paddle, then urgent operative exploration must be undertaken. The vascular pedicle can be compressed or kinked. In addition, the skin paddle can be inset under too much tension. It is critical to confirm the thoracodorsal pedicle continuity before committing to flap harvest.

2. Flap necrosis can occur but is a rare finding with the LDMF, as the blood supply to the muscle and skin paddle are extremely robust if harvested correctly. Partial flap necrosis requires operative debridement and closure as typically this will result in exposure of the implant if not appropriately addressed.

3. Complications related to the prosthetic device such as capsule formation, infection, migration, and rupture could all occur. Prosthetic infection is treated with culture-specific antibiotics but a low threshold for a removal must be considered especially in patients who have had previous radiation therapy or are undergoing chemotherapy. Creating a stable submuscular pocket at the time of the initial breast reconstruction prevents migration of the breast implant. Capsular contracture over a TE or permanent implant can occur and is treated by performing a partial or complete capsulectomy to recreate a soft tissue envelope around the implant. Adjuvant radiotherapy can lead to fibrosis of the skin envelope and potentially increase capsular contracture around the prosthetic implant.

4. Brachial plexus injuries occur from improper padding or positioning of the patient during the operative procedure. The axilla must be padded appropriately and care must be taken not to hyperextend the arm during dissection.

RESULTS

The LDMF is an extremely reliable and robust option for unilateral or bilateral breast reconstruction. There are many indications for this flap, especially in combination with a prosthetic device for immediate or delayed breast reconstruction. The most common indications we have found for this flap are for thin patients without appropriate abdominal wall tissue, obese patients who with implants alone would not have appropriate projection and whose abdomens represent potential areas of surgical morbidity, and patients whose abdomen cannot be used secondary to previous surgery. In addition, in smokers whose mastectomy flaps can become compromised becomes a relatively ideal candidate when well-perfused tissue harvested from the back is placed over prosthetic devices and under challenged mastectomy flaps. Common uses for this flap are for the partial, unilateral, and bilateral mastectomy defects. Surgical technique is straightforward, results are predictable, and the postoperative course is protracted relative to free tissue transfer from the abdominal wall, which can potentially affect core muscle strength and lead to bulge and hernia formation on the abdominal wall. The following three cases represent examples of the use of the LD flap with or without the skin paddle for breast reconstruction.

Case 1: This patient is a 47-year-old woman with a sarcoma of the left breast. Adjuvant radiotherapy was planned for this patient regardless of whether the patient was to undergo a partial or complete mastectomy. In addition, she had significant scarring on her abdominal wall from previous laparotomies, precluding the use of an abdominal wall-based flap. The flap was harvested with a skin paddle to be deepithelialized to fill the dead space and secure the flap into the defect (Fig. 30.4A–G). The figures show the patient preoperatively with an "X" over the upper lateral portion of the left breast where the tumor is located. The LDMF markings are shown clearly on the back. The

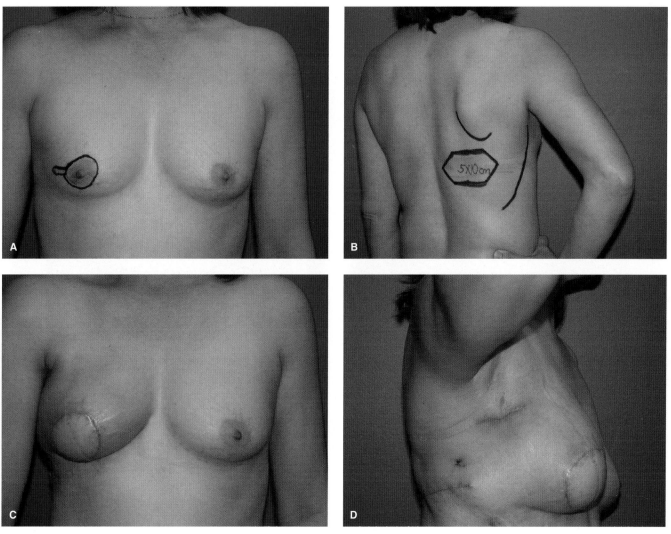

Figure 30.5 **A.** Frontal view of a patient before undergoing a skin-sparing mastectomy. **B.** The tip of the scapula, skin paddle, and the lateral border are marked preoperatively in a standing position. **C.** Postoperative result following immediate breast reconstruction with a latissimus dorsi myocutaneous flap and submuscular saline 300 cc–filled implant. **D.** Lateral view of the patient showing well-healed donor site and axillary incisions.

Part VII: Breast Reconstruction

deepithelialized flap is tunneled through the axillary incision and then placed into the left breast defect. Postoperative views show excellent symmetry to preoperative findings. The donor site incisions are well healed and placed within the bra line.

Case 2: The patient is a 48-year-old woman with right breast cancer who underwent a skin-sparing mastectomy through a periareola incision along with a sentinel lymph node biopsy (Fig. 30.5A–D). The mastectomy defect was reconstructed with a pedicled LDMF plus a 300 cc saline implant placed submuscularly. The LD muscle was sutured to the lateral chest wall in addition to the pectoralis major muscle to create appropriate anatomic contour and an ideal submuscular pocket. Postoperative views show excellent symmetry with well-healed and inconspicuous donor site incisions.

Case 3: This is a 57-year-old woman with a right breast cancer desiring a left prophylactic mastectomy (Fig. 30.6A–D). She had a previous abdominoplasty and circumferential body lift, precluding the use of an abdominal wall-based flap. The patient underwent bilateral LDMFs with immediate insertion of submuscular TEs. The TEs were later changed to permanent saline implants. Postoperative views reveal excellent symmetry with well-healed inconspicuous donor site scars.

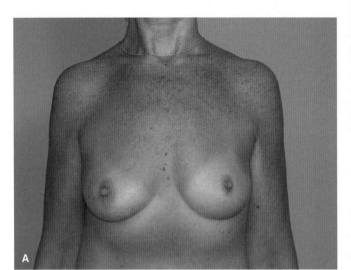

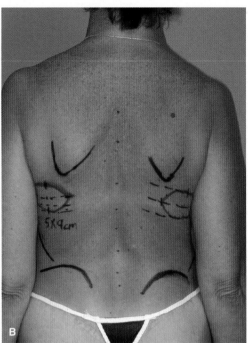

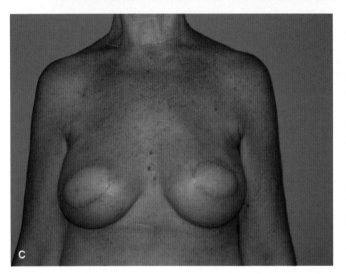

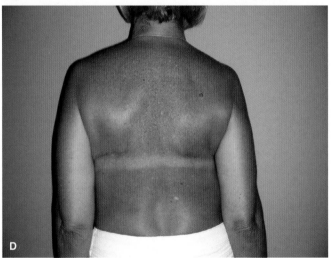

Figure 30.6 A. Frontal view of a patient before undergoing bilateral skin-sparing mastectomies and immediate reconstruction with bilateral LDMFs plus saline implants. **B.** Preoperative markings showing the tip of the scapula, iliac crest, and the skin paddle of latissimus dorsi muscle. **C.** Postoperative results showing excellent contour and symmetry of the reconstructed breasts. The skin paddles will be used for nipple reconstruction in a staged procedure. **D.** Back view of the patient revealing well-healed donor site scars in the bra line.

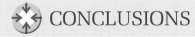 CONCLUSIONS

Breast reconstruction using the LDMF is an extremely versatile tool for the plastic and reconstructive surgeon. The ability to harvest tissue from the back and transfer this tissue in a pedicle fashion without a microvascular anastomosis offers a convenient and relatively quick type of procedure for both immediate and delayed breast reconstruction. The ability to offer this flap with a simultaneous insertion of a TE or permanent or postoperative adjustable implant further enhances the aesthetical perfection of this reconstructive procedure.

Favorable outcomes along with patient satisfaction are experienced with the LDMF for breast reconstruction. Total flap loss is low with this flap as compared with 5%

accepted rates for abdominal wall tissue transfer. Donor site morbidity typically found as donor site seromas can be managed in an outpatient setting. Patient satisfaction with this type of breast reconstruction is extremely high.

Autologous breast reconstruction using the LDMF with or without and implant is an extremely valuable and versatile tool. Patients who require small volumes for immediate and delayed breast reconstruction typically can be reconstructed with the LDMF alone. However, patients requiring larger volumes of tissue are typically reconstructed with the LDMF and a prosthetic implant in combination. Aesthetic outcomes are extremely natural, with the results closely approximating that of autologous tissue reconstruction from the abdominal wall. If properly selected and applied soundly in autologous breast reconstruction, this flap will yield highly predictable and outstanding results.

Suggested Readings

Bostwick J. Latissimus dorsi flap reconstruction. In: Bostwick J, ed. *Plastic and Reconstructive Breast Surgery*. St. Louis, MO: Quality Medical Publishing, 2000:867–974.

Chang DW, Youssef A, Cha S, et al. Autologous breast reconstruction with the extended latissimus dorsi flap. *Plast Reconstr Surg.* 2002;110:751–759.

Disa JJ, McCarthy CM, Mehrara BJ, et al. Immediate latissimus dorsi/prosthetic breast reconstruction following salvage mastectomy after failed lumpectomy/irradiation. *Plast Reconst Surg.* 2008; 121(4):1279–1287.

Hernanz F, Regano S, Redondo-Figuero C, et al. Oncoplastic breast-conserving surgery: analysis of quadrantectomy and immediate reconstruction with latissimus dorsi flap. *World J Surg.* 2007; 31(10):1934–1940.

Hammond DC. Latissimus dorsi flap breast reconstruction. *Clin Plast Surg.* 2007;34(1):75–82.

Kronowitz SJ, Robb GL, Youssef A, et al. Optimizing autologous breast reconstruction in thin patients. *Plast Reconstr Surg.* 2003; 112(7):1768–1778.

Kronowitz SJ, Kuerer HM. Advances and surgical decision-making for breast reconstruction. *Cancer.* 2006;107(5):893–907.

Maxwell GP. Iginio Tansini and the origin of the latissimus dorsi musculocutaneous flap. *Plast Reconstr Surg.* 1980;65:686–692.

McCraw JB, Maxwell GP, Horton CE. Reconstruction of the breast following mastectomy. *Acta Chir Belg.* 1980;79:131–133.

McCraw JB, Papp C, Edwards A, et al. The autogenous latissimus breast reconstruction. *Clin Plast Surg.* 21(2):279–288.

Munhoz AM, Montag E, Fels KW, et al. Outcome analysis of breast conservation surgery and immediate latissimus dorsi flap reconstruction in patients with T1 to T2 breast cancer. *Plast Reconstr Surg.* 2005;116(3):741–752.

Munhoz AM, Aldrighi C, Montag E, et al. Periareolar skin-sparing mastectomy and latissimus dorsi flap with biodimensional expander implant reconstruction: surgical planning, outcome, and complications. *Plast Reconstr Surg.* 2007;119(6):1637–1649.

Olivari N. The latissimus flap. *Br J Plast Surg.* 1976;29:126–128.

Olivari N. Use of thirty latissimus dorsi flaps. *Plast Reconstr Surg.* 1979;64(5):654–661.

Spear SL, Boehmler JH, Taylor NS, et al. The role of the latissimus dorsi flap in reconstruction of the irradiated breast. *Plast Reconstr Surg.* 2007;119(1):1–9.

Tarantino I, Banic A, Fischer T. Evaluation of late results in breast reconstruction by latissimus dorsi flap and prosthesis implantation. *Plast Reconstr Surg.* 2006;117(5):1387–1394.

31 Autologous Reconstruction: Gluteal Flap Breast Reconstruction

Michael R. Zenn

 ## INDICATIONS/CONTRAINDICATIONS

Indications

Autogenous tissue reconstruction of the breast by utilizing gluteal tissues is indicated in any woman with a partial or complete deformity of the breast. There must be adequate tissue in the gluteal area to match the requirements for breast reconstruction. Gluteal tissues are a solid second or third choice for autologous breast reconstruction after abdominal-based tissue reconstructions (transverse rectus abdominis myocutaneous (TRAM), deep inferior epigastric perforator (DIEP), superficial inferior epigastric artery (SIEA)) or possibly back tissues (latissimus flaps). Although abdominal-based flaps are usually more popular for donor site cosmetic reasons, patients without sufficient abdominal tissue or previous abdominal surgery are often ideally suited for gluteal reconstruction. This often includes patients requiring bilateral reconstruction such as prophylactic mastectomy patients who do not have adequate tissue in the abdomen for two reconstructions. Patients seeking gluteal flap reconstruction as a general rule wish to avoid the use of synthetic implants. They are willing to accept a scar in a location that is well hidden and not easily visible to themselves.

Advantages
- Faster recovery than with abdominal flaps (TRAM, DIEP).
- No risk of abdominal hernias or bulges.
- Good projection of the reconstruction.
- There is less postoperative discomfort than with abdominal-based flaps.

Contraindications
- Patients who are in poor health who would be at risk for a prolonged surgical procedure under a general anesthesia.

■ Extreme obesity where the blood supply to the buttock tissues may be hard to localize and capture in the flap (body mass index > 30).
■ Lack of recipient site inflow vessels (internal mammary artery, thoracodorsal artery).

Relative Contraindications

■ Smokers, because of the vasoconstrictive effects of nicotine, who have higher incidence of wound healing problems, especially at the donor site.
■ Inadequate tissue for reconstruction.
■ Previous surgery in the area of the gluteus.
■ Large breast reconstructions (larger than a C cup).
■ Unwillingness to have scar or deformity of the gluteal area.
■ Patients who will be having postoperative radiation therapy as part of their cancer care. In this case, reconstruction will be delayed until after radiation to avoid radiation damage to the reconstructed breast.

PREOPERATIVE PLANNING

Workup for gluteal flap surgery for breast reconstruction starts with a thorough history and physical examination taking into account potential for local, regional, and metastatic disease. Areas of previous surgery or injury at the donor or recipient sites should be closely examined. From the general medical standpoint, patients should be screened for poorly controlled diabetes, cardiac disease, pulmonary disease, and renal disease. These procedures are major undertakings and do not warrant unnecessary morbidity. Remember, patients can always forego a lengthy and possibly risky surgery and use an external prosthesis. A history of smoking is not an absolute contraindication but does say something about the patient's ability and willingness to take an active role in her care and do something to ensure success. Although smoking does not cause gluteal flap failures, the vasoconstrictive effects of nicotine have been shown to cause necrosis of mastectomy flaps and buttock wound healing problems. Chronologic age is probably less important that physiologic age. As a general rule, these procedures are not offered to patients in their 70s or older.

The issue of radiation therapy as part of the patient's adjuvant therapy deserves special mention. It has been shown convincingly that radiation of a soft tissue reconstructive flap can potentially cause adverse effects on that tissue that include firmness, distortion, pain, and even failure of the reconstruction. It is for this reason that patients who require radiation for their cancer care should have their gluteal flaps delayed, preferably 6 months or more after their radiation treatment. Reconstruction in the irradiated chest wall field has the same success rate as in a nonirradiated case but has the advantage of placing soft, supple, nonirradiated tissue on the chest for a more durable reconstruction. It should be noted that once a patient has been irradiated, contracture and induration of the chest wall skin may increase skin requirements for reconstruction, making the gluteal flap less useful or limiting its ultimate size.

Finally, preoperative evaluation should include evaluation of the contralateral breast in cases of unilateral reconstruction. Ultimately, the goal of reconstruction is to enable a patient to achieve symmetry in clothes. Absolute symmetry out of clothes is unrealistic and, if present, will not stand the test of time as each breast mound will respond differently to physiologic and physical changes over time. For patients with large or ptotic breasts, there should be a willingness for contralateral surgery for symmetry to best match the configuration of the gluteal flap reconstruction. This would include mastopexy or breast reduction. In a bilateral reconstruction, it is somewhat easier to match sides since the composition of the breast reconstructions will be similar. With that said, matching in clothes remains the standard.

No studies need to be performed preoperatively to evaluate the recipient site or the donor site vessels. Because of the extensive nature of this procedure, bilateral cases are performed only if two microsurgeons are available. Most surgeons will do one side at a time, separated by 4 to 6 months.

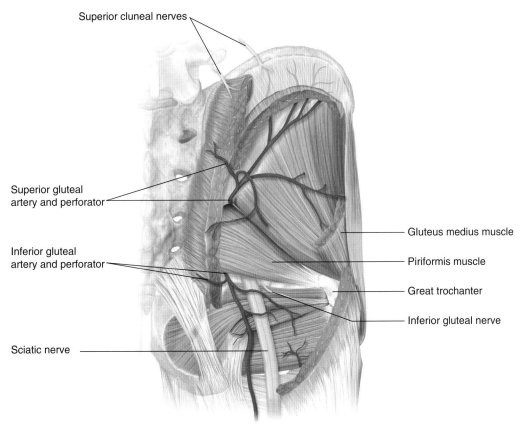

Superior cluneal nerves

Superior gluteal
artery and perforator

Inferior gluteal
artery and perforator

Sciatic nerve

Gluteus medius muscle

Piriformis muscle

Great trochanter

Inferior gluteal nerve

Figure 31.1 The anatomy of the superior and inferior gluteal vessels. Note the piriformis muscle in relation to the two vascular systems.

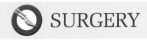 SURGERY

Relevant Anatomy

Gluteal tissues can be carried on one of two vascular supplies: the superior gluteal artery or the inferior gluteal artery (Fig. 31.1). Gluteal-based flaps were first described as myocutaneous flaps where a block of tissue from the buttock was carried with underlying gluteus maximus muscle and the gluteal blood vessels. This is no longer practiced as the muscle is unnecessary for vascular supply of the buttock skin and fat. These flaps are based on the perforating vessels of the inferior and superior gluteal arteries, so-called perforator flaps. The SGAP (superior gluteal artery perforator) and IGAP (inferior gluteal artery perforator) flaps are the current standard for gluteal-based flaps. Which flap is used is determined by the distribution of excess fat and skin in that particular patient. Both flaps have the advantage of a longer pedicle length than their muscle-bound relative since the dissection of the intramuscular course adds to the ultimate length of the pedicle, facilitating microsurgery. By not harvesting muscle with the flap, the SGAP and IGAP flaps also minimize morbidity by maintaining muscle strength and integrity.

SGAP flaps are much more commonly performed than IGAP flaps for the following reasons:

1. Improved donor site aesthetic. The incision and tissue removal is similar to a buttock lift and leaves the buttock with good contour.
2. Adequate pedicle length. Since gluteal muscle is not taken, the ultimate length of the perforating blood vessels off the superior gluteal artery are more than adequate for reanastomoses and placement of the flap in the proper position. This was the limiting factor to using superiorly based gluteal flaps when muscle was included.
3. The inferior gluteal artery is intimately associated with the posterior femoral cutaneous nerve supplying sensation to the posterior thigh and the motor nerve to the

entire gluteus muscle (inferior gluteal nerve). By avoiding these completely, one limits the potential morbidities caused by their injury.

With all that said, the IGAP should be entertained in those patients whose fat and skin distribution is mainly in the lower buttock area.

Relevant muscles in this area are as follows:

1. The gluteus maximus muscle. The gluteus maximus is quadrangular in shape. It originates from the bony pelvis and inserts into the gluteal tuberosity of the femur. It is a powerful extensor and is important in activities such as standing from a squatting position, heel walking, and climbing stairs. Perforating vessels of the superior and inferior gluteal artery perforate this muscle, supplying the overlying skin and fatty tissue.
2. The piriformis muscle lies beneath the gluteus muscle. It arises from the sacrum and inserts into the greater trochanter. The superior gluteal vessels emerge superior to it and the inferior gluteal vessels inferior to it.

There are multiple perforators from each vessel through the muscle but only one perforator is required to ensure vascularization of the flap. Cutaneous nerve supply to the buttock is via the nervi clunii superioris, which are branches of the lumbar nerves. They can be identified at the superior margin of the gluteal artery perforator flap and, if found large enough, can be raised with the flap to innervate the gluteal flap and give sensation to reconstruction.

Surgical Marking

Markings for the gluteal flap are made in the standing position and then confirmed intraoperatively. Marking of the superior gluteal flap employs the rule of "thirds" (Fig. 31.2). The posterior superior iliac spine and the prominence of the greater trochanter of the femur are palpated and marked. A line drawn between these points and divided into thirds will

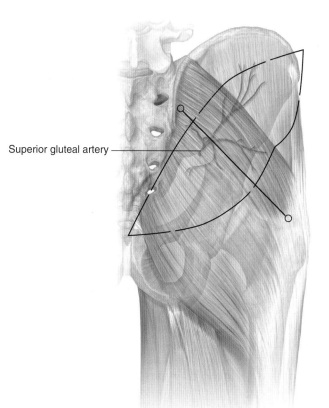

Superior gluteal artery —

Figure 31.2 "Rule of thirds." A line drawn between the posterior superior iliac spine and the prominence of the greater trochanter of the femur these points and divided into thirds will denote the expected location of the superior gluteal artery at the junction between the upper and middle third.

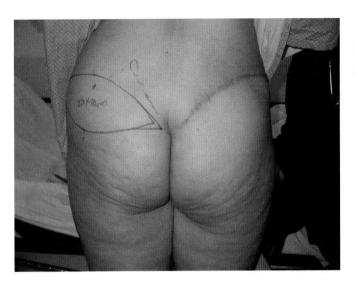

Figure 31.3 Clinical case with the markings utilizing the rule of thirds. This patient is 4 months after the contralateral side, and the scar location and quality can be seen.

denote the expected location of the superior gluteal artery at the junction between the upper and middle third. The location of the piriformis muscle can be found by drawing a line from the posterior superior iliac spine to the coccyx. A new line drawn from the midpoint of this line to the trochanter will show the position of the piriformis muscle, helping to differentiate between the superior and inferior gluteal perforating vessels.

When the patient is positioned in the operating room, a handheld Doppler probe can be used to search for and confirm perforators in these areas. The skin design can then be marked on the buttock, including within it the identified perforators (Fig. 31.3). The skin design can be up to 30 cm in length and 10 to 12 cm in width and still allow closure of the buttock without tension. The axis of the flap is made slightly oblique or horizontal in position to best hide the ultimate scar and to effectively lift the buttock area, improving its aesthetic.

For immediate breast reconstruction, a lateral position can be employed and a two-team approach can be used. The oncologic team can perform the mastectomy while the reconstructive team harvests the ipsilateral gluteal flap. In delayed cases, a supine–prone strategy is employed in which the recipient site is first prepared supine. Once adequate vessels are found for reconstruction, the wound is temporarily closed and the patient is changed to a prone position for harvest of the flap. Once harvested, the flap is placed on the back table and the donor site is quickly closed. The patient is returned to the supine position for the microscopic anastomosis and insetting of the flap.

Since these cases are long and in unnatural positions, exquisite care must be taken to pad the patient appropriately to prevent pressure-related problems.

Recipient Site

Prior to the final flap dissection, the recipient site is prepared. In the case of immediate reconstruction, the thoracodorsal system is evaluated first as it is normally exposed already from any axillary lymph node dissection (Fig. 31.4). If deemed inadequate or if they have not yet been dissected, the internal mammary system is evaluated first as this recipient location facilitates shaping and accommodates even short pedicle lengths (Fig. 31.5). Perforators from the internal mammary are evaluated first. If deemed inadequate, a portion of the pectoralis major muscle and the third rib can be removed with exposure of the internal mammary artery and vein. The inframammary fold also is checked at this point and reinforced with zero silk suture if it has been detached. With delayed reconstruction, the old mastectomy plane is reestablished. If there has been previous radiation, skin may be tight, and a bisecting of the lower flap is often helpful in developing the pocket and securing the inframammary fold. This skin ultimately will be resected with placement of the gluteal flap. Should there be any compromise or problems with the flap, the skin is not sacrificed until the very end of the inset so that closure can be obtained.

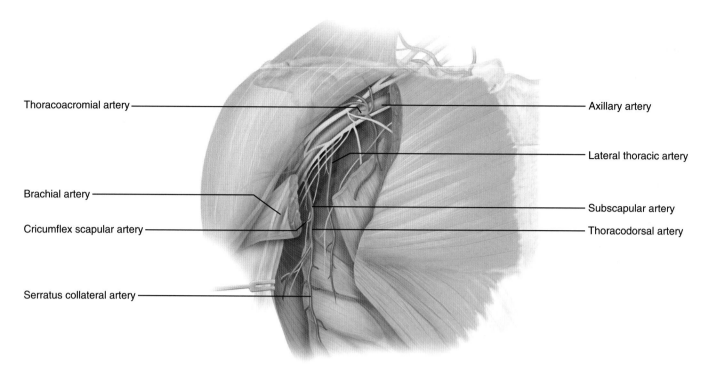

Thoracoacromial artery

Brachial artery

Cricumflex scapular artery

Serratus collateral artery

Axillary artery

Lateral thoracic artery

Subscapular artery

Thoracodorsal artery

Figure 31.4 If axillary lymph node dissection has been done, the thoracodorsal or serratus branch of the thoracodorsal vessels can be used for recipient vessels.

Figure 31.5 More commonly, the third or fourth rib is resected to expose the internal mammary artery (IMA) and internal mammary vein (IMV) for recipient vessels. Only rarely are two ribs resected (as pictured) and sometimes large perforators through the pectoralis are present and no rib resection is required.

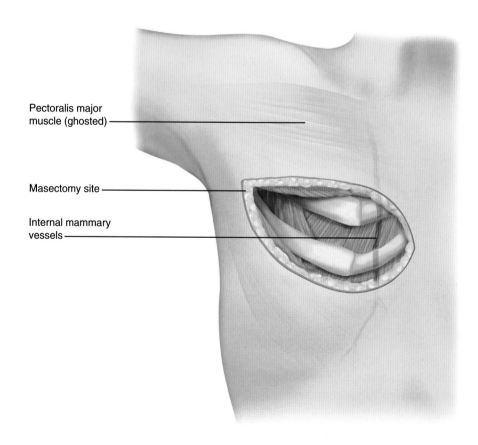

Pectoralis major muscle (ghosted)

Masectomy site

Internal mammary vessels

Flap Dissection

Skin incisions are made and dissection is beveled to include the necessary amount of fat based on the preoperative plan and tissue needs for breast reconstruction. Ultimately, the usable amount of skin and fat is limited by the need to close the buttock and prevent deformity. Dissection proceeds down directly to the gluteus maximus muscle fascia (Fig. 31.6A). Since the perforating vessels are medially based, the flap is quickly elevated from lateral to medial until the first perforator is found (Fig. 31.6B). Laterally, the dissection will begin over the fascia lata, and the gluteal fatty tissue is dissected off this until the muscle is encountered. It is easiest to identify and dissect the perforators from the subfascial plane, so once the gluteus muscle is identified, the fascia is incised and carried with the flap. It is also helpful to progress with flap elevation along the direction of the muscle fibers as the perforators are then easily seen and potential damage to them minimized. Although multiple perforators may be encountered, one large or two smaller perforators are all that are required to carry the flap (Fig. 31.6C). If two perforators are close and can be lined up from the same break in the muscle, both are dissected and used (Fig. 31.6).

Once these perforators are identified, dissection from the medial aspect is then performed to identify all potential perforators and to isolate the tissue on the desired pedicle. If an innervated flap is desired, dorsal branches of the lumbar segmental nerves must be identified in the superior medial area of the flap, and then these are traced back to their origin. A single large branch is all that is required, and this can be coapted to the forth intercostal nerve if it has been identified in the recipient site. As dissection

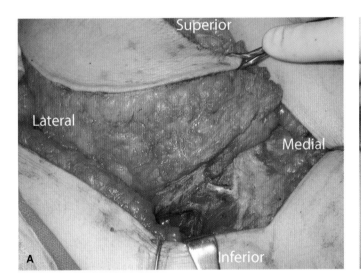

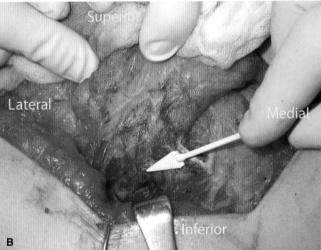

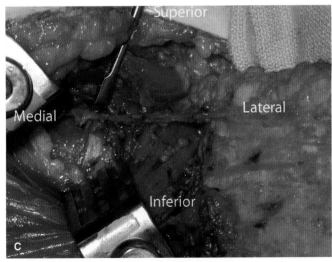

Figure 31.6 **A.** Initial dissection. **B.** Further dissection into the muscle and initial identification of perforator at the location shown by arrow and confirmed with Doppler probe. **C.** Final dissection of the perforator through the muscle to the foramen, maximizing vessel length and diameter.

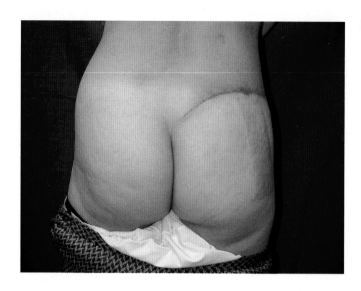

Figure 31.7 Donor site at 3 months.

proceeds through the muscle, self-retaining retractors are used to maintain an optical window to follow the vessels down to their origin. Multiple side branches are encountered, and these are divided and controlled with vascular clips. Vessels are prone to spasm during this dissection and are irrigated with a vasodilating solution (lidocaine, papaverine, thorazine). Much of the dissection can be performed with bipolar cautery to minimize bleeding and to maintain a bloodless field. All fascial attachments to the gluteus medius, the gluteus minimus, and the piriformis muscles need to be released to follow the vessels course to its origin at the foramen. Once below the level of the muscles, loose areolar tissues surrounding the vessels can be gently dissected with a pushing motion by using a Kittner dissector. Dissection should be followed down to the foramen to ensure adequate pedicle length and also to maximize arterial diameter. Pedicle length typically ranges from 8 to 10 cm, arterial diameter at the foramen measures 1 to 2.5 mm. Typically, the comitans veins can be quite large, up to 4 mm in size. Careful dissection is critical to avoid deep bleeding, which can obscure pedicle dissection, shorten the final pedicle length, and lengthen the procedure. Pedicle length of the flap is usually 7 to 12 cm.

Once the vessels are completely isolated and the flap perfused, 5,000 units of heparin are given, and after 10 minutes, the artery and the vein are divided and the flap is placed back on the table in cool gauze. Donor site irrigation and hemostasis is then accomplished. Donor site closure includes undermining of the skin flaps; reapproximation of the split gluteal muscle with absorbable sutures and placement of a suction drain over the muscle as donor site seroma is a possible complication (Fig. 31.7). The suction drain placed should exit laterally so the patient does not sit on it postoperatively. Defatting of the lateral and medial dog-ears is also performed. Scarpas fascia is reapproximated with 0 Vicryl suture. Skin is closed with Vicryl suture in the dermis and running 3-0 monocryl as a subcuticular suture. A compression garment is recommended for up to 4 weeks postoperatively. This takes tension off the closure and minimizes the risk of seroma.

Recipient Site/Flap Inset

The flap is then placed on the chest to best accomplish breast reconstruction. In the case of immediate reconstruction, the microsurgery can be performed while buttock closure is occurring, but the patient must still be reprepped and draped in the supine position for final shaping and inset. In the delayed situation, flap inset is performed in the supine position after the donor site has been closed and the patient has been turned and appropriately padded. The operating microscope is used to reanastomose the artery and the vein. Arterial anastomosis is usually accomplished using 9-0 interrupted nylon suture. Venous anastomosis is performed using a venous coupler or by a running anastomosis (Fig. 31.8). Any mismatch in vessel size should be managed to prevent postoperative thrombosis. This can be accomplished with a venous coupler or by tapering the larger venous cuff with a running suture prior to anastomosis. Once the anastomoses

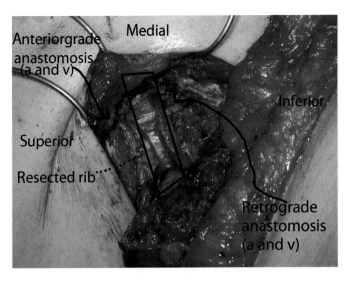

Figure 31.8 This figure demonstrates the use of the IMA and IMV for recipient site. In this case, two pedicles of a free TRAM were reconnected: one anterograde, one retrograde. The veins are reconnected with couplers, seen as small silicone disks in the photograph. Arteries are handsewn under the microscope with 9-0 or 10-0 suture. The gluteal artery perforator flap requires only one arterial reconnection and one venous connection.

are performed and the clamps are removed, perfusion of the flap is evaluated. Doppler probes are placed directly on the arterial and venous anastomoses for postoperative monitoring. These are easily removed usually 2 weeks postoperatively in the office. Care is taken to ensure no kinking or compression of the pedicle occurs during the closure and the Doppler probes assist in monitoring the signals throughout this process. Mastectomy skin flaps can be trimmed as needed, and portions of the gluteal flap can be deepithelized. The flap is positioned horizontally to recreate the breast shape. Unlike abdominally based tissues, which are much less fibrous in nature, fullness of the superior reconstruction is often sacrificed to maintain adequate projection and breast shape in the inferior pole. Secondary fat grafting can be used if it is needed to correct this. The flap is fixed to the chest wall and pectoral fascia by using 0 Vicryl suture (Fig. 31.9).

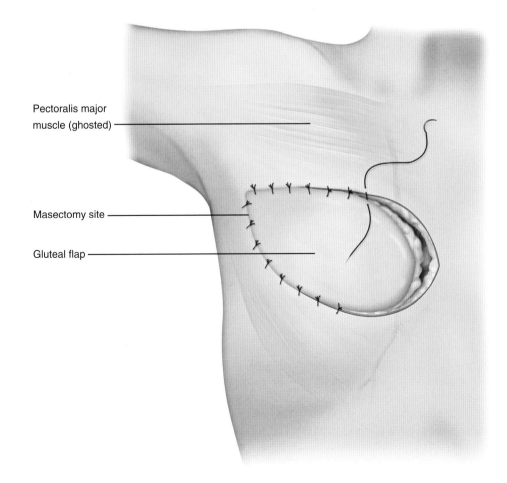

Figure 31.9 Once the flap is positioned on the chest, the fat and fascia are secured superiorly to the pectoralis fascia with absorbable suture. This prevents descent of the flap in the immediate postoperative period.

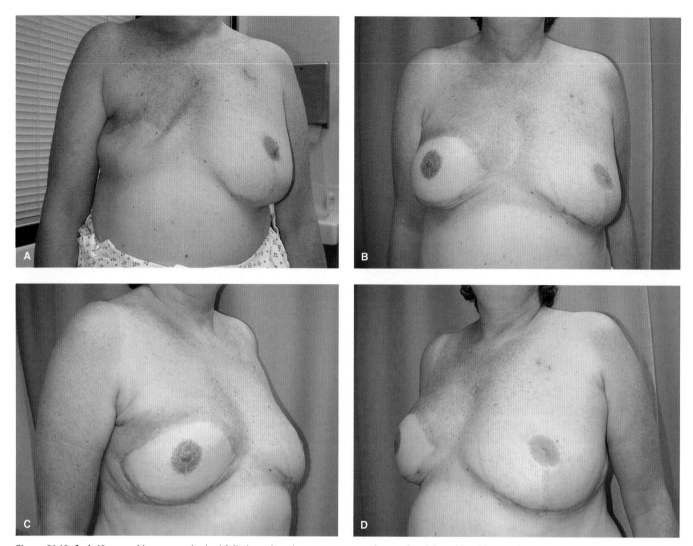

Figure 31.10 A. A 48-year-old woman who had failed previous breast reconstruction on the right, with a history of chest wall irradiation. **B.** Anteroposterior view 9 months after superior gluteal artery perforator flap for salvage and breast reduction on the left for symmetry. **C.** Right oblique view. **D.** Left oblique view.

Exaggerated projection in the lower pole of the reconstruction and a hollowness in the upper reconstruction is frequently observed in these flaps. After obtaining the desired shape, a drain is placed through a separate lateral incision, and skin closure is performed in layers (Figs. 31.10 and 31.11).

POSTOPERATIVE MANAGEMENT

Patients are extubated in the operating room and transferred to the recovery room. Unilateral reconstruction may range from 6 to 8 hours, and recover room stays are 1 to 2 hours. Patients will then be transferred to the floor where they will be monitored by nursing staff who are familiar with flaps. Doppler probes will be checked hourly as will any available skin paddle for capillary refill time for the first 48 hours. The patient remains nil per os for the first night and then is advanced to a regular diet as tolerated. By postoperative day 1, patients are moving to a chair, and by day 2, they are ambulating. Most patients are discharged from the hospital on postoperative day 3. Deep vein thrombosis prevention begins in the operating room with sequential compression devices. Intraoperative heparin is used for the flaps, and this is transitioned on postoperative day 2 to an aspirin once a day. Aspirin is continued for the first month. Care is taken postoperatively to avoid any pressure on the flaps. Patients may sit in a chair or lie supine in the bed. They are not allowed to be in the prone or lateral position for the first 2 months.

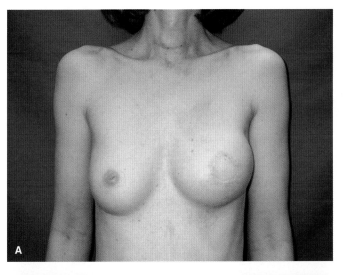
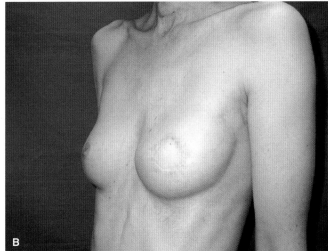
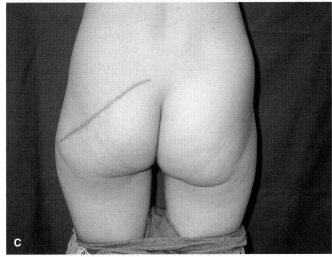

Figure 31.11 A. A 36-year-old woman 7 months postoperative after a left breast reconstruction with a SGAP flap (anteroposterior view). **B.** Oblique view **C.** Donor scar and minimal deformity at 7 months.

Seroma should be expected in gluteal reconstructions and drains can often be left in 2 to 3 weeks. In spite of this, aspiration in the office may be necessary as the area is rich in lymphatics and there is motion in this area with regular ambulation.

Patients are usually seen at 4 months for evaluation of the result and for planning of revisional surgery, which is almost always necessary in a gluteal flap.

Revisions

During the first 4 months, the shape of the reconstructed breast may not match the contralateral breast. This is in large part due to the fibrous nature of the fatty tissue and the fact that it cannot safely be distributed in the first operation. In the revisional procedure performed at 4 months, further shaping of the breast mound can be performed with a combination of the liposuction and flap advancement, especially in areas that have not received radiation. Fat grafting is an alternative to fill in areas of ridges that need further rounding to give a normal appearance. In many cases, the shape and size of the natural breast cannot be matched exactly but the gluteal flap may have allowed the patient to have a reconstruction when otherwise an implant reconstruction would have been impossible. One must also keep in mind that matching is a snapshot in time and that over time, in a unilateral reconstruction, the two breasts will age differently because of their different composition. In this scenario, patients should anticipate further revision of the natural breast to continue to match the reconstructed breast. When bilateral reconstruction is performed with gluteal flaps, it is anticipated the flaps will age similarly and these revisions would be less necessary. Revisions at the donor site are also needed to revise scars

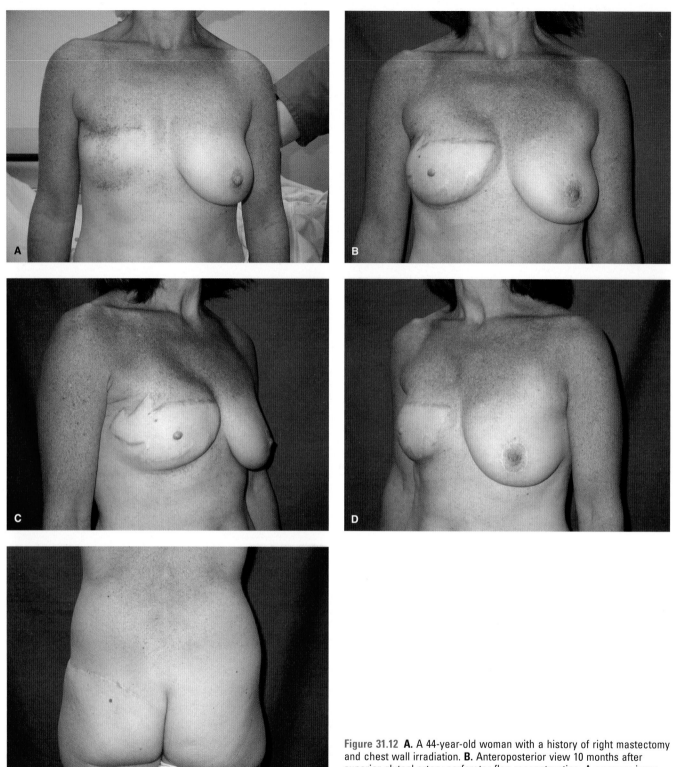

Figure 31.12 A. A 44-year-old woman with a history of right mastectomy and chest wall irradiation. **B.** Anteroposterior view 10 months after superior gluteal artery perforator flap reconstruction. A common issue after irradiation with gluteal flaps is the lack of skin to use in the reconstruction. Here the inelastic irradiated skin is incorporated into the reconstruction and shaped with Z-plasties. **C.** Right oblique view. **D.** Left oblique view. **E.** Donor site scar and minimal deformity at 10 months.

TABLE 31.1	Gluteal Flap Complications
Major Complications	**Minor Complications**
• Flap loss—partial or complete • Bleeding • Infection • Nerve injury • Deep vein thrombosis • Pneumothorax from rib removal • Pulmonary embolism • Myocardial infarction • Death	• Scar • Contour deformity • Asymmetry • Pain • Seroma at the donor site

or to fill out the deformities if present. In general, the IGAP flaps require more donor site revision. Although the scar may lie within the gluteal crease, this can present more of an overall shape problem and prevent the wearing of certain clothes due to the conspicuous nature of the scar and the flattening of the lower buttock. Many of these patients will require contralateral procedures to balance the buttocks. While this might be true with the superiorly based flaps, the buttock lift provided is usually more aesthetic.

Revisional surgeries can often be combined with contralateral breast procedures to make the shapes more symmetric. This may include breast reduction, breast lift, or breast augmentation as needed. Procedures including nipple reconstruction and nipple areolar tattooing are performed only after the surgeon and the patient are happy with the mound reconstruction. It may require a series of revisions to get to a point where the patient is happy enough that nipple reconstruction can be performed. Nipple reconstruction is performed in standard fashion either with a nipple graft or a local tissue rearrangement to build projection (see Chapter 33). This can easily be accomplished if it lies within the skin paddle of the gluteal flap. Nipple reconstructive procedures are performed 4 months after the last revision, and tattoo follows 2 months afterward (see Fig. 31.12A–E).

COMPLICATIONS

Fortunately, major complications with gluteal surgery are rare (see Table 31.1). Total flap loss is on the order of 2% in centers routinely performing microsurgical flaps. Partial loss, sometimes referred to as *fat necrosis*, is also less likely in gluteal flaps than in abdominal-based flaps due to the improved vascularity and lack of distinct zones of perfusion as seen in the abdomen. Fat necrosis can be seen in 5% of cases and usually requires a revision in the operating room if the area does not completely resolve on its own. Nerve injuries can be a result of pressure injury from improper padding or from surgical division, especially in dissection of the IGAP flap, so especial care must be taken to preserve the posterior femoral cutaneous nerve and the inferior gluteal nerve. Pneumothorax requiring a chest tube is rare as the pleural cavity is not entered to expose the mammary vessels and if entered inadvertently no damage to the underlying lung parenchyma occurs so no air leak is present. Deep vein thrombosis and pulmonary embolism should be treated prophylactically, with intermittent compression boots and heparin when indicated. Myocardial infarction and death should be limited with proper patient selection. Minor complications including scars, contour abnormalities, pain, and seroma can be seen with any type of breast reconstruction and are not uncommon.

PEARLS AND PITFALLS

In the case of unilateral reconstruction, be careful when considering contralateral buttock recontouring such as liposuction or buttock lift. This will be valuable tissue for reconstruction if a second reconstruction is required. Try to emphasize with patients that fit in clothes is the goal and if they can get by without contralateral procedures it is in their best interest. If the difference is too noticeable, these procedures can be done, and the patient must be made aware that this donor site would no longer be available for future reconstruction.

RESULTS

Gluteal-based flaps for breast reconstruction (SGAP, IGAP) are an accepted method of autogenous breast reconstruction (see Figs. 31.10 and 31.11). Especially in cases where the abdomen is not available or is inadequate for breast reconstruction, the gluteal area is a natural second choice. Proper patient selection and proper informed consent will ensure the best possible results and the happiest of patients.

Suggested Readings

Allen RJ, Guerra AB, Erhard HA, et al. Superior gluteal artery perforator flap. In: Blondeel PN, ed. *Perforator Flaps: Anatomy, Technique, and Clinical Applications.* St. Louis, MO: Quality Medical Publishing, 2006:486–497.

Allen RJ, Tucker C. Superior gluteal artery perforator free flap for breast reconstruction. *Plast Reconstr Surg.* 1995;95(7):1207–1212.

Blondeel PN. The sensate free superior gluteal artery perforator (S-GAP) flap: a valuable alternative in autologous breast reconstruction. *Br J Plast Surg.* 1999;52:185–193.

Blondeel PN, Ali R, Hamdi M. The superior gluteal artery perforator flap in breast reconstruction. In: Spear SL, ed. *Surgery of the Breast, Principles and Art.* 2nd ed. Philadelphia, PA: Lippincott Williams & Wilkins, 2006:856–865.

Blondeel PN, Demuynck M, Mete D, et al. Sensory nerve repair in perforator flaps for autologous breast reconstruction: sensational or senseless? *Br J Plast Surg.* 1999;52(1):37–44.

Blondeel PN, Landuyt KV, Hamdi M, et al. Soft tissue reconstruction with the superior gluteal artery perforator flap. *Clin Plast Surg.* 2003;(30):371–382.

Boustred AM, Nahai F. Inferior gluteal free flap breast reconstruction. *Clin Plast Surg.* 1998;25(2):275–282.

Codner MA, Nahai F. The gluteal free flap breast reconstruction: making it work. *Clin Plast Surg.* 1994;21:289–296.

Della Croce FJ, Sullivan SK. Application of the superior gluteal artery perforator free flap for bilateral simultaneous breast reconstruction. *Plast Reconstruct Surg.* 2005;116:87–104.

Fujino T, Harasina T, Aoyagi F. Reconstruction for aplasia of the breast and pectoral region by microvascular transfer of a free flap from the buttock. *Plast Reconstr Surg.* 1975;56(2):178–181.

Goodwin MD, Chang BW. Breast reconstruction—superior gluteal artery perforator (SGAP) flap. In: Nahabedian MY, ed. *Cosmetic and Reconstructive Breast Surgery.* Philadelphia, PA: Saunders Elsevier, 2009:67–82.

Guerra AB, Allen RJ, Levine JL, et al. Inferior gluteal artery perforator flap. In: Blondeel PN, ed. *Perforator Flaps: Anatomy,* *Technique, and Clinical Applications.* St. Louis, MO: Quality Medical Publishing, 2006:500–511.

Guerra AB, Metzinger SE, Bidros RS, et al. Breast reconstruction with gluteal artery perforator (GAP) flaps: a critical analysis of 142 cases. *Ann Plast Surg.* 2004;52(2):118–225.

Kankaya Y, Ulusoy MG, Oruç M, et al. Perforating arteries of the gluteal region. *Ann Plast Surg.* 2006;56:409–412.

Koshima I, Moriguchi T, Soeda S, et al. The gluteal perforator-based flap for repair of sacral pressure sores. *Plast Reconstr Surg.* 1993; 91(4):678–683.

Roche NA, Van Landuyt K, Blondeel PN, et al. The use of pedicled perforator flaps for reconstruction of lumbosacral defects. *Ann Plast Surg.* 2000;45(1):7–14.

Serletti JM. Pedicle TRAM, free TRAM and perforator flaps. In: Guyuron B, ed. *Plastic Surgery: Indications and Practice.* Philadelphia, PA: Saunders Elsevier, 2009:247–259.

Shaw WW. Superior gluteal free flap breast reconstruction. *Clin Plast Surg.* 1998;25(2):267–274.

Shaw WW. Breast reconstruction by superior gluteal microvascular free flaps without silicone implants. *Plast Reconstr Surg.* 1983; 72(4):490–501.

Taylor GI, Palmer JH. The vascular territories (angiosomes) of the body: experimental study and clinical applications. *Br J Plast Surg.* 1987;40(2):113–141.

Verpaele AM, Blondeel PN, Van Landuyt K, et al. The superior gluteal artery perforator flap: an additional tool in the treatment of sacral pressure sores. *Br J Plast Surg.* 1999;52(5):385–391.

Windhofer C, Brenner E, Moriggl B, et al. Relationship between the descending branch of the inferior gluteal artery and the posterior femoral cutaneous nerve applicable to flap surgery. *Surg Radiol Anat.* 2002;24(5):253–257.

Zenn MR. Control of breast contour by the use of Z-plasty in the irradiated breast reconstruction. *Plast Reconstruct Surg.* 2003; 112(1):210–214.

Zenn MR, Millard JA. Inferior gluteal flap harvest with sparing of the posterior femoral cutaneous nerve. *J Reconstr Microsurg.* 2006; 22:509–512.

32 Secondary Reconstruction: Reduction Mammoplasty, Mastopexy, and Breast Augmentation

Nolan Karp

When choosing a method of breast reconstruction, it is often possible to select a technique that will closely match the contralateral breast in size and shape. Other times, the method chosen will require alteration of the contralateral breast to achieve symmetry. Some patients may even request surgery on the normal breast for either cosmetic or functional reasons. In patients with very large breasts, mammograms following breast reduction surgery will be easier to interpret. The timing of the symmetry procedure and the technique chosen should not interfere with either the patient's cancer treatment or future monitoring of the contralateral breast.

Available techniques include breast reduction, mastopexy, augmentation, or a combination of these techniques. Not only is the selection of technique important but also its timing is critical to achieving the best cosmetic results.

INDICATIONS/CONTRAINDICATIONS

Breast Reduction

Breast reduction is most often required when patients have breasts larger than a C cup. It is extremely difficult to achieve symmetry in these large, usually ptotic, breasts by any reconstructive technique. When tissue expansion is chosen, the degree of expansion required would often result in extreme thinning of the overlying skin and sufficient ptosis is usually impossible to attain. In the ptotic patient, autologous tissue reconstructive techniques are preferable, assuming there is adequate donor site tissue available. Breast reduction is best performed as a secondary procedure after flap reconstruction or at the time of permanent implant placement after tissue expander reconstruction. Breast reduction techniques all result in some internal breast scarring postoperatively. These mammographic changes are well understood and do not interfere with interpretation. When breast reduction is performed, it is important to choose a technique that has a low risk for fat necrosis. When fat necrosis occurs within the breast, it can pose diagnostic problems, usually requiring biopsy. Liposuction is avoided in breast reduction due to potential distortion of the internal architecture of the breast, which may make future mammographic interpretation more difficult. This is particularly important in the group of patients who have had cancer in the other breast.

Mastopexy

Mastopexy is often required when significant ptosis exists in the contralateral breast since breast symmetry is the goal of reconstruction. Mastopexy, similar to breast reduction, is best performed as a secondary procedure. Available mastopexy procedures either reshape the skin or internally reshape the breast mound. Internal architectural distortion should be minimized in these patients if possible. It is best to avoid mastopexy techniques that extensively reshape the breast gland. In general, long-term results have been very similar for both internal reshaping procedures and dermal procedures.

Breast Augmentation

Usually breast augmentation is useful in small-breasted women who have undergone implant reconstruction and need additional upper breast fullness in the normal breast to achieve symmetry. Augmentation will always interfere with future mammograms, making it difficult to visualize all of the breast tissue when an underlying implant is present. When the implant is small, placed subpectorally, and remains soft, the degree of mammographic distortion is minimal. The use of saline implants placed underneath the pectoralis muscle has significantly reduced the incidence of capsular contracture and subsequent firmness of the breast. When augmentation is being considered, carefully documented consultations with the oncologic surgeon and mammographer are important. Augmentation is best performed at the time of final implant placement to achieve best symmetry.

When symmetry procedures are necessary, all issues must be discussed with the patient and other treating physicians before deciding on the method of breast reconstruction. The need for contralateral breast surgery may alter the choice of technique chosen for the breast reconstruction.

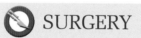 SURGERY

Breast Reduction

The vast majority of the breast reductions performed for symmetry after contralateral breast reconstruction can be done with the short scar vertical technique. Occasionally, in patients with very large or very ptotic breasts Wise-pattern or anchor-type scar (inverted-T) reductions are required.

Our method of short scar breast reduction is based in part on the technique described by Hall-Findlay with some modifications as previously described by the author. Briefly, the patient is marked in the standing position, with the new nipple position marked at the level of the inframammary fold, matching the location of the nipple of the reconstructed breast. The outline of the future nipple–areolar complex is designed by utilizing a mosque pattern, and the medial and lateral extent of resection are marked with a breast displacement technique. These lines are curved gently and connected to a point 2 to 4 cm above the inframammary fold, depending on the size of the breast. The medially based pedicle is designed from 6 to 10 cm in width, again depending on the size of the breast, with part of the pedicle within the mosque pattern. The nipple–areolar circumference is usually marked with a 42-mm diameter cookie cutter (Fig. 32.1).

The operation begins by deepithelializing the pedicle, followed by elevation of a thin inferior flap to the chest wall fascia and subsequent resection of the inferior pole of the

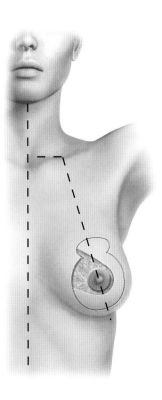

Figure 32.1 The markings and operative plan for medial pedicle breast reduction.

breast from just deep to the subcutaneous plane to the level of the pectoralis fascia. Breast tissue is resected laterally and medially according to the desired breast size and to allow rotation of the medially based dermoglandular pedicle. Care is taken to leave the inferior pole "empty" while leaving the superior pole largely intact. This is especially important when matching an implant reconstruction on the other side (Fig. 32.2).

Figure 32.2 Resection of tissue and rotation of pedicle.

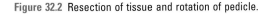

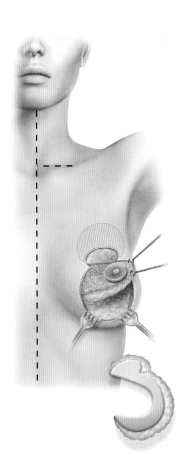

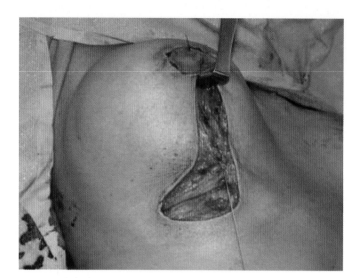

Figure 32.3 Pedicle in position and pillar sutures being placed. The entire bottom of the breast is empty.

After insetting the areola, the parenchyma of the medial pedicle is sutured to the tissue of the lateral "pillar" (Fig. 32.3). These pillar sutures are critical for setting the ultimate breast shape. The patient is then placed in a sitting position, and the breasts are assessed for size, shape, and symmetry. The patient is returned to the supine position and adjustments to the pillar sutures and additional resection performed as necessary. At this point, liposuction may be used as an adjunctive contouring technique; it is especially useful for removal of axillary breast tissue in obese patients. Hemostasis is then obtained and closed suction drains are placed. Finally, the skin incisions are closed in layers. The patients are usually sent home the same day without any external breast support.

Mastopexy

The type of mastopexy procedure performed is dictated by the nature of the deformity. Patients with minor degrees of ptosis are frequently treated with periareolar (concentric) mastopexy procedures. Periareolar mastopexy is also often the procedure of choice when breast augmentation is combined with mastopexy. As the volume of the breast is increased by the implant, the need and degree of the mastopexy procedure becomes less. As the ptosis worsens, vertical mastopexy with a lollipop-type incision or conventional mastopexy with inverted-T incision might be indicated.

Periareolar (Concentric) Mastopexy

Since mastopexy is a cosmetic procedure, patient acceptance of the scars has always been a limiting factor. The periareolar mastopexy method has the least amount of scarring. The main problem with periareolar mastopexy procedures has been spread of the scar with time. The development of permanent purse-string sutures has helped solve this problem. The use of purse-string sutures to close a circular wound was first described in plastic surgery in 1985. Spear et al. in 1990 described three rules to mark the patient having concentric mastopexy that seemed to produce more predictable aesthetic results (Fig. 32.4). The rules are as follows: (1) the outer concentric circle must be drawn not to exceed the original areola diameter by more than the original areola diameter exceeds the inner concentric circle diameter, (2) the diameter of the outer circle should never be more than twice the diameter of the inner circle, and (3) the final areola size should be an average of the inner and outer concentric circles.

Following these rules and placing a permanent purse-string suture has made periareolar mastopexy a viable choice when minimal lift or repositioning of the nipple is required to achieve symmetry.

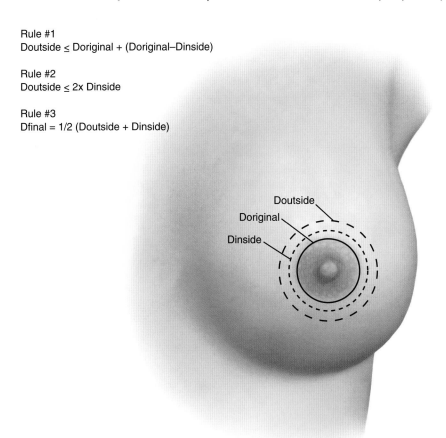

Rule #1
Doutside ≤ Doriginal + (Doriginal−Dinside)

Rule #2
Doutside ≤ 2x Dinside

Rule #3
Dfinal = 1/2 (Doutside + Dinside)

Doutside
Doriginal
Dinside

Figure 32.4 Spear rules. Illustrative markings of the three concentric circles for the Spear rules in mastopexy design. *D* refers to the diameter of the labeled circles.

Vertical Incision Mastopexy

The periareolar mastopexy techniques are limited by the amount of tissue manipulation and nipple–areolar movement that is possible. Some patients require more tissue rearrangement or skin resection than can be achieved with concentric mastopexy techniques.

The vertical mastopexy is performed with a periareolar scar and a vertical limb. The vertical limb is on a barely visible part of the breast, usually heals well, and is rarely an issue with the patient. Unlike the inframammary incision, which can often be seen medially or laterally, the vertical is never seen in bathing suits or clothing as long as it is kept above the inframammary fold.

Vertical mastopexy procedures are not new, and Lassus and Lejour have been performing these procedures since the 1960s. The Lassus and Lejour mastopexy procedures are similar in many ways. In both cases, the blood supply to the nipple is based on a superior pedicle. Skin is resected in the lower portion of the breast, and a central pedicle of tissue is developed on the basis of the superior blood supply. This central tissue is sutured in an elevated fashion to the pectoralis fascia. The result is longer lasting because the breast shape is based on tissue rearrangement and suturing and not on skin resection alone (Fig. 32.5).

Daniel Marchac developed a technique that is similar to those developed by Lassus and Lejour except that he places a small transverse scar at the bottom of the breast at the end of the case. This scar eliminates some of the excess skin associated with the Lassus and Lejour techniques. The patient's breast shape is better at the end of the case, but the price is a short transverse scar.

In mastopexy surgery, the most difficult problem is maintaining upper pole fullness and preventing recurrent ptosis. Biggs and Graf have developed a procedure that creates an inferior chest wall flap that is repositioned in the upper part of the breast. This flap is passed under a loop of pectoralis muscle and sutured in place in the elevated position. The Biggs–Graf technique is performed most commonly with a vertical incision, but an L-shaped incision or an inverted-T incision can also be used (Fig. 32.6).

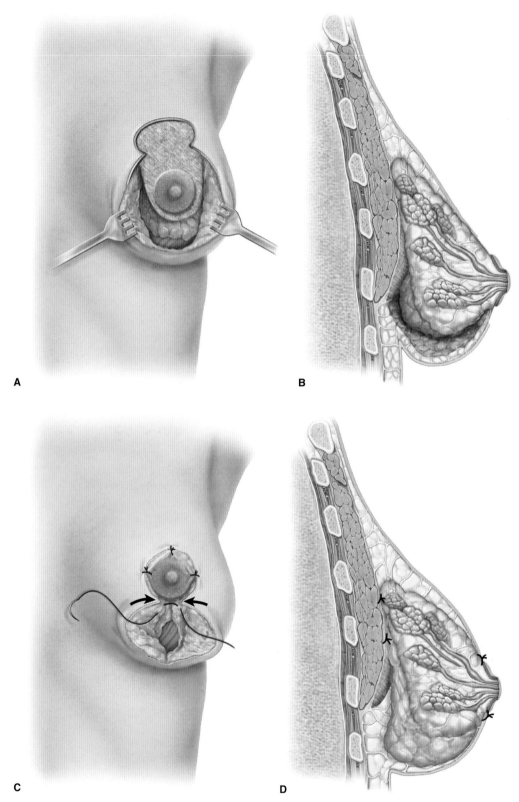

Figure 32.5 Lejour and Lassus method. **A.** Mobilization of the central pedicle. **B.** Central pedicle rotated into elevated position. **C.** Glandular pillars sutured together. **D.** Configuration of the breast at the end of the case.

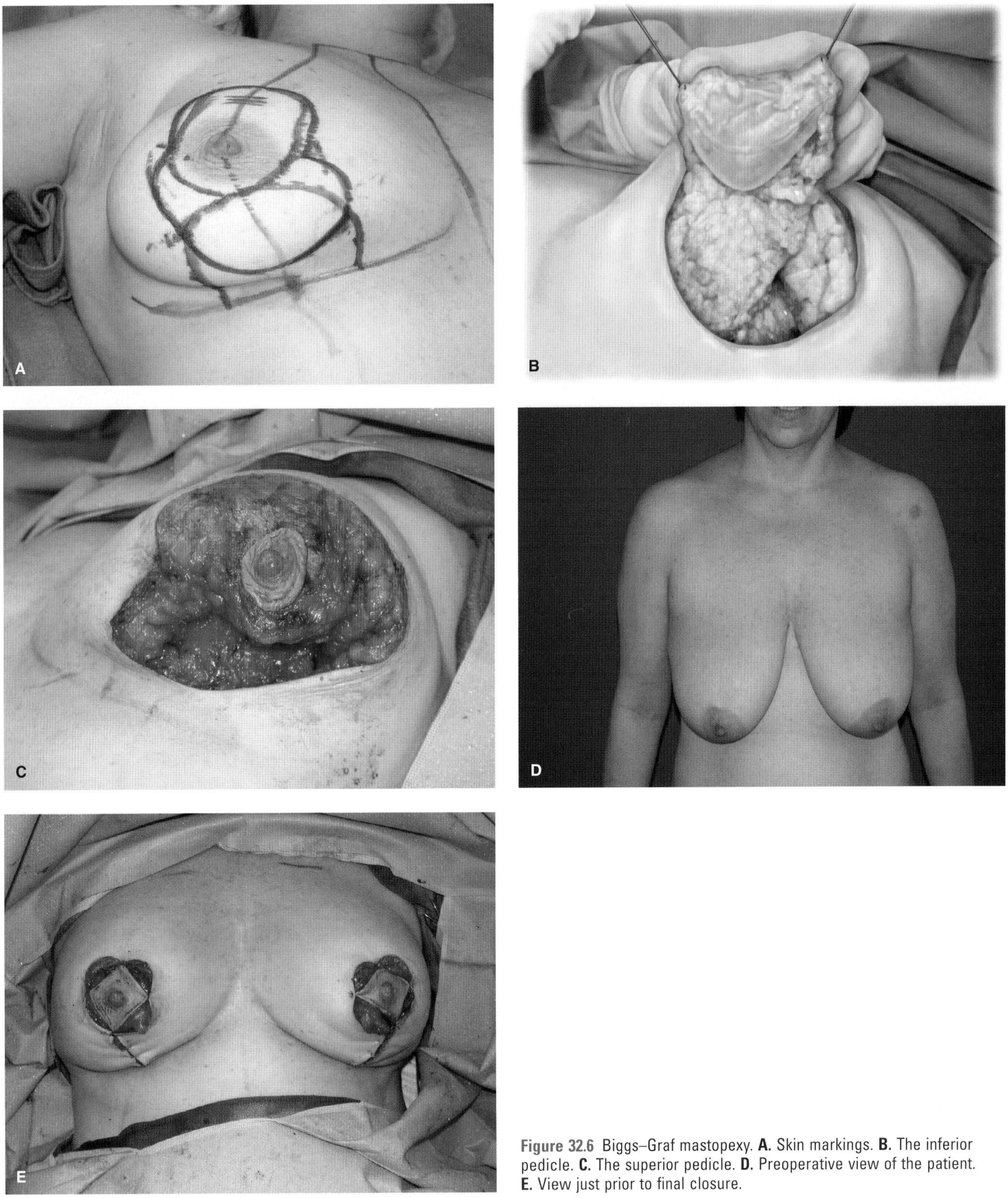

Figure 32.6 Biggs–Graf mastopexy. **A.** Skin markings. **B.** The inferior pedicle. **C.** The superior pedicle. **D.** Preoperative view of the patient. **E.** View just prior to final closure.

The blood supply to the nipple–areolar complex is based on a superior dermal pedicle. The inferior chest wall flap blood supply is through the chest wall. The nipple–areolar position is marked at the level of the inframammary fold and the superior pedicle is designed. The shape of the breast is based, once again, on tissue rearrangement and suturing, not on skin resection.

Inverted-T Mastopexy Procedures

In cases with severe ptosis or that require extensive nipple–areolar repositioning, inverted-T mastopexy procedures are performed. The original inverted-T procedures for mastopexy involved skin resection with extensive skin undermining and minimal parenchymal resection. The theory behind this procedure was that keeping the skin and breast in continuity contributed to a longer lasting result.

Unfortunately, the skin-only mastopexy is frequently followed by recurrent ptosis. Several authors have suggested repositioning and suturing of the breast parenchyma in addition to skin resection as a solution to this problem. These operations were based on the pedicle breast reduction procedures or the Biggs/Graf–type mastopexy.

The mastopexy techniques that incorporate tissue rearrangement and suturing seem to have longer lasting results than skin resection–alone mastopexy procedures. The principle is to empty the bottom of the breast, and then reposition the tissue in the upper pole of the breast. An empty space is created in the lower pole of the breast that allows pillar sutures to be applied and the breast narrowed and reshaped. The skin is allowed to redrape and has no role in the ultimate shape of the breast.

Augmentation and Augmentation Mastopexy

Breast ptosis is caused by a relative excess of skin envelope for the amount of breast tissue that is present. The procedures to decrease the skin envelope and rearrange and reposition the breast volume have been discussed earlier. Another option is to increase the breast volume with breast augmentation. This will often help correct the skin–breast volume disparity. Breast augmentation is frequently combined with mastopexy. The augmentation procedure usually decreases the size and scope of the mastopexy procedure.

In an augmentation mastopexy procedure, the mastopexy may be as small as a periareolar skin excision to reposition the nipple–areolar complex or as large as an anchor scar mastopexy with glandular rearrangement. The extent of the procedure depends on the needs of the particular patient.

The simplest augmentation mastopexy procedure involves resection of an ellipse (also called *crescent*) of skin above the areola to raise the nipple–areolar position relative to the inframammary fold. The most that the nipple–areolar complex can be raised with this type of procedure is approximately 2 cm. If the areola shape is an issue, then the procedure should be converted to a concentric mastopexy to redistribute the tension around the entire areola circumference.

When modest skin tightening or repositioning of the nipple–areolar complex is required, the full concentric mastopexy might be indicated. If the two circles of the mastopexy are truly concentric, then there will be no nipple elevation. To elevate the nipple, the outer circle must encompass more skin above the nipple than below.

The pocket for the implant is created either through the periareolar cut or through part of the mastopexy incision, and the implant is usually placed in the subpectoral position. After implant placement, the marks are reevaluated in the sitting position. Only then are the final incisions for mastopexy performed (Fig. 32.7).

In the case of concentric mastopexy, the outer circle markings are confirmed and incised. The guideline for marking concentric mastopexies was established by Spear and has been discussed earlier. A nonabsorbable purse-string suture is placed in the dermis of the outer circle. There is usually some pleating in the incision that resolves within 1 and 2 months. The permanent suture helps keep the scar narrow and the areola from enlarging.

Vertical scar augmentation mastopexy is usually used to correct moderate degrees of breast ptosis and allows greater ability to move the nipple–areolar complex and

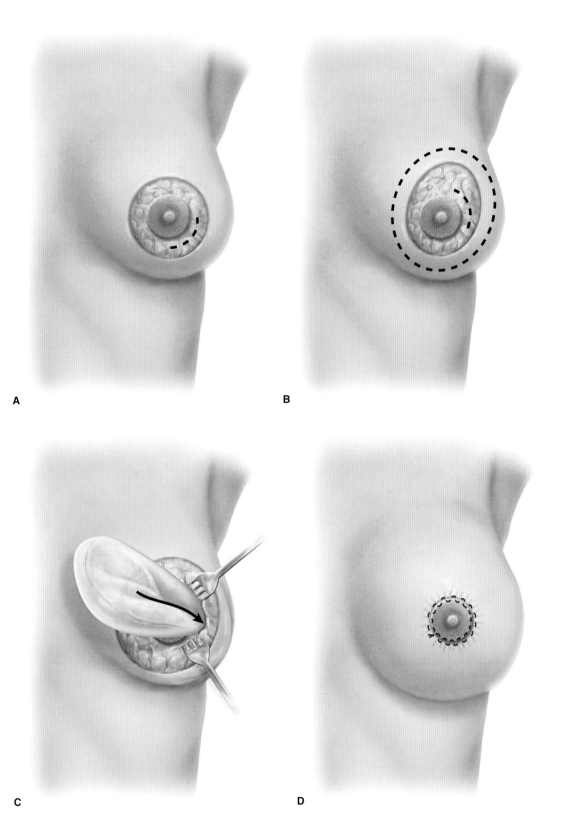

A

B

C

D

Figure 32.7 Periareolar mastopexy and augmentation. **A.** Skin resection. **B.** Area undermined. **C.** Insertion implant. **D.** Final closure.

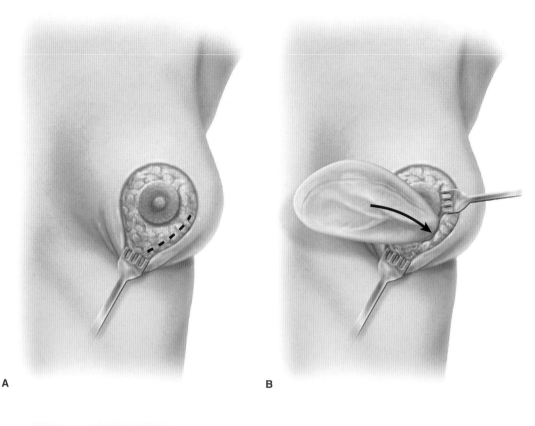

A

B

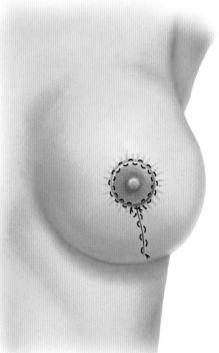

C

Figure 32.8 Vertical mastopexy and augmentation. **A.** Skin resection. **B.** Insertion implant. **C.** Final closure.

remove excess skin. Occasionally, a small piece of breast tissue at the bottom of the breast is excised to correct ptosis. Relocation of tissue at the bottom of the breast to the top of the breast is less important than in mastopexy alone because the implant is being used (Fig. 32.8).

Inverted-T scar augmentation mastopexy is rarely indicated. In these cases, the ptosis is so severe and the implant size is not enough to allow adequate skin resection by using the vertical or periareolar techniques. This procedure allows maximal control of the nipple–areolar position, skin removal, and breast shaping. The major drawback is the scarring. Augmentation mastopexy patients are no different than other aesthetic patients. They desire maximal improvement with minimal scarring. Some patients will accept a lesser result to avoid longer scars.

There is a common misconception in augmentation mastopexy patients that the implant should be placed in the submammary position. This offers the patient less surgery and less postoperative pain. While subpectoral implant placement is associated with more postoperative pain, the incidence of capsular contracture, implant palpability, and excess upper pole fullness is less. Currently, in the United States, augmentation mastopexy patients are allowed to have either saline- or silicone-filled breast implants. Silicone implants placed in the submuscular position have a lower incidence of capsular contracture than those placed in the submammary position.

When the implant is placed in the subpectoral position, approximately 50% of the implant is covered with muscle. The partial muscle coverage allows as much flexibility in shaping when compared with subglandular implant placement. At the same time, mammography is more accurate, and the chance of upper pole visibility is less. The augmentation mastopexy population tends to be older and have thinner soft tissue than the breast augmentation population. The ability to perform mammograms and the issues of upper pole fullness are real issues in this group.

Augmentation mastopexy is much more challenging than either breast augmentation or mastopexy alone. The patient's goals and desires need to be carefully addressed, and the scars and limitations of the procedures discussed.

Postoperative Care

All breast reduction patients and most mastopexy patients have closed suction drains placed during surgery. A supportive surgical bra is used for 3 to 4 weeks after the drains are removed. Tape strips are placed on the incisions at surgery and left in place on for at least 2 to 3 weeks. Patients begin normal daily activities in a few days. Lower body exercise is allowed in 1 to 2 weeks. Upper body exercise is allowed in 3 to 4 weeks. Patients may shower as soon as the drains are removed.

Complications

There were no cases of partial or complete nipple loss on the contralateral side in patients having symmetry procedure after ipsilateral reconstruction. The return of nipple sensibility is excellent and appears to be similar in patients who have undergone breast reduction, mastopexy, or augmentation. There are occasional (less than 1%) cases of hematoma or cellulitis requiring hospital admission or reoperation. Drains are used in most cases, but after drain removal, occasionally seromas might develop. These are treated in the office with aspiration and have never required reoperation.

⟿ PEARLS AND PITFALLS

- Most breast reductions for symmetry can be performed as short scar/vertical procedures. The inverted-T–type incision should be rarely used.
- Mastopexy by using internal architecture manipulation should be minimized in breast cancer patients.
- Breast augmentation for symmetry should be performed in the subpectoral plane when possible. This decreases the risk for capsular contracture, implant palpability, and excess upper pole fullness. Mammography, in this high-risk group, is also easier.
- No matter what techniques are used, in unilateral reconstruction with contralateral symmetry procedure, aging may require further revisions over time.

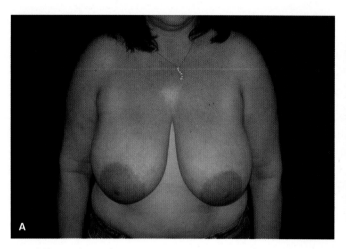

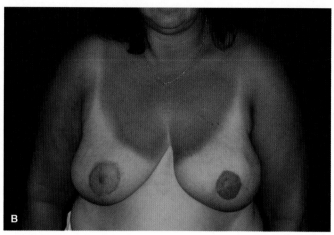

Figure 32.9 Patient with left implant reconstruction and right breast reduction. **A.** Preoperative. **B.** Postoperative.

⚛ RESULTS

Symmetry procedures are safe and effective. The breast shape is achieved by a technique or a combination of techniques that achieve maximal symmetry with the reconstructed breast (Figs. 32.9 and 32.10). Over time, the reconstructed breast and the contralateral breast may become asymmetric. This is more likely if the method of reconstruction is different from what is done in the contralateral breast. For example, a breast with an implant reconstruction will tend to stay in position and have little ptosis. A contralateral breast that consists of breast parenchyma, even after breast reduction or mastopexy, is likely to drop with time. Skin resection alone is not a factor in breast shape in the long term. Subsequent procedures may be required to correct these ongoing asymmetries over time. On the other hand, an autologous reconstruction matched with a contralateral breast that is reduced or lifted is unlikely to become significantly asymmetric with time.

With vertical breast reduction, the breasts tend to bottom out less and, therefore, revisions are less likely.

I never leave the operating room with a breast shape I am not happy with. I never rely on time or settling to achieve the desired result. I will do whatever it takes to have a good shape at the end of the case.

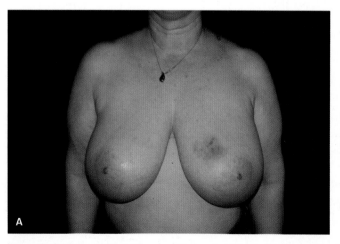

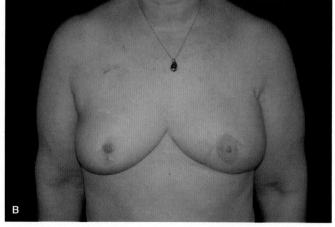

Figure 32.10 Patient with left free muscle-sparing free transverse rectus abdominis myocutaneous reconstruction and right breast reduction. **A.** Preoperative. **B.** Postoperative.

Early results with short scar breast reduction show breasts that are rounder and more aesthetic than those reduced with the inferior pedicle technique. The patient satisfaction is excellent. Younger patients are more accepting of breast reduction surgery with the shorter scar.

CONCLUSIONS

Secondary procedures are frequently performed to enhance the result of the primary breast reconstruction procedure. These procedures are best performed as a subsequent procedure. This provides the best chance for an optimal surgical result. Ideally, the need for the secondary procedures should be discussed with the patient as part of the initial consultation. When properly performed, these procedures can raise the overall result of the breast reconstruction to a much higher level.

Suggested Readings

Graf R, Biggs TM. In search of better shape in mastopexy and reduction mammoplasty. *Plast Reconstr Surg.* 2002;110:309.

Hall-Findlay E. A simplified vertical reduction mammaplasty shortening the learning curve. *Plast Reconstr Surg.* 1999;104:748.

Hall-Findlay E. Vertical breast reduction with a medial pedicle. *Aesthetic Surg J.* 2002;22:185.

Karp NS. Mastopexy and mastopexy augmentation. In: *Grabb and Smith's Plastic Surgery.* 6th ed. Philadelphia, PA: Lippincott Williams & Wilkins; 2007; 585–592.

Karp NS. Medial pedicle/vertical breast reduction made easy: the importance of complete inferior glandular resection. *Ann Plast Surg.* 2004;52:458.

Lassus C. Update on vertical mammaplasty. *Plast Reconstr Surg.* 1999;104:2289.

Lejour M. *Vertical Mammoplasty and Liposuction of the Breast.* St. Louis, MO: Quality Medical Publishing; 1993.

Marchac D, de Olarte G. Reduction mammoplasty and correction of ptosis with a short inframammary scar. *Plast Reconstr Surg.* 2002; 110:309.

Peled IJ, Zagher U, Wexler MR. Purse-string suture for reduction and closure of skin defects. *Ann Plast Surg.* 1985;14:465.

Spear SL, Giese SY, Ducic I. Concentric mastopexy revisited. *Plast Reconstr Surg.* 2001;107:1294.

Spear SL, Kassan M, Little JW. Guidelines in concentric mastopexy. *Plast Reconstr Surg.* 1990;85:961.

33 Secondary Reconstruction: Nipple–Areolar Reconstruction

Albert Losken

Introduction

Creation of the nipple–areolar complex often represents completion of postmastectomy breast reconstruction. Although this is considered a relatively minor procedure, its importance cannot be overstated. The nipple represents a natural break point in the breast and is a well-defined anatomic landmark contributing significantly to the final aesthetic outcome. Nipple reconstruction will often transform a nondescript mound into a breast, highlighting both shape and symmetry. Despite potential loss of projection and the fact that nipple function (erogenous sensation and lactation) is not preserved, the majority of women still choose to reconstruct the nipple–areolar complex, further emphasizing the importance of this procedure. Patients feel better with their breast reconstruction following completion of nipple reconstruction, and studies have demonstrated greater patient and partner satisfaction with nipple reconstruction (1–3). Many different options exist when it comes to technique that is probably testament to the fact that we are yet to identify the ideal method of nipple reconstruction. The technique chosen needs to be reliable, easy to perform, and versatile, with sufficient long-term projection.

INDICATIONS/CONTRAINDICATIONS

Nipple reconstruction is essentially indicated whenever there is an absence of the nipple due to congenital reasons, or more commonly following mastectomy for the treatment of breast cancer. Since it is a minor procedure that can be performed under local anesthesia, there are really no absolute medical contraindications; however, it does require reconstruction of a breast mound with reasonable shape and symmetry with the opposite side before attempting to reconstruct the nipple. The main reason why nipple reconstruction would not be performed is related to patient choice. Some patients will chose to defer nipple reconstruction for various reasons.

⟩ PREOPERATIVE PLANNING

Appropriate preoperative planning is crucial. Many variables need to be taken into consideration prior to reconstruction of the nipple. Incorrect placement of the new nipple no matter how good the actual nipple looks results in an unfavorable outcome. Patient desires and expectations need to be discussed. Important anatomic considerations include the position of the nipple on the breast, size, color, texture, and areola shape.

Timing

Immediate nipple reconstruction at the time of formal breast reconstruction is possible in select situations (4,5). Women with relatively small, nonptotic breast who undergo a skin-sparing or areola-sparing mastectomy and autologous reconstruction and do not require adjustment of the opposite breast are reasonable candidates for immediate nipple reconstruction. Other situations when immediate nipple reconstruction is reasonable include bilateral autologous breast reconstruction when nipple position is easily determined and reproduced at the time of reconstruction. However, since the position of the reconstructed breast mound is often unpredictable, the vast majority of nipples are reconstructed secondarily once the final shape has been established. This is often approximately 3 months following the reconstruction; however, it is delayed longer in the setting of adjuvant therapy. Another reason for performing nipple reconstruction at a secondary stage is that the patient is then able to participate in deciding on the most appropriate nipple position.

Additional Procedures

Nipple reconstruction is often performed once the final shape and symmetry has been achieved. It is reasonable to perform nipple reconstruction with minor adjustments in shape and size made to the reconstructed breast (Fig. 33.1). Minor adjustments to the contralateral breast also make it possible to predict desired nipple position on the reconstructed breast. However, whenever major revisions are required to improve symmetry and shape or when adjustments are required on both sides, it becomes preferable to defer nipple reconstruction.

Nipple Position

Although we often have little control over the potential for loss of nipple projection, appropriate positioning of the reconstructed nipple is arguably even more important

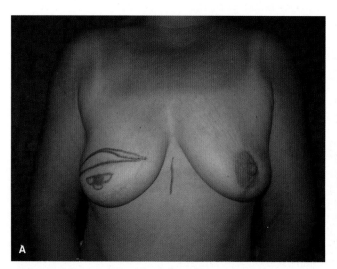 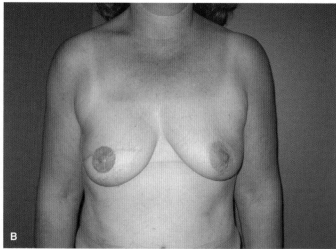

Figure 33.1 A. This 49-year-old women previously underwent a right transverse rectus abdominis myocutaneous flap reconstruction and a simultaneous contralateral mastopexy. Her right breast was slightly more ptotic than the now-stable left one. **B.** She had a minor revisional lift on the right at the time of nipple reconstruction and is shown with good symmetry at completion of areola tattoo.

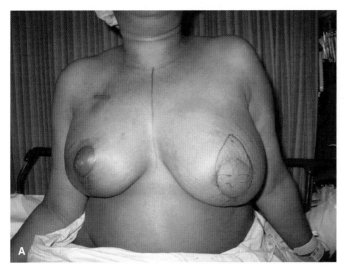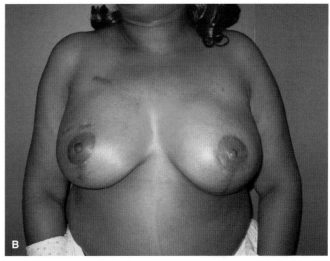

Figure 33.2 **A.** A left mastopexy-type revision of the transverse rectus abdominis myocutaneous flap was performed at nipple reconstruction to improve shape and symmetry. The nipple is reconstructed within the skin island, which is then elevated on a large central mound. The flap is debulked at the same time. **B.** She is shown 6 m postoperatively.

and is something that is completely within our control. A poorly positioned nipple, even if it has the best shape and projection, is considered a failure and significantly affects final shape and symmetry. Secondary correction of position is often difficult and with expander reconstruction essentially requires removal and reconstruction in a different location if possible. The nipple–areolar complex position can be adjusted primarily or secondarily similar to a mastopexy-type technique when a skin island is present following skin-sparing mastectomy (Fig. 33.2).

Anatomy

The normal nipple position is approximately 19 to 21 cm from the sternal notch or mid-clavicular line. Other measurements include approximately 9 to 11 cm from the mid-point of the sternum and 8 cm from the nipple to the inframammary fold. Areola diameter varies; however, it is typically in the range of 42 to 45 cm.

Marking

Nipple position is determined preoperatively with the patient in the standing position. When the skin island following skin-sparing mastectomy and autologous reconstructions is aesthetically located on the breast mound, the nipple position is typically marked in the center of the skin island. Implant reconstruction and delayed reconstruction will often require more measurements and calculation. Unilateral reconstruction requires matching the reconstructed nipple with the contralateral nipple position. This is easiest when the breast mounds are fairly symmetric and the opposite nipple is appropriately positioned on the breast mound. It is more challenging when adjustments to the contralateral breast mound are indicated and the new nipple position needs to be anticipated on the basis of the proposed position of the contralateral nipple following adjustment (Fig. 33.3). It is important to measure the position with two coordinates (Fig. 33.4). The midline of the chest is marked, and the distance from the contralateral nipple to the midline is measured and recreated on the reconstructed side. A second measurement from higher up on the midline or from the sternal notch to the nipple is also measured and confirmed on the opposite side before finalizing proposed position. A triangle is essentially created with two equal measurements on each side. The ideal nipple position following bilateral reconstructions is often determined on the basis of the shape of the breast mound and breast meridian. Placing the nipple too medial or too high is a mistake. Patient input is often helpful; round stickers can be placed temporarily and easily repositioned to determine appropriate position.

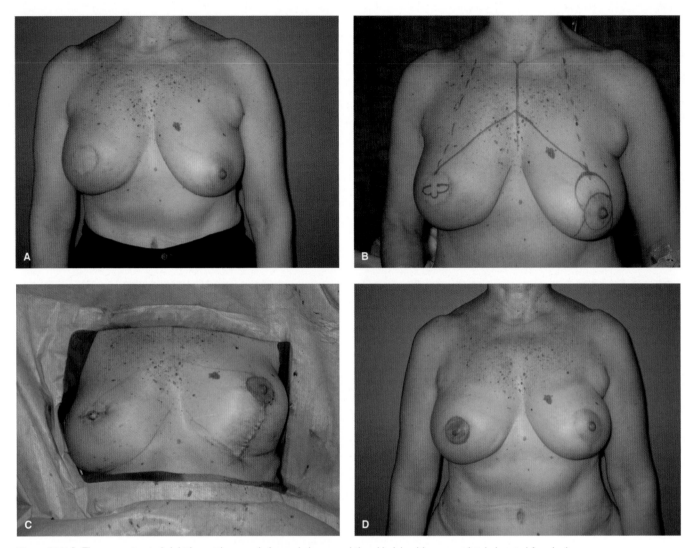

Figure 33.3 **A.** The reconstructed right breast has good size and shape, and the skin island is appropriately located for nipple position. A minor adjustment is required to the left breast. **B.** It is important to mark appropriately preoperatively with accurate measurements because the intraoperative symmetry is often inaccurate. **C.** Intraoperative nipple positions. **D.** Her final result is shown 1 year postoperatively with appropriate nipple symmetry.

Figure 33.4 Nipple position is typically marked and measured on two axis points: one from the sternal notch and another from the midline at the level of the nipple.

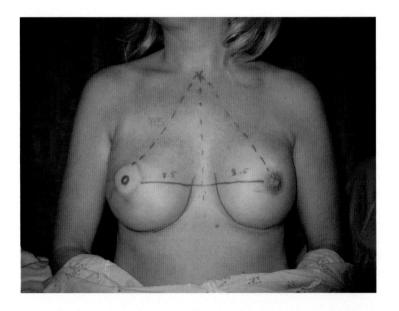

Once the nipple position has been determined and marked with a circle, the type of flap design is drawn out. The flap markings are adjusted depending on the size and shape of the contralateral nipple.

Technique

Although numerous techniques have been described, the two basic methods include local flaps and a composite graft.

Local Flaps

Local flaps are more popular since women are often hesitant to interfere with the opposite normal nipple. Local flaps are essentially all variants of the same principle, whereby random flaps are designed relying on the subdermal plexus, and wrapped in unique designs to create projection. Some of the techniques include the quadrapod flap, skate flap, dermal fat flap, double-opposing–tab flap, S flap, Anton–Hartrampf star flap, C-V flap, and the T and H flaps (6–14). Choice of technique is mainly determined by surgeon preference and comfort. Evidence-based comparisons in the literature are sparse, making claims of one techniques superiority to others difficult (15). One expected outcome that all local flap techniques have in common is loss of nipple projection. Although this is difficult to quantify, on average, a 50% reduction can be expected usually within the first few months. Modifications are continually being performed in an attempt to improve long-term projection.

The skate flap is another local flap option that is designed on the future areola base leaving an area that typically requires a skin graft for coverage. Once nipple position is determined, the axis for the skate flap is designed by drawing a line tangential to the nipple base. This axis should be rotated to avoid including the mastectomy scar within the wings or body of the skate flap. The length of this base tangent is approximately three times the diameter of the nipple circle. The height of the body is approximately twice the height of the opposite nipple erect. Curved lines are then drawn between the ends of the base tangent to the apex of the flap. The ellipsoid margins are incised, raising the two wings starting thin and becoming thicker. The central third of the base tangent is not incised to maximize flap perfusion. The wings of the skate flap receive their blood supply from intradermal vessels and the central pedicle. When the base is reached, the remaining wedge of skin is elevated with underlying subcutaneous tissue equivalent to the nipple's diameter. The central pedicle is raised and wrapped with the lateral wings to create the nipple. The pointed tip configuration can be avoided by amputating the tip distally and closing it primarily or in a purse-string manner. The donor site is either closed primarily or covered with a full-thickness skin graft harvested from the groin or other suitable area (Fig. 33.5).

The C-V flap is an evolution of the skate flap and is the author's preferred technique. It is a simple technique that essentially involves one C-flap and two V-flaps. The position of the desired nipple is marked with a circle. Two horizontal lines are marked on either side of the circle (Fig. 33.6). These parallel lines are usually approximately a centimeter apart and would result in 1 cm of projection. The width of these flaps determines the projection. The upper line is longer to create the V-portion that allows primary closure without contour distortion. The C-flap is then marked inferiorly (if a superiorly based flap is chosen). The C-flap donor site creates a circular base for insetting the V-flaps. The diameter of the C-flap will be similar to that of the final nipple diameter. It is important not to make this half circle too wide or too large since this will flatten the nipple. The pedicle is kept approximately a centimeter wide. It is important to maximize the blood supply by preserving the subcutaneous tissues and subdermal plexus at the level of the pedicle. Adjustments are made to the markings depending on the size of the contralateral nipple. However, most of the time, the nipple is made as large as possible and twice as big as the opposite nipple to allow for anticipated loss of projection. The flaps are then infiltrated with lidocaine and epinephrine. The incisions are made full thickness with a 15C blade. The V-flaps are elevated with some subcutaneous fat. The C-flap is elevated and the flap is back-cut toward the pedicle only

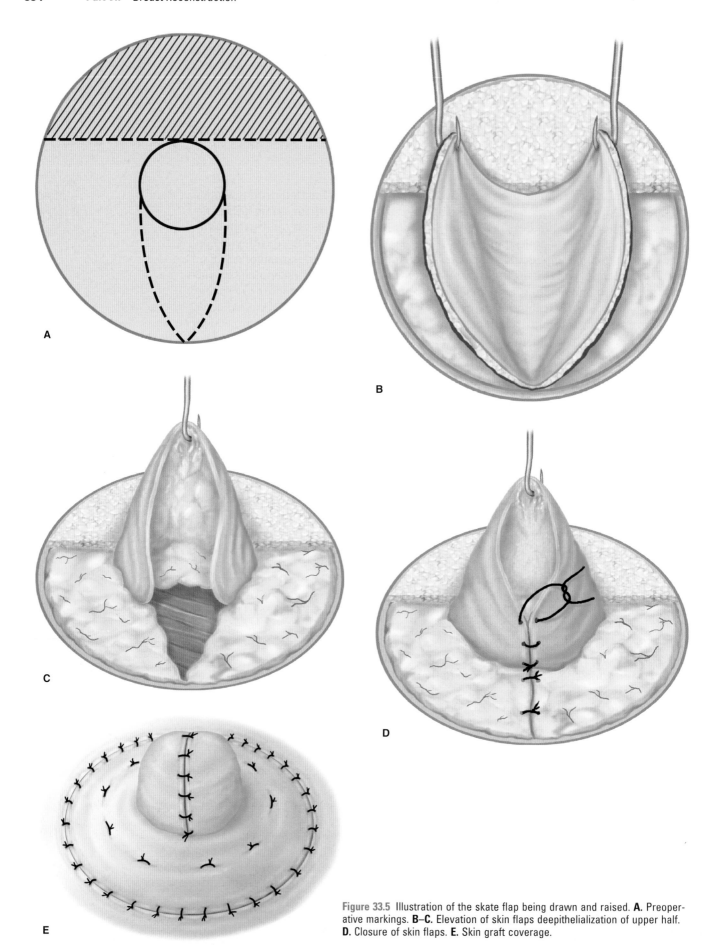

A

B

C

D

E

Figure 33.5 Illustration of the skate flap being drawn and raised. **A.** Preoperative markings. **B–C.** Elevation of skin flaps deepithelialization of upper half. **D.** Closure of skin flaps. **E.** Skin graft coverage.

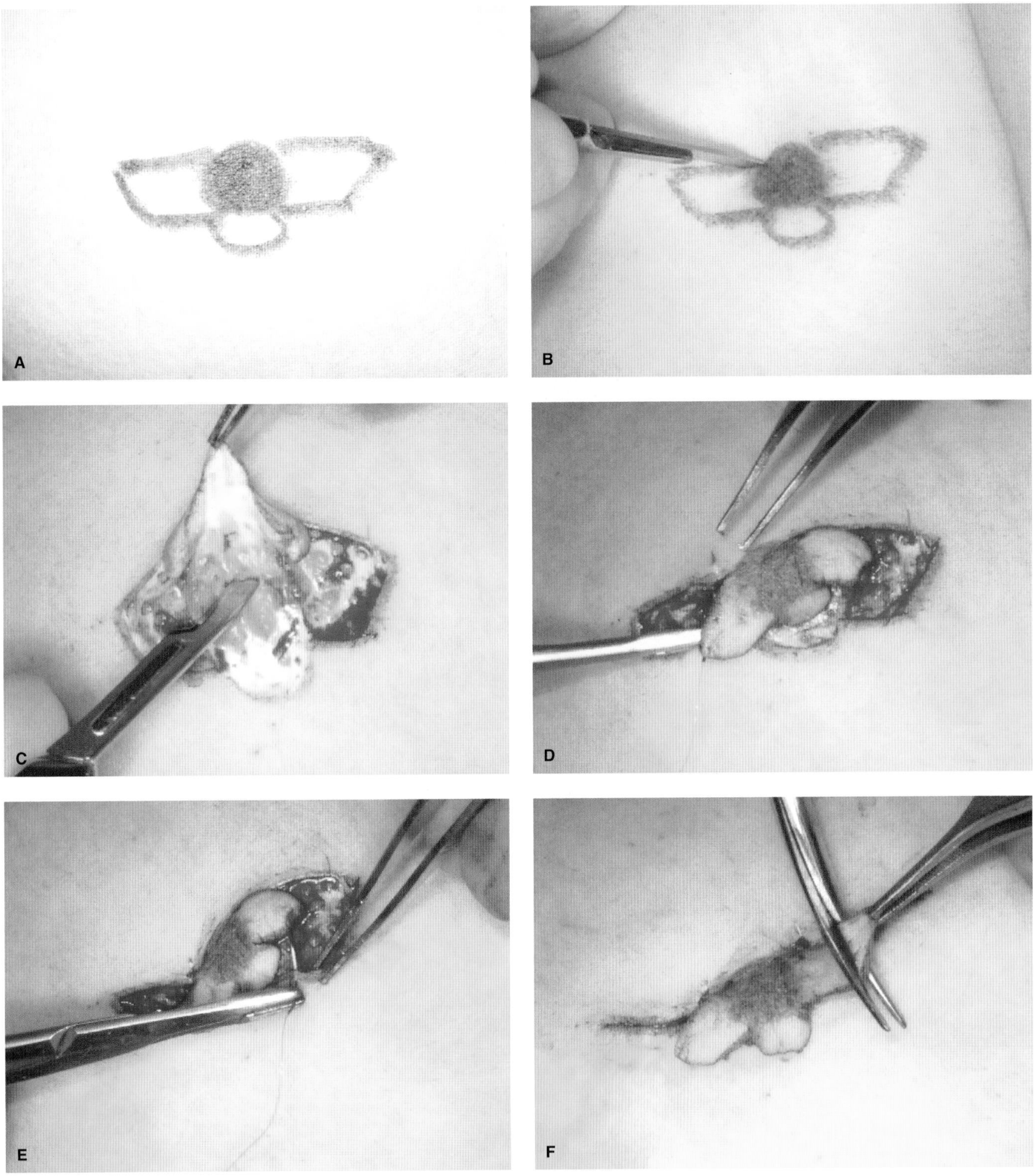

Figure 33.6 A. The C-V flap is marked with a generous superiorly based pedicle. **B.** The width of the V-flaps determines nipple height and the circumference of the C-flap determines nipple diameter. **C.** The flaps are incised in a full-thickness fashion and are elevated, preserving the central attachments as much as possible. They are released to allow unrestricted elevation of the C-flap. **D–F.** The donor sites are closed and the tips of the V-flaps are excised. (*continued*)

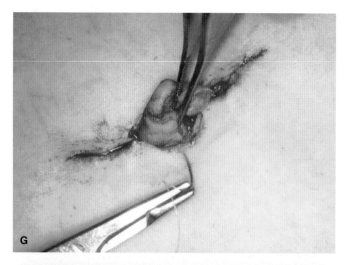

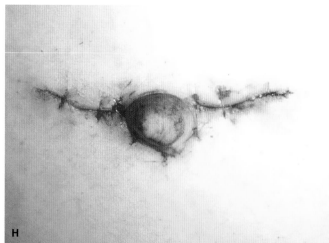

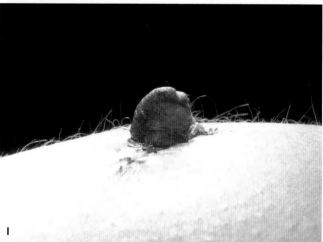

Figure 33.6 (*Continued*) **G.** A three-point stitch
is placed at the base of the nipple and the C-
flap is secured on top. **H–I.** Closure of skin.

as much as is required to lift the nipple up 90 degrees unrestricted. Since the dermis
is often thicker following latissimus dorsi reconstruction, the skin flaps are kept thinner than usual. After minimal undermining if necessary, the V-flap donor site is closed
with resorbable sutures. The tips of the V-flaps are then trimmed square to maintain the
even 1-cm height. The flaps are wrapped around and sutured inferiorly at the 6 o'clock
position to the middle of the C-flap donor site, which serves as a nipple defining stitch.
The C-flap is then placed on top as a cap.

Adjustments are made following implant reconstruction when the nipple is located
at the level of the mastectomy scar. The C-flap is often located on the other side of the
horizontal scar and subsequently deepithelialized and used as the base. The V-flaps are
then created (without the horizontal components) and rotated around each other without trimming the ends (Fig. 33.7).

When areola reduction is desired, the periareola incision is marked using a modified skate flap technique (16,17) (Fig. 33.8). An inner more oval-shaped incision is
marked around the proposed nipple reconstruction. The nipple position is marked and
a skate design is drawn with the horizontal lines being taken out to the circle. The oval-
shaped inner marking becomes a circle once the nipple flaps are lifted. The size of the
oval depends on the desired areola diameter. The inner and outer incisions are made,
and the rim of excess skin is removed. The nipple reconstruction is performed as
described earlier, however, without the V- tips. The ends of the flaps are trimmed appropriately for size. The donor sites are closed primarily. The periareola skin flaps are then
undermined minimally and a purse-string suture is used to reduce the size of the areola to the desired diameter. This is then sutured to the inner circle.

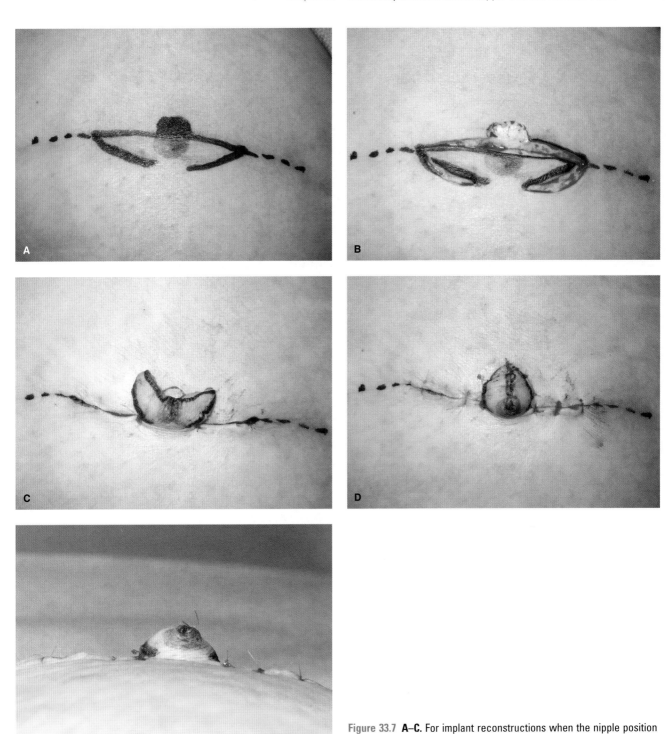

Figure 33.7 A–C. For implant reconstructions when the nipple position is at the horizontal scar, the C-flap is deepithelialized and left down as a base. **D–E.** The V-flaps are rotated around for projection.

Technical Modifications to Improve Outcome

1. Wide base to ensure adequate blood supply
2. Overcorrect projection
3. Establishing a stable base for the new nipple. This can be achieved by deepithelializing the C-flap or by raising the C-flap in the subdermal plane.
4. The tips of the flaps can be deepithelialized and tucked within the core of the construct rather than resecting them if additional volume is required.
5. Purse-string–type areola closures
6. Soft tissue fillers for projection.

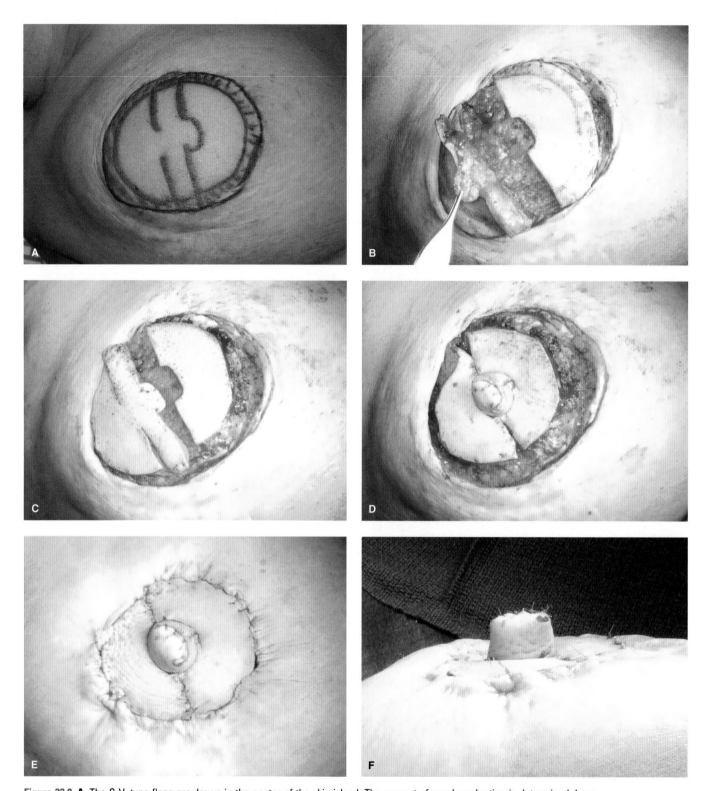

Figure 33.8 A. The C-V–type flaps are drawn in the center of the skin island. The amount of areola reduction is determined, keeping in mind that the skin island is going to be reduced even more once the flaps are raised. **B–C.** The flaps are elevated in a full-thickness fashion, and the rim of skin is removed circumferentially. **D–E.** The nipple is reconstructed, and the outer circle is closed in a purse-string fashion to the size of the proposed areola diameter. **F.** Projection is shown from the lateral view.

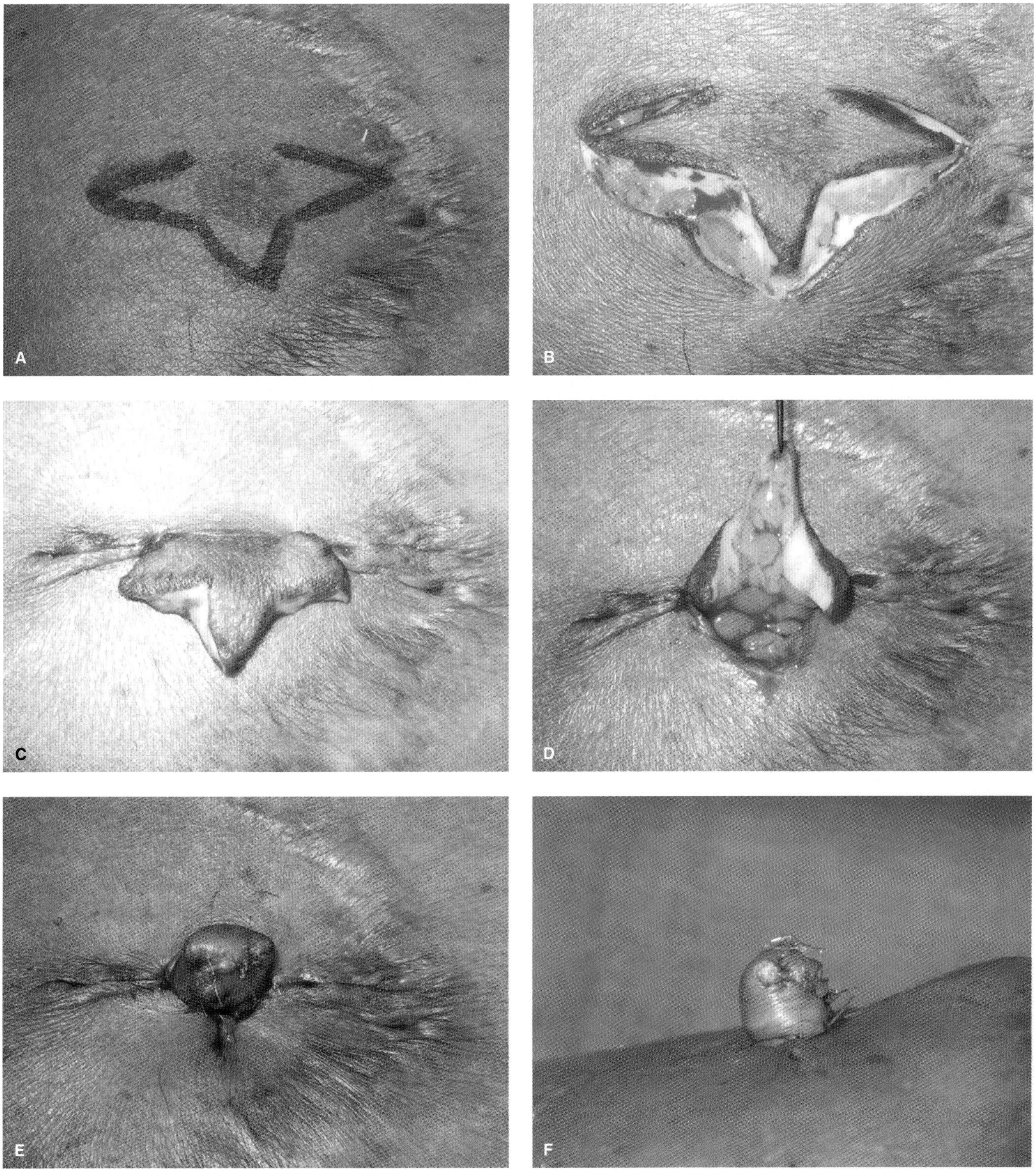

Figure 33.9 A–D. The modified star flap is demonstrated and elevated in the usual fashion. **E–F.** The donor sites are chosen and the flaps are wrapped for projection.

The modified star flap employs three triangular flaps that are rotated around to create projection, and it remains a popular approach. Once the nipple position has been determined on the breast mound, a 1 to 1.5 cm base is chosen, usually caudal. The two lateral flaps are then drawn, approximately 1.5 to 2 cm in length. The apex flap is similarly drawn. The flaps are elevated in a full-thickness fashion, including underlying fat when additional volume is desired. The donor sites are undermined and closed primarily. The lateral flaps are rotated and interdigitated with the apex flap being placed on top as a cap (Fig. 33.9).

Composite Grafts

Composite grafts are another option for nipple reconstruction, with the most common technique being free nipple grafting from the opposite nipple being the most common. This can be used as a primary nipple reconstruction when the contralateral nipple is large, or secondarily to augment a flattened local flap.

Nipple-Sharing Technique

When the opposite nipple is of adequate size and the patient is accepting, it is a natural donor site and provides good tissue match. The surgeon can carefully control the amount of tissue removed and restored (18,19). The new nipple matches the normal nipple perfectly with regard to color and texture, but both nipples are approximately one-half the size of the original. Once the position of the neonipple has been determined, a small circle is deepithelialized, or skin flap is elevated. The nipple graft is harvest with an 11 blade in a horizontal, vertical, or wedge orientation (Fig. 33.10). The donor site is closed with 5-0 resorbable sutures. The graft is then sutured down on the reconstructed breast, ensuring sufficient surface contact for graft revascularization. Graft immobilization is performed using a bolster-type dressing and left on for 10 to 14 days. Excellent long-term projection is observed once the graft is revascularized. The major factor limiting popularity of this technique is hesitance on the patient and surgeon to violate the contralateral, normal breast.

Other composite grafting techniques have included *ear lobule, labia grafts, mucous membrane, umbilicus,* or *toe pulp* with fair results (20–27). Once again, loss of nipple projection has been a major concern. Of all the composite flaps described, only the opposite nipple technique has yielded fairly consistent results and is still often utilized today.

Nipple Augmentation

Nipple augmentation techniques have been described in an attempt to maintain projection. Numerous sources exist including bone, cartilage, fat, allografts, and even hydroxyapatite crystals (23,28,29,30). This can be performed at the time of initial nipple reconstruction if the opposite nipple is large and the patient desires additional volume that a local flap could not achieve. These essentially involve placing additional material within a local flap in order for revascularization to occur. The majority of nipple augmentation techniques are being used at a secondary procedure when loss of projection has occurred, and an additional 4 to 5 mm is desired.

Areola Reconstruction

Many options exist for areola reconstruction, ranging from simple to complex. *Skin grafts* provide a more textured areola reconstruction, however, at the expense of a donor site. Use of the labium minus was first suggested by Milton Adams in 1949 for areola reconstruction and remained a popular technique during that time (21). This provided very similar color and texture. Millard proposed a split-skin graft from the opposite side for areola reconstruction (31). The opposite areola is an acceptable donor site when a contralateral reduction mammoplasty or mastopexy is planned. Skin grafts from the upper inner thigh were also used; however, they were generally abandoned because they left a painful donor site. Local flap techniques that harvest surrounding epidermal elements, such as the skate flap, often require wound coverage with a nonspecialized skin graft and creation of an areola at the same setting. The texture is acceptable; however, tattooing is often required postoperatively for color match. Ultraviolet light was used in the past to hyperpigment the skin graft areola.

Intradermal tattooing without grafting is a safe and effective nonsurgical procedure that gives resemblance of an areola (32). This is usually performed approximately 2 to 3 months following nipple reconstruction. When placed on the transverse rectus abdominis myocutaneous (TRAM) skin island or mastectomy skin flaps, it can be performed with little or no local anesthesia. Colors are chosen on the basis of the contralateral areola or patient preference in bilateral reconstructions. Overcorrection is often required in anticipation of color fade. Adequately matching areola size and shape is equally

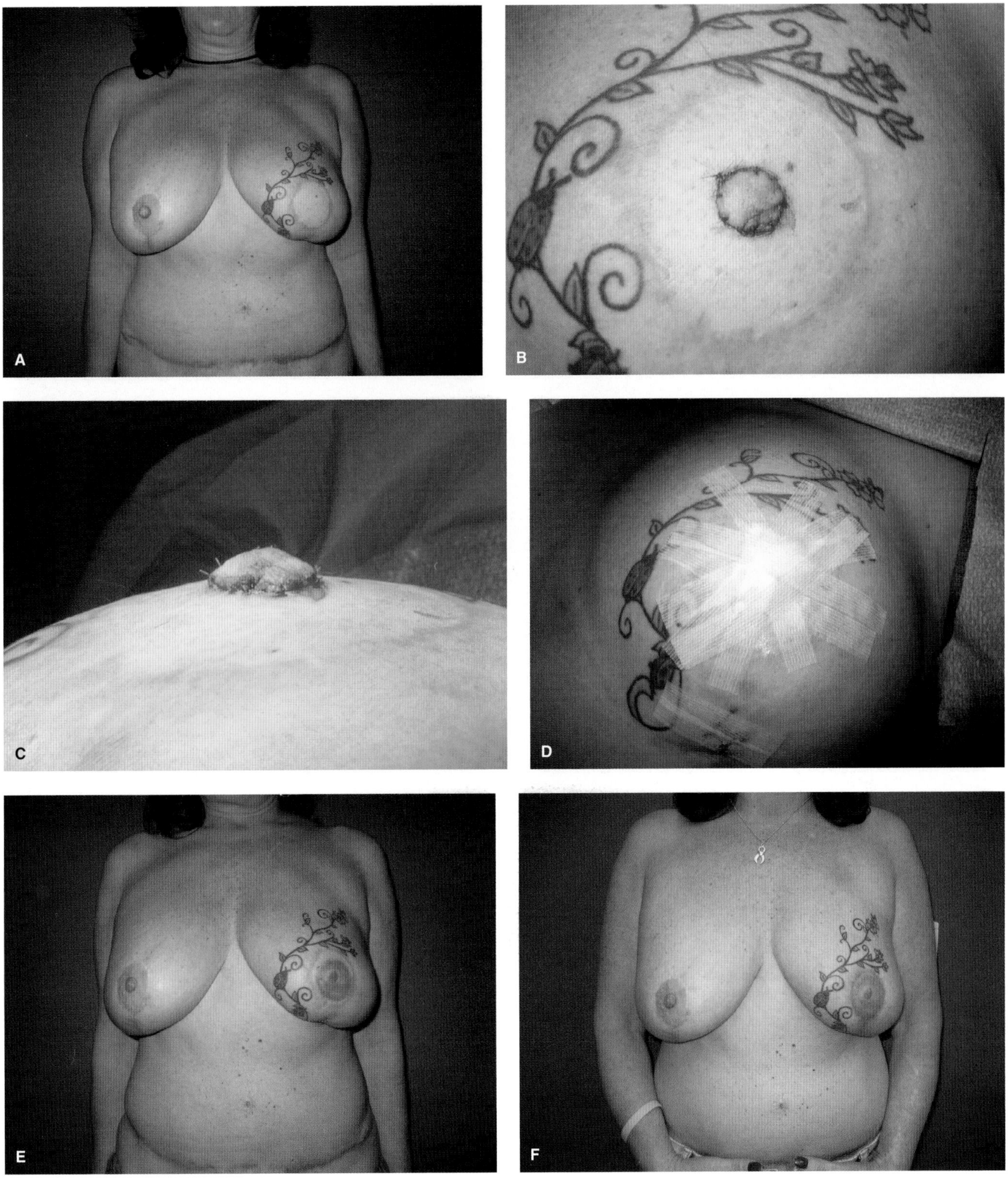

Part VII: Breast Reconstruction

Figure 33.10 A–C. A nipple-sharing technique is used to reconstruct the left nipple following transverse rectus abdominis myocutaneous flap reconstruction. **D.** The bolster dressing is applied for graft immobilization. **E–F.** The size of the skin island following areola tattoo was distracting and she underwent areola reduction using the periareola mastopexy technique and revision to the lower pole scar.

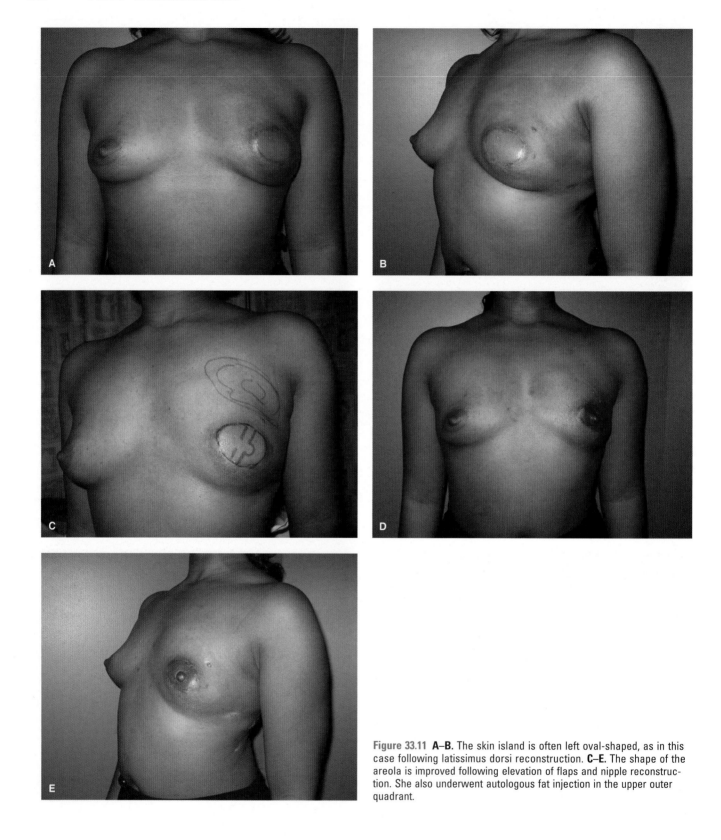

Figure 33.11 A–B. The skin island is often left oval-shaped, as in this case following latissimus dorsi reconstruction. **C–E.** The shape of the areola is improved following elevation of flaps and nipple reconstruction. She also underwent autologous fat injection in the upper outer quadrant.

important in reconstruction of the nipple–areolar complex. This procedure requires a skilled technician who can work with the patient to find an acceptable color match to the contralateral nipple, with the understanding that the ink's intensity will fade somewhat with time. It is safe, effective, and eliminates the need for additional procedures with own donor-site morbidities. Spear noted an 84% satisfaction rate at a mean of 25 months post-tattooing, with 10% requiring a touch-up (32). Long-term results at our institution revealed a 62% satisfaction rate on the pigmentation analogue scale for those who underwent tattooing, and only 14% requested retattooing for fading (6). Adequately matching areola size and shape is equally important in reconstruction of the nipple–areolar complex. When a skin island is present, it is often preferable to have the size of the skin island identical to that of the contralateral areola. A circle within a circle is often distracting and should be avoided. This can be corrected at the time of nipple reconstruction by using the mastopexy-type areola reduction technique (Fig. 33.11). Otherwise, it could be corrected secondarily with a purse-type mastopexy areola reduction (Fig. 33.10).

POSTOPERATIVE MANAGEMENT

It is important that a protective dressing be applied postoperatively to avoid compression or sheer forces on the reconstructed nipple. Various designs have been used, including a stack of 4 × 4 gauze pads with a hole in the middle, the hub of a 10 cc syringe, or special custom-made nipple guards. These are kept on for the first month. Free nipple grafts require a bolster-type dressing to be left on for the first 10 to 14 days, followed by a nonocclusive dressing for another few weeks.

Outcome

Evidence-based comparisons in the literature is sparse, making claims of one techniques superiority to others difficult (15). One expected outcome that all local flap techniques have in common is loss of nipple projection (6).

Projection

Loss of nipple projection seems to be the only constant in this rapidly evolving field. Historically, a 50% reduction in projection has been the quoted figure for most techniques. Recent reports have focused on evaluating long-term projection by using various local flaps. Shestak and Nguyen demonstrated better long-term projection with the skate and star flap than the bell flap, with the major decrease occurring in the first 3 months (33). Kroll demonstrated better projection with the tab flap than the star flap (10). Others have shown that 41% of intraoperative projection is present at 2 years when using the star flap (34). They were able to calculate a predictable change in projection by adjusting the length of the flap. Expanded skin is thought to be thinner and it undergoes atrophy more, contributing to a greater loss of nipple projection. The authors presented similar results at 5-year follow-up in a smaller series (6). Modifications are continually being performed in an attempt to improve long-term projection. Banducci et al. (35) reported a 71% decrease in projection at an average follow-up of 38.7 months by using the Anton–Hartrampf star technique. A mean nipple projection of 2.5 mm was reported using the modified skate flap following implant reconstruction in 422 reconstructions at an average follow-up of 44 months (36). Overcorrection at the time of nipple reconstruction is recommended to allow for loss of projection with time, regardless of which technique is used.

Complications

Complications following nipple reconstruction are relatively rare. We recently reviewed outcome following 255 nipple reconstructions by using the C-V technique and demonstrated a complication rate of 3%, which included tip necrosis and some wound dehiscence (Fig. 33.12). Although patients were generally found to be satisfied with the nipple reconstruction (3.8/5), projection (3.2/5), symmetry (4.2/5), and tattooing (3.2/5), the most common complaint was for more nipple projection (38% of patients). Tissue expander reconstruction had the lowest satisfaction, likely because of the thin nature of the skin flaps. Latissimus dorsi reconstructions results in the most satisfied

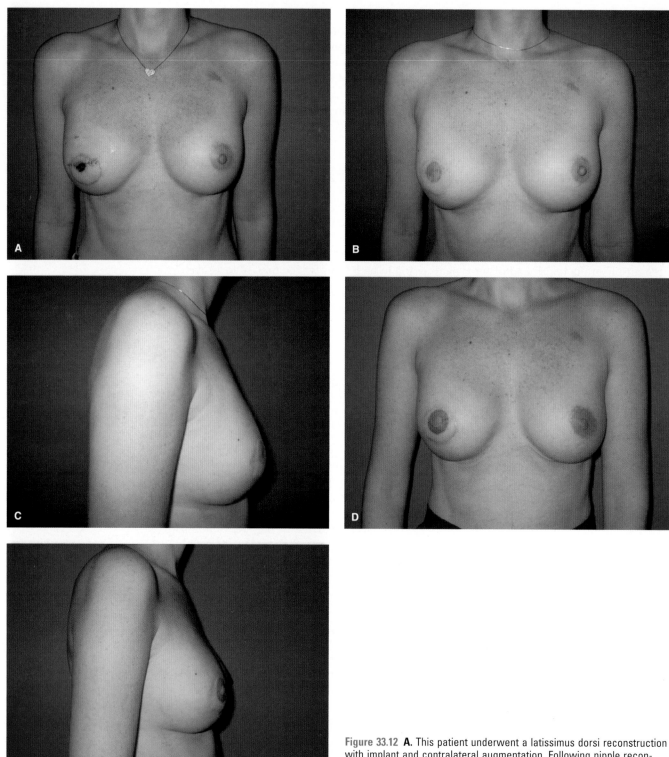

Figure 33.12 A. This patient underwent a latissimus dorsi reconstruction with implant and contralateral augmentation. Following nipple reconstruction, she had flap tip necrosis. **B–C.** She lost a significant amount of projection, which was corrected using a free nipple graft from the opposite breast. **D–E.**

patients following nipple reconstruction; however, they were more likely to have issues such as tip necrosis. Since the skin flaps are relatively thick, it is important not to close the nipple too tight in an attempt to maximize volume (37).

Sensation

The return of sensation has always been an interesting topic in breast reconstruction. Liew et al. documented a 76% objective return in pain, temperature, and touch sensation in the reconstructed free TRAM tissue (38). Sensory return in the reconstructed nipple is thought to occur via nerve in-growth into the flap from the mastectomy bed (39,40). As the local flap techniques are based on either native skin (as in skin-sparing mastectomies) or autologous flap tissue, it is not unreasonable to expect a small amount of sensory return at long-term evaluation.

Malposition

Nipple–areolar malposition is most commonly caused by placing the reconstruction on an unstable or incompletely reconstructed breast mound. This asymmetry is often difficult to correct and can be prevented by allowing the reconstruction enough time to heal adequately and the breast mound to develop its final shape.

Patient Satisfaction

Improvement in overall patient satisfaction of both the breast mound and nipple–areolar reconstruction remains the primary challenge for the reconstructive surgeon. Although patient satisfaction with the reconstructive process is high, patients continue to express dissatisfaction with the loss of nipple projection, poor color match, asymmetry in size and shape, and texture and position of the reconstructed nipple–areolar complex. Even with the most modern reconstructive techniques, loss of nipple projection remains the leading complaint by patients, with 19% and 14% of patients reporting less than satisfactory results in two recent studies (3,6). Patient satisfaction with the entire breast reconstruction process was greater than 80% in both studies.

Future Considerations

The ideal solution to nipple reconstruction would be a method that replaces soft tissue projection that is maintained, without donor-site morbidity or associated risks experienced with allogenic implants. The ability to engineer cartilage or other tissues into precise shapes and sizes is possible and might have implications for nipple reconstruction in the future. Tissue-engineered nipple reconstruction has been described in animal models using autologous chondrocytes over a biodegradable copolymer (41). The human nipple shape was created by injecting a polymer seeded with autologous chondrocytes. The biodegradable copolymer was then used as a scaffold to guide growth. Long-term results, safety, and maintenance of the trophism concepts for soft tissue generation need to be confirmed in animal models prior to human applications.

CONCLUSION

Reconstruction of the nipple–areolar complex remains a critical part of postmastectomy breast reconstruction with both physical and psychological benefits. Many options exist in the form of local flaps or composite grafts, and although loss of long-term projection is a common complaint, patients are generally satisfied with the results.

References

1. Lipa JE, Addison PD, Neligan PC. Patient satisfaction following nipple reconstruction incorporating autologous costal cartilage. *Can J Plast Surg.* 2008;16:85–88.
2. Wellisch DK, Schain WS, Noone RB, et al. The psychological contribution of nipple addition in breast reconstruction. *Plast Reconstr Surg.* 1987;80:699–704.
3. Jabor MA, Shayani P, Collins DR, et al. Nipple-areolar reconstruction: satisfaction and clinical determinants. *Plast Reconstr Surg.* 2002;119:457–463.
4. Williams EH, Rosenberg LZ, Kolm P, et al. Immediate nipple reconstruction of a free TRAM flap breast reconstruction. *Plast Reconstr Surg.* 2007;120:1115.
5. Delay E, Mojalla A, Vasseur C, et al. Immediate nipple reconstruction during immediate autologous latissimus breast reconstruction. *Plast Reconstr Surg.* 2006;112:964.
6. Losken A, Mackay GJ, Bostwick J. Nipple reconstruction using the C-V flap technique: a long-term evaluation. *Plast Reconstr Surg.* 2001;108:361.
7. Little JW III, Munasifi T, McCulloch DT. One-stage reconstruction of a projecting nipple: the quadrapod flap. *Plast Reconstr Surg.* 1983;71:126–132.
8. Little JW. Nipple–areolar reconstruction. In: Habal MB, et al., eds. *Advances in Plastic and Reconstructive Surgery*; vol 3. Chicago, IL: Year Book Medical Publishers; 1987:43.
9. Hartrampf CR, Culbertson JH. A dermal-fat flap for nipple reconstruction. *Plast Reconstr Surg.* 1984;73:982–986.
10. Kroll SS, Hamilton S. Nipple reconstruction with the double opposing tab flap. *Plast Reconstr Surg.* 1989;84:520.
11. Cronin E, Humphreys D, Ruiz-Razura A. Nipple reconstruction: the S-flap. *Plast Reconstr Surg.* 1988;81:783.
12. Anton M, Eskenazi LB, Hartrampf CR. Nipple reconstruction with local flaps: star and wrap around flaps. *Perspect Plast Surg.* 1991;5:67–78.
13. Chang WHJ. Nipple reconstruction with a T-flap. *Plast Reconstr Surg.* 1984;73:140–143.
14. Hallock GG, Altobelli JA. Cylindrical nipple reconstruction using an H flap. *Ann Plast Surg.* 1993;30(1):23–26.
15. Momeni A, Becker A, Torio-Padron N, et al. Nipple reconstruction: evidence-based trials in the plastic surgery literature. *Aesthetic Plast Surg.* 2008;32:18.
16. Hammond DC, Khuthaila D, Jane K. The skate flap purse-string technique for nipple-areolar complex reconstruction. *Plast Reconstr Surg.* 2006;120(2):399–406.
17. Weinfeld AB, Somia N, Codner MA. Purse-string nipple-areolar reconstruction. *Ann Plast Surg.* 2008;61(4):364.
18. Tyrone JW, Losken A, Hester TR. Nipple-areolar reconstruction. *Breast Dis.* 2002;16:117–122.
19. Bostwick J III. *Plastic and Reconstructive Surgery of the Breast.* 2nd ed. St. Louis, MO: Quality Medical Publishing; 2000.
20. Wexler MR, O'Neal RM. Areola sharing to reconstruct the absent nipple. *Plast Reconstr Surg.* 1973;51:176.
21. Adams M. Labial transplant for loss of nipple. *Plast Reconstr Surg.* 1949;5:295.
22. Muruci A, Dantas JJ, Norgueira LR. Reconstruction of the nipple-areolar complex. *Plast Reconstr Surg.* 1978;61:558.
23. Brent B, Bostwick J. Nipple-areolar reconstruction with auricular tissues. *Plast Reconstr Surg.* 1977;60:353.
24. Silsby JJ. Nipple reconstruction. *Plast Reconstr Surg.* 1976;57:667–668.
25. Gruber RP. Method to produce better areola and nipples on reconstructed breasts. *Plast Reconstr Surg.* 1977;60(4):505–513.
26. DeCholnoky T. Breast reconstruction after radical mastectomy: formation of missing nipple by everted navel. *Plast Reconstr Surg.* 1966;38(6):577.
27. Klatsky SA, Manson PN. Toe pulp free grafts in nipple reconstruction. *Plast Reconstr Surg.* 1981;68:245.
28. Eo S, Kim SS, Da Lio AL. Nipple reconstruction with C-V flap using dermofat graft. *Ann Plast Surg.* 2007;58(2):137.
29. Cheng MH, Rodriquez ED, Smartt JM, et al. Nipple reconstruction using the modified top hat flap with banked costal cartilage graft: long-term follow-up in 58 patients. *Ann Plast Surg.* 2007;59(6):621.
30. Garramone CE, Lam B. Use of Alloderm in primary nipple reconstruction to improve long term nipple projection. *Plast Reconstr Surg.* 2007;119:1163.
31. Millard DR Jr. Nipple and areola reconstruction by split-skin graft from the normal side. *Plast Reconstr Surg.* 1972;50(4):350–353.
32. Spear SL, Convit R, Little JW III. Intradermal tattoo as an adjunct to nipple-areolar reconstruction. *Plast Reconstr Surg.* 1989;83:907.
33. Shestak KC, Nguyen TD. The double opposing periareola flap: a novel concept for nipple-areolar reconstruction. *Plast Reconstr Surg.* 2007;119:473.
34. Few JW, Marcus JR, Casa LA, et al. Long-term predictable nipple projection following reconstruction. *Plast Reconstr Surg.* 1999;104(4):1321–1324.
35. Banducci DR, Le TK, Hughes KC. Long-term follow-up of a modified Anton-Hartrampf nipple reconstruction. *Ann Plast Surg.* 1999;43(5):467–470.
36. Toni Z, Anu A, Cordeiro P. Surgical outcomes and nipple projection using the modified skate flap for nipple-areolar reconstruction in a series of 422 implant reconstructions. *Ann Plast Surg.* 2009;62(5):591.
37. Otterburn D, Losken A. An outcome evaluation following postmastectomy nipple reconstruction using the C-V flap technique. *Ann Plast Surg.* 2010;64(5):574–578.
38. Liew S, Hunt J, Pennington D. Sensory recovery following free TRAM flap breast reconstruction. *Br J Plast Surg.* 1996;49(4):210–213.
39. Lapatto O, Asko-Seljavaara S, Tukianen E, et al. Return of sensibility and final outcome of breast reconstruction using free transverse rectus abdominis musculocutaneous flaps. *Scand J Plast Reconstr Surg.* 1995;29(1):33–38.
40. Place MJ, Song T, Hardesty RA, et al. Sensory reinnervation of autologous tissue TRAM flaps after breast reconstruction. *Ann Plast Surg.* 1997;38(1):19–22.
41. Cao LC, Lach E, Kim TH, et al. Tissue-engineered nipple reconstruction. *Plast Reconstr Surg.* 1998;102(7):2293–2298.

Index

Note: Page locators followed by f and t indicates figure and table respectively.

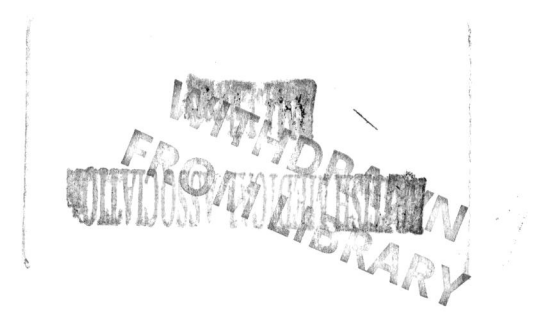